OXFORD MEDICAL PUBLICATIONS

Emergencies in Sports Medicine

Published and forthcoming titles in the Emergencies in ... series:

Emergencies in Adult Nursing
Edited by Philip Downing

Emergencies in Anaesthesia, Second Edition
Edited by Keith Allman, Andrew McIndoe, and Iain H. Wilson

Emergencies in Cardiology, Second Edition
Edited by Saul G. Myerson, Robin P. Choudhury, and Andrew R.J. Mitchell

Emergencies in Children's and Young People's Nursing
Edited by Edward Alan Glasper, Gillian McEwing, and Jim Richardson

Emergencies in Clinical Medicine
Edited by Piers Page and Greg Skinner

Emergencies in Clinical Radiology
Edited by Richard Graham and Ferdia Gallagher

Emergencies in Clinical Surgery
Edited by Chris Callaghan, J. Andrew Bradley, and Christopher Watson

Emergencies in Critical Care
Edited by Martin Beed, Richard Sherman, and Ravi Mahajan

Emergencies in Mental Health Nursing
Edited by Patrick Callaghan and Helen Waldock

Emergencies in Obstetrics and Gynaecology
Edited by S. Arulkumaran

Emergencies in Oncology
Edited by Martin Scott-Brown, Roy A.J. Spence, and Patrick G. Johnston

Emergencies in Paediatrics and Neonatology
Edited by Stuart Crisp and Jo Rainbow

Emergencies in Palliative and Supportive Care
Edited by David Currow and Katherine Clark

Emergencies in Primary Care
Chantal Simon, Karen O'Reilly, John Buckmaster, and Robin Proctor

Emergencies in Psychiatry
Basant K. Puri and Ian H. Treasaden

Emergencies in Respiratory Medicine
Edited by Robert Parker, Catherine Thomas, and Lesley Bennett

Emergencies in Sports Medicine
Edited by Julian Redhead and Jonathan Gordon

Emergencies in Trauma
Aneel Bhangu, Caroline Lee, and Keith Porter

Head, Neck and Dental Emergencies
Edited by Mike Perry

Medical Emergencies in Dentistry
Nigel Robb and Jason Leitch

Emergencies in Sports Medicine

Edited by

Dr Julian Redhead

FRCP, FCEM, MFSEM

Consultant in Emergency Medicine
Imperial College Healthcare NHS Trust
London, UK

Dr Jonathan Gordon

FRCS, MSc, FCEM, MFSEM

Consultant in Emergency Medicine
Victoria Infirmary
Glasgow, UK

OXFORD
UNIVERSITY PRESS

OXFORD
UNIVERSITY PRESS

Great Clarendon Street, Oxford OX2 6DP

Oxford University Press is a department of the University of Oxford.
It furthers the University's objective of excellence in research, scholarship,
and education by publishing worldwide in

Oxford New York

Auckland Cape Town Dar es Salaam Hong Kong Karachi
Kuala Lumpur Madrid Melbourne Mexico City Nairobi
New Delhi Shanghai Taipei Toronto

With offices in

Argentina Austria Brazil Chile Czech Republic France Greece
Guatemala Hungary Italy Japan Poland Portugal Singapore
South Korea Switzerland Thailand Turkey Ukraine Vietnam

Oxford is a registered trade mark of Oxford University Press
in the UK and in certain other countries

Published in the United States
by Oxford University Press Inc., New York

© Oxford University Press 2012

The moral rights of the authors have been asserted
Database right Oxford University Press (maker)

First published 2012

All rights reserved. No part of this publication may be reproduced,
stored in a retrieval system, or transmitted, in any form or by any means,
without the prior permission in writing of Oxford University Press,
or as expressly permitted by law, or under terms agreed with the appropriate
reprographics rights organization. Enquiries concerning reproduction
outside the scope of the above should be sent to the Rights Department,
Oxford University Press, at the address above

You must not circulate this book in any other binding or cover
and you must impose the same condition on any acquirer

British Library Cataloguing in Publication Data
Data available

Library of Congress Cataloging in Publication Data
Library of Congress Control Number: 2011943540

Typeset by Cenveo, Bangalore, India
Printed in China
on acid-free paper through
Asia Pacific Offset

ISBN 978–0–19–960267–4

10 9 8 7 6 5 4 3 2 1

Oxford University Press makes no representation, express or implied, that the
drug dosages in this book are correct. Readers must therefore always check the
product information and clinical procedures with the most up-to-date published
product information and data sheets provided by the manufacturers and the most
recent codes of conduct and safety regulations. The authors and the publishers
do not accept responsibility or legal liability for any errors in the text or for the
misuse or misapplication of material in this work. Except where otherwise stated,
drug dosages and recommendations are for the non-pregnant adult who is not
breastfeeding.

Preface

Participation in sport and exercise at all levels is recognized as a factor in increasing the medical well being of participants. With the Olympics due in 2012 it is expected that increasing numbers of the population will participate in organized activities.

Healthcare professionals will be expected and encouraged to provide medical care during these events. It is important that these professionals are adequately prepared to provide this care.

A number of excellent courses are available for healthcare professionals to acquire and practice their skills. This text should be viewed as an accompaniment to these courses and to provide immediate access to reliable information at the patients side. The text covers all aspects of the emergencies likely to be encountered and gives important information as to their immediate treatment.

Sport and Exercise Medicine became recognized as a speciality in 2005 with the establishment of a faculty in 2006. Higher specialist training in the speciality began in 2007, with trainees undertaking a 4 year specialist training programme.

The majority of the chapters have been written by trainees within the new speciality, allowing expertise from many different sports to be represented.

We would like to thank them all for their hard work in completing the chapters. We would also like to thank our colleagues within the Emergency Departments for their patience in allowing us to complete the book. The book is dedicated to our wives, Lucy and Julie, and children, Georgina, William, Kate, and Megan.

Acknowledgements

We wish to thank Dr Carl Waldmann for his input and advice for Chapter 9, Head Injuries, and acknowledge Ellen McDougall RGN, Nurse Paralympics GB for the section on autonomic dysreflexia within Chapter 19, Athletes with a disability.

Contents

Contributors *xi*
Symbols and abbreviations *xiii*

1	Planning and preparation	1
2	General approach to the injured or unwell athlete	11
3	Cardiorespiratory arrest	17
4	Athletes with pre-existing conditions	33
5	Collapse during exercise	51
6	Altitude sickness	65
7	Sudden cardiac death in sport	77
8	General medical emergencies	89
9	Head injuries	113
10	Airway injuries	129
11	Maxillofacial injuries and infection in sports medicine	137
12	Spinal injuries	153
13	Thorax	163
14	The abdomen	175
15	Pelvic trauma	195
16	Upper limb injury	209
17	Lower limb injury	227
18	Paediatrics	251
19	Athletes with a disability	271

20 Aggressive patients — 277
21 Breaking bad news — 283
22 Communication — 291

Index *303*

Contributors

Fiona Burton
ST6 Emergency Medicine
Victoria Infirmary
Glasgow
UK

Eva M. Carneiro
First Team Doctor
Chelsea FC
London
UK

Susan Daisley
Consultant Emergency Medicine
Victoria Infirmary
Glasgow
UK

Sarah Davies
Specialist trainee in Sport and Exercise Medicine
London Deanery
London
UK

Julie Gordon
Consultant in Emergency Medicine
Crosshouse Hospital
Kilmarnock
UK

Peter L Gregory
The New Dispensary
Warwick
UK

Jonathan Hanson
Consultant in Sport and Exercise medicine, Scottish Rugby Union.
Department of Emergency
Dr Mackinnon Memorial Hospital
Broadford
Skye
UK

Courtney Kipps
Principal Clinical Teaching Fellow and Honorary Consultant in Sport and Exercise Medicine
University College London
London
UK

Pria Krishnasamy
Speciality Registrar in Sport and Exercise Medicine
London Deanery
London
UK

Jonathan Lacey
Anaesthetic Trainee
Imperial School of Anaesthesia
London
UK

Nina Maryanji
ST 6 Royal Infirmary
Glasgow
UK

Yvonne Moulds
SpR Emergency Medicine
Ayr Hospital
Ayr
UK

Shabaaz Mughal
Club Doctor, Tottenham Hotspur Football Club
Sport & Exercise Medicine
Consultant Physician
Whipps Cross University Hospital
London
UK

James Noake
Specialist trainee in Sport and Exercise Medicine
London Deanery
London
UK

Noel Pollock
Consultant in Sport & Exercise Medicine
UK Athletics London Medical Officer
Hospital of St John and St Elizabeth
London
UK

John Rogers
Consultant in Sport & Exercise Medicine
Endurance Medical Officer UKA
UKA National Performance Centre
Loughborough University
Loughborough
UK

Richard Seah
Senior Registrar in Sport & Exercise Medicine
Royal National Orthopaedic Hospital NHS Trust
Stanmore
Middlesex
UK

Kevin Thomson
Consultant in Emergency Medicine
Victoria Infirmary
Glasgow
UK

Eleanor Tillett
Honorary Consultant Sport & Exercise Medicine
University College London Hospital
London
UK

Symbols and abbreviations

⚠	warning
☙	controversial topic
▶▶	don't dawdle
▶	important
♀	female
♂	male
#	fracture
ℳ	website
A&E	Accident & Emergency
ABC	airway, breathing, circulation
ABPI	ankle–brachial pressure index
AC	acromio-clavicular
ACE-I	angiotensin converting enzyme inhibitors
ACL	anterior cruciate ligament
ACS	acute coronary syndrome
AD	autonomic dysflexia
ADH	anti-diuretic hormone
AED	automated external defibrillator
AF	atrial fibrillation
ALS	advanced life support
AMS	acute mountain sickness
AMPLE	allergy, medications, past medical history, last eaten, events preceding
AP	anteroposterior
AS	ankylosing spondylitis
ATLS	advanced trauma life support
AV	atrioventricular
AVPU	Patient alert, Patient responds to verbal stimulus, Patient only responds to painful stimulus, Patient is unresponsive
bd	twice daily
BLS	basic life support
BM	blood glucose monitor
BNF	British National Formulary
BNFC	British National Formulary for Children
BP	blood pressure
CAD	coronary artery disease

CPR	cardiopulmonary resuscitation
CRP	c-reactive protein
CSF	cerebrospinal fluid
CT	computed tomography
CXR	chest X-ray
DIPJ	distal interphalangeal joint
DKA	diabetic keto-acidosis
DMARDs	disease modifying anti-rheumatic drugs
DPL	diagnostic peritoneal lavage
DVT	deep venous thrombosis
EAC	exercise-associated collapse
EAH	exercise-associated hyponatraemia
ECG	electrocardiogram
ECHO	echocardiogram
ED	Emergency Department
EIA	exercise-induced asthma
ERCP	endscopic retrograde cholecystic pancreatogram
ESR	erythrocyte sedimentation rate
ET	Endo-tracheal
FAST	focused assessment with sonography for trauma
FBC	full blood count
FDP	Flexor digitorum profundus
FDS	Flexor digitorum superficialis
FOOSH	fall onto an outstretched hand
GCS	Glasgow Coma Scale
GI	gastrointestinal
GMC	General Medical Council
GTN	glyceryl trinitrate
HACE	high altitude cerebral oedema
HAPE	high altitude pulmonary oedema
HATI	human tetanus immunoglobulin
Hb	haemoglobin
HCM	hypertrophic cardiomyopathy
HIV	human immunodeficiency virus
HOCM	hypertrophic obstructive cardiomyopathy
IBD	Inflammatory bowel disease
IgE	immunoglobin E
IHD	ischaemic heart disease
IM	intramuscular
ITP	idiopathic thrombocytopenic purpura

ITU	intensive therapy unit
IV	intravenous
JVP	jugular venous pressure
LAT	lignocaine, adrenaline, and tetracaine
LIF	left iliac fossa
LMA	laryngeal mask airway
LOC	loss of consciousness
LV	left ventricle
MCL	medial collateral ligament
MD	muscular dystrophy
MDU	Medical Defence Union
MI	myocardial Infarction
MILS	manual in-line immobilization
MRI	magnetic resonance imaging
MS	multiple sclerosis
MTP	metatarso-phalangeal
NAI	non-accidental injury
NCEPOD	National Confidential Enquiry into Patient Outcome and Death
NP	nasopharyngeal
NPA	nasopharyngeal airway
NSAID	non-steroidal anti-inflammatory drug
OGTT	oral glucose tolerance test
OP	oropharyngeal
OPA	oropharyngeal airway
OPT	orthopantomogram
ORIF	open reduction internal fixation
$PaCO_2$	partial pressure of CO_2
PaO_2	partial pressure of O_2
PCL	posterior collateral ligament
PEA	Pulseless electrical activity
PEF	peak expiratory flow
PEFR	peak expiratory flow rate
PIPJ	proximal interphalangeal joint
PMHx	past medical history
po	by mouth
pr	per rectum
PTE	pulmonary embolism
PU	pass urine
RA	rheumatoid arthritis

RBC	red blood cell count
RIF	right iliac fossa
RTA	road traffic accident
RTP	return to play
RUQ	right upper quadrant
SAH	subarachnoid haemorrhage
SARS	severe acute respiratory syndrome
SBP	systolic blood pressure
SC	subcutaneous
SCAT	Sport Concussion Assessment Tool
SCD	sudden cardiac death
SIGN	Scottish Intercollegiate Guidelines Network
SOB	shortness of breath
STI	soft tissue injury
SUFE	slipped upper femoral epiphysis
SVT	supraventrular tachycardias
TB	tuberculosis
VF	ventricular fibrillation
VT	ventricular tachycardia
WADA	world antidoping agency
WBC	white blood cell count
WBGT	wet bulb globe temperature index

Chapter 1

Planning and preparation

Introduction 2

CHAPTER 1 **Planning and preparation**

Introduction

To fail to prepare is to prepare to fail.

This adage is relevant not only to sporting success, but also when considering planning of medical cover for a sporting event. This chapter outlines the major issues to consider when preparing to cover a sporting event focusing particularly on anticipation and planning for the management of life- and limb-threatening sporting emergencies together with common accident and emergency presentations in a pre-hospital sporting setting.

'There is no place for a token medical presence at sporting events'. This statement issued by the MDU (Medical Defence Union, UK) illustrates the change in attitude over recent years with regard to doctors covering all standards and levels of sporting competition. In previous years, many doctors, physiotherapists, and allied health professionals would volunteer to cover a range of sporting events despite inadequate training, equipment, and personnel. With the development of sport and exercise medicine as a specialty in its own right, the bar is now set considerably higher for doctors and physiotherapists covering these events. The risk of being sued if things go wrong is significant. More importantly, all medical personnel covering sporting events have an ethical responsibility and duty of care to the participants to be properly trained and to make sure they have access to the necessary emergency equipment.

There are many things to take into consideration when agreeing to cover a sporting event and we will cover each one in turn:

Type of sport

Clearly, the type of sport being covered will influence the nature and frequency of injuries seen, and the medical cover, personnel, and equipment required.

In sports, such as motorsport and horse racing, for example, participants are more likely to sustain significant traumatic injuries and there is a requirement to provide personnel and equipment to manage a range of life- and limb-threatening emergencies.

In sports like rugby and football (soccer, American, Gaelic, Australian Rules), again, significant and minor trauma is commonly seen, although athletes also frequently present with over-use type injuries and acute muscle, tendon, and ligamentous injuries.

Sports such as professional boxing and martial arts may see an increased incidence of bleeding and head injuries, whilst diving, rugby, and equestrian see a higher incidence of spinal injuries.

Other sports such as cricket, golf, tennis, swimming, and track and field events, the incidence of life- and limb-threatening emergencies is significantly less. In these non-contact sports, a broad range of over-use type injuries are more commonly seen, but this is not to say that the more significant traumatic/orthopaedic and life-threatening problems do not also occur.

At any sporting event, sudden cardiac events can occur, both in the athletes themselves, but more commonly in excited support staff and spectators. Anaphylaxis may also be encountered in any sport.

⚠ It is important that the doctor or allied health professional covering the event is familiar with the rules of the sport they are covering.

Participants
Clearly, coverage of child, adult, and elderly sporting events will expose the sports medicine practitioner to pathology specific to that age group, and this needs to be accounted for in planning.

When possible, it is extremely useful to have carried out or have access to medical screening data of participants prior to the event. For example, athletes with a previous history of diabetes, epilepsy, cardiac problems, or a history of anaphylactic emergencies should be considered and potential emergencies planned for in advance. Knowledge of the past medical history is particularly important if travelling with a team, and the need for vaccination should also be considered when travelling.

Covering disabled sporting events carries unique challenges and these will be discussed in 📖 Chapter 19.

Responsibilities
When agreeing to cover an event, it is important to make clear from the outset what your responsibilities are. Are you there to cover the athletes only, the spectators/crowd, or both? Are you specifically attached to one team or side? Who is looking after your team's support staff? What other medical personnel will be present? What is their background and experience?

Depending on the size of the event, there will usually be separate first aid or medical cover for spectators. In the UK this is often provided by St John's Ambulance volunteers. At smaller events, where there is no specific doctor to cover spectators you may also be expected to treat people on the sideline. For larger events, it is the responsibility of the doctor covering the sporting event to inform the local A&E department in writing well in advance that the event is taking place. It is useful to reconfirm this closer to the time and to discuss the level of medical cover for the event with one of the senior A&E doctors.

Depending on the nature of the injury, illness, or medical complaint it is sometimes necessary for the doctor covering the athletes to help assess and treat someone from the crowd. One should be wary of being drawn into these situations as it can, in turn, leave the athletes on the field of play uncovered and we would discourage medical personnel specifically covering athletes from getting involved with the crowd unless absolutely necessary, e.g. life-threatening emergency where your help is required.

Venue

It is important to arrive early to look around and get a feel for the venue if you have not worked there before. It is useful to know where various key places and personnel are should you be called to give assistance off the field of play. Key areas to find well in advance of competition are ambulance access, all medical/physio areas, warm-up areas, antidoping rooms, media area, access points to the field of play. Covering events at large stadiums brings its own unique challenges.

The Taylor report was produced by Lord Taylor of Gosforth in the aftermath of the Hillsborough disaster in 1989. In this tragic incident at a football stadium in Sheffield, England, 96 Liverpool FC fans lost their lives. The Taylor report laid out recommendations for safety at sports grounds with specific advice regarding emergency medical cover for the crowd. This was followed by the publication of the Gibson report in 1990. This report stated that, when the number of spectators is expected to be greater than 2000, a doctor trained in advanced first aid is required to be present. The Taylor report recommended that at events where a crowd greater than 5000 is expected, a fully equipped ambulance should be present. It is important to be aware of any major incident plans. We would recommend clarifying what medical cover is in place for the crowd in advance when agreeing to cover athletes/participants at any sporting event.

Environmental conditions

Environmental conditions are an important consideration when planning to cover an event. Of particular concern are the risks of exercising in hot and cold conditions, and of exercising at high altitudes.

Exercising in high temperatures for long periods of time (e.g. marathons, triathlons) increases the risk of conditions such as heat stroke, exercise-associated collapse, and hyponatraemia. Heat stroke and hyponatraemia are medical emergencies, and adequate planning and preparation is crucial in preventing, identifying, and managing these conditions. The wet bulb globe temperature index (WBGT) is used in sport to determine how safe it is to exercise in warm conditions. It takes into account a variety of factors including air temperature, humidity, solar and ground radiation, and wind speed. It is recommended that endurance events should not be held when the WBGT exceeds 28°C. In cooler countries like the UK, the WBGT is not yet widely used at endurance sporting events, even though the above pathologies still occur. Cancelling an event due to adverse environmental conditions can initially bring much criticism both from organizers and participants who have put months into preparation, but ultimately it may be necessary to save lives.

In October 2007, the Chicago marathon was cancelled mid-run due to temperatures soaring to 31°C with one runner dying and hundreds admitted to hospital. In terms of preventative measures, educating participants well in advance on adequate conditioning, acclimatization, cooling, and appropriate rehydration strategies is important. Regular drink and first aid stations are essential. Medical support covering endurance events should be well trained and equipped to deal with emergencies peculiar to hot conditions. Many mass participation endurance events now issue doctors covering the event with rectal thermometers and have point of care analysers at the finish lines to measure serum sodium concentrations. Cold ice baths should be available at the finish for rapid cooling of participants with heat stroke.

Exercising in the cold brings a different set of challenges. Cold pathologies, such as hypothermia and frostbite are more likely to be seen in winter and water-based sports, such as cross-country skiing, mountain climbing, swimming, triathlon, wind surfing, and scuba diving. Endurance events where participants are exposed to milder temperatures for long periods of time with inadequate clothing can also be problematic, e.g. Ironman triathlon.

Hypothermia is defined as a core body temperature of 35°C or lower. As with heat pathologies, it is important that the covering doctor has an adequate thermometer if they are to correctly identify and monitor this condition. We would recommend the use of a low reading rectal thermometer for this purpose. Passive and active rewarming methods should be available when there is a risk of hypothermia, e.g. dry blankets, space blankets, hot drinks, hot air blankets, and the application of heat packs to the torso, axillae, and groin. Again, education of participants well in advance on preventative strategies and written guidance for well-trained medical staff is an essential part of planning.

We will discuss the management of environmental emergencies in more detail in Chapter 5.

Medical personnel required

Demand on medical services from previous similar event coverage will help guide the organizing medical officer when planning the number of doctors, physiotherapists, paramedics and ambulance technicians, nurses, first aiders, and sports massage therapists required.

It is important to take into account the expected number of participants and available epidemiological literature when planning medical cover. At larger national and international sporting events, teams often have their own doctors and physiotherapists who work alongside medical staff responsible for the event.

A co-ordinated multidisciplinary team approach is an important part of event coverage. It is useful to meet the different members of the team before the event starts to make introductions and raise any concerns.

We would strongly recommend practicing emergency scenarios with the different members of the team before the event starts, e.g. spinal injury, fracture dislocation of ankle, anaphylaxis, cardiac arrest, etc. This serves several purposes—it refreshes emergency care skills, it helps clarify people's roles, it familiarizes staff with the medical equipment they may need to use, and it helps people who may have never met before interact and get to know each other.

CHAPTER 1 **Planning and preparation**

Transportation

Imagine trying to carry a 16-stone rugby player with a badly sprained ankle 200 m to the warmth of the nearest dressing room and one soon understands the importance of assistance with transport. Simple items such as a stretcher or a set of crutches to transfer a casualty from the field of play should be readily available.

For time-critical emergencies, an ambulance should be sought to transport the athlete/patient to the most appropriate medical facility or hospital. Larger sporting events will usually have a fully equipped ambulance and paramedics in attendance at the venue. It may seem like common sense, but the covering medical personnel should know the emergency service number relevant to the country they are working in (i.e. 999 in UK). One should be ready to provide an accurate address and be able to give relevant information about the casualty to the ambulance control centre. If one is working in an area where it is likely to take a significant length of time to transport a casualty to hospital then they should be proficient in providing advanced life support in a pre-hospital setting.

To save valuable time, it is often useful to have someone at the entrance to the sporting venue to meet and direct the ambulance to the casualty.

Communication

As with working in any medical specialty, the practice of good communication skills can make the difference between a happy, competent, and well co-ordinated team of professionals and a disorganized, inefficient, and ineffective shambles! When covering certain sports, e.g. horse racing, motorsport, medical staff may be large distances apart and effective communication devices are crucial.

A charged mobile phone with good network signal coverage is one of the most useful items to have in your possession when covering a sporting event. It is useful to exchange mobile numbers with other medical personnel and key officials covering the event. Many larger events will also have walkie-talkies (hand-held radio transceivers) for medical staff and officials. In noisy venues with large crowds it is useful to have an earpiece connection or even headphones. It is important to test these devices before usage to make sure one is using the correct channel and that the volume is adequate.

Equipment and medication

Items will vary depending on the practitioner's own preference, the type of sport covered, local supplies, number of participants, and duration of event coverage. Pitch side doctors and physiotherapists will often carry a small grab bag (Fig. 1.1) with commonly used emergency equipment and medication. It is important to be mindful of the world antidoping agency (WADA) code and its banned substance list when preparing medication supplies for a sporting event. The following list is neither prescriptive nor exhaustive.

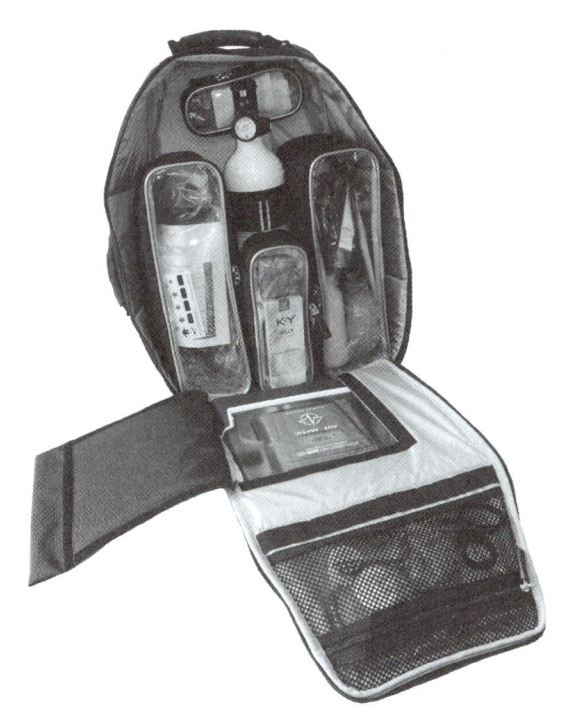

Fig. 1.1 Pitch side resuscitation bag—'Sportpromote'.

- Effective means of communication with paramedics—own mobiles and walkie talkies
- Designated first aid or treatment room with the ability to provide privacy for the casualty
- Automated external defibrillator (AED)—defibrillator
- Emergency equipment including oro- and nasopharyngeal airways, laryngeal mask apparatus, O_2, Entonox®, bag valve mask, range of cervical collars, spinal board, selection of intravenous (IV) cannulae, fracture splints
- IV fluids (normal saline 1 L) IV giving sets, selection of cannulae, and venflon skin fixers
- Resus pocket masks
- EpiPen® or generic alternative (or adrenaline 1:1000 solution 1 mg in 1 mL—1 ampoule)
- Otoscope/ophthalmoscope
- Stethoscope
- Sphygmomanometer

CHAPTER 1 **Planning and preparation**

- Mirror
- Thermometer
- Blood glucose testing meter
- British National Formulary (BNF)/BNF for Children (BNFC)
- Bottles of water for rehydration and cleaning
- Peak flow meter
- Salbutamol inhalers
- Compatible spacer device
- Beclometasone inhaler
- Portable nebulizer
- Salbutamol nebules
- Ipratropium bromide nebulizer solution
- Prednisolone tablets
- Beclometasone spray
- Paracetamol
- Codeine
- Ibuprofen
- Diclofenac
- Voltarol Emulgel®
- Loperamide
- Metoclopramide po
- Metoclopramide—10 mg 2-mL amp for injection
- Gaviscon® liquid
- Omeprazole
- Broad spectrum antibiotics
- Benzylpenicillin 600 mg for intramuscular (IM) injection—Crystapen® 2 vial GP pack
- Hydrocortisone 1% cream
- Strepsils® or other throat lozenges
- Disposable tongue depressors
- Urinalysis Multistix®
- Fluorescein eye drops 1%
- Tetracaine eye drops 1%
- Ear drops—Otomize®
- Bandages, slings/triangular bandage, sterile gauze pads, cling film, providone-iodine, dressing packs, dressings—dry, moist, and non-stick
- Scalpels
- Needles—greens, blues and orange
- 2, 5, and 10-mL syringes
- Suture kits
- 3/0, 4/0 and 5/0 sutures
- Steri-strips®
- Staple suture pack
- Anti-tetanus prophylaxis
- Nasal plugs
- Sterets
- Lidocaine 1%
- Bupivicaine 0.5%
- Range of Tubigrip® sizes
- Variety of tapes
- Collar and cuff

- Chlorphenamine for injection 10 mg/mL
- Cetirizine or other antihistamine
- Hydrocortisone for injection—Efcortesol® 5-mL ampoule
- Diazemuls® 5 mg/mL—2 mL ampoule
- Diazepam rectal tube 2.5 mL (10 mg) tube
- Saline or water for injection—10 mL
- GlucoGel® gel
- Glucagon for injection 1 mg
- Glucose for IV injection 20%, 50 mL
- Bib clearly identifying role
- Identification with assured access to all areas
- Bag for kit
- Vinyl or latex examination gloves
- Injury reporting sheets with carbon copy paper
- Sharps disposal bins
- Clinical waste bags
- Heavy gauge scissors
- Emergency cricothyroidotomy kit
- Morphine sulphate for intravenous injection—10 mg/mL × 10 (this will need to written on a separate script and kept in a locked case). It requires secure storage outside of competition times and if carried should be obtained using form FP10CDF
- Naloxone 2 mL (800 mcg) prefilled syringe
- Glyceryl trinitrate (GTN) spray 400 mcg/dose
- Aspirin 300 mg
- Adrenaline 1 in 10,000—1 mg in 10 mL for injection
- Hyoscine butylbromide
- Ice bags
- Dental kit
- Sport concussion assessment tool (SCAT) card

You will need to ensure you are familiar with all the equipment you take with you or are provided with at the event, i.e. AED. Remember that controlled drugs, whilst useful, are also potentially problematic (i.e. keeping secure, passing through airport security) and you should give serious consideration to such issues when travelling abroad.

In terms of getting your own kit together it is perhaps easier to think about what you require to manage your patient with respect to the airway, breathing, circulation (A, B, C), and break down the other items into either the medical or surgical items you will need. Keeping these different items in 3 separate smaller bags within 1 large bag will help to ensure you have everything to hand when you need it.

Do not be too concerned about bringing complex items of kit at the expense of remembering the simple things, i.e. gloves, sharps bins, etc.

Documentation

Documentation in a sporting context may be difficult, with many consultations taking place in a public place where writing detailed notes and recording medical information electronically may simply not be possible. The use of hand-held electronic devices that link to computers can be useful for the more IT literate practitioner. It is often necessary to document consultations many minutes or even hours after the assessment took place, and some form of *aide memoire*, such as a notepad, is often helpful. Most professional sports clubs now use encrypted online electronic medical records, which can be accessed and added to from anywhere in the world with Internet access.

In the medico-legal age we now work in, good documentation is increasingly important. In emergencies, good documentation is particularly important for communicating with medical staff taking over care in a hospital setting. Injury reporting sheets, as used by paramedics, with sections for primary and secondary surveys together with carbon copy paper are useful for this purpose.

Headed note paper and a prescription pad are also useful.

Security/identification
At major championships, participants, officials, and medical staff are issued with accreditation passes. These will usually have numbers to signify which areas can be accessed. It is important to check that you will be able to access any area where your assistance may be needed. This usually means access all areas, although this is not always possible. In life-threatening emergencies (particularly in foreign countries where language barriers can be a problem) one may need to get access to a competitor quickly to ensure proper medical care is established. It is useful to plan for these eventualities in advance and anything that easily identifies you as medical personnel is usually all that is needed. In the current political climate, large sporting events can be a target for terrorists and it is useful to be familiar with any major incident plans.

Indemnity
Medical staff covering sporting events should discuss their indemnity cover with their defence organization in advance to make sure they are covered for any potential legal action. National governing bodies in sport may also be able to offer advice in this difficult area. In professional sport, indemnity insurance can prove costly, but should never be ignored.

Further reading
Allen M (2000). Medical officers at sporting events. *Journal of the Medical Defence Union*, **16**:8–9.

Gibson RM (1990). *Report of the Medical Working Party*. HMSO, London.

Lord Justice Taylor (1990). *Final Report into the Hillsborough Stadium Disaster*. HMSO, London.

www.sportpromote.co.uk/medical-bag.

Chapter 2

General approach to the injured or unwell athlete

Introduction *12*

Introduction

Proper planning prevents poor performance.

Doctors and other healthcare professionals will be called upon to deal with both traumatic and medical emergencies. The general principles in the treatment of these patients are the same. Often there will be little or no information available to the attending professional, and so the priorities must be to restore the patient's vital functions first, and then, when time allows a more detailed head to toe assessment can be carried out.

The assessment, by definition, must be rapid and accompanied by action. It must also be thorough and miss nothing out. The prioritized assessment, which was first comprehensively described in the advanced trauma life support course, lends itself to the treatment of the critically ill patient, but should also be used in the initial assessment of all patients. This chapter will give an overview of the assessment but details will also be available in subsequent chapters.

Preparation

- Ensure you have equipment available to you to deal with the emergencies you might encounter
- Ensure that you are familiar with any equipment provided at an event
- Ensure you are familiar with evacuation routes for casualties
- Ensure you are aware of local facilities to continue the treatment of your patients and how to access them in an emergency
- Ensure that you regularly practice scenarios for the conditions you are likely to encounter, ideally with the other healthcare resources you will usually have available
- Ensure all personnel involved in treating a patient are aware of the principles of initial assessment and management, as well as the potential resources involved in the care of these patients
- Ensure that you understand when it is safe or appropriate to approach a patient while on the field of play. It is often best to discuss this with any official, ensuring that emergency care can be delivered in a safe environment and in a timely manner.

Rapid assessment and synchronous resuscitation

Obtain a brief history from the patient, relatives, or witnesses. This can be done while beginning to assess the patient. The mnemonic AMPLE is useful in this regard.
- **A**—allergies
- **M**—medication
- **P**—past medical history
- **L**—last meal
- **E**—events leading up to the need for medical help.

Check whether the patient is conscious

Always approach a patient involved in trauma as if they may have a cervical spine injury. Before talking to the patient hands should be placed around the head to provide in line immobilization of the neck. This is best provided by approaching a prone patient from their head end. Approaching from the side

and calling to a patient is likely to provoke the reaction of turning the head, which may exacerbate a spinal injury.
- If the patient is conscious then introduce yourself and reassure the patient. Patients who survive critical situations will often remember calm words directed to them for a long time afterwards
- If the patient is unconscious call for help and continue the assessment
- Ensure that you have allocated a single person to call an ambulance, asking them to confirm to you when this has been achieved
- Initially check to see if the patient is breathing. If they are not breathing then proceed directly to treat them for cardiac arrest—detailed in 📖 Chapter 3.

A: assess the airway
- If the patient is able to speak normally, then the airway is patent. Ensure that the voice is not 'hoarse', or that stridor is present from upper airway obstruction, or injury
- If stridor or hoarseness is present, then urgent transfer to an emergency department (ED) is indicated. The patient should be kept calm and given high flow oxygen. Do not attempt to examine the throat. No surgical airway is indicated in a conscious patient
- If the patient is unconscious then the airway can be opened by a jaw thrust manoeuvre:
  - Direct visualization of the oral cavity can be made and suction, if available, used to clear any secretions/blood, etc.
  - Keep the tip of the suction catheter under direct vision at all times
  - Large objects can be removed from the mouth, such as mouth guards, but no blind finger sweeps should be undertaken
  - Ensure enough personnel are available to log roll the patient in the event of vomiting—ensure they understand their individual role in the event of requiring a log roll.

B: assess the breathing
- Count the respiratory rate and assess the effort required in breathing, such as pain, extramuscular use (in-drawing, recession, tracheal tug, etc.)
- Examine the chest for abnormal movement patterns such as asymmetrical chest movement or evidence of a flail segment
- Check for tenderness
- If possible listen to the chest for additional sounds such as wheeze or absence of sounds suggestive of a pneumothorax. If a pneumothorax is suspected check for evidence of tension by ensuring the trachea is central suggesting no abnormal mediastinal shift
- For treatment of chest injuries see 📖 Chapter 3; however, the majority of chest injuries are treated initially with high flow oxygen only
- If a tension pneumothorax is suspected then it can be relieved by a needle decompression, if the practitioner has been trained in the procedure.

In the athletic population it is appropriate to treat all patients with a potential chest injury with high flow oxygen.

C: assess the circulation
- Feel the pulse and count the rate
- If the radial pulse is palpable then it may be assumed that the systolic Blood Pressure (BP) is over 90 mmHg. If a pulse is not palpable then intravenous fluids (IV) may be beneficial and simple manoeuvres such as raising the legs would be appropriate, depending on the injuries to the pelvis, or lower limbs
- Examine for distended neck veins. If they are distended then consider a diagnosis of tension pneumothorax if other signs are present:
  - Evidence of chest injury
  - Respiratory distress
  - Reduced breath sounds
  - Hyper-resonance to the chest on the affected side.

Shock can be divided into 5 mechanisms
- Hypovolaemic
- Neurogenic (due to spinal injury and characterized by decreased blood pressure, but a normal or slow heart rate)
- Obstructive (e.g. tension pneumothorax)
- Cardiogenic
- Septic.

In sports medicine the first three are the most likely. It must be remembered that athletes have a large cardiac reserve and will often have a bradycardic resting pulse. In these circumstances a 'normal' heart rate may be indicative of early 'shock'.

The treatment of shock includes applying pressure to external bleeding points, IV fluids if the radial pulse is absent, raising the legs if appropriate, giving high flow oxygen via a non re-breath mask (one with a reservoir bag).

D: assess neurological disability
This is best assessed using the AVPU scale:
- **A**—patient alert
- **V**—patient responds to verbal stimulus
- **P**—patient only responds to painful stimulus
- **U**—patient is unresponsive.

If the patient is alert but has suffered a head injury then further analysis for concussion should be carried out using an appropriate scoring system (see p.116).

Always assume a neck injury, and protect the cervical spine unless you have clinically examined, and cleared any possible injury.

E: expose the patient
Always ensure that all potential injuries have been excluded. This is best done by a rapid head to toe examination as indicated by the injury pattern. Ensure the patient remains warm.

Continuing evaluation of the patient
- If the patient's condition deteriorates always reassess the patients ABCDE, and treat appropriately
- Arrange for evacuation of the patient to an appropriate medical area while awaiting further assistance from the ambulance service or other appropriate medical care
- Evacuation of the patient should be carried out assuming a spinal injury whenever appropriate. The log roll of the patient is an essential element of this process and whenever possible the team likely to be involved in this manoeuvre should practice together prior to the event.

The log roll
This is an important manoeuvre in the care of any patient with a suspected spinal injury, including an unconscious patient. This involves 4 personnel to carry out the roll and at least one person to examine the patient or manoeuvre extraction equipment into place.

Person 1
This person provides in line immobilization of the cervical spine. They are also in charge of the whole manoeuvre and therefore have additional responsibilities.
- Ensure safety of the patient at all times
- Ensure all personnel are briefed as to the mechanism of the roll
- Ensure all staff have correct hand positions
- Ensure all staff are briefed as to the correct instructions for the roll. This is often best expressed by 'ready, brace, roll'—where the manoeuvre starts on the instruction roll
- Ensure the patient is briefed.

Person 2
Ensure the arms are placed across the chest, and then position hands so that one is placed on the opposite shoulder to where this person is placed, and the other on the pelvis.

Person 3
One hand is placed on the pelvis next to person 2 hand (sometimes they cross hands for stability). The other is placed under the patients opposite thigh.

Person 4
One hand is placed under the thigh next to person 3 hand. The other hand is placed under the opposite calf. All hands should be placed on bony areas for stability.

Extremity trauma

This will also be covered in subsequent chapters, but the principles of treatment are:
- Check for a pulse
- If obvious deformity and a pulse is palpable then do not attempt reduction unless trained to do so
- If obvious deformity and no pulse, then if the practitioner feels comfortable in gently reducing the area to an anatomical position, this can be attempted. If a pulse is regained then splint the limb in that position. If no pulse is achieved then ensure that medical personnel summoned are aware of the absence of a pulse
- Splint the limb—this is usually achieved through the use of a box splint, although vacuum splints may also be used. It is important to practice with the equipment available prior to an event
- If the wound is open, i.e. a breach of the skin has occurred, then a clean dressing should be placed over the area. If possible a photograph should be taken, so that other attending practitioners can review the wound without removing the dressing
- Analgesia should be provided. This is often best given by the use of Entonox®, or opiates if monitoring is available.

Entonox®

This is a 50:50 mixture of NO and O_2. It is delivered through a patient demand valve. It provides analgesia, but does not render the patient unconscious. It has a short half-life, so constant inhalation while in pain will be necessary.

Contraindications to use:
- Head injury
- Chest injury
- Suspected injury due to diving to depths.

Relative contraindications to use
- Patients where air may be trapped in an organ, e.g. post some ophthalmological operations, sinusitis, etc.
- In a cold environment it is necessary to mix the gases, which will separate under 4°C. This involves inversion of the bottle at least three times.

Opiates

- Fentanyl 'lollipops' are increasingly being used in the pre-hospital environment
- They provide excellent analgesia without the need for IV access
- Patients must have appropriate monitoring available and be trained in their use
- Storage of the drug must comply with regulations regarding the storage of controlled drugs.

Chapter 3

Cardiorespiratory arrest

Basic life support: an introduction *18*
Adult basic life support *20*
Paediatric basic life support *26*
Adult advanced life support *28*
Planning for critical care incidents at sporting events *31*

Basic life support: an introduction

The most recent European Resuscitation Council Guidelines were published in October 2010. The key message from these guidelines remains the provision of effective CPR and early defibrillation where available.

These guidelines do not fundamentally change from the greater emphasis on chest compressions that was the basis of the 2005 guidelines. The aim is making these as uninterrupted as possible. The ratio of compressions to ventilations therefore remains 30:2.

- Once CPR has started it should not stop unless the victim shows signs of life, such as return of consciousness, in addition to a return of normal breathing
- Within a sports setting, there is also the potential of concurrent trauma and so manual in-line immobilization (MILS) should be carried out to protect the cervical spine during resuscitation attempts if injury is suspected:
  - This will not be possible with only 1 provider of life support
  - If MILS is interfering with quality of resuscitation, and the risk of neck injury is considered to be low then it may be discarded
- On field cardiac arrest classically occurs as an 'off the ball' syncopal collapse
- Recent high profile cases such as Marc Vivian Foe, Miklos Feher, and Antonia Puerta continue to highlight the issue of sudden cardiac death:
  - They demonstrate the need to ensure adequate training of pitchside medical staff in life-support, as well as access to appropriate medical kit including defibrillators
  - The case of the collapse of Evander Sno who was successfully defibrillated at the pitchside also shows the invaluable benefit to be gained by being trained in life support and having the appropriate kit.

Remember that basic life support (BLS) is only basic in terms of the levels of kit required to perform it. It is a vital part of the cardiac arrest management and you should be familiar with the algorithms so that you are comfortable in performing it.

Adult basic life support

This is based upon the European Resuscitation Guidelines 2010. Follows an ABC approach (Fig. 3.1):
- Check safe to approach
- Speak to casualty 'Are you alright?'
- Stimulate the casualty for responsiveness through gentle shaking, but if a potential spinal injury is suspected consider a very gentle stimulus above and below the clavicle.

Outcome 1: patient responds
Leave him where he is unless he is in danger. Try to find out what's wrong. Reassess regularly.

Outcome 2: no response
- Shout for help and turn patient onto their back. Pay some consideration to the chance of a potential spinal injury when moving the athlete, but not if it interferes with ongoing management
- If still no response:
  - Call for help
  - Ensure an ambulance has been called and an AED requested
  - Ensure you have access to your resuscitation equipment.
- **A** Open the airway via head tilt, chin lift, or jaw thrust
- **B** Place your cheek above the casualty's mouth:
  - Look (at the chest)
  - Listen (for breathing)
  - Feel (breath on your cheek) for normal breathing for *no more* than 10 s. If you have any doubt then act as if *not* normal
- **C** Those who are skilled at palpating the carotid pulse can do so whilst assessing breathing. Otherwise look for signs of circulation, such as the athletes colour and normal breathing.

Outcome 1: patient breathing normally
- Place patient to the recovery position
- Await ambulance
- Reassess breathing regularly.

Outcome 2: not breathing normally
- Ensure an ambulance has been called/requested, leave the patient as a last measure to contact help
- If the casualty is not breathing normally, assume there is no circulation and commence cardiac compressions at a ratio of 30 compressions to 2 rescue breaths and at a rate of compression of 100–120/min
- Continue until:
  - The patient shows signs of a regaining consciousness *and* starts to breathe normally
  - Until more skilled help arrives
  - Until you are exhausted.

ADULT BASIC LIFE SUPPORT

```
UNRESPONSIVE?
      ↓
Shout for help
      ↓
 Open airway
      ↓
NOT BREATHING NORMALLY?
      ↓
   Call 999
      ↓
  30 chest
compressions
      ↓
2 rescue breaths
30 compressions
```

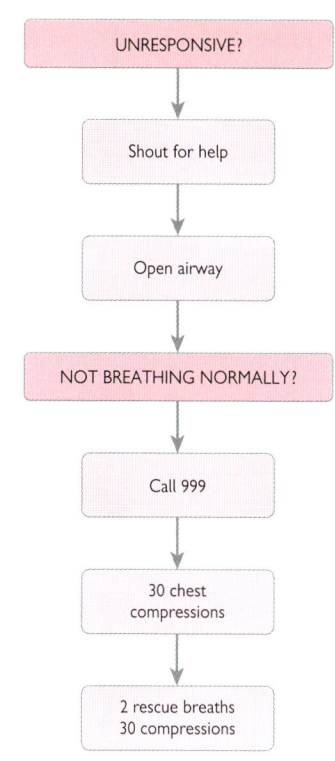

Fig. 3.1 Adult basic life support algorithm. Reproduced with the kind permission of the Resuscitation Council (UK).

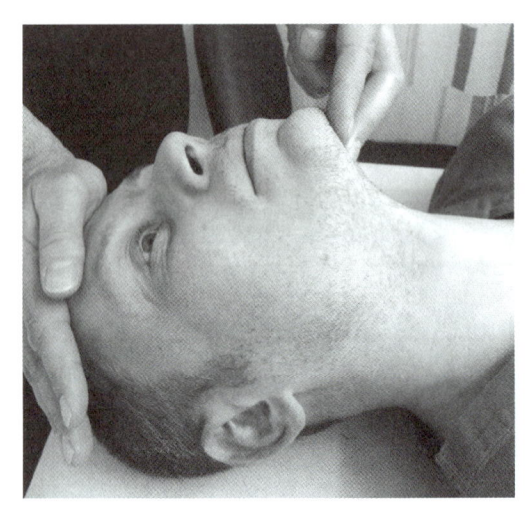

Fig. 3.2 Head tilt, chin lift.

Head tilt, chin lift
- Unsuitable in suspected c-spine injury.
- Place one hand across the forehead and two fingers of the other under the point of the chin.
- Lift up under the chin and support the forehead – 'Sniffing the morning air' position—see Fig. 3.2.

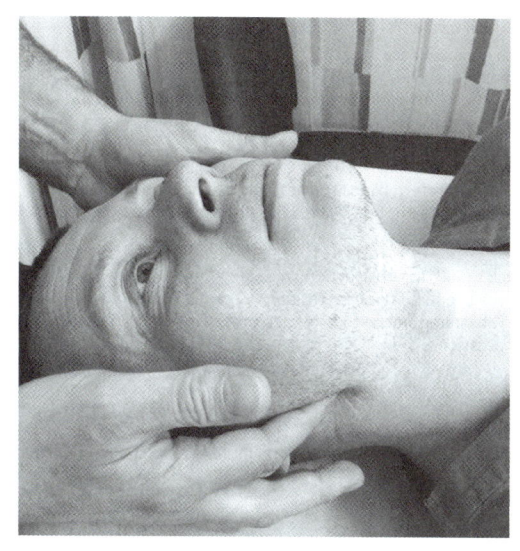

Fig. 3.3 Jaw thrust.

Jaw thrust
- Not recommended for lay individuals
- Place both thumbs on the zygomas with the fingers behind the angles of the mandible
- Lift the mandible forward thus elevating the tongue away from the soft palate—see Fig. 3.3.

Cardiac compressions
- Ratio of 30 compressions: 2 breaths
- Kneel by the side of the victim
- Place the heel of one hand in the centre of the chest with the other hand upon it
- Press firmly down 5–6 cm. Allow full recoil of chest after compression
- Return hands to starting position without losing contact with the chest
- Repeat 30 times
- Perform compressions at a rate of 100–120/min.

Rescue breaths
- Pinch nose with the index finger and thumb of the hand resting on the patient's forehead
- Allow mouth to open, but maintain chin lift
- Form a seal around victim's lips with your mouth
- Blow steadily into mouth
- Watch chest rise for 1 s. (This is shorter than in previous guidelines)
- Repeat and return hands to chest compression position, thereby minimizing interruptions. The 2 breaths should take no more than 5 s.

What if the chest doesn't rise on rescue breaths?
- Check mouth for obstruction
- Is there adequate neck extension?
- Do not attempt more than two breaths before returning to compressions.

Tired
- Evidence suggests the quality of compressions falls in tired rescuers, so swap after 2 min
- *Compression only:* perform cardiopulmonary resuscitation (CPR) at a rate of 100–120/min
- Entirely reasonable for those unwilling to do mouth to mouth ventilation.

Risk to rescuer from mouth to mouth resuscitation
- Very small
- Occasional report of tuberculosis or severe acute respiratory syndrome (SARS)
- No HIV transmission reported
- Consider use of a pocket mask with valve.

Upon arrival of a defibrillator
- Connect pads to patient and shock *immediately* if advised.
- **Note:** 2° min of CPR are no longer performed before defibrillating in the case of an unwitnessed arrest out of hospital.

Drowning
Five initial rescue breaths followed by 1 min of chest compressions is recommended *before* going to get help.

Paediatric basic life support

The main difference between the cardiac arrest suffered by a child compared with an adult is that the aetiology is usually primarily cardiac in adults whereas in children it is more commonly respiratory resulting in a secondary cardiac arrest (see Fig. 3.4).

Initial assessment is along the same A, B, C guidelines as for the adult.
- Check safe to approach
- Speak to casualty 'Are you alright?'
- Stimulate the casualty for responsiveness through gentle shaking, but if a potential spinal injury is suspected consider a very gentle stimulus above and below the clavicle.

Outcome 1: patient responds
- Leave him where he is unless he is in danger
- Try to find out what's wrong
- Reassess regularly.

Outcome 2: no response
- Shout for help and turn patient onto their back. Pay some consideration to the chance of a potential spinal injury when moving the athlete, but not if it interferes with ongoing management.
- If still no response:
  - Call for help
  - Ensure an ambulance has been called
  - Ensure you have access to your resuscitation equipment
- Upon confirming arrest give 5 initial rescue breaths before starting compressions
- If you are on your own, perform 1 min of CPR *before* going for help
- Ratio of 15 compressions: 2 breaths
- Compress the chest by *at least* one-third of its depth. This is a subtle difference to highlight and reassure that it is safe to compress a child's chest.
  - Use two fingers for an infant under 1 year
  - Use one or two hands for a child over 1 year as needed to achieve depth of compression. Rate is at least 100, but not greater than 120/min
- If you are struggling to achieve ventilations then consider foreign body or repositioning of the child's head or neck to a more 'neutral' position compared to the 'sniffing the morning air' position used in adults
- A standard defibrillator can be safely used for children over 8 years of age:
  - Between the ages of 1 and 8 years paediatric pads or mode if available on the AED should be used if possible. If not available then use the AED as it comes.
  - For an infant under 1-year-old, if no other manually adjustable defibrillator is available then an AED should still be used if the rhythm is shockable.

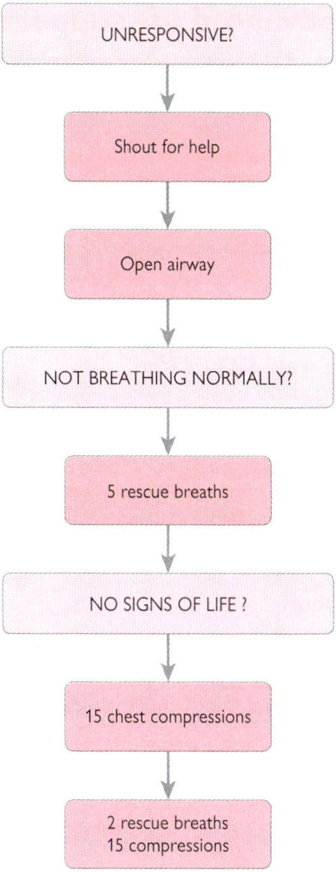

PAEDIATRIC BASIC LIFE SUPPORT

```
UNRESPONSEIVE?
     ↓
Shout for help
     ↓
Open airway
     ↓
NOT BREATHING NORMALLY?
     ↓
5 rescue breaths
     ↓
NO SIGNS OF LIFE ?
     ↓
15 chest compressions
     ↓
2 rescue breaths
15 compressions
```

Fig. 3.4 Paediatric basic life support. Reproduced with the kind permission of the Resuscitation Council (UK).

Adult advanced life support

- Initially follows the BLS algorithm, but rather than continuing to exhaustion, there is reassessment at 2 min intervals. The difference is to intervene with early defibrillation and possibly drug therapy if appropriate
- The crux of advanced life support (ALS) is deciding if the rhythm is shockable (ventricular fibrillation, ventricular tachycardia) or non-shockable (asystole or pulseless electrical activity) whereupon a separate limb of the algorithm develops for each (Fig. 3.5)
- 2 min of 30 compressions to 2 ventilations roughly equates to 10 breaths, i.e. 5 cycles of 30:2
- CPR should continue even while the defibrillator is charging, thus minimizing the loss of compressions pre-shock.

Automated external defibrillator

- This device is capable of analysing the underlying cardiac rhythm and advising the user whether to deliver a shock to attempt to re-store normal circulation
- They come in a variety of complexities, but are very reliable and a safe way of partially skilled users performing defibrillation. Training is *not* required in order to use these
- AED should be requested at the same time that the ambulance is called.

Abnormal rhythms

Ventricular fibrillation (VF)
- Random uncoordinated myocyte activity
- Always fatal unless defibrillated.

Ventricular tachycardia (VT)
- The beat is being led by ventricular muscle rather than the natural pacemaker of the heart—the sinoatrial node
- A rhythm of varying degrees of organization, so it may or may not provide a blood pressure
- An inefficient rhythm that will eventually decay to VF.

Asystole
- No electrical activity in the heart
- Cannot be defibrillated
- Has a very poor outcome.

Pulseless electrical activity (PEA)
- Normal electrical activity of the heart is uncoupled from its mechanical action
- Usually a complex cause that needs to be addressed
- A non-shockable rhythm.

Drugs

Delivery should be intravenous (IV). If IV access is unavailable then the intraosseous route is recommended. The tracheal route is no longer recommended.

Adrenaline 1 mg
- 1 in 10,000 IV. 10 mL = 1 mg
- Given in the shockable side of the ALS algorithm immediately after the third shock and every 3–5 min thereafter
- Works as a powerful peripheral vasoconstrictor, thus promoting blood flow to vital organs
- In the non-shockable side of the algorithm it is given immediately, then every 3–5 min.

Amiodarone 300 mg
Given at the same time as adrenaline after the 3rd shock.

Atropine 3 mg IV
No longer routinely recommended in asystole or PEA.

Prolonged or non-shockable arrests
Consider the '4H's and 4T's' and address these issues as necessary.
- *Hypothermia:* caused by immersion or exposure
- *Hyper/hypokalaemia:* think medication (diuretics)
- *Hypoxia:* common in general population and children
- *Hypovolaemia:* recent trauma or occult bleeding?
- *Thromboembolic disease:* recent flight?
- *Toxins:* recreational drugs?
- *Tamponade:* recent chest trauma?
- *Tension pneumothorax:* recent trauma or chest pain?

Advanced airway management
- Most airways will be managed with effective basic manoeuvres and a bag valve mask
- Equipment such as a nasopharyngeal airway (NPA) or an oropharygeal airway (OPA) are useful tools
- In ALS, endotracheal intubation is the 'gold standard' method of addressing hypoxia
- However, intubation is a complex skill that needs to be performed frequently to ensure safe insertion; it is thus out of the scope for many sports medicine practitioners
- An intermediate stage of airway management involves the laryngeal mask airway (LMA)—effectively a 'hands-free' face mask that is inserted to sit on top of the glottis
- LMAs need little skill or practice to use and are a useful tool in the sports setting. A more modern variant is the i-gel thermogel device.

Key advanced life support points/ changes
- Minimize interruptions to chest compressions. Rhythmic compression maintains coronary perfusion pressure during diastole. This pressure falls rapidly when compressions cease. Continue chest compressions whilst waiting for the defibrillator to charge. Each minutes delay in defibrillation results in a 10% decreased chance that resuscitation will be successful
- Compress the chest 5–6cm at a rate of 100–120 per min
- Rescue breaths take 1 s to inflate the chest
- Atropine is no longer recommended.

30 CHAPTER 3 Cardiorespiratory arrest

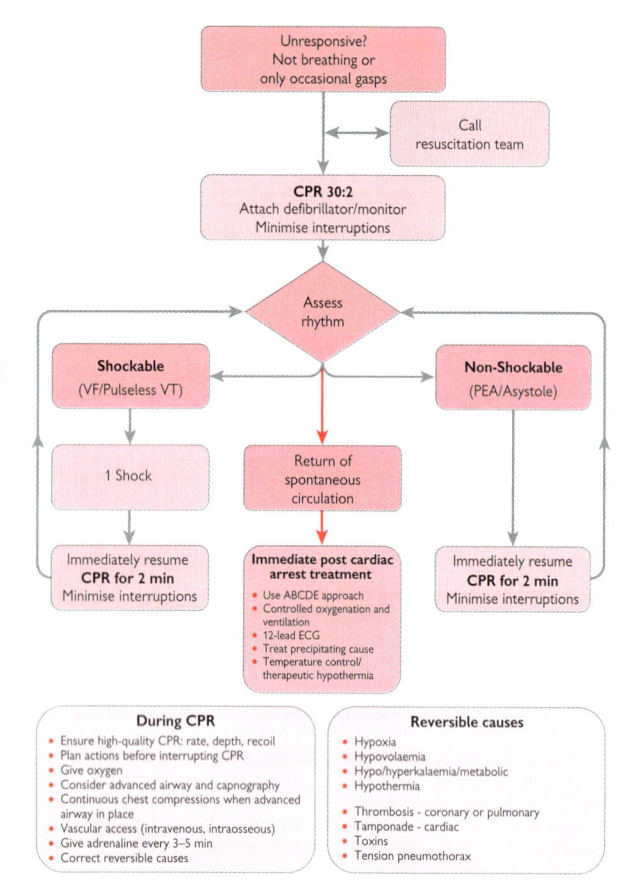

```
                    Unresponsive?
                    Not breathing or
                    only occasional gasps
                           ↕                    Call
                                           resuscitation team

                         CPR 30:2
                 Attach defibrillator/monitor
                    Minimise interruptions

                         Assess
                         rhythm

      Shockable                              Non-Shockable
    (VF/Pulseless VT)                        (PEA/Asystole)

         ↓                Return of                  ↓
      1 Shock          spontaneous
                        circulation

         ↓                   ↓                       ↓
   Immediately resume   Immediate post cardiac    Immediately resume
   CPR for 2 min        arrest treatment          CPR for 2 min
   Minimise             • Use ABCDE approach      Minimise interruptions
   interruptions        • Controlled oxygenation
                          and ventilation
                        • 12-lead ECG
                        • Treat precipitating cause
                        • Temperature control/
                          therapeutic hypothermia
```

During CPR	Reversible causes
• Ensure high-quality CPR: rate, depth, recoil	• Hypoxia
• Plan actions before interrupting CPR	• Hypovolaemia
• Give oxygen	• Hypo/hyperkalaemia/metabolic
• Consider advanced airway and capnography	• Hypothermia
• Continuous chest compressions when advanced airway in place	• Thrombosis - coronary or pulmonary
• Vascular access (intravenous, intraosseous)	• Tamponade - cardiac
• Give adrenaline every 3–5 min	• Toxins
• Correct reversible causes	• Tension pneumothorax

Fig. 3.5 Adult advanced life support algorithm. Reproduced with the kind permission of the Resuscitation Council (UK).

Planning for critical care incidents at sporting events

- There are now many courses in the UK that provide sports pre-hospital critical care skills. (E.g. Remo/Area/Immofp/Phtcc/Scrumcaps/Sportpromote)
- All these courses advise that availability of critical care kit and appropriate training to use it should be an essential part of match day planning
- Remember that the guidelines suggest attempted defibrillation should occur within 3 min of a cardiac arrest, therefore having a defibrillator locked in someone's car is insufficient!
- Critical care kit needs to be in the immediate vicinity of where athletic activity is taking place and skill updates need to be frequently repeated by all members of the wider medical team.

Further reading

Resuscitation Council.

శ www.resus.org.uk.

Chapter 4

Athletes with pre-existing conditions

Diabetes mellitus *34*
Respiratory *36*
Neurological and neuromuscular disorders *38*
Cardiovascular conditions *42*
Arthritis *48*
Female athlete triad *49*

Diabetes mellitus

▶▶ For the management of hypoglycaemia and diabetic keto-acidosis (DKA) see 📖 p.92.

- Diabetes is a chronic condition characterized by a lack of endogenous insulin. This results in chaotic blood glucose levels
- Diabetes occurs in approximately 4% of the UK population. There has been a notable increase in diagnosed cases in the last 10 years, although this varies widely depending on different population groups
- Approximately 10–15% of diabetics are insulin dependent with 85–90% either dietary or tablet controlled
- Exercise is important in the diabetic population due to the secondary effects diabetes has on end organ disease and its association with such conditions as ischaemic heart disease, hypertension, and peripheral vascular disease
- As a team clinician you may be called to treat someone who is suffering the effects of diabetes who is either known to be diabetic, or presenting for the first time
- A history of lethargy, polyuria, and polydipsia are classically described symptoms for someone presenting with diabetes. More subtle presentations such as recurring skin infections should also raise the possibility of the diagnosis
  - Always test blood sugar in an athlete in whom you suspect diabetes may be a possibility or the cause of the symptoms presenting to you
  - Capillary blood glucose testing kits are readily available and relatively inexpensive, but may provide you with vital information about your athlete
- Usual blood glucose is 4–6 mmol/L though this can increase to 8 mmol/L after meals
- A fasting venous blood glucose of >7 mmol/L is suggestive of diabetes, as is a random blood sugar of >11.1 mmol/L
  - Diagnosis should not be made on the basis of just one blood test especially if there are no specific symptoms
  - Remember the stress response can elevate blood glucose
  - If in doubt, the diagnosis is confirmed using a 2 h glucose tolerance test where blood sugar will be >11.1 mmol/L.

Impaired glucose regulation

This condition is important as it may lead eventually to diabetes, but is managed in the first instance using dietary advice and exercise. It is usually diagnosed where fasting glucose is <7 mmol/L, but oral glucose tolerance test (OGTT) is >7.8 mmol/L, but <11.1 mmol/L.

'Gestational diabetes' encompasses both gestational impaired glucose tolerance and gestational diabetes mellitus. Diagnostic criteria are as above and should be reviewed post-partum.

World Antidoping Agency

Insulin remains a prohibited substance on the World Antidoping Agency WADA's checklist and as such any athlete diagnosed with insulin dependent diabetes must have a therapeutic use exemption certificate competed in accordance with WADA regulations.

Diabetes and exercise

The benefits of exercise on the secondary effects of diabetes such as peripheral and cardiovascular disease is well recognized. It will help in weight loss and promote increased insulin sensitivity. However, glycaemic control can become harder to manage especially in prolonged exercise as glucose stores deplete.

The main aims of diabetic management are to:
- Allow the individual to enjoy life as normally as possible, taking as much responsibility for their disease management as they can. For the athlete, the aims are exactly the same
- The goal is to provide as much education as possible, encouraging the patient to pre-empt the symptoms they are likely to experience such as dehydration and hypoglycaemia by keeping well hydrated and taking enough carbohydrates
- General advice includes taking a carbohydrate snack prior to exercise if the blood sugar level is <5.5 mmol/L. It is a balancing act that may also involve reducing the dose of insulin on days of heavy exercise, and increasing the number of times that the blood glucose is taken
- Self-testing may need to occur, before, during as well as after exercise
- Keeping a stock of easily absorbed carbohydrate readily to hand is vital, and encouraging the athlete to take responsibility for bringing this with them helps to reinforce their autonomy over their disease.

Foot care

Even small wounds affecting the toes can become significant issues with the increased incidence of infection in diabetics. This is compounded by the effects of peripheral vascular disease and neuropathy.
- Regular inspection of footwear, both training and competing can help to minimize the risks of wounds developing
- Good simple foot hygiene and nail care is also vital
- If in doubt refer the athlete to a podiatrist, chiropodist, or back to the diabetic team caring for them.

Diabetes and infection

The aim is to prevent infections from developing, but when they do then insulin requirements will increase. Even in the face of decreased carbohydrate consumption, it is likely you will need to increase the insulin dose.
- Best advice is to be guided by increasing the frequency of monitoring
- Even when appetite is decreased it is important to still try to maintain a reasonable carbohydrate load—even via fluids such as milk and glucose loaded drinks
- Watch out for signs of dehydration especially in the face of vomiting or diarrhoea. Assess for impending ketoacidosis suggested by hyperventilation, tachycardia, and ketotic smell from the athletes breath
- If available test urine for signs of ketones. If in doubt refer to hospital for assessment, intravenous fluid resuscitation, and sliding scale of insulin.

Respiratory

▶▶ For the management of status asthmaticus please refer to 📖 p.94.

Asthma

Asthma is a lower respiratory condition characterized by a triad of:
- Bronchoconstriction
- Increased mucous production
- Mucosal swelling due to inflammation.

This results in shortness of breath, wheeze, and cough, which may be worse at night especially in children. Asthma, like diabetes, is documented to be on the increase and it is highly possible that you will be asked to care for an athlete who suffers from this condition. Early identification of athletes under your care who suffer from asthma is important to ensure you understand their condition prior to any acute episode.
- What inhalers do they take?
- Any previous hospital admissions?
- Any previous intensive therapy unit (ITU) admissions?
- What precipitants are they aware of, particularly non-steroidal anti-inflammatories. Is it exercise induced?
- What is their usual peak flow?

An athlete may present to you with an acute episode of shortness of breath and wheeze heralding a sudden exacerbation or there may be a more gradual deterioration in a patient in whom asthma is either known or suspected, but who has not responded to treatment.

Asthma sufferers participate in sport at all levels up to and including at an elite level. The benefits of exercise should be explained to sufferers who should be reassured and encouraged to participate in an exercise programme.

Exercise induced asthma (EIA)

This condition is characterized by bronchoconstriction induced by histamine release brought about by exercise. The vast majority of patients with asthma will suffer from EIA, although the condition can occur in the general population without a demonstrable diagnosis of asthma at rest.
- In patients reticent to participate in exercise because of the symptoms of EIA, reassurance and a graded exercise programme should be utilized
- Salbutamol should be taken prior to commencing exercise
- An exercise prescription may be useful in such patients to tailor an individual programme.

World Antidoping Agency

Salbutamol and salmeterol are the only two beta-2 agonists not prohibited as long as the manufacturers recommended therapeutic regime is not exceeded.
- Maximum dose of salbutamol is 1600 mcg per 24 h.
- All glucocorticoids are prohibited irrespective of route of administration. See ⌁ www.wada-ama.org.

Neurological and neuromuscular disorders

Specific medical issues can arise in individuals with neurological and neuromuscular disorders. This chapter aims to cover issues around epilepsy, cerebral palsy, Parkinson's disease, multiple sclerosis, and muscular dystrophy. Cerebrovascular disease and head injury is covered in Chapter 9 and spinal injury is covered in Chapter 12.

Epilepsy

Epilepsy is a relatively common condition and is characterized by recurrent unprovoked seizures due to abnormal electrical discharges within the brain. Classified as generalized or partial.

- *Generalized:* here, the epileptic activity involves both halves of the brain. Consciousness is always lost
  - *Grand mal:*
  - Tonic-clonic
  - Clonic
  - Myoclonic
  - *Petit mal:* usually in children. Otherwise known as 'absence' seizures.
- *Partial:* the epileptic activity involves part of the brain
  - Simple—no loss of consciousness
  - Complex—may partly lose consciousness or be unable to remember aspects of the fit.

A partial seizure may progress to a generalized seizure and this is then known as a secondary generalized seizure. Epileptic seizures increase the risk of trauma, fracture, dislocations, burns, and pneumonia due to aspiration. Medical conditions that can predispose to seizures include hypotension, diabetes mellitus, liver, and kidney disease, electrolyte imbalance such as hyper- or hyponatraemia, hypercalcaemia, and alcohol withdrawal.

Main considerations
- Seizure control
- Risk of bodily harm
- Avoidance of seizure precipitating factors. This include stress, sleep deprivation, alcohol, irregular food, and drug intake.

⚠ For the management of seizures notably status epilepticus please refer to pp.98–99.

- Injury rates for athletes suffering from seizures is not reported as being increased in comparison to athletes who do not suffer from seizures
- However, certain sports may need to be avoided in athletes whose seizure control is poor, such as motorsport
- Caution should always be exercised in the case of known seizure sufferers who should not be allowed to swim without direct supervision and appropriate support
- It is important to be aware of the medications taken by athletes in your care who suffer from seizures, as well as the side effects of the drugs they take

- One of the commonest reasons for seizures in someone already on treatment is sub therapeutic levels of the anticonvulsant +/− poor compliance. It is possible that a decrease in their performance may be related to a side effect of their anticonvulsant treatments.

Cerebral palsy

Cerebral palsy encompasses a group of physical disabilities that appear in infancy or early childhood (see Table 4.1 for a medical classification). The disabilities result from damage to areas in the brain, which can cause loss of balance and posture control, abnormal muscle tone and spinal reflexes, disturbance in sensation, perception, cognition, and communication.

Table 4.1 Medical classification of cerebral palsy

Category	Site of injury	Presentation
Pyramidal	Cortical system	Spastic, hyper-reflexia, 'clasp-knife', hypertonia, prone to contractures
Extrapyramidal	Basal ganglia and cerebellum	Athetosis, ataxia, 'lead-pipe' rigidity, chorea
Mixed	Combination of above	Combination of above

Considerations
- Cardiorespiratory fitness levels can be low in individuals with cerebral palsy, and hence caution may be needed to monitor heart rate, blood pressure (BP) and lactate responses
- Lower peak physiological responses (10–20%)
- Lower mechanical efficiency due to added energy to overcome muscle tone
- Fatigue and stress can increase symptoms of athetosis and spasticity
- Caution with regards to medications as seizures are common in cerebral palsy, anti-spasmodics, and muscle relaxants used can cause drowsiness and lethargy.

Management
- Physical screening
- Monitor/be aware of dysrhythmias or BP changes
- Be aware of concomitant cognitive, visual, hearing, and speech difficulties
- Do not assume decreased cognitive ability in the presence of drooling or decreased quality of verbal skills.

Parkinson's disease

Parkinson's disease is a chronic progressive disorder involving the extrapyramidal system that regulates muscle reflexes. It is commonly known to consist of a triad of symptoms; rigidity, akinesia (or bradykinesia) and resting tremor. It is thought the reduction of neurotransmitter, dopamine, which is produced in the basal ganglia results in symptoms such as resting tremor, bradykinesia, rigidity, and gait and postural abnormalities.

Relevance to exercise and sport
- Autonomic nervous system dysfunction is common
- Thermal regulation can be difficult to manage with excessive sweating common and fluid losses related to this contributing to dehydration
- Altered heart rate and BP responses
- Movement disorders and muscle rigidity may result in increased oxygen consumption
- Side effect of medications:
  - Levodopa/carbidopa can cause exercise bradycardia, transient peak dose tachycardia and dyskinesia
  - Selegeline can be associated with dyskinesia
  - Some medications are associated with cardiac dysrhythmias
  - Postural Instability can cause balance problems or falls.

Due to paucity of research in this area, general assessment, and management of the athlete with specific consideration to the following is recommended:
- ABC
- Postural issues
- Monitor heart rate and BP
- Cardiac monitor/electrocardiogram (ECG) if suspicion of arrhythmias.

Multiple sclerosis

Multiple sclerosis affects female more than males by a ratio of 2–3:1 and is thought to be an autoimmune condition that affects the myeline sheaths in the neurons in the central nervous system. This results in various symptoms, most notably, spasticity, incoordination, impaired balance, muscle weakness, sensory deficits, autonomic dysfunction of the cardiovascular system, heat sensitivity, and tremor. Exercise in patients with multiple sclerosis (MS) is particularly helpful in maintaining flexibility, cardiovascular fitness as well as helping to prevent secondary complications such as osteoporosis.

Relevance to exercise and sport
- Altered heart rate and BP responses due to cardiovascular autonomic dysfunction
- Heat intolerance
- Sensory loss
- Adequate hydration (urinary frequency, urgency, and incontinence is common, and hence, some individuals may limit fluid intake).

The following general assessment and management is recommended:
- ABC
- Monitor heart rate and BP
- Cardiac monitor/ECG if suspicion of arrhythmias
- Assessment of hydration status—oral/IV fluid as necessary.

Muscular dystrophy

Muscular dystrophy (MD) characterized by progressive muscle weakness, affecting predominantly the skeletal muscles. There are different types of MD namely:
- Duchenne MD
- Becker MD
- Fascio-scapulo-humeral
- Limb girdle
- Myotonic dystrophy.

Depending on the type of dystrophy, symptoms can be mild and progress slowly or progress rapidly causing severe muscle weakness, functional disability, and loss of ability to walk.

The following conditions may occur in individuals with muscular dystrophy:
- Severe muscle weakness, functional disability
- Cognitive delay
- Premature cataracts
- Swallowing problems
- Cardiac conduction block
- Gastrointestinal dysmotility
- Impaired glucose tolerance.

The following general assessment and management is recommended:
- ABC
- Monitor heart rate and BP
- Cardiac monitor/ECG if suspicion of arrhythmias
- Assessment of hydration status—give oral/IV fluid as necessary
- Monitor for muscle cramps. If increasing muscular pain post-exercise especially in the presence of dark urine consider referral to hospital for assessment of possible myoglobinuria secondary to rhabdomyolysis.

Cardiovascular conditions

Cardiovascular disease
Cardiovascular disease in this section will encompass both coronary artery disease (CAD) and conduction disturbances.

Coronary artery disease
CAD encompasses a spectrum of conditions that have the similar pathophysiology of coronary artery narrowing due to atherosclerotic plaques causing myocardial ischaemia.
- Complete obstruction of blood flow to the myocardium leads to myocardial infarction.
- Individuals with CAD are considered to be at high risk of developing life-threatening situations as the cracking of atherosclerotic plaques, with the subsequent formation of platelet aggregation and thrombosis, can cause cardiac events.

Symptoms of CAD include:
- Chest pain
- Palpitations
- Shortness of breath
- Dizziness
- Referred pain to the neck or left arm pain
- Collapse.

Assessment and management of any individuals presenting with suspected coronary artery disease should include the following:
- ABC
- Oxygen via facemask
- Monitor heart rate and BP
- IV access
- *Nitrate:* sublingual if blood pressure is adequate
- Cardiac monitor/ECG
- Call the ambulance
- If there is access to emergency facilities, IV opiate analgesia can be administered at a titrated dose (by trained medical professional)
- In situations of cardiac arrest, resuscitation guidelines should be followed as described in p.21.

Conduction disturbances
Conduction disturbances or arrythmias are common in individuals with coronary artery disease, although they can occur in isolation as either congenital or acquired conditions. Among the common arrythmias encountered in this group are:
- Heart blocks, frequent ectopics, and atrial fibrillation
- Supraventricular tachycardia is a common arrythmia found in the younger population, i.e. without CAD
- The danger with all arrythmias is progression to ventricular fibrillation or asystole.

In the event of an arrythmia, assessment and management should be based on identifying the cause and establishing if the arrythmia is new or a known occurrence, which is controlled with treatment. Clinical evaluation of the patient should be as follows:

- ABC
- Oxygen via facemask
- Monitor heart rate and BP
- Cardiac monitor/ECG
- Depending on the arrythmia and its presentation, i.e. new vs. old, controlled vs. uncontrolled, further evaluation, and referral may be necessary
- If in doubt, call the ambulance to transfer to Accident & Emergency (A&E) for further evaluation.

⚠ For the management of supraventricular tachycardias (SVT) arrhythmias see 📖 p.108.

Hypertension

According to the latest British Hypertension Society Guidelines (BHS-IV, 2004), classification of BP levels are as shown in Table 4.2.

Individuals are usually on drug treatment if they have sustained Grade 2 hypertension (>160/100 mmHg) or Grade 1 hypertension with any com-

Table 4.2 Classification of blood pressure levels

Category	Systolic blood pressure (mmHg)	Diastolic blood pressure (mmHg)
Blood pressure		
Optimal	<120	<80
Normal	<130	<85
High normal	130–139	85–89
Hypertension		
Grade 1 (mild)	140–159	90–99
Grade 2 (moderate)	160–179	100–109
Grade 3 (severe)	≥180	≥110
Isolated systolic hypertension		
Grade 1	140–159	<90
Grade 2	≥160	<90

Data from Williams, B., Poulter, N.R., Brown, M.J., et al. (2004). The BHS Guidelines Working Party. British Hypertension Society Guidelines for Hypertension Management—BHS IV: summary. *Br Med J* **328:** 634–40.

plications. These include target organ damage or if there is an estimated 10-year risk of cardiovascular disease ≥20% despite lifestyle advice.

Considerations on assessment of individuals with hypertension are:
- Heart rate and BP measurement

Chapter 4 Athletes with pre-existing conditions

- BP is usually elevated in individuals that exercise. However, in individuals with hypertension, the absolute level of systolic BP attained during exercise is usually higher due to an elevated baseline level
- Another caution is that these patients maybe on anti-hypertensive treatment; sometimes 2–3 combinations at once. Classes of drugs generally used are angiotensin-converting enzyme inhibitors (ACE-I), angiotensin-II receptor blockers, betablockers, calcium channel blockers, thiazide diuretics, and alphablockers
- Betablockers and to a lesser degree, calcium channel blockers (diltiazem and verapamil) reduce the heart rate response to submaximal and maximal exercise
- Dihydropyridine calcium channel blockers may increase heart rate response to exercise
- Betablockers also reduce the resting BP and the rise of BP from baseline level when exercising
- Alphablockers, calcium channel blockers, and vasodilators may cause post-exertional hypotension
- Diuretics may result in serum potassium abnormalities which may predispose to exercise-induced arrhythmias.

Hence, the following symptoms or signs should prompt further assessment:
- Chest pain
- Dizziness
- Collapse
- Shortness of breath out of proportion to the level of exercise.

When exercising, BP should be maintained below systolic <220 mmHg and diastolic <105 mmHg.

Individuals should not exercise if resting BP is systolic >200 mmHg or diastolic >115 mmHg.

Management
- Stop exercising
- ABC
- Administer oxygen via facemask
- Monitor heart rate and BP
- Cardiac monitor/ECG if there is access
- Depending on the presentation, further assessment, and treatment may be needed with transfer to the hospital if symptoms are not controlled or if further assessment is necessary.

Peripheral vascular disease

Peripheral vascular disease is caused by atherosclerotic lesions in the arteries of the limbs which restrict blood flow distally to the peripheries. A common symptom is intermittent claudication which can present as a cramp or ache in the muscles resulting from exercise. It is typically relieved with rest.

Assessment should include:
- Measures of claudication pain times from history
- Peripheral pulse examination and capillary refill testing (<2 s is normal)
- Ankle–brachial pressure index (ABPI)
- Assess whether coronary artery disease is present.

Management will depend on findings from history and clinical examination:
- ABC
- If distal limb ischaemia is suspected, exercise should be stopped and further referral to a specialist centre or A&E is advised
- Concomitant CAD should be actively sought and treated.

Heart failure

Heart failure refers to the inability of the myocardium to adequately pump blood and hence oxygen and nutrients to the metabolizing tissues in the body. This could be due to systolic dysfunction, diastolic dysfunction, or both.
- Heart failure results in decreased cardiac output during exercise and in severe cases at rest
- There is compensatory ventricular volume overload, mismatch of ventilation to perfusion in the lung, impaired vasodilatation, and renal insufficiency leading to sodium and water retention.

Typically, individuals with heart failure would be on drugs to control their symptoms and progression of disease. These include ACE-I, diuretics, angiotensin receptor blockers or betablockers.

Symptoms of heart failure include:
- Shortness of breath
- Fatigue
- Reduced exercise tolerance
- Peripheral oedema.

Exercise in these individuals also cause different physiological responses:
- Reduced cardiac output due to a drop in ejection fraction and/or stroke volume
- Abnormal blood distribution
- High peripheral resistance
- Exertional hypotension
- Predisposition to arrhythmias.

Hence, assessment and management should include:
- ABC
- Oxygen via face mask
- Heart rate and BP monitoring
- Cardiac monitor/ECG if available
- Intravenous access if not haemodynamically stable
- Consider treatment with diuretics or sublingual GTN if haemodynamically compromised
- Transfer to hospital.

Hypertrophic obstructive cardiomyopathy

Hypertrophic obstructive cardiomyopathy (HOCM) is primarily a disease of the cardiac muscle where the myocardial fibres become hypertrophied and disarrayed. It is thought to be the commonest cause of sudden death in athletes.

Prodromal symptoms may occur in HOCM. However, in many cases, sudden death may the first presentation of this condition. Symptoms and risk factors that should be looked out for are:
- Exertional dyspnoea
- Chest pain
- Palpitations
- Pre-syncope or syncope
- Family history of sudden cardiac death.

In the event of symptoms during exercise in an undiagnosed individual, further investigation will be needed. This includes:
- ECG
- Echocardiography with Doppler
- Further cardiological referral and evaluation if indicated.

In the event of cardiac arrest or collapse, assessment and management should be followed as described in Chapter 3.

⚠ Arthritis

Rheumatoid arthritis and ankylosing spondylitis

Rheumatoid arthritis (RA) affects females more commonly than males, whilst the opposite is true of ankylosing spondylitis (AS). In RA, onset is usually insidious with stiffness of joints notably in the morning, and increasing pain, and swelling.

- Disease progression eventually leads to deformity of the affected joints commonly affecting the wrist, fingers, and feet
- AS affects the spine and results in back pain
- Rest is appropriate when flare ups of both diseases occur, but exercise is very useful in helping to keep the joints from becoming stiff
- Contact sports should be avoided and swimming is generally accepted as being the exercise most appropriate to minimize impact on joints, whilst providing cardiovascular exercise
- Most athletes with RA will be familiar with the differing medications they will take varying from non-steroidal anti-inflammatories through to steroids and disease modifying anti-rheumatic drugs (DMARDs) such as gold, methotrexate, and penicillamine
- Side effects of these drugs are common and can be debilitating for the patient.

Other issues such as anaemia related to the chronicity of the disease itself, or as a direct side effect of the medications may complicate the management of these patients.

- Rheumatoid patients are more likely to suffer from strokes or myocardial infarctions as part of the systemic effects of the inflammation
- Management of most acute presentations is no different in the rheumatoid patient than in the unaffected population
- Exceptions to this include the management of potential cervical spine injuries which can occur with relatively minimal trauma. This should be suspected in anyone with either RA or AS who complains of neck pain after *any* injury
- Both conditions predispose the patient to spinal injury
  - Management differs because the usual technique of spinal immobilization involving lying the patient flat and applying a spinal collar may convert the injury into an unstable one due to the pathological effects of the diseases on the spine
  - The patient should instead lie as flat *as can be tolerated,* a collar applied *if tolerated,* tape, and blocks applied to the each side of the head.

❶ Under no circumstances should anyone with rheumatoid arthritis or ankylosing spondylitis be forced to lie flat wearing a semi-rigid collar if this worsens their symptoms in any way.

Female athlete triad

The female athlete triad is known to consist of a triad of
- Amenorrhoea
- Osteopenia
- Eating disorders.

Potential complications encountered in this group include collapse due to hypoglycaemia and stress fractures. If stress fractures occur in long bones of the limbs, serious consequences of blood loss may occur.
- Menstrual irregularities can occur due to the combination of exercise intensity and low body weight due to the effect on hypothalamic hormones that control the hypothalamic-gonadal axis
- Delayed menarche, oligomenorrhoea, and amenorrhoea in the years of potential maximal bone mineralization is thought to be associated with lower rate of bone mineral secretion and with increased risks of osteoporotic fractures later in life
- Fracture of the long bones due to normal stresses is a rare, but is a potential complication in the exercising population, especially if there is a history of osteopenia
- However, fractures can occur in all bones where there is impact on exercise, especially due to overuse. Most commonly, this will be bones in the ankle, foot, tibia, and the femur
- General assessment and management will depend on the presentation.
  - Consider ABC
  - Administer oxygen via facemask
  - Beware of cervical spine trauma in the case of a distracting injury. Management with manual in-line stabilization, cervical collar, and spinal board should be followed. This is described further in Chapter 12
  - IV access
  - Check BP and heart rate
  - Splint the involved area from the joint above to the joint below
  - Check for neurovascular status of the limb involved
  - Ensure systolic BP >80 mmHg. IV fluids may be given to keep systolic BP above this level
  - Transfer to hospital
  - In the case of stress fractures involving the pars interarticularis, it is important to exclude any lower limb neurology.

Further reading
Williams, B., Poulter, N.R., Brown, M.J., et al. (2004). The BHS Guidelines Working Party. British Hypertension Society Guidelines for Hypertension Management—BHS IV: summary. *Br Med J* **328**: 634–40.

Chapter 5

Collapse during exercise

Definitions *52*
Principles of assessment *53*
Exercise-associated collapse *54*
Heatstroke *56*
Hypothermia *58*
Exercise-associated hyponatraemia *62*

Definitions

As well as the common causes of collapse familiar to most medically-trained personnel, athletes are also at risk of collapse from causes that may specifically relate to their particular exercise, such as trauma or extremes of heat:
- Exercise-associated collapse
- Hypothermia
- Heatstroke
- Exercise-associated hyponatraemia
- Cardiac arrest
- Hypoglycaemia
- Anaphylaxis
- Trauma
- Other medical conditions
- Orthopaedic injuries.

Principles of assessment

- Early symptoms and signs may be non-specific and the basic life-support principles of Airway, Breathing, Circulation (A, B, C) must always be attended to first (see 📖 pp. 13–14).
- Loss of consciousness or indeed *any* alteration of mental state (drowsiness, confusion, disorientation, irrational behaviour, aggression, seizures, etc.) suggests a high likelihood of severe hypoglycaemia, hyponatraemia, hyperthermia, or hypothermia.
- Rectal temperature is the only reliable method of assessing core temperature in the field.
- Hydration status is a useful indicator of dehydration, or conversely, hyponatraemia due to fluid overload. For example, from skin turgor, dry mucus membranes, or the inability to spit, through to oedema or puffiness.
- Blood sodium and glucose levels should be checked.
- Site of collapse is an important indicator of severity. Collapse before finishing the event suggests serious illness.

Assessment of the collapsed athlete

- **A:** Airway
- **B:** Breathing
- **C:** Circulation including pulse rate, rhythm, character, and systolic BP
- **D:** Disability or mental status
- **E:** Environment (rectal temperature)
- **F:** Fluid status including change in body weight
- **G:** Blood glucose and sodium
- **H:** History including site of collapse

Accurate diagnosis is vital to ensure that serious causes of collapse are appropriately treated. Except in the case of trauma or cardiac insufficiency, where standard advanced life support (ALS)/advanced trauma life support (ATLS) protocols apply, treatment with intravenous fluids should not be instituted until serum sodium has been checked.

Exercise-associated collapse

Exercise-associated collapse (EAC) is the inability to stand or walk unaided as the result of light-headedness, faintness, dizziness, or syncope. EAC is one of the most common reasons for admission to the medical tent at endurance events and classically presents after finishing the event.

EAC is related to postural hypotension that develops upon finishing exercise. Inactivation of the calf muscle pump and subsequent pooling of blood in the legs causes a reduced atrial filling pressure and syncope.

Assessment
- **A:** normal
- **B:** normal
- **C:** postural hypotension (>20 mmHg drop in systolic BP supine to standing). BP and pulse rate normal in supine position
- **D:** usually normal, may have transient loss of consciousness (LOC) during syncope but rapidly resolves in the supine, legs up position
- **E:** ≤39°C
- **F:** normal or dry[1]
- **G:** normal blood glucose and sodium
- **H:** collapse after cessation of exercise.

Treatment
- Place athlete in the Trendelenburg position (supine and head-down, with legs and pelvis elevated)
- Oral fluids.

---

[1] Fluid loss due to sweating, diarrhoea, and vomiting, may contribute to EAC, but there is no evidence that athletes with EAC are any more dehydrated than their non-collapsing counterparts in the same race.

Heatstroke

⚠ Heatstroke can be fatal. The diagnosis of heatstroke is made in anyone with symptoms or signs of organ dysfunction, most commonly altered mental status (including collapse, drowsiness, confusion, etc.) and a rectal temperature >41°C. See Box 5.1 for causes of heat gain and loss.

- Cerebral hyperthermia may lead to hypothalamic failure and loss of thermoregulatory control accelerating the process. Myoglobin release due to rhabdomyolysis can cause renal failure and hyperkalaemia
- Hyperthermia causes suppression of cardiac function leading to reduced cardiac output which may progress through tissue hypoxia, metabolic acidosis to organ dysfunction and multi-system organ failure
- Athletes may remain symptom-free despite rectal temperatures ≤40.5°C. Above this temperature, symptoms tend to occur and an athlete may collapse.

Assessment
- **A:** normal
- **B:** normal, but may be hyperventilating
- **C:** hypotension, tachycardia
- **D:** altered mental state
- **E:** >41°C
- **F:** normal or dry. Sweating may be present, but its absence does not exclude the diagnosis
- **G:** normal blood glucose and sodium
- **H:** presentation may be during or after the event.

Treatment
- Rapid whole body cooling through cold- or ice-water immersion. Alternatively ice-packs to the groin, axillae, and neck may be used
- Close observations and cooling should continue until rectal temperature has reduced, mental status has returned to normal, and cardiovascular function is stable
- Slow recovery or prolonged unconsciousness indicates that hospital admission is required
- Patients may be discharged home from the medical tent if
  - There has been rapid recovery *and*
  - Rectal temperature does not increase in the first hour after cessation of active cooling.

Box 5.1 Heat gain and loss in exercise

Heat gain
- *Endogenous:* muscle activity and metabolism
- *Exogenous:* environmental

Heat loss in exercise
- In low environmental temperatures (below body temperature), heat is lost through convection and radiation from the skin, with some contribution from conduction. During exercise and when environmental temperature ≥ body temperature sweating allows much more effective heat loss through evaporation.
- In humid conditions however, evaporation is reduced and cooling becomes less effective. An athlete may be unable to lose heat during exercise in high temperature and high humidity environments and so begin to overheat, even in relatively short-distance races and in seemingly cool conditions. Exercise in such situations becomes dangerous.
- The wet bulb globe temperature (WBGT) index takes into account the humidity as well as solar and ground radiation in combination with air temperature and wind speed. The American College of Sports Medicine has produced guidelines for the amount of exercise that can be safely carried out in hot conditions based on the WBGT.

Hypothermia

Hypothermia is defined by a core temperature <35°C. It occurs when body heat losses exceeds heat generated.
- Peripheral sensory nerves relay information on temperature to central receptors in the hypothalamus, which responds by stimulating shivering to generate body heat
- The receptors in the skin are more sensitive to the rate of change in temperature than the actual temperature
- A rapid drop in temperature, for example falling into cold water, is felt more acutely than a slow decrease
- Thus a gradual drop in temperature may not be accompanied by a sense of cold and shivering may not be initiated.

⚠ The athlete may therefore not be aware of the cold.

Athletes are at risk of hypothermia when they are unable to generate enough body heat to keep the body warm. This may occur in relatively warm temperatures!

Risk factors
- *Exhaustion:* slow moving, unable to generate body heat through activity
- Hypoglycaemia impairs shivering
- Inadequate clothing or protective equipment
- *Rain:* increases heat loss through convection
- *Cold wind:* wind chill factor effectively reduces the temperature and increases heat loss through evaporation
- *Accident or injury:* leaving athlete exposed
- *Immersion in cold water:* much greater heat loss through convection.

Physiological effects
- Peripheral vasoconstriction to reduce body heat losses and to protect core temperature. This underlines the importance of measurement of core body temperature (with a rectal thermometer) rather than peripheral temperature (oral, tympanic, or axillae)
- Reduced cardiac output. Myocardial depression and impaired electrical conduction combined with reduced circulating volume as a result of fluid loss from sweating and respiration during exercise
- Cardiac arrhythmias. Impaired electrical conduction leading to decreased heart rate initially with prolonged segments on electrocardiogram (ECG). ST segment J-waves may be evident, suggesting hypothermia. Atrial fibrillation (AF) and ventricular fibrillation (VF) may occur. AF may settle with rewarming
- Hyperventilation is a cold-induced reflex and may exacerbate dehydration and heat loss.

Neurological changes
- Involuntary shivering initially, later muscle rigidity
- Hyper-reflexia initially, diminished or absent reflexes in severe hypothermia

- Dysarthria, slow reaction time, impaired co-ordination, and delayed cerebration due to delayed nerve conduction
- Amnesia progressing through confusion and drowsiness to loss of consciousness.

Assessment of hypothermia

Classified into mild, moderate, and severe hypothermia dependent upon symptoms and temperature, although symptoms may vary from person to person. (Table 5.1)

Table 5.1 Assessment of hypothermia

	Mild	Moderate	Severe
A	Normal	Normal, Can develop bronchospasm	Normal, Can develop pulmonary oedema
B	Tachypnoea	Tachypnoea	Hypoventilation
C	Tachycardia	Tachycardia	Hypotension, bradycardia, arrhythmias (including VF), asystole
D	Subjective feeling of cold, shivering, Amnesia, dysarthria, apathy, signs of withdrawal	Reduced shivering, Fatigue, drowsiness, confusion, poor judgment	Muscle rigidity Inappropriate behaviour, reduced level of consciousness
E	33–35°C, cold conditions, rain, and/or wind	31–32°C, cold conditions, rain, and/or wind	<3°C, cold conditions, rain, and/or wind
F	Urinary urgency[*]	Dehydration	Dehydration
G	Normal	Normal to low	Normal to low
H	During or after event, inadequate clothing or protection, accident or injury, immersion		

[*] Peripheral vasoconstriction temporarily induces an increase in central blood volume, which causes a cold diuresis, contributing to dehydration.

Treatment of hypothermia

Mild
Active rewarming: warm clothes, warm sweet drink, hot packs to torso, or hot tub.

Moderate
- *Passive rewarming only in the field setting:* remove from cold environment, remove wet clothes, insulate
- *Transfer to hospital for active rewarming:* continual cardiovascular monitoring for hypotension and arrhythmias.

Severe
- Passive rewarming only in the field setting, *but* handle the patient as little as possible to avoid risk of precipitating ventricular fibrillation
- Transfer to intensive care for active rewarming.

Further notes
- Space blankets do not prevent further heat loss. In established hypothermia, continuing heat loss is primarily through convection, not radiation
- Avoid further exercise. Glycogen depletion through exercise will prevent shivering
- Apply hot packs to torso only, as peripheral rewarming increases peripheral blood flow reducing central blood volume. This may lead to cardiovascular collapse. Hot tubs provide hydrostatic support so help to maintain blood pressure
- Remove a hypothermic patient from cold water in the horizontal position. Loss of hydrostatic pressure from the water may precipitate hypotension and cardiovascular collapse.

❶ At very low temperatures, signs of life may be difficult to detect. Death cannot be determined until after rewarming.

A person is not dead until 'warm and dead'.

CHAPTER 5 **Collapse during exercise**

☼ **Exercise-associated hyponatraemia**

Exercise-associated hyponatraemia (EAH) is a rare, but preventable cause of death in endurance exercise.

- EAH should be considered a possible diagnosis in anyone with altered mental status including seizures or unconsciousness during or after an endurance event. Core temperature will be normal. Seizures may also be the initial presentation
- EAH is a dilutional hyponatraemia caused by fluid intake in excess of body fluid losses during or in the first 24 h after exercise. Inappropriate anti-diuretic hormone (ADH) release during exercise may be an additional contributing factor
- Relative hyponatraemia in the vascular compartment causes an osmotic fluid shift into adjacent tissues, which manifests itself as puffiness and oedema peripherally, but centrally as cerebral and pulmonary oedema
- Early signs and symptoms are non-specific (nausea, vomiting, puffiness, bloating) and may be confused with those of dehydration. In a similar fashion, lack of urination, more commonly attributed to dehydration, may be a sign of ongoing renal impairment due to ADH
- More severe cases may develop signs of central nervous system dysfunction such as confusion, aggression, seizure, stupor, or coma.

Pulmonary and cerebral oedema, if untreated, will cause death.

Risk factors
- ♂>♀
- Long distance event (usually >4 hr)
- Consumption of more than 3 L of fluid
- Weight gain during the race
- Low body mass index
- Slow race pace.

Assessment
- **A:** normal
- **B:** normal, but tachypnoea and hypoxia may develop with pulmonary oedema
- **C:** normal, well filled
- **D:** normal in early EAH, altered mental state as severity increases
- **E:** ≤39°C
- **F:** normal or overloaded.[1] A history of copious fluid consumption during or after the event may be available, but cannot be relied upon, especially if confused. Little or no urination suggests renal dysfunction
- **G:** serum sodium <135 mmol/L. Normal glucose
- **H:** collapse during or up to 24 h after the event.

---

[1] Observe for facial and peripheral puffiness or oedema. Also look for tight rings, watchstraps, socks, etc.

Treatment
- Alert and orientated individuals and sodium <135mmol/L (mild-moderate EAH):
  - Give salty snacks or salty broth
  - Observe closely
  - No oral fluids until onset of urination
- Any evidence of altered mental state or pulmonary oedema and sodium <135mmol/L (severe EAH):
  - Administer oxygen
  - Administer 100 mL IV bolus of 3% salt which may be repeated up to 3 times at 10-min intervals if required
- Hypotonic or isotonic solutions (including 0.9% salt) are contra-indicated
- May require hospital admission to receive further treatment including ventilatory support, especially if slow to improve.

Notes
Weight gain during exercise is a valid marker of fluid overload. Runners should expect to lose up to 2% body weight over the course of a marathon due to carbohydrate/substrate utilization.
- Therefore, even neutral weight balance and weight loss <2% are indicators of fluid overload
- Urgent sodium level must be obtained and catheterization may be undertaken to aid assessment of renal function.

Prevention
- Avoid excessive drinking during exercise. Encourage ad libitum drinking—rely on your thirst telling you when to drink. It is a very sophisticated and accurate mechanism
- Weigh athletes before and after training runs in different weather conditions drinking the fluids available at the race in order to better understand how their body reacts to fluid. Neutral weight balance or weight gain on runs >21 miles suggests they have drunk too much
- Avoid excessive drinking after exercise. The risk of EAH remains present for several hours afterwards
- Sodium-containing sports drinks do not prevent EAH if they are consumed excessively. They too are hypotonic or isotonic and will contribute to the inherent dilution of EAH.

Chapter 5 Collapse during exercise

Further reading

Almond, C.S., Shin, A.Y., Fortescue, E.B., et al. (2005). Hyponatremia among runners in the Boston Marathon. *N Engl J Med* **352**: 1550–6.

Armstrong, L.E., Casa, D.J., Millard-Stafford, M., et al. (2007). American College of Sports Medicine position stand. Exertional heat illness during training and competition. *Med Sci Sports Exer* **39**(3): 556–72.

Castellani, J.W., Young, A.J., Ducharme, M.B., et al. (2006). American College of Sports Medicine position stand. Prevention of cold injuries during exercise. *Med Sci.Sports Exer* **38**(11): 2012–29.

Hew-Butler, T., Ayus, J.C., Kipps, C., et al. (2007). Statement of the Second International Exercise-Associated Hyponatremia Consensus Development Conference, New Zealand. *Clin J Sport Med* **18**(2): 111–21.

Holtzhausen, L.M., Noakes, T.D., Kroning, B., et al. (1994). Clinical and biochemical characteristics of collapsed ultra-marathon runners. *Med Sci Sports Exer* **26**(9): 1095–101.

Noakes, T. (2001). Exercise in the heat. In: Bruckner, P., Khan, K. (eds) *Clinical Sports Medicine*, 2nd edn. Sydney: McGraw-Hill Australia Pty Ltd. 798–806.

Noakes, T. (2001). Exercise in the cold. In: Bruckner, P., Khan, K. (eds) *Clinical Sports Medicine*, 2nd edn. Sydney: McGraw-Hill Australia Pty Ltd, 807–15.

Roberts, W.O. (1994). Assessing core temperature in collapsed athletes: what's the best method? *Physician Sportsmed.* **22**(8):49–55.

Roberts, W.O. (2007). Exercise-associated collapse care matrix in the marathon. *Sports Med* **37**(4–5): 431–33.

Speedy, D.B., Noakes, T., Holtzhausen, L.M. (2005). Exercise associated collapse: postural hypotension, or something deadlier? *Physic Sportsmed* **31**(3): 23–9.

Chapter 6

Altitude sickness

Altitude sickness 66
Acute mountain sickness 68
High altitude cerebral oedema 71
High altitude pulmonary oedema 72
Who is at risk? 74

Altitude sickness

What goes up must come down

Barometric pressure falls linearly with increasing altitude. The oxygen concentration of air remains constant at 21%, regardless of altitude. Consequently, the partial pressure of oxygen in ambient air reduces proportionately with increasing altitude (Fig. 6.1). It is this hypobaric hypoxia that leads to the spectrum of medical conditions commonly referred to as altitude sickness.

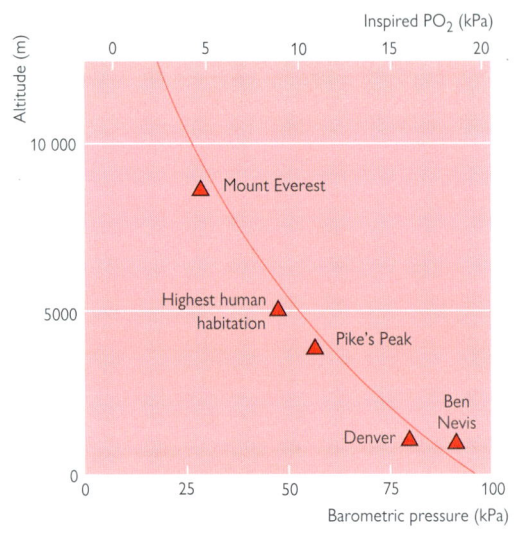

Fig. 6.1 The effect of altitude on the partial pressure of oxygen. Reproduced from Johnson et al., *Oxford Handbook of Expedition and Wilderness Medicine*, 2008, with permission from Oxford University Press.

Definition of altitude
- *High altitude:* 1500–3500 m
- *Very high altitude:* 3500–5500 m
- *Extreme altitude:* above 5500 m.

Altitude sickness

Altitude sickness is an umbrella term used to describe the following three acute conditions:
- Acute mountain sickness (AMS) occurs in 50–70% of those ascending to above 3500 m
- High altitude cerebral oedema (HACE) occurs in around 1% of people ascending to 4000–5500 m

- High altitude pulmonary oedema (HAPE) occurs in around 2% ascending to 4000–5500 m.

AMS and HACE are thought to involve the same cerebral pathology and represent the mild and life-threatening ends of the spectrum, respectively. HAPE, a pulmonary illness, may present independent of AMS. It is important to highlight. However, all three conditions manifest from the same hypoxic insult and there is therefore frequent concurrence with significant clinical overlap.

Normal physiology in response to altitude

In order to survive at altitude the body must acclimatize by employing a multi-system response:

- *Respiratory*: increased minute ventilation to improve oxygenation (known as the hypoxic ventilatory response). Consequent lowering of $PaCO_2$ results in a respiratory alkalosis
- *Renal*: increased excretion of bicarbonate ions and retention of H^+ ions compensates the development of alkalosis and allows further increases in ventilation. This adaptation explains the polyuria often experienced at altitude
- *Cardiovascular*: increased heart rate, cardiac output, and vasoconstriction of pulmonary vasculature attempt to improve gaseous exchange and delivery of oxygenated blood to tissues
- *Haematological*: in response to the low PaO_2 there is increased hemoglobin production to improve the oxygen-carrying capacity of the blood
- *Neurological*: cerebral blood flow has been shown to increase significantly during ascent to high altitude.

Prevention

- Avoid rapid ascension to altitudes above 2000–2500 m
- Ascend slowly with stops at intermediate altitudes
- Avoid vigorous exercise on the first few days of arrival
- Acetazolamide (125 mg–250 mg twice daily (bd)) beginning 48 hr before ascent to altitude and continued for 5 days has been shown to be beneficial in prevention of symptoms.

Differential diagnoses (Table 6.1)

Table 6.1 Differential diagnoses of altitude sickness

Acute mountain sickness	High altitude pulmonary oedema
Dehydration	Pulmonary embolus
Hypoglycaemia	Infection
Hypothermia	Myocardial infarction
Hyponatraemia	
Cerebral infection	
Space occupying lesion	
Stroke	

Acute mountain sickness

More than half of people ascending to an altitude of 3500 m will suffer AMS. Although often not an emergency in itself it is imperative to be able to recognize and manage AMS appropriately to avoid life-threatening sequelae, such as HACE/HAPE.

Typical onset
- Altitudes between 2500–3500 m (high altitude)
- Within 4–24 hr of ascent to altitude.

Symptoms
See Table 6.2.
Headache (frontal/generalized) plus at least one of:
- Nausea
- Vomiting
- Dizziness
- Lethargy/listlessness
- Sleep disturbance.

Table 6.2 Lake Louise Symptom Score for AMS. A score of 3–5 is considered diagnostic of mild/moderate AMS. A score >6 is diagnostic of severe AMS

Symptoms	Severity	Points
Headache	No headache	0
	Mild headache	1
	Moderate headache	2
	Severe headache, incapacitating	3
Gastrointestinal	No gastrointestinal symptoms	0
	Poor appetite or nausea	1
	Moderate nausea or vomiting	2
	Severe nausea or vomiting	3
Fatigue and/or weakness	Not tired or weak	0
	Mild fatigue/weakness	1
	Moderate fatigue/weakness	2
	Severe fatigue/weakness, incapacitating	3
Dizziness/ lightheadedness	Not dizzy	0
	Mild dizziness	1
	Moderate dizziness	2
	Severe dizziness, incapacitating	3

Table 6.2 *Continued*

Symptoms	Severity	Points
Difficulty of sleeping	Slept as well as usual	0
	Did not sleep as well as usual	1
	Woke up many times, poor night's sleep	2
	Unable sleep	3

Reproduced from UIAA Medical Commission Consensus Statement No. 2: Emergency Field Management of Acute Medical Sickness, High Altitude Pulmonary Oedema, and High Altitude Cerebral Oedema, 2009, with permission from the International Climbing and Mountain Federation (UIAA)

Management (mild/moderate) (see Fig. 6.2)
- Rest and avoid further ascent
- Ensure patient remains well hydrated
- Symptomatic treatment (anti-emetics, simple analgesia), although it is usually self-limiting
- Descend if symptoms worsen or do not improve within 24 hr
- Only consider continuing ascent once patient is symptom free.

Management (severe)
- Rest
- Descend (at least 500 m)
- Symptomatic treatment (anti-emetics, simple analgesia)
- Acetazolamide (250 mg bd)
- Consider dexamethasone (8 mg, then 4 mg every 6 hr).

If descent is not possible
- Oxygen
- Portable hyperbaric chamber (e.g. Gamow Bag).

Note: distinguishing severe AMS and HACE can be difficult. If in doubt, treat as HACE.

CHAPTER 6 **Altitude sickness**

HACE
- Severe headache
- Incoordination
- Behaviour change
- Hallucination
- Ataxia
- Disorientation
- Confusion
- Lower consciousness

HAPE
- Breathing difficulty
- Reduced exercise tolerance
- Cough, sometimes "Wet"
- Blood stained sputum

Headache → Simple pain-killer → **AMS** Headache + one of following
- Loss of appetite
- Nausea
- Vomiting
- Lethargy
- Sleep disturbance
- Dizziness

Descend oxygen

Dexamethasone 8 mg initially (orally or IM/IV if unconscious) then 8 mg/6 hrs

Gamow Bag

Descend oxygen
Sit upright
Keep warm
Nifedipine 20 mg SR/6 hrs
Gamow Bag

Stop further ascent rest
Simple pain-killers
antiemetic

No improvement → Descend continue treatment → Worsens

Descend oxygen

Diamox 2 × 250 mg per day

Dexamethasone 4 mg every 6 hrs oral or IM/IV

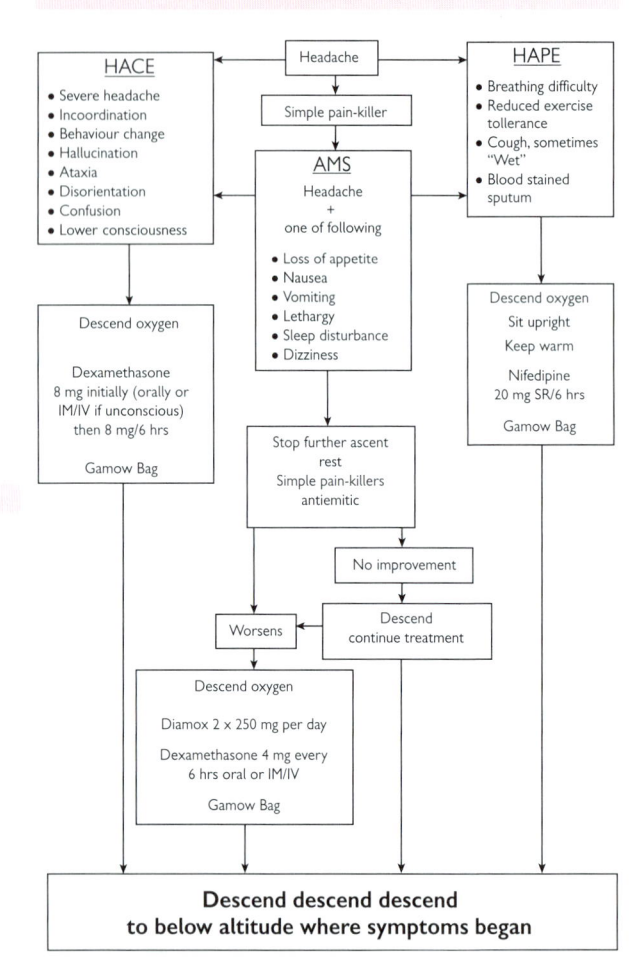

Gamow Bag

Descend descend descend to below altitude where symptoms began

Fig. 6.2 Management flow chart for altitude sickness. Reproduced from UIAA Medical Commission Consensus Statement No. 2: Emergency Field Management of Acute Medical Sickness, High Altitude Pulmonary Oedema, and High Altitude Cerebral Oedema, 2009, with permission from the International Climbing and Mountain Federation (UIAA).

High altitude cerebral oedema

HACE represents the extreme of AMS and is a rare and life threatening emergency. It is a clinical diagnosis defined by the development of altered mental status and/or ataxia in a patient with AMS (or HAPE).

Typical onset
- Altitudes between 4000 and 5500 m (very high altitude)
- 1–3 days after ascent to altitude.

Symptoms/signs
- Headache refractory to simple analgesics
- Nausea
- Vomiting
- Dizziness
- Ataxia (heel-to-toe walking is a sensitive field test)
- Cognitive impairment, e.g. confusion, irrational behaviour
- Coma.

Management (Fig. 6.2)
- Organize urgent descent or evacuation
- Portable hyperbaric chamber if descent not possible
- Oxygen
- Dexamethasone (8 mg, then 4–8 mg every 6 hr)
- Acetazolamide (250 mg bd)
- If symptoms do not improve with the above consider alternative diagnoses (see Table 6.2).

High altitude pulmonary oedema

HAPE is the most common cause of death from altitude-related illness.

Typical onset
- Altitudes between 4000 and 5500 m (very high altitude)
- 1–3 days after ascent to altitude (typically the 2nd night).

Symptoms/signs
- Worsening dyspnoea on exertion, becoming symptomatic at rest
- Tachypnoea
- Persistent cough, becoming productive of frothy/bloody sputum
- Severe fatigue and exercise intolerance
- Crackles/wheeze in at least one lung field
- Tachycardia
- Cyanosis
- Fever (often leading to misdiagnosis of chest infection).

Management (Fig. 6.2)
- Increasing oxygenation is the highest priority in HAPE
- Organize urgent descent or evacuation
- Use a portable hyperbaric chamber if descent not possible
- Oxygen
- Keep upper body upright to minimize effects of oedema
- Avoid exertion (raises pulmonary arterial pressure)
- Prevent cold/hypothermia (raises pulmonary arterial pressure)
- Nifedipine slow release:
  - 20 mg, repeated every 6–8 hr if necessary
  - Effects should be evident after 15 min
- Acetazolamide (250 mg bd)
- Salmeterol (can help clearance of alveolar fluid)
- The use of diuretics is not beneficial in the treatment of HAPE
- If symptoms do not improve consider alternative diagnoses (see Table 6.2).

Note: if you are unsure whether someone is suffering HAPE or HACE, then treat empirically (severe HAPE can often trigger HACE) by organizing descent (or hyperbaric chamber), oxygen, dexamethasone, nifedipine, and acetazolamide.

Pathophysiology

The exact pathophysiology involved in altitude sickness remains very much unclear.
- *AMS/HACE:* hypoxaemia initiates a vasodilatory response that results in increased cerebral blood flow. The increased capillary pressure (possibly combined with worsened capillary permeability) eventually leads to the development of cerebral oedema.
- *HAPE:* vasoconstriction of the pulmonary circulation following hypoxic insult leads to pulmonary hypertension. This is responsible for the development of the non-cardiogenic, hydrostatic pulmonary oedema seen in HAPE.

Drugs

Acetazolamide (Diamox®)
- Carbonic anhydrase inhibitor
- Accelerates acclimatization by promoting bicarbonate diuresis and providing respiratory stimulus (see p.67)
- It does not mask the symptoms of altitude sickness
- Often used prophylactically if sufficient acclimatization will not be possible or person is at high risk of developing AMS:
  - Start 1 day before ascending to altitude
  - Continue for 2 days once at maximum altitude
- *Side effects:* tingling in extremities, altered taste, polyuria.

Dexamethasone
- Potent steroid
- Improves cerebral oedema
- Drug treatment of choice in HACE/AMS
- Does not accelerate acclimatization (unlike acetazolamide)
- *Can mask AMS:* do *not* ascend whilst taking dexamethasone
- *Side effects:* rebound AMS if suddenly withdrawn, mood changes, hyperglycaemia, dyspepsia.

Nifedipine
- Calcium-channel blocker
- Reduces pulmonary artery pressure
- Drug treatment of choice in HAPE (variable results)
- May be prescribed for prophylaxis of HAPE in recurrent sufferers
- *Side effects:* reflex tachycardia, hypotension.

Who is at risk?

Everyone is at risk of developing altitude sickness regardless of sex, age, fitness level, and race; it is notoriously unpredictable.

Risk factors for altitude sickness
- Previous history of altitude sickness (most relevant)
- Fast ascent to high altitude
- Higher altitude
- Dehydration
- Strenuous exercise at altitude (most relevant to HAPE)
- Ignoring early symptoms
- Gaining more than 300–500 m in sleeping altitude per day (relevant at altitudes greater than 3000 m)
- Some research shows young people (<50 years old) and men may be more susceptible (though this may be a reflection of the more aggressive ascent profiles used by these groups)
- Removal/destruction of carotid body (e.g. due to surgery or radiotherapy) will affect the ability to initiate an hypoxic ventilatory response and hence acclimatization
- Pre-existing pulmonary hypertension will increase risk of HAPE.

Note: smoking, hypertension, coronary artery disease (CAD), asthma, and mild chronic obstruction pulmonary disease do not appear to affect susceptibility to high-altitude illness. Physical fitness is not protective.

Key learning points
- Consider everyone to be at risk of altitude sickness
- There is significant individual variation in clinical presentation
- Illness at altitude is altitude sickness until proven otherwise
- Have a low threshold to diagnose and treat as HACE or HAPE
- Do not ascend with symptoms of AMS
- Descend urgently if symptoms worsen or HACE/HAPE develop
- Descent is the key to treatment; other measures (drugs, hyperbaric chambers) are intervening measures that buy you time
- Acetazolamide does not mask symptoms
- Never ascend whilst on dexamethasone
- If symptoms do not improve on descent, review your diagnosis
- Adopt a conservative ascent profile to prevent altitude sickness.

Aetiology

In the over 35's, ischaemic heart disease is, by far, the commonest cause. There are a number of causes in under 35's.

Congenital

Hypertrophic cardiomyopathy (HOCM)
- Leading cause of death in 36% of cases
- Predisposition to supraventricular and ventricular arrhythmias
- *Clinical signs:*
  - Jerky pulse
  - Double apex beat
  - Fourth heart sound
  - Ejection systolic murmur
  - Abnormal ECG in 90%
  - Characteristic echocardiograph features
- *Adverse prognostic signs:*
  - Family history sudden death
  - Autosomal dominance inheritance
  - Ventricular tachycardia (VT) episodes
  - Young age of symptom onset

Idiopathic concentric left ventricle (LV) hypertrophy
- Associated with athletic training
- Increased incidence in black athletes
- ECHO changes reduce with deconditioning over 6 month period.

Anomalous coronary artery origins
Left coronary travels between aorta and pulmonary trunk from right coronary sinus, compressed frequently at high heart rates—fall in coronary perfusion pressure—leading to chest pain, syncope, or sudden death.
- *Investigations:*
  - Changes may be found on resting electrocardiogram (ECG)
  - Stress ECG testing
  - Coronary angiography

Long QT
- QT prolonged to more than 0.44 s corrected for heart rate
  - Increased risk ventricular arrhythmias
  - Episodes associated with stress and exercise
  - Treated with betablockers, sympathectomies, or pacemakers

Wolff-Parkinson White
- Short PR interval—less than 0.12 s
- Delta wave on ECG gives appearance of wide QRS
- Accessory pathways lead to atrial arrhythmias and possible VF
- Surgical ablation of the pathway maybe required

Arrhythmnogenic right ventricular dysplasia
- Right ventricular cardiomyopathy
- Leads to ventricular arrhythmias
- High incidence in Northern Italy.

Aortic rupture
- Marfan syndrome is a connective tissue derangement leading to increased incidence of aortic dissection and rupture
  - Congenital—autosomal dominant
  - Musculoskeletal, ocular, and cardiovascular abnormalities
  - Patients appear tall with long slender limbs, high arched palette, and visual problems

Valvular disease
Can be congenital, acquired, or degenerative.
- Aortic stenosis
  - Management depends on presence of symptoms: chest pain, breathlessness, syncope
  - If moderate then restriction of sporting activity suggested.

Acquired

Post-viral cardiomyopathy
- Viral illness leading to lymphocytic infiltration of the heart muscle, leading to reduction of cardiac function and potential arrhythmias
- Athletes with a pyrexia should be rested

Ischaemic heart disease
- Resting ECG may not show any abnormality
- Stress ECG, cardiac computed tomography (CT), or cardiac angiography investigations of choice.

Presentation

The presentation of a patient with risk factors for sudden cardiac death maybe subtle.

Over 35-year-olds

In the over 35-years-old age group, the classical presentation of exertional angina may not be present, but should always be asked about in a patient prior to undertaking exercise. Other risk factors for ischaemic heart disease should be sought including:
- Diabetes
- Smoking
- Hypercholesterolaemia
- Family history
- Hypertension
- Previous history of ischaemia, valvular, or structural heart disease.

The resting ECG may not be helpful and more specific tests are often required to exclude the possibility of hidden cardiac disease.

Under 35-year-olds

In this age group symptoms of syncope, chest pain, unexplained shortness of breath, palpitations, or dizziness should always be taken seriously and a full assessment performed which should include:
- A full history
- A cardio-respiratory clinical examination
- ECG
- Then an echocardiograph if indicated or the symptoms are recurrent.

Sometimes a coach may identify an athlete as being overly 'tired' or having reduced exercise tolerance. Although vague, such subtle symptoms should also be considered as potentially originating from an occult cardiac cause. The examination for a potential cardiac cause should be included as part of the investigation of this patient.

Screening

Veneto experience in northern Italy
- Screen every competitive athlete in general population at school age
- Abnormality means exclusion from sport
- Based on 25 years of data
- 90% reduction in death from hypertrophic cardiomyopathy (HCM)
- Not repeated elsewhere, e.g. Northern Europe.

Screening tools
- *Family history:* good for autosomal dominant HCM/ischaemic heart disease (IHD)
- *Symptoms and sign:* the majority of deaths have no preceding signs or symptoms. However, any should be investigated fully
- *ECG:*
  - International Olympic Committee & European Heart Association recommend ECG screening, although the American Heart Association do not
  - ECG changes are sometimes difficult to interpret due the 'normal' changes associated with the athletic heart. If there is any doubt then a cardiology expert opinion should be sought to report the ECG
  - 2010 European ECG criteria are associated with improved specificity, but preserved sensitivity than 2005 criteria
- *Other—echocardiogram (echo)/magnetic resonance imaging (MRI):*
  - Less useful as screening tool for large population
  - 1 in 500 athletes screened will have an abnormal ECHO but it should be remembered that the prevalence of SCD is variably reported
  - Hypertrophied 'athletic heart' can mimic HCM on echocardiogram (ECHO).

The outcome of a screening programme may have significant effects with ethical issues affecting both athlete and clinician. There are potential insurance, mortgage, and employment implications for the athlete of having a diagnosis made, even though there is a very small risk of death.

Screening for a team
Advantages
- Possibly easier to fund
- Easier to control population group
- Access to specialist sports cardiology opinions
- Easier access to more advanced investigations
- Perceived by public and athletes that screening will reduce/prevent on-field sudden cardiac death (SCD).

Disadvantages
- Cardiac screening will not prevent all on-field SCD due to some of the unscreenable acquired causes (e.g. IHD/post-viral myocarditis/variable penetrance of HCM)
- Time-intensive as informed consent is required

- *Ethical issues:*
  - A player may not want to be screened
  - A player may wish to ignore the advice given following the screening programme
  - Informed consent is required.

2010 Recommendations for interpretation of 12-lead electrocardiogram in the athlete (Table 7.1)

Table 7.1 Classification of abnormalities of the athlete's electrocardiogram

Group 1: Common and training-related ECG changes	Group 2: Uncommon and training-unrelated ECG changes
Sinus bradycardia	T-wave inversion
First-degree AV block	ST-segment depression
Incomplete RBBB*	Pathological Q-waves
Early repolarization	Left atrial enlargement
Isolated QRS voltage criteria for left ventricular hypertrophy	Left-axis deviation/left anterior hemiblock
	Right-axis deviation/left posterior hemiblock
	Right ventricular hypertrophy
	Ventricular pre-excitation
	Complete LBBB or RBBB*
	Long- or short-QT interval
	Brugada-like early repolarization

*RBBB, right bundle branch block; LBBB, left bundle branch block.

Reproduced from Corrado D, Pellicia A et al. Recommendations for interpretation of 12-lead electrocardiogram in the athlete, *European Heart Journal*, 2010, **31**(2): pp. 243–59, by permission of European Society of Cardiology.

Management

Sudden cardiac death

Anticipation of an event is important. Access to a defibrillator and other equipment to aid basic life support (BLS) is vital.

Regular updates and simulation training should be undertaken by any health care professional involved in sport. Preparation for a cardiac event on the field of play, or in the crowd, should be anticipated and planned for.

The minimum requirements for equipment would include:
- Defibrillator, regularly serviced and up to date with latest support software
- Pocket ventilation device
- Airway support devices, e.g. oropharyngeal airway.

Other equipment will depend on the expertize of the heath care professional. (see p.18).
- The approach should be the same as for any 'collapsed' patient, although early defibrillation is important as the most likely arrhythmia will be ventricular in origin
- Unfortunately, survival to discharge in the under 35-years athletic group is still poor, despite high quality cardiopulmonary resuscitation (CPR) and early defibrillation. This may possibly be due to the genetic nature of serious cardiac pathology.

Prevention

Exercising and viral illness
- If pyrexial, avoid strenuous exercise
- If apyrexial and symptoms in one system only (e.g. coryza), normal activity is permitted
- If apyrexial and symptoms in two or more systems (e.g. coryza, cough, myalgia), no 'vigorous' activity is permitted.

Pre-sudden cardiac death pathology and treatments
- *Hypertrophic cardiomyopathy:*
  - Calcium antagonists/beta blockers
  - Septal myectomy
  - Implantable defibrillator
- *Anomalous coronary artery origins:* surgical re-implantation
- *Ion channelopathies:*
  - Wolff–Parkinson–White syndrome—radiofrequency ablation of ac-cessory pathways
  - Long Q–T syndrome—drugs, genetic counselling, implantable defibrillators.

Further reading

Corrado, D., Basso, C., Schiavon, M., et al. (1998). Screening for hypertrophic cardiomyopathy in young athletes. *N Engl J Med* **339**(6): 364–9.

Corrado, D., Basso, C., Schiavon, M., et al. (2008). Pre-participation screening of young athletes for prevention of SCD. *J Am Coll Cardiol* **52**(24): 1981–9.

Corrado, D., Pelliccia, A., Bjørnstad, H.H., et al. (2005). Cardiovascular preparticipation screening of young competitive athletes for prevention of sudden death: proposal for a common Euro-pean protocol. *Eur Heart J* **26**: 516–24.

Corrado, D., Pellicia, A., Heidbuchel, H., et al. (2010). Recommendations for interpretation of 12-lead electrocardiogram in the athlete. *Eur Heart J* **31**(2): 243–59.

Drezner, J.A. (2008). Contemporary approaches to the identification of athletes at risk for sudden cardiac death. *Curr Opin Cardiol* **23**(5): 494–501.

Eckart, R.E., Scoville, S.L., Campbell, C.L., et al. (2004). Sudden death in young adults: a 25-year review of autopsies in military recruits. *Ann Intern Med* **141**(11): 829–34.

Harmon, K.G., Irfan, M.A., Klosner, D., et al. (2011). Incidence of cardiac death in National Collegiate Athletic Association athletes. *Circulation* **123**: 1594–600.

Maron, B.J., Doerer, J.J., Haas, T.S., et al. (2009). Sudden deaths in young competitive athletes: analysis of 1866 deaths in the United States. *Circulation*, **119**(8): 1085–92.

Maron, B.J., Pelliccia, A., Spataro, A., et al. (1993). Reduction in left ventricular wall thickness after deconditioning in highly trained Olympic athletes. *Br Heart J* **69**: 125–8.

Maron, B.J., Thompson, P.D., Ackermann, M.J., et al. (2007). Recommendations and considerations related to preparticipation screening for cardiovascular abnormalities in competitive athletes. *Circulation* **115**: 1643–55

Maron, B.J., Thompson, P.D., Ackerman, M.J., et al. (2007). Recommendations and considerations related to pre-participation screening for cardiovascular abnormalities in competitive athletes: 2007 update: a scientific statement from the American Heart Association Council on Nutrition, Physical Activity, and Metabolism: endorsed by the American College of Cardiology Foundation. *Circulation* **115**: 1643–55. (Consensus statement from the American Heart Association advocating use of a patient/family history and physical exam for the preparticipation evaluation, and reaffirming position against universal ECG screening in athletes.)

Wilson, M.G., Basavarajaiah, S., Whyte, G.P., et al. (2008). Efficacy of personal symptom and family history questionnaires when screening for inherited cardiac pathologies: the role of electrocardiography. *Br J Sports Med* **42**: 207–11.

Chapter 8

General medical emergencies

Diabetes mellitus *90*
Acute exacerbations of asthma *94*
Anaphylaxis *96*
Seizures *98*
Acute onset shortness of breath *100*
Chest pain emergencies *102*
Emergency causes of headache *106*
Palpitations *108*

Diabetes mellitus

While *hyper*glycaemia is rarely a pitch-side emergency, *hypo*glycaemia can cause brain damage or death, but fortunately is easily treatable.

Hypoglycaemia

Occurs when blood sugar is less than 3 mmol/L (but treat if less than 4 mmol/L and symptomatic).

Hypoglycaemia is usually caused by inadequate carbohydrate intake, excessive exercise, oral hypoglycaemic drugs or excessive insulin administration. It may also be the result of faulty glucose readings.

▶ Any athlete found unconscious should be assumed to be hypoglycaemic until proven otherwise. Likewise, any athlete who becomes aggressive and agitated should have hypoglycaemia excluded as a cause for their presentation.

Look for signs/symptoms such as:
- Sweating, anxiety, pallor, hunger tremor, *progressing to*
- Cold peripheries (driven by the sympathetic nervous system), tachycardia, headache, and dizziness, *progressing to*
- Confusion, behavioural change (such as aggressiveness and agitation), slurred speech, focal neurological deficit (due to neuroglucopaenia).

Ultimately, there will be loss of consciousness and possible seizure activity. Management depends on the conscious level of the athlete, with the aim to prevent progression from a mild episode to a severe one.

▶ Ask for help and do not leave the athlete alone.
- If alert and co-operative, repeat the blood glucose
- Provide a rapidly-acting carbohydrate, such as a concentrated sugar drink, sweet tea, and sweets or chocolate
- An alternative is to administer 30–50 g oral glucose gel, such as Glucogel® (40% dextrose gel). This may be more appealing to the athlete who is less co-operative and reluctant to drink
- Follow this up by administering a more sustained release of carbohydrate, such as bananas or sandwiches
- In athletes who are unconscious, assess and manage the airway, breathing, and circulation (A, B, Cs) as described in 📖 pp.13–14
- Medical management involves an IV injection of glucose and/or an intramuscular (IM) injection of glucagon. Glucose can be administered in varying concentrations. Aim to give 25 g by either 125 mL of 20%, 250 mL of 10%. Flush the cannula with saline, as concentrated dextrose is highly irritating to veins. Patients should regain consciousness or become coherent within a few minutes, although complete recovery may lag by up to an hour
- Repeat the blood glucose measurement and transfer to a place of safety, such as hospital, for readings to be repeated hourly until they become stable
- If the athlete has over-dosed on long-acting insulin or an oral hypoglycaemic drug, set up 500 mL 5–10% dextrose IV infusion to run over 5 h for transfer to hospital.

Note: There is no place for buccal glucose solutions in the unconscious or fitting patient:
- Some blood glucose readers may not be particularly accurate in assessing low blood sugars—if an athlete presents with symptoms, but a low end of normal BM then treat as for a mild hypo.
- If an athlete has a low sugar, but is asymptomatic, repeat the reading.
- If still low then assume asymptomatic hypoglycaemia and treat without waiting for symptoms to occur.
- Remember glycogen stores may be low especially in an athlete who has been exercising for a long period of time. In this situation, glucose is preferable to glucagon.

Considerations for the doctor
Review the athlete's current medication, inspecting all drugs taken.
- Consider other, much rarer causes of hypoglycaemia, including acute liver failure and acute alcohol consumption
- Recurrent hypoglycaemia may herald diabetic kidney disease. Poor kidney function reduces the need for insulin, which is partially metabolized by the kidney
- Betablockers mask the warning signs of hypoglycaemia
- Individuals with well-controlled diabetes are more at risk of hypoglycaemia and are less sensitive to developing signs/symptoms. These individuals develop neurological signs early with fewer warning signs
- Is there any possibility that the episode may have been self-inflicted?

Considerations for the insulin-dependent athlete
Different types of exercise in different environmental conditions can have variable effects on glucose. Advice should include:
- When exercising away from home, remember to carry carbohydrates that provide short-term energy, such as glucose drinks and fruit, as well as long-acting energy, such as nuts and wholemeal bread
- Carry out training when blood glucose is above fasting level, but not high. 1–2 h after a meal is ideal
- Develop the habit of measuring your blood glucose before, during (where practical) and after exercise. This gives a better understanding of personal carbohydrate and insulin requirements; which can be tailored to avoid detrimental fluctuations in blood glucose levels
- Athletes need approximately 15–30 g glucose for every 30 min of high intensity exercise
- Prolonged exercise (>2 h) usually necessitates regular carbohydrate consumption throughout to avoid hypoglycaemia
- Symptoms of dehydration can be mistaken for low blood sugars. Ensure you consume plenty of fluids before, during and after exercise
- Remember that after intensive exercise, your blood glucose may continue to drop for several hours
- Carbohydrate ingestion after exercise restocks your muscle stores and prevents low blood glucose
- Try not to drink alcohol after you exercise as it lowers blood glucose levels further and exacerbates dehydration.

Hyperglycaemia

Hyperglycaemia occurs in diabetics due to acute illness, steroids, and faulty testing. Hyperglycaemia in non-diabetics may be caused by glucose intolerance in the context of acute illness, such as infection or myocardial infarction; steroids, and faulty readings.

Do not over-react to mildly raised blood glucose (e.g. 12 mmol/L) on a single test. Diabetic ketoacidosis (DKA) or hyper-osmolar complications may take days to develop.

Diagnosis of DKA involves:
- Hyperglycaemia (usually >14 mmol/L) in association with
- Metabolic acidosis
- Ketones in blood and urine.

In the majority of cases, you will not have access to blood tests. Even if you have access to urine testing for ketones the athlete is usually so dehydrated they will struggle to provide a sample of urine for testing.

Metabolic acidosis should be strongly suspected in a patient who has an ongoing high respiratory rate that cannot be attributed to any other cause as they try to blow off the acid that has built up. There may be a smell of ketones on the athletes breath—similar to nail polish (caused by acetone).

- Assess A, B, Cs and check the blood glucose
- Measure blood pressure (BP) and check for urinary ketones if possible
- Organize transfer to hospital for insulin sliding scale and to prevent progression to DKA if:
  - Blood glucose remains elevated and urinary ketones are positive
  - The blood glucose is >20 mmol/L
  - The athlete is hypotensive or unwell, e.g. drowsy, confused, gastrointestinal (GI) upset (abdominal pain, nausea, or vomiting)
- Set up 1000 mL IV saline for transfer to hospital. The rate of infusion should be adjusted according to level of dehydration and presence of cardiac disease.

▶ In managing DKA, the mainstay of treatment is fluid resuscitation— do not commence on IV or subcutaneous (SC) insulin pre-hospital.

Hyperglycaemia hyperosmolar state is a condition usually occurring in patients with Type 2 diabetes and is rarely seen in the young athlete who is far more likely to present with DKA. In this condition there is marked hyperglycaemia without acidosis or ketones. Treatment is again to correct the associated dehydration and does not involve insulin first line.

Considerations for the doctor

Non-insulin dependent diabetics may require insulin to maintain blood glucose control during episodes of acute illness.

Individuals with blood glucose >20 mmol/L are more at risk of DKA during intensive exercise. This is because the hormone response to exercise (glucagons, catecholamines, growth hormone, and glucocorticosteroids) is counter-regulatory to insulin at a time when there is already a lack of circulating insulin. This can rapidly increase blood glucose levels.

True laboratory glucose measurements are often higher and are more accurate than pitch-side capillary readings.

Acute exacerbations of asthma

There are athletes with asthma who train and compete within all sporting disciplines without significant impedance to their activities. Athletes who participate in outdoor sports are more likely to be exposed to common triggers, such as pollen and grass, although indoor arenas also harbour allergens, such as chalk dust or chlorine.
- The classic presentation is wheeze, breathlessness, and cough
- Exercise-induced asthma (EIA) due to airway mucosa irritation by dry and/or cold air is increasingly recognized in athletes
  - Presentation is with a combination of classic symptoms towards the end and after vigorous exercise
  - Typically these episodes resolve quickly and without concern
  - Acute asthma attacks are relatively common and usually resolve with inhalation of a short-acting beta-2 agonist
  - Rarely, an attack is severe and the athlete rapidly deteriorates; in this potentially life-threatening situation, prompt recognition and management is crucial.

It is always important to bear in the mind the differential diagnosis associated with the presentation of shortness of breath.
- Anaphylaxis
- Pneumothorax
- Pulmonary embolism
- Pulmonary oedema—especially associated with altitude
- Pneumonia.

These are all important to consider, especially the diagnosis of anaphylaxis, which can be more common in patients who have asthma.
- A panic attack is not an acceptable diagnosis unless all other causes of shortness of breath have been carefully considered and excluded by careful history and examination.
- Clinical examination and peak expiratory flow (PEFR; either as a percentage of the patient's known best, or estimated from their height and age) are vital in classifying the severity of the attack, and thus allowing appropriate pre-hospital treatment and referral to hospital.

The aim is to classify the exacerbation into 1 of the 3 subgroups below as detailed by the British Thoracic/SIGN Guidelines of 2008.

Classification of acute asthma

Moderate exacerbation
- Increasing symptoms
- PEF between 50–75% of best or predicted
- No features of acute severe asthma.

Severe exacerbation
Any *one* of:
- PEF 33–50% of best or predicted
- Respiratory rate ≥ 25/min

- Heart rate ≥ 110/min
- Inability to complete sentences in one breath.

Life-threatening exacerbation
Any one of:
- PEF <33% or unable to carry out
- Silent chest with feeble respiratory effort
- Cyanosed
- Bradycardic or hypotensive
- Exhausted
- Decreased GCS (anything <15).

Other indicators, such as blood gases are clearly not appropriate in the pre-hospital setting but will detect rising CO_2 levels, which is a pre-terminal finding.

Oxygen saturations may be monitored with the use of a portable saturation probe. Anything less than 92% while breathing air is indicative of a life-threatening exacerbation.

Treatment of acute asthma

- Sit the athlete up to aid lung expansion and reassure
- Assess and classify the athlete into one of the 3 categories as above. Note that peak expiratory flow rate (PEFR) is vital
- Note past medical history; risk of severity increases with past history of hospital admission for asthma, ventilation, >3 types of asthma drugs, and repeated presentations to Emergency Department
- If PEFR is 75% or more, and there are no features of a moderate exacerbation then the management starts with inhaled bronchodilators (e.g. salbutamol, terbutaline) and reassess, including PEFR
- If there are any features of a moderate, severe, or life-threatening exacerbation, *then commence oxygen at as high a flow rate as possible—ideally 15 L/min via non-rebreathable facemask (CO_2 retention is never an issue at this stage.)*
- Commence nebulized beta-2-agonist, i.e. salbutamol 5 mg driven by oxygen, rather than air
- In severe asthma or asthma where there has been a poor response to the initial nebulizer consider continuous nebs and also add ipratropium bromide 0.5 mg to the beta-2-agonist
- In all cases of acute asthma give po prednisolone 50 mg for 5 days
- If there is no significant clinical response to bronchodilator therapy, or any of the following are present:
  - Unable to complete sentences in one breath
  - PEFR <50% of best or predicted
  - Respiratory rate >25 min
  - Heart rate >120 bpm *(NB. Beta-2-agonists may cause tachycardia)*
  - Hypotensive (systolic blood pressure (SBP) <100 mmHg)
  - Feeble breath sounds or 'silent chest'
  - Cyanosis or O_2 saturations <92%
  - Arrange urgent transfer to Emergency Department.
- Exhaustion, confusion, or coma may require intubation to assist breathing and maximize oxygenation. This should be only be attempted by those adequately trained and competent in a pre-hospital setting.
- Note that routine prescription of antibiotics is unnecessary.

Anaphylaxis

Anaphylaxis is an immunological mediated systemic response resulting from the second exposure of a patient to an allergen with which they have already had previous sensitization (Fig. 8.1). It is a Type 1 immunoglobulin E (IgE)-mediated response.
- An *anaphylactoid* reaction is clinically indistinguishable from anaphylaxis, but is not the result of an immune mediated response
- Common allergens include nuts, strawberries, stings, and non-steroidal anti-inflammatories, such as diclofenac or ibuprofen.

An athlete may or may not have previously suffered from anaphylaxis, and thus may or may not be aware of the symptoms to look out for, or the treatments they require. Being aware as a team clinician that any of your athletes have allergies and the extent of these allergies is paramount in allowing you to consider the diagnosis and administer treatment.

Clinical manifestations
- *Airway:* swelling of tongue or mucosal surfaces, i.e. lips
- *Stridor:* hoarse voice
- *Breathing:* wheeze, increased respiratory rate
- *Circulation:* tachycardia, hypotension, increase capillary refill time
- *Skin:* flushed, itchy, urticaria
- *GI:* diarrhoea, vomiting.

Distinguishing between allergy and anaphylaxis
Anaphylaxis should be immediately suspected and treated if there is:
- Rapid progression of symptoms
- Skin or mucosal changes in association with either,
  - Airway compromise, *and/or*
  - Respiratory compromise, *and/or*
  - Circulatory compromise, i.e. decreased BP

That is, adrenaline IM is only required in the presence of a compromise of A, B, or C.

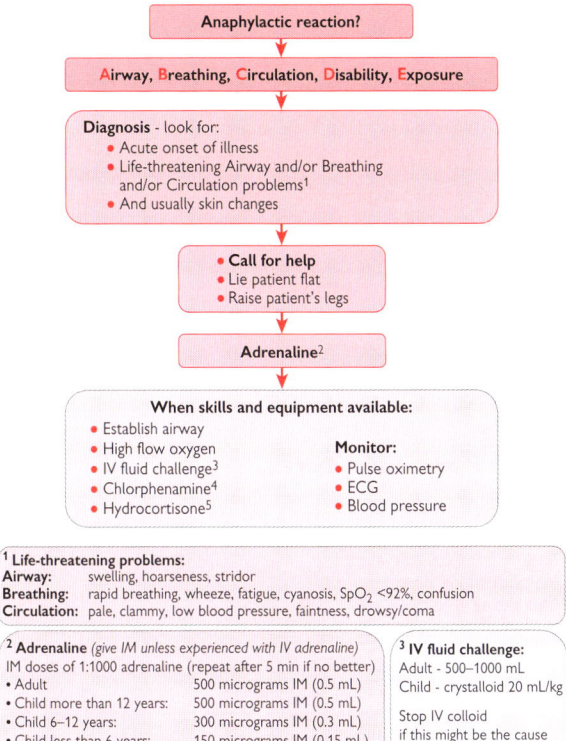

ANAPHYLAXIS

Anaphylactic reaction?

↓

Airway, **B**reathing, **C**irculation, **D**isability, **E**xposure

↓

Diagnosis - look for:
- Acute onset of illness
- Life-threatening Airway and/or Breathing and/or Circulation problems[1]
- And usually skin changes

↓

- **Call for help**
- Lie patient flat
- Raise patient's legs

↓

Adrenaline[2]

↓

When skills and equipment available:
- Establish airway
- High flow oxygen
- IV fluid challenge[3]
- Chlorphenamine[4]
- Hydrocortisone[5]

Monitor:
- Pulse oximetry
- ECG
- Blood pressure

---

[1] **Life-threatening problems:**
Airway: swelling, hoarseness, stridor
Breathing: rapid breathing, wheeze, fatigue, cyanosis, SpO_2 <92%, confusion
Circulation: pale, clammy, low blood pressure, faintness, drowsy/coma

[2] **Adrenaline** (give IM unless experienced with IV adrenaline)
IM doses of 1:1000 adrenaline (repeat after 5 min if no better)
- Adult: 500 micrograms IM (0.5 mL)
- Child more than 12 years: 500 micrograms IM (0.5 mL)
- Child 6–12 years: 300 micrograms IM (0.3 mL)
- Child less than 6 years: 150 micrograms IM (0.15 mL)

Adrenaline IV to be given **only by experienced specialists**
Titrate: Adults 50 micrograms; Children 1 microgram/kg

[3] **IV fluid challenge:**
Adult - 500–1000 mL
Child - crystalloid 20 mL/kg

Stop IV colloid if this might be the cause of anaphylaxis

	[4] **Chlorphenamine** (IM or slow IV)	[5] **Hydrocortisone** (IM or slow IV)
Adult or child more than 12 years	10 mg	200 mg
Child 6–12 years	5 mg	100 mg
Child 6 months to 6 years	2.5 mg	50 mg
Child less than 6 months	250 micrograms/kg	25 mg

Fig. 8.1 Anaphylaxis algorithm. Reproduced with the kind permission of the Resuscitation Council (UK).

Seizures

(See 📖 also p.38)

Focus of management of epilepsy or seizures of any aetiology is clearly prevention. When a seizure occurs, the management is prescriptive. Being prepared is vital—ensure you have access to the correct equipment, including a mobile phone.

- Status epilepticus is defined as seizure activity ongoing for more than 30 min, or repeated seizures without consciousness being regained
- It is a life-threatening condition with a high mortality, the rate of which increases with the increasing duration of the seizure.

Management aims

- Maintain an airway
- Terminate the seizure if not self-terminated within 2 min
- Identify potential reversible causes namely *hypoglycaemia*.

⚠ Remember that cardiac arrest caused by ventricular fibrillation may present as a short-lived seizure. Check for a pulse in all patients suffering from a seizure.

When to phone an ambulance

- Status epilepticus
- Seizure lasting longer than 5 min
- Athletes first seizure
- Seizure as a result of injury
- Injury resulting from seizure
- Multiple seizures.

Medications

There are a number of medications belonging to the benzodiazepine family that can be used to terminate seizures.

All members of the benzodiazepine family have a similar side-effect profile, such as respiratory depression and hypotension. The extent of these effects varies between drugs, but being familiar with these effects is paramount, as is having the correct equipment to deal with them.

Management of seizures

- Maintain airway. Use a naso- or oropharyngeal airway if tolerated. (The latter may be impossible to insert due to teeth clenching)
- Administer 15 L of oxygen as available
- Check for a pulse
- If fitting for more than 2 min:
  - Obtain IV access and check a blood glucose monitor (BM)
  - Administer either lorazepam 4 mg IV or diazepam 10 mg IV (buccal or intranasal route of benzodiazepine administration may be more appropriate)
- Phone an ambulance if fitting for more than 5 min

- If still fitting after 10 min
  - Administer second dose of benzodiazepine
  - *Ensure ambulance has been called.*

Acute onset shortness of breath

The presenting complaint of shortness of breath (SOB) raises the potential of many differential diagnoses. The ability to distinguish between these causes is usually based on a sound clinical history and examination findings, with very little routinely required in terms of immediate investigations. PEFR and oxygen saturations are the exceptions, and can be very helpful pitchside.

- Asthma (see p.94)
- Anaphylaxis (see p.96)
- Simple pneumothorax (see p. 169)
- Tension pneumothorax (see p. 170)
- Pulmonary embolism (PTE)
- Pulmonary oedema
- Pneumonia
- Metabolic acidosis.

Pulmonary embolism

Very unusual presentation to a team clinician but may be seen as a result of a deep venous thrombosis (DVT) that migrates from the lower leg to the lungs. May present suddenly as a cardiac arrest or over the course of a few weeks with episodes of SOB, with or without chest pain that appear to settle spontaneously.

- Look for evidence of a DVT with a history directed at assessing risk factors such as previous DVT, lower limb immobilization in cast, recent flight
- Examination should look for calf swelling and tenderness
- The chest will usually yield little in terms of examination, with normal lung fields a common finding
- Saturations will typically be low and may be difficult to pick up if the patient is shocked
- Administer high flow oxygen as soon as possible
- Obtain IV access and commence fluids if shocked
- Immediately transfer to hospital for ongoing management and investigations.

Pulmonary oedema

The most likely presentation to the team physician will be of either pulmonary oedema induced at altitude (see p.72) or as an acute episode of left ventricular failure in the case of a more elderly patient.

If clinically suspected by history such as previous episodes, onset when lying flat, associated chest pain, or by examination, such as tachycardia, bilateral crepitations, patient cold, and clammy, lower leg oedema, then apply high flow oxygen, obtain IV access and administer furosemide. Nitrates are likely to be required and can be given as long as systolic BP is maintained above 90 mmHg.

Pneumonia

Unusual to present hyper-acutely with sudden shortness of breath, and more common to present with a progression of symptoms including SOB in association with cough (which usually becomes productive in the case of bacterial pneumonias), pyrexia, general malaise, anorexia, pleuritic chest pain, rigors.

- Examination may reveal crepitations, tachypnoea, tachycardia, and decreased saturations
- Hospital referral will be required in anyone who is hypotensive, saturations <94%, significant co-morbidity or deterioration despite treatment with oral fluids, anti-pyretics, such as paracetamol, and antibiotics in the case of clinical bacterial pneumonia
- Antibiotics should be prescribed according to local policy, i.e. amoxicillin as first line primary care treatment.

Metabolic acidosis

It is worth remembering that someone who becomes progressively SOB may not actually be suffering from a primary respiratory problem and instead may be suffering from a buildup of acid.

- The acidosis is best cleared from the body by blowing off carbon dioxide via the lungs—resulting in an increase in the respiratory rate
- In the young the most common cause of metabolic acidosis is DKA (see p.92) or renal failure resulting in uraemia
- Pointers to the diagnosis may be from the history—especially in diabetics with a ketotic odour
- Patients will usually have a clinically clear chest and are likely to saturate at 99–100% unless peripherally shut down
- Note that in the case of a PTE, where the chest may again also be clear, the saturations are almost certainly highly likely to be abnormal
- Other causes of metabolic acidosis include toxins such as aspirin, and the potential of an overdose (accidental or deliberate) should also be considered
- Treatment is directed to reversing the cause of the acidosis though this should begin by maximizing oxygen uptake with high flow oxygen and fluid resuscitation good first line measures especially when the diagnosis is in doubt
- Transfer to hospital will always be required in these patients.

Chest pain emergencies

There are many potential causes of chest pain from problems that affect the skin (such as shingles) through the musculoskeletal system (such as muscular tear, costochondritis, fractured ribs) and finishing with the vital organs—lungs (including pleura) heart, and mediastinum.
- Pain may also radiate from other structures such as those of the upper abdomen, notably the stomach
- A thorough history and examination should allow the causes of chest pain to be narrowed down, and hopefully a firm diagnosis made.

▶▶ If you are unclear of the cause of chest pain then assume it to be significant, and seek assistance and transfer to hospital.

Many of the potentially life-threatening causes of chest pain have been discussed elsewhere in the book most notably in the pre-ceding pages of this chapter.

The pre-hospital key to diagnosis lies firmly in the history and to a lesser extent on examination. A structured approach to assessment should always be thoroughly carried out and regardless of the aetiology of the pain. A similar pre-hospital treatment plan can be commenced.

Pain can be categorized in many ways, but one of the easiest involves dividing into either pleuritic or non-pleuritic, where pleuritic pain is classically sharp in nature and worsened by breathing.

This is not set in stone, i.e. pericarditis may not be pleuritic in nature but it is worth considering the different causes in this manner to be clear in your mind what you are assessing for.

Potential pleuritic causes of chest pain
- Pneumothorax (📖 pp.169–71)
- Pulmonary Embolism
- Pneumonia
- Pericarditis (+/– Myocarditis)
- Musculoskeletal.

Pericarditis
- Inflammation or infection of the pericardium can result in fluid accumulating in the pericardial sac. At a critical volume, this fluid prevents the heart from contracting resulting in cardiogenic shock. The volume necessary to cause tamponade will vary depending on the length of time it takes to accumulate
- Pericarditis typically causes a sharp pain that may worsen with movement and potentially with breathing. The pain is classically worsened when lying flat and eased when sitting forward
- Pericarditis may result from viral infections, but tuberculosis (TB) should also be considered especially in anyone presenting with a secondary pericardial effusion
- Assessment may reveal very little though a pericardial rub should be looked for at the left lower sternal edge. Muffled heart sounds, raised jugular venous pressure (JVP) and hypotension (Beck's triad) would suggest cardiac tamponade necessitating immediate transfer to hospital

- Management of anyone with pericarditis involves maximizing oxygenation with high flow oxygen and supplying analgesia. Assessment in hospital should be carried out to allow an ECG to be undertaken to confirm the diagnosis and an echocardiogram (ECHO) performed to exclude an effusion.

Musculoskeletal
- Note that musculoskeletal causes of pain, whilst very common are diagnoses of exclusion made after every other cause has been considered
- In the case of trauma, anyone in whom you truly suspect fractured ribs should be closely monitored and consideration made to refer for X-ray—not to diagnose the rib fracture, but to exclude concomitant underlying lung pathology, such as pneumothorax
- Pre-hospital management, common to all of the above conditions involves commencing high flow oxygen and analgesia to the patient
- Specific treatments may need to be administered, such as decompressing a tension pneumothorax or administering antibiotics
- Entonox® is not an appropriate analgesic agent in these cases, as oxygenation should be maximized.

▶▶ Anyone with abnormal observations and pleuritic chest pain will require referral to hospital.

Non–pleuritic causes of chest pain
- Myocardial infarction (MI) or acute coronary syndrome (ACS)
- Aortic Dissection
- Pancreatitis
- Gastritis.

Myocardial infarction/acute coronary syndrome
This is an unusual presentation for a young athlete, although certain drugs (such as anabolic steroids and cocaine) can predispose the patient to suffering from an MI/ACS. It will more commonly present in the older athlete who may or may not have risk factors for ischaemic heart disease, such as smoking, hypertension, or a past history of angina.
- Pain is classically described as tightness, heaviness, crushing pain that may radiate to either arm or the neck.
- There may be associated shortness of breath, sweating, or nausea.
- Pain that lasts for longer than 15 min and is of this nature should be assumed to be a result of an MI/ACS and an ambulance phoned for the patient.
- The distinction between an MI/ACS is not important in the pre-hospital setting as treatment with oxygen, aspirin, sublingual nitrate, and IV opiate if available is the basis for treating both conditions.

CHAPTER 8 **General medical emergencies**

Aortic dissection
Again, an unusual presentation (incidence not clear as failure to initially diagnose the condition occurs in up to a third of cases), although commoner in some sports, such as basketball in which there is a higher incidence of athletes with Marfans syndrome.
- This condition along with others such as Ehlers–Danlos, syphilis, and hypertension predisposes the aorta to a weakness in the medial layer of the vessel
- It is this weakness that results in a tear in the intima and resulting dissection of the aorta
- Pain will depend on which aspect of the aorta is affected and it may change in position as the tear evolves
- Anterior chest pain may be found in ascending or aortic root dissections, with neck pain in arch dissection
- Pain from the descending aorta is classically described as tearing interscapular pain.

▶ Pain usually *maximal at onset*, which may help to distinguish from MI/ACS.
- Examination should assess for pulse including both radial arteries.
- Assess BP in both arms although it should be remembered that it can be normal to have differences of up to 20 mmHg between arms.
- BP maybe high or low, with hypotension a poor prognostic indicator.
- Listen to heart sounds for murmurs or muffled sounds that might suggest an associated effusion or tamponade.
- Listen to the chest for evidence of an effusion.
- Pre-hospital treatment involves oxygenating and supplying analgesia with immediate transfer of the patient to the nearest hospital.

Emergency causes of headache

- Headache is a common symptom that may occur as the result of many different pathologies both benign as well as life-threatening
- Most people will experience a headache significant enough to require analgesia at some point in their lives
- It is a common complaint and the key to identifying the life-threatening causes usually lies with taking an adequate history
- Best thought of as divided into traumatic and non-traumatic causes.

Traumatic causes
- Subdural haematoma (p.125)
- Extradural haematoma (p.125)
- Concussion (p. 122).

The history in these cases is usually evident with respect to trauma. The lucid interval prior to deterioration in conscious level is still an unfortunate classic presentation of an extra-dural and is the reason that serial neuro-observation should be routinely performed after every head injury and for a period not less than 24 h.

Non-traumatic causes
- Subarachnoid haemorrhage
- Meningitis/encephalitis
- Hypertensive crisis
- Temporal arteritis.

Certain 'red flags' in the history may help to point towards the cause of a life-threatening headache.
- Sudden onset—highly suggestive of subarachnoid headache (SAH)
- Most severe headache ever (SAH)
- Described as 'like being hit on the back of the head with a baseball bat' (SAH)
- Associated with a syncopal episode (SAH)
- Sudden onset of severe upper neck pain without palpable tenderness and good range of movement (SAH)
- Photophobia (SAH or meningitis)
- Neck stiffness (meningitis)
- Purpuric rash (meningitis)
- Associated fever (meningitis)
- Temporal headache (consider temporal arteritis especially if over 40 years old).

Subarachnoid haemorrhage
- Usually the result of rupture of a berry aneurysm or arteriovenous (AV) malformation
- Incidence varies between countries but is about 10:100,000/year
- Anyone who volunteers the information of pain like 'being hit on the back of the head' should be assumed to have a SAH until proven otherwise
- Involves admission to hospital for CT scan +/– lumbar puncture

- There may be vomiting in association with the occipital headache
- Mortality approaches 50%
- Key to treatment is identification and emergent referral to hospital.

Meningitis/encephalitis
- May be viral or bacterial
- May occur in isolation or together therefore treatment usually involves antibiotics and antivirals IV
- Symptoms may be rapid in onset (i.e. <24 h) in about 25% with the potential for a rapid deterioration in condition unless treated with antibiotics quickly
- Symptoms may be fairly non-specific, making diagnosis difficult
- Pyrexia, headache, vomiting, photophobia, and neck stiffness are classic textbook signs that may also be found in a number of other conditions making diagnosis difficult in times of influenza outbreak for example:
  - Bacterial meningitis can be caused by many different organisms including *Neisseria meningitidis* and *Strep pneumonia*. Pneumococcal meningitis has the highest incidence of mortality
  - Pre-hospital management involves pain relief, antiemetic, anti-pyretics, IM benzylpenicllin, and IV fluids if necessary.

Hypertensive crisis
It is common for BP to rise in response to pain. As such, an elevated BP may be a normal physiological finding in a patient suffering from headaches caused by migraines, for example:
- In contrast, someone who is suffering from a headache brought about by uncontrolled BP must be identified and treated in the hospital setting
- Usually in this setting the systolic BP will be >220 mmHg
- Refer immediately to hospital anyone who has symptomatic high BP.

Temporal arteritis
- Unusual under the age of 40 years
- Affects females more than males
- Important as a cause of headache associated with irreversible blindness
- Headache may be sudden and located to the temporal area
- Pain may be felt when combing the hair
- Hospital referral is necessary for erythrocyte sedimentation rate (ESR) and biopsy though treatment may commence with steroids in suspected cases without blood or biopsy test results.

Palpitations

- Palpitations are a relatively common complaint. They are described as an awareness of a forceful and usually fast heart beat
- There are many causes of palpitations but the aim is distinguishing the benign ('skipped beat') from the life-threatening tachyarrythmias
- Palpitations may occur as an isolated symptom or may be associated with symptoms of syncope, chest pain, shortness of breath, or dizziness
- Any association with syncope mandates an immediate hospital assessment
- Chest pain will also usually result in a hospital admission though this may be avoided in an athlete who is known to suffer recurrent supraventricular tachycardias (SVT) and whose symptoms terminate with cessation of the SVT
- It is important to try to distinguish the rate and rhythm of the palpitations, the regularity of their onset as well as any precipitating or relieving factors
- History and examination are key.

History

- Is this an awareness of a 'skipped' beat, multiple beats, or a sustained episode of the heart racing?
- If racing then for how long?
- Are there any associated symptoms as described above?
- How often has this happened before?
- Is there anything you can do to make them stop?
- Have you had any previous cardiac history?
- Are you on any medications?
- Is there any family history of cardiac disease or sudden death?
- Is there a history of alcohol or cocaine abuse?

Remember iatrogenic causes of arrhythmias, such as over doseage of local anaesthetic.

Examination

This is based around the ABC principles described in Chapter 2.
Check the pulse for evidence of a tachycardia with a rate above 100 bpm.

- Is it regular or irregular?
- What is the volume of the pulse?
- The blood pressure?
- Is the patient shocked or clinically well?

Investigation

- The ability to obtain a 12-lead ECG or even a rhythm strip should confirm the clincal findings with respect to the actual heart rate if caught in time
- It will also allow you to classify the tachycardia as either an SVT or VT
- Maximal heart rate is usually considered to be around 220 bpm minus age and it is highly unlikely that a sinus tachycardia would present at a rate greater than this.

Management of palpitations

See Fig. 8.2.
- Management is based on identifying the underlying driver for the tachycardia as either SVT or VT and treating the patient on the basis of their cardiovascular status
- A controlled pulse with occasional ectopic beats can usually be managed with simple reasssurance
- If you do not have access to an ECG then vagal manouevres may be performed on a stable patient with a tachycardia
- This will have no effect on VT, but may cardiovert an SVT
- Remember to check for a carotid bruit prior to performing carotid massage
- Any athlete suffering from palpitations will require a full cardiology work up including ECG and ECHO
- Blood tests may also be useful in identifying any electrolyte abnormalities, such as hypomagnesia, which may predispose to recurrent arrythmias.

110 CHAPTER 8 **General medical emergencies**

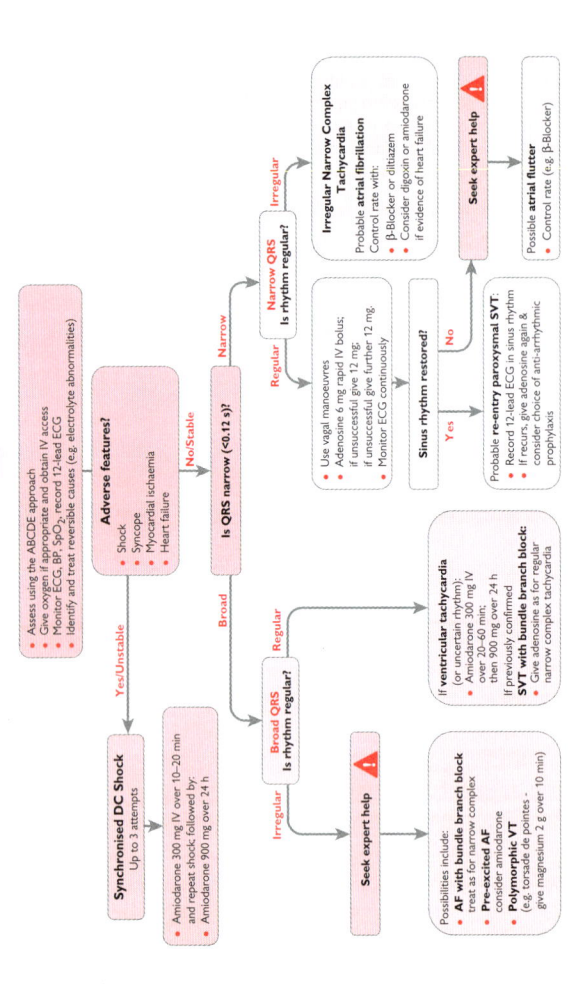

Fig. 8.2 Algorithm for management of tachycardia. Reproduced with the kind permission of the Resuscitation Council (UK).

Further reading

British Thoracic Guidelines/Scottish Intercollegiate Guidelines Network (2008, revised 2011). Available at: www.sign.ac.uk/pdf/qrg101.pdf.

Resuscitation Council. Available at: www.resus.org.uk.

Chapter 9
Head injuries

Background *114*
Pitchside equipment and pre-event preparation *115*
Pitchside assessment of head injury *116*
Minor head injury management *118*
Significant head injury management *120*
Concussion management *122*
Subdural haematoma *125*
Extradural haematomas *125*
Diffuse cerebral swelling *125*
Intracerebral haematomas *126*
Scalp injuries *126*

Background

Head injury is common in contact sports ranging from minor injury with no neurological deficit through varying degrees of concussion to traumatic brain injury. The pitchside practitioner must be competent in assessment and management of head injuries with awareness of sequelae.

- In a recent National Confidential Enquiry into Patient Outcome and Death (NCEPOD) report 'Trauma: who cares' it was noted that in the UK, traumatic brain injury accounts for 15–20% of deaths between the ages of 5 and 35 years, with an incidence of 9 per 100,000 per year
- Outcome after head injury depends upon the initial severity of injury and also the extent of any subsequent complications and how these are managed
- Most of the patients who attend hospital after a head injury do not develop life-threatening or disabling complications in the acute stage. However, in a small, but important group of patients, outcome is made worse by a failure to either detect promptly or to deal adequately with complications
- There is a growing body of evidence that secondary insults occur frequently and exert a profound, adverse effect on out-come from severe head injury. It is therefore recommended that hypotension (systolic blood pressure (SBP) <90 mmHg) and hypoxia (PaO_2 <8 kPa) must be scrupulously avoided or treated immediately to avoid worsening outcome.

Pitchside equipment and pre-event preparation

Equipment
- Oxygen with reservoir bag mask
- Suction apparatus
- Airway adjuncts
- Full length spinal board with body and head straps
- Adjustable size cervical collar.

Pre-event preparation
- Contact local hospital to inform of event, ensure hospital has computed tomography (CT) scanning facilities available. Identify your nearest neurosurgical unit
- Assess ambulance provision at the event. Are paramedics needed? Is the team proficient in the log roll technique. Are they aware of their roles and responsibilities with a designated lead?
- Try to practice scenarios pre-event with medical and pitchside team
- Be aware of and make adjustments according to environmental conditions
- Ensure efficient access from pitch to medical room/ambulance for injured player
- Ensure all staff are aware of location of equipment and evacuation procedures.

Pitchside assessment of head injury

- The pitchside practitioner must watch the sporting event in order to witness the mechanism of any injury, in a head injury particular attention is paid to any loss of consciousness
- Should the practitioner need to enter the field of play, they must ensure a safe approach
- This will usually involve ensuring that the match officials have stopped the play or event
- It is useful to have introduce yourself prior to the event and ensure that an agreement is reached as to how this will occur
- The approach to the patient will be the same as for any injured player (see Chapter 2).
  - **A:** airway
  - **B:** breathing
  - **C:** circulation
  - **D:** disability (assessed using the Glasgow Coma Scale or the AVPU) measure of response
  - **E:** exposure/environment.

AVPU scale
- A: Alert
- V: Responsive to Vocal stimuli only
- P: Responsive to Pain stimuli only
- U: Unresponsive.

Glasgow Coma Scale
Eye opening
- 4 Spontaneous
- 3 Verbal commands
- 2 Pain
- 1 None.

Best motor response
- 6 Obeys
- 5 Localizes
- 4 Withdraws
- 3 Abnormal flexion posturing
- 2 Abnormal extension posturing
- 1 None.

Best verbal response
- 5 Orientated
- 4 Disorientated or confused
- 3 Inappropriate words
- 2 Incomprehensible sounds
- 1 None

Potential cervical spine injuries

If loss of consciousness, assume C-spine injury:
- ABCDE + oxygen (12–15 L of 100% with reservoir bag) + C-spine immobilization. This can be carried out manually in the first instance. During transfer, 'triple immobilization' should be carried out, with a correctly sized rigid neck collar, sandbags (or equivalent) to either side of the head, and tape placed over the forehead and sandbags and attached to the extraction device, and the same replicated over the chin
- If evidence of airway obstruction, jaw thrust manoeuvre should be performed and/or an airway adjunct inserted after being correctly sized
- The patient should be log-rolled onto an extraction device, e.g. a long board or 'scoop' stretcher
- If the patient vomits then a log roll manoeuvre will be required to turn them onto their side.

If there is no loss of consciousness:
- Assessment of head injury and C-spine can be performed. Following injury player should be held in manual in line stabilization in supine position whilst assessment is carried out
- Practitioner must assess for any sign of gross neurological deficit including visual disturbance
- Player must be fully conscious, alert, and orientated in order to clear the C-spine:
  - Ask regarding neck pain and palpate cervical spine for tenderness or step deformity
  - Assess limb movement and ask regarding any paraesthesia or anaesthesia
  - Gently allow mobilization of the neck stopping and instituting immobilization if there is any pain and or resistance.

The Nexus guidelines (see Box 9.1) provide a validated guideline for the clearance of cervical spine injury (for further information see p.158).

Box 9.1 The NEXUS clinical criteria for c-spine clearance

1. The absence of tenderness at the posterior midline of the cervical spine
2. The absence of a focal neurological deficit
3. A normal level of alertness
4. No evidence of intoxication
5. Absence of clinically apparent pain that might distract the patient from the pain of a cervical spine injury

ⓘ Minor head injury management

For the purposes of this chapter a minor head injury is classified as one which had neither loss of consciousness nor neurological deficit evident. Principals of management are the same as all head injuries with a primary survey—ABCDE in the first instance. This is followed by clearance of the C-spine, assessment of neurological function, Modified Maddock's questions (Box 9.2), and gradual return to upright position and then fluid replacement.

- Answering any question incorrectly is suggestive of concussion and mandates removal from the pitch
- Whether the athlete stays on the pitch or is removed, continual reassessment is recommended. If the player continues the practitioner must watch their movements closely and ask regarding symptoms at breaks in play and at half-time and full-time
- If it is decided to remove from play a decision needs to be made regarding transfer to hospital. Should there be any neurological deficit or C-spine injury suspicion then player must be sent for further investigation and management
- If player is deemed unable to continue yet no suspicion of traumatic brain injury then player must be monitored by practitioner for at least the first hour post injury and then followed up with head injury advice
- Beware distracting injuries such as scalp laceration and ensure you fully access the potential head and neck injury first. Ensure all wounds are fully cleaned and explored prior to closure.
  - Reassess at end of game with full neurological examination and Maddock's questions.
  - Ensure the player is monitored for at least the 1st hour post-injury.
  - When the patient is discharged from your care they must have a responsible adult to monitor them for the next 24 h.
  - Information should be provided to the patient and carer, and backed up with written advice for them to follow (Box 9.3). This should include information on treatment of a minor head injury
- It is imperative to keep thorough medical notes of the injury and management
- It is useful to have head injury advice sheets readily available to give to the player having explained the process with their responsible adult who will be with them for the next 24 h
- These should contain contact details of club medical staff to ensure any deterioration is reported and appropriate management instigated
- The head injury advice sheet should also contain information about symptoms the player may experience (see Box 9.4). The development of any of these symptoms mandates urgent medical reassessment.

Box 9.2 Modified Maddock's questions

1. At what venue are we?
2. Which half is it?
3. Who scored last?
4. What team did we play last week?
5. Did we win the last game?

Box 9.3 Home with head injury advice

- 'Brain rest'
- No alcohol
- Minimize stimulants, e.g. TV, computer
- Ensure patient is not alone over first 24 hr
- Do not drive
- Ensure adequate hydration

Box 9.4 Signs of significant head injury

Include:
- Progressively worsening headache
- Repeated vomiting
- Visual disturbance
- Excessive drowsiness, irritability or altered personality
- Dizziness, loss of balance, or convulsions
- Blood or clear fluid, leaking from the nose or ear
- New deafness in one or both ears
- Unusual breathing patterns
- Loss of use of part of the body
- Confusion, strange behaviour, any problems understanding or speaking

Significant head injury management

A significant head injury is classified for the purposes of this chapter, as injury causing witnessed loss of consciousness and/or neurological deficit on examination (see Box 9.4 for signs of significant head injury).

Management, as with all head injuries, begins with the primary survey:
- ABCDE + oxygen (12–15 L 100% with a reservoir bag)
- C-spine immobilization should be instigated if there is loss of consciousness as practitioner cannot clear a C-spine in an unconscious player
- In an unconscious player's airway compromise may require a jaw thrust, as well as airway adjuncts
- If the player suffers a seizure it is important to maintain in line immobilization as much as possible, however, with violent movements this will need to be gentle support, rather than rigid immobilization. Likewise oxygen therapy should be continued even in violent movements by placing mask in close vicinity to airway
- If possible full neurological assessment should be instigated. Signs and symptoms requiring hospital transfer for CT to exclude cerebral pathology include:
  - Depressed GCS below 14, which continues after initial presentation
  - Focal neurological signs
  - Suspicion of skull fracture, open or depressed
  - Signs of fracture at base of skull (haemotympanum, 'panda' eyes, cerebrospinal fluid leakage from ears or nose, Battle's sign)
  - Significant progressive headache, excessive drowsiness, visual disturbance, repeated vomiting
  - Post-traumatic seizure
  - Amnesia of events more than 30 min prior to injury.

It is recommended to call ahead with status update of injured player to hospital. Having established links pre event the hospital will be aware of event and possibility of injuries being brought in.

It is imperative to once again ensure thorough documentation of the injury and subsequent management, it is also important to communicate clearly with the player if applicable and with paramedics, ambulance staff, and the member of your medical team who may accompany player to hospital if transfer is to occur.

⚠ Concussion management

At the International Conference on Concussion in sport, held in Zurich in 2008, a consensus statement was produced that defined concussion as: 'a complex pathophysiological process affecting the brain, induced by traumatic biomechanical forces. Several common features that incorporate clinical, pathological, and biomechanical injury constructs that may be utilized in defining the nature of a concussive head injury include:

- Concussion may be caused either by a direct blow to the head, face, neck, or elsewhere on the body with an 'impulsive' force transmitted to the head
- Concussion typically results in the rapid onset of short-lived impairment of neurological function that resolves spontaneously
- Concussion may result in neuropathological changes, but the acute clinical symptoms largely reflect a functional disturbance, rather than a structural injury
- Concussion results in a graded set of clinical symptoms that may or may not involve loss of consciousness. Resolution of the clinical and cognitive symptoms typically follows a sequential course; however, it is important to note that in a small percentage of cases, post-concussive symptoms may be prolonged
- No abnormality on standard structural neurological imaging studies is seen in concussion.

The suspected diagnosis of concussion can include one or more of the following clinical domains:

- *Symptoms:* somatic (e.g. headache), cognitive (e.g. feeling like in a fog) and/or emotional symptoms (e.g. lability).
- *Physical signs:* e.g. loss of consciousness, amnesia
- *Behavioural changes:* e.g. irritability
- *Cognitive impairment:* e.g. slowed reaction times
- *Sleep disturbance:* e.g. drowsiness.'

The complexity of the definition demonstrates the complexity of the condition.

- ⚠ It is important to appreciate that consciousness may still be retained and that imaging studies will be normal
- During pitchside assessment of head injury brief neuropsychological tests that assess attention and memory function have been shown to be practical and effective to diagnose concussion. Such tests include the Maddock's questions
- Concussion may be immediately apparent and necessitate removal from play or it may present post-event with the player having continued to play on. It is important to repeat the Maddock's questions as part of the practitioner's full neurological assessment following head injury if a player has continued
- If concussion is diagnosed this will mandate a graded return to play to allow symptom resolution. Further tools to assess concussion include the Sport Concussion Assessment Tool (SCAT)

- Baseline neuropsychological testing (e.g. Impact, Cog Sport) can aid as an indicator of return to play, allowing comparison of cognitive function against the players own healthy baseline
- Symptom resolution is, however, the key to return to play
- ⚠ The cornerstone of concussion management is physical and cognitive rest until symptoms resolve and then a graded programme of exertion prior to medical clearance and return to play
- Typical resolution of symptoms is achieved in 7–10 days in 80–90% of cases. In some sports there are guidelines and minimum time restrictions set for return to player, e.g. RFU 21 days depending on medical supervision
- Graded return to activity is in various stages with at least 24 h between each stage, if symptoms recur at any stage then the protocol dictates dropping back to the last asymptomatic stage and then progressing once more. An important consideration in return to play is that concussed athletes should not only be symptom-free but also should not be taking any pharmacological agents/medications that may mask or modify the symptoms of concussion
- A detailed concussion history taken at baseline while the player is healthy provides important information in the event of a concussion. It is important to ascertain the severity of impact/injury, return to play time (Box 9.5), and frequency of concussive episodes
- There is little evidence to suggest that repetitive head injuries result in 'second impact syndrome' (rapid, severe cerebral oedema following head injury sustained, whilst still symptomatic from previous concussion) or cumulative damage. Indeed, it seems more likely that there is a genetic predisposition to concussion incidence and/or outcome (i.e. some athletes may be more prone to concussion and take longer to recover from them)
- Where an athlete has a history of previous concussions medical staff may proceed with extra caution when making return to play decisions.

Box 9.5 Graduated return to play (RTP) protocol

- Rehabilitation stage
- Functional exercise at each stage of rehabilitation
- Objective of each stage

Stage 1
- No activity
- Complete physical and cognitive rest
- Recovery

Stage 2
- Light aerobic exercise
- Walking, swimming, or stationary cycling, keeping intensity at 70% maximum predicted heart rate. No resistance training
- Increase heart rate

Stage 3
- Sport-specific exercise
- Sport specific drills. No head impact activities
- Add movement

Stage 4
- Non-contact training drills
- Progression to more complex training drills. May start progressive resistance training
- Exercise, co-ordination, and cognitive load

Stage 5
- Full contact practice
- Following medical clearance participate in normal training activities
- Restore confidence and assess functional skills by coaching staff

Stage 6
- Return to play
- Normal game play

Subdural haematoma

The traumatic injury causes blood to be released into the subdural space. This is classically due to rupture of the bridging cerebral veins.
- There is usually a brief loss of consciousness and period of confusion. It is more common in the older athlete
- As the mass increases further symptoms will develop. These will depend on the location of the haematoma, but can be quite subtle with increasing headache or vomiting, being the only early symptoms
- The injury may be associated with a substantial soft tissue injury to the head and possible associated cranial vault fracture, but these do not have to be present
- Late features of intracranial pressure increase from the mass may include ipsilateral third nerve palsy
- Prognosis from an acute subdural event will often depend more on damage to the cerebral parenchyma from the force of injury, rather than the presence of a subdural bleed itself.

Extradural haematomas

This results from a direct blow to the skull. This causes deformation of the skull and tearing of the vessels associated with the extradura. It is commonly associated with fractures in adults, but is also seen in children due to the flexibility of the skull.
- 50% of the bleeding is associated with the middle meningeal artery
- 33% are associated with venous bleeds
- Fractures of the skull can also lead to mass effect from accumulating blood
- The patient will usually present with an injury associated with loss of consciousness
- The patient may then appear to return to normal
- However after a variable period of time, symptoms of raised intracranial pressure will start usually with headaches or vomiting
- Sometimes the presentation can be dramatic with a patient proceeding from apparent normal consciousness to deeply unconscious in a matter of minutes
- Prompt surgical evacuation is required for all expanding extradural haematomas.

Diffuse cerebral swelling

- This can occur after only minor head injuries and children appear to be particularly at risk
- There is rapid cerebral swelling leading to a rise in the intracranial pressure. The mechanism for this is not well understood
- Treatment is the same for all types of brain injury with an ABCDE approach.

Intracerebral haematomas

- These can occur in response to a direct blow or from movement of the brain within the skull vault (leading to the coup and conta-coup injury patterns)
- Signs and symptoms will depend on the location of the injury within the brain parenchyma.

Scalp injuries

The scalp is made up of five distinct layers
- **S**: skin
- **C**: connective tissue
- **A**: aponeurosis
- **L**: loose areolar tissue
- **P**: periosteum

The scalp has an excellent blood supply and can allow an extra-cranial haematoma to expand readily. Patients can lose a large amount of blood through a scalp wound leading to hypotension, which is a poor prognostic sign for an intracranial injury.

Remember, however, to exclude other causes of blood loss, which you should assess for as part of the circulation assessment. Treatment to prevent blood loss will initially consist of direct pressure. Suturing will also help to control haemorrhage. This usually requires a large curved needle.

The evaluation of a scalp wound should include palpation for a possible depressed fracture, identification, and removal of foreign bodies and careful cleaning with copious amounts of water.

When closing the wound the aponeurosis must be closed with interrupted sutures and then the skin closed over it. However, in an emergency all layers can be closed together. For minor injuries to the scalp, glue can be a quick and effective alternative.

During a sporting event, sutures are often placed quickly to prevent blood loss and to return the player to the field of play as soon as possible. On these occasions it is appropriate to remove the sutures after completion of the sport and to ensure thorough wound exploration and cleaning prior to repeating the suture of the wound for best cosmetic effect.

Further reading

Advanced Resuscitation and Emergency Aid course (2009). Available at: www.remosports.com/area-courses.

National Institute for Health and Clinical Excellence (NICE) (2007). *Head Injury Guide*. NICE, London.

(2008). Consensus Statement on Concussion in Sport. 3rd International Conference on Concussion in Sport, Zurich, November.

England Hockey: Concussion Policy Statement and Management Guidelines.

National Confidential Enquiry into Patient Outcome and Death (2007). *Trauma: Who Cares?* NCEPOD, London.

Chapter 10

Airway injuries

Introduction *130*
What constitutes an airway injury? *131*
How might an airway injury present? *132*
Managing airway injuries *134*

Introduction

Life-threatening airway injuries are very rare. However, it is important to be aware that they are significantly more frequent in those sports in which blunt or crush trauma can occur, e.g. a clothes-line tackle in rugby, or blows from the fists or feet in martial art disciplines, or those that involve high speed projectiles, e.g. hockey (stick or ball).

What constitutes an airway injury?

Airway injury can potentially occur at any point in the respiratory tract. However, there are 2 key zones particularly at risk:

Face (oral and nasal cavities)
- Soft tissue swelling may result in immediate or delayed airway obstruction
- The tissues have a rich blood supply therefore persistent bleeding puts airway at risk of occlusion, e.g. severe epistaxis
- Fractures of the facial bones (nose, zygoma, maxilla, and mandible) can result in distortion of normal anatomy and encroachment on the airway, particularly when grossly displaced; they are also associated with significant bleeding that is difficult to control
- In bilateral fractures of the mandible the anterior segment has the potential to shift backwards, causing the tongue to block the airway (see p.146).

Neck (larynx and trachea)
- Soft tissue swelling with or without cartilaginous fractures can result in obstruction.
- Fractures of the larynx can occur, leading to rapid distortion of the airway and associated bleeding resulting in partial or complete airway obstruction.
- Recurrent laryngeal nerve injury may lead to vocal cord dysfunction or paralysis.

In any neck injury it is necessary to consider the possibility of a cervical cord injury or damage to the carotid vessels such as a dissection—often presenting with a history of neck injury and neurological symptoms.

How might an airway injury present?

Facial soft tissue trauma, with associated bleeding and swelling, is usually easy to recognize. If an injury is not immediately apparent, suspect airway trauma in a player complaining of:
- Dyspnoea
- Hoarseness
- Neck pain or laryngeal tenderness
- Haemoptysis
- Difficulty or pain on swallowing or talking
- Stridor—harsh inspiratory noise.

If there is immediate or impending loss of airway the player will be extremely agitated and in respiratory distress, making intervention very difficult. It is unlikely they will be co-operative! Invariably the player will become rapidly cyanosed and unconscious if the airway is not restored.

If the player is unconscious, indicators of potential airway compromise include:
- Abnormal, high-pitched inspiratory, or expiratory sounds (stridor/stertor)
- Epistaxis
- Haematoma or bruising
- Neck swelling or subcutaneous emphysema
- Loss of anatomical landmarks and/or bony crepitus (suspect an acute fracture).

Managing airway injuries

As with any trauma patient, a systematic assessing airway, breathing, and adequacy of circulation (A, B, C) approach should be followed along with c-spine immobilization (spinal injuries often co-exist with airway trauma). Supplementary high flow oxygen should also be administered via a non-rebreathable reservoir mask.

'Walking wounded' players with a suspected airway injury should be immediately withdrawn from play. It is crucial to appreciate that the onset of signs and symptoms may be delayed and progressive, therefore loss of patency of the airway may occur precipitously. A single examination is not sufficient.

A player who may have sustained a facial fracture or has persistent epistaxis despite first line interventions (e.g. direct sustained pressure, ice application, nasal packing, and topical adrenaline) should be referred to hospital for further assessment.

Basic manoeuvre

Jaw thrust
Fingers are placed behind the angle of the jaw and the jaw is drawn forward away from the face, allowing soft tissues to be pulled away from the back of the throat (see p.23).

Airway adjuncts

(Only if patient unconscious or gag reflex is absent, e.g. GCS <8.)
- Nasopharyngeal (NP) airway (avoid if suspicion of basal skull fracture or there is nasal deformity and/or heavy bleeding):
  - Size estimation roughly by diameter of player's little finger
  - Lubricate tip, then insert with bevel facing inwards, parallel to palate, rotating gently as it is advanced.
- Oropharyngeal (OP) airway:
  - Size from angle of mandible to incisors
  - Insert with concave surface upwards, then rotate 180° once soft plate encountered or under direct vision using a torch and tongue depressor.

Advanced airway management

This requires specialist equipment and training in its use:
- *Laryngeal mask airway (LMA):* technically easy to insert, but doesn't protect from aspiration of stomach contents
- *Endo-tracheal (ET) intubation:* ideally whilst maintaining in-line immobilization.

Attempting to insert a more definitive airway should not delay transfer to hospital if basic techniques are permitting adequate gas exchange.

Surgical airway techniques

Often a last resort, but may be the only option remaining if the airway compromise is not corrected by the methods described above. Again, requires specific training and a degree of expertise.

- *Percutaneous needle cricothyroidotomy:*
  - Large bore cannula inserted into trachea though the cricothyroid membrane; oxygen tubing then attached with either a small hole made in it or 3-way valve attached
  - Allow expansion of lungs with 1 s flow on, then deflation with 4 s of flow off
  - Permits oxygenation, not ventilation, therefore CO_2 retention occurs rapidly.
- *Surgical cricothyroidotomy:* commercially available kits, e.g. Portex Minitrach II®. Permits ventilation, either spontaneously or artificially with bag and valve apparatus.

Chapter 11

Maxillofacial injuries and infection in sports medicine

Introduction *138*
Anatomy *139*
Principles of managing maxillofacial injuries *140*
Soft tissue injuries *142*
Dental injuries *144*
Maxillofacial fractures *146*
Medical maxillofacial emergencies *150*

Chapter 11 Maxillofacial injuries and infection

Introduction

> My face is so pretty, you don't see a scar, which proves I'm the king of the ring by far (Muhammed Ali).

Maxillofacial soft tissue and bony injuries are very common in athletes despite the recommended use of dental guards and face shields in contact sports, such as rugby and soccer. The rise in participation of contact sports, coupled with increasing pressure on individuals to maintain cosmetic appearances, have resulted in rising public perception of physical beauty demanding no imperfection, and so it is important that patients with disfiguring injuries are treated to obtain the best possible outcome, both anatomically and cosmetically.

- The treating physician must be at the forefront of up-to-date management of maxillofacial injuries and infections sustained during sporting activity
- Maxillofacial injuries sustained by sportsmen (and women) vary from simple cuts and abrasions to dental injuries and severe facial fractures requiring life-saving airway support measures, and subsequent surgical fixation
- The ABC with cervical spine control assessment (as detailed in Chapter 2) must be used in all patients with maxillofacial injuries, as they are often associated with head and cervical spine injury
- The mechanism of maxillofacial injuries is generally direct impact from an external source (another player, sports equipment, the local environment, or hard surfaces)
- Forces exerted during such injuries can lead to shear, compression, friction, or traction of the soft tissues and associated structures.

⚠ As with all injuries and infection, it is assumed that the reader will perform thorough wound cleaning in extensive or heavily contaminated wounds, and human tetanus immunoglobulin (HATI) in tetanus prone wounds, and as such this will not be discussed further in this chapter.

Anatomy

- The anterior aspect of the face is bordered superiorly by the frontal bones, laterally by the temporal bones, and inferiorly by the muscles of the neck
- The facial skeleton consists of nine bones: four paired (nasal, zygomatic, maxilla, palatine, and the mandible)
- The nasal bones and zygomatic arches are prominent facial features, and, therefore, most commonly injured during facial trauma
- The nasal, frontal, and maxillary sinuses form part of the facial skeleton, and are also easily damaged in facial trauma due to being thin walled
- Motor innervation of the face is by the five main branches of the facial nerve (CN VII) as it traverses through the parotid gland, and sensory innervation by the three branches of the trigeminal nerve (CN V) The infra-orbital nerve (CN V^2) passes through the infra-orbital foramen and supplies the skin on the lateral side of the nose, the upper lip, the lower eyelid, and damage to this nerve is a good indicator of underlying zygomatico-orbital fractures.

Principles of managing maxillofacial injuries

History
- Obtain details of the mechanism of injury
- Was the athlete unconscious?
- Can they remember what happened?
- Complaints of pain, altered vision and paraesthesia must be clearly documented at the outset
- This will allow a focused assessment and may tie pathologies together such as the diplopia and cheek numbness found in an infra-orbital fracture
- In addition, a targeted medical, drug, and tetanus vaccination history should be taken, and drug allergies noted. Being aware of the athlete's past history prior to an injury occurring saves time and distraction.

Examination
- Initially assessed with the airway, breathing, circulation (ABC) approach and the cervical spine must not be overlooked—see Chapter 2
- Ensure that the airway is secure and safe before proceeding to examine injuries, and if there is any indication of immediate or potential airway compromise, seek advice and support from a colleague who can manage the airway as a matter of urgency— see p.129
- The face is extremely vascular and even minor injuries may result in significant bleeding, which need to be treated quickly with irrigation and haemostatic measures (local compression or sutures) to enable thorough examination of the wound
- Initial visual inspection must take into account facial asymmetry from the front, side, and skyline views of the face. Palpate superiorly, from the frontal bones and proceed inferiorly and laterally, feeling for bony steps or crepitus
- Always examine the oral cavity for soft tissue, bony, and dental injuries, which may not be apparent externally

▶▶Document all missing and damaged teeth, and their whereabouts—if necessary you will need to ensure they are not located in the airway
- Note all areas of swelling, as this may indicate underlying injury
- The size, shape, location, and depth of lacerations needs to be clearly documented, and all wounds must be explored to exclude a foreign body (this may need to be performed under general anaesthetic, depending on the severity and complexity of the wound)
- Finally a systematic assessment of motor and sensory function of the cranial nerves supplying the face must be carried out to investigate whether there is associated nerve damage, which may require urgent repair. This is especially important in those with injuries potentially involving the facial nerve (Table 11.1) or the orbital area affecting the trigeminal nerve.

Table 11.1 Rapid assessment of facial nerve motor function

Facial nerve branch	Test of motor function
Frontalis	Look up/frown
Zygomatico-temporal	Screw up eyes
Buccal	Twitch nose
Mandibular and cervical	Purse the lips

Soft tissue injuries

Abrasions
- Need to be thoroughly cleaned and all debris removed. Use a toothbrush if necessary to reduce the risk of infection and 'tattooing', particularly prevalent if the injury is due to contact with a tarmacadam or gravel surface
- Depending on the extent of injury this may need to be performed in the Emergency Department or even in the theatre in extensive injuries. Topical local anaesthetic in the form of lignocaine, adrenaline, and tetracaine (LAT) gel is useful here.

Haematomas
- Painful, but the vast majority will settle over a few days without intervention
- Be wary of expanding haematomas in locations that may compromise the airway or pulsatile haematomas overlying vascular structures, such as the temporal artery
- These will need review to exclude underlying vascular injury, such as a false aneurysm
- In these rare circumstances of progressive swelling overlying a blood vessel, do not aspirate, but compress and refer to hospital.

Subperichondral haematomas to the ear, often caused by blunt injury, may cause a cartilage deformity known as 'cauliflower ear'.
- This should be treated with fine needle aspiration or small incision followed by a compression dressing
- This management can be delayed until the end of the match but can be managed thereafter and the sooner the better
- Depending on experience this may be possible to perform in a sterile environment in or around the changing facilities—if in doubt refer to the hospital for formal treatment.

Lacerations
- Clean all wounds to minimize contamination and explore for foreign bodies prior to closure
- Depending on the location and size of the wound, formal closure may be delayed until after the match, i.e. eyebrow
- If in doubt obtain soft tissue X-rays for glass or metal contaminated wounds
- Simple lacerations can be closed with 5.0 or 6.0 nylon sutures. Due to the very vascular nature of the face, most lacerations tend to heal very well
- Very deep wounds, those with complicated irregular margins, or on delicate areas of the face should be referred to the appropriate specialty for formal closure
- Missed foreign bodies will usually result in infected wounds or wounds that fail to heal. If X-ray is normal then ultrasound at a later date can be useful.

Eye

- Simply asking the athlete if he can see ok is a highly useful starting point
- Ask about blurring of vision and diplopia, and check both pupils are reacting normally with no blood in the anterior chamber (hyphaema)
- Are the eye movements normal?
- Remember the assessment is about ensuring normal eye function
- The eyeball should also be fully examined for penetrating injuries, and an assessment of visual acuity, and CN II-IV and VI-VII is mandatory
- Any penetrating injury, damage to the tarsal plates, eyelid margins, lacrimal system, or the canthi should be referred to ophthalmology for further management
- Those individuals with nerve damage should be referred to the maxillofacial or plastic surgical teams for microsurgical repair
- Lacerations involving the eyebrow should be closed by alignment of the brow borders by a clinician experienced enough to manage the wound
- Do not shave eyebrow hair at wound edges as its re-growth is unpredictable. Simple eyelid lacerations can be closed as outlined above.

Mouth

- Lip lacerations involving the vermilion border should be carefully closed, as a 1-mm step in the vermilion border is visible at conversational distances
- Only carry out this procedure if you are familiar with the techniques involved—this can be done in a sterile environment in or around the changing facilities if required
- Simple intra-oral lacerations that are not full thickness should be managed by oral hygiene measures and do not require formal closure
- Full thickness intra-oral lesions that extend through to the external skin may be managed by suturing the external skin wound, leaving the intra-oral wound to heal by secondary intention with good oral hygiene
- Larger, full thickness, penetrating wounds should be referred for formal closure
- Intra-oral or full thickness wounds involving the mid-cheek should be carefully examined for parotid duct damage, as this may require referral for stenting or repair.
- Tongue lacerations will generally heal with good hygiene and do not require closure
- However, full thickness anterior lacerations, which involve the margins of the tongue, may result in a bifid tongue, so will require referral for specialist repair.

⚠ Dental injuries

- Contact sports can result in significant dental injury, which may or may not be associated with soft tissue injury and facial fractures
- Teeth can be fractured, mobilized (loosened), subluxed, or avulsed
- If possible, ask the patient to run their tongue over their teeth and check for new chips or missing teeth
- Missing teeth and fragments must be located, if not with the patient
- Ensure that associated soft tissue injuries are explored for teeth and fragments, and if necessary perform a chest X-ray to exclude the possibility of inhalation
- If you can feel or see steps in-between the teeth suspect an underlying maxillary or mandibular injury.

Fractured teeth

Do not require emergency medical management, but may cause significant pain due to exposure of the dentine, pulp, and dental nerve. Mobilized or subluxed teeth should be gently put back into normal position when possible, and then splinted appropriately.

Displaced teeth

Must be gently manipulated back into the correct position and then splinted pending urgent dental assessment. In children where only the milk teeth are involved reassurance should be given to the parents.

Avulsed teeth

- If brought in with the patient, should be gently cleaned with saline or water to remove debris—care should be taken to hold the tooth by the crown, as damaging the periodontal ligament remnants on the roots will discourage successful re-implantation
- The socket should be gently irrigated, and the tooth slowly, but firmly re-implanted (if possible) until it sits in alignment with the other teeth
- The patient must then bite down on swabs for at least half an hour
- If the tooth cannot be re-implanted (e.g. if there is associated mandibular fracture or the alveolus is damaged), it must be immersed in milk, cool tap water, or isotonic saline pending repair
- If the patient is able, the tooth can also be placed in the buccal vestibule of the mouth, between the cheek and gums, whilst *en route* to a dentist.

Dentoalveolar injuries

- This involves fracture of the bone and associated teeth, and must be treated as an open fracture
- Consider tetanus prophylaxis and antibiotic cover
- All dental injuries will require urgent dental review by the athlete's own dentist
- Dental injuries in association with alveolar and mandibular fractures need to be referred to the maxillofacial surgeons for appropriate immediate treatment.

Maxillofacial fractures

The most common fractures in sporting injuries are of the nasal, zygomatic, orbital, and mandibular bones. Less commonly the frontal and maxillary bones will be affected when there have been high velocity injuries.

Nasal fractures
- The most common injury to the face
- The patient may have uni- or bilateral epistaxis, which may require haemostatic measures from external compression to posterior nasal packing using nasal tampons or balloon catheters
- External compression will resolve most bleeding at the pitchside:
  - If it has not subsided in under a couple of minutes then a nasal tampon is a useful second step, but effectively prevents the athlete from returning to competition in most sporting situations
  - If the bleeding is controlled pitchside and the athlete returns to play then at the end of the play examine the nose, ideally with a nasal speculum and a light source, or even an auroscope in the dressing room
  - In patients with nasal injuries, those with a septal haematoma may progress to cartilage necrosis if this is not drained over the next 12–24 h. A septal haematoma resembles a blue-red swelling originating from the septum.
- Fractures can be referred to Ear, Nose, and Throat (ENT) department after 5–7 days, allowing the swelling to settle so the extent of the fracture can be fully assessed
- At that point, any significant cosmetic deformity or nasal airway defect can be surgically corrected
- Do not delay further as operative fixation will be hampered by any delay more than 7 days
- Cerebrospinal fluid (CSF) rhinorrhoea, often seen as a 'tramline' of blood, edged by clear fluid indicates damage to the naso-ethmoidal area and warrants urgent CT imaging (see p.113).

Zygomatic (cheekbone) fractures
- Patient may have significant swelling over the flattened zygomatic bone
- Those with lateral and inferior orbital wall damage may have altered infra-orbital nerve sensation, peri-orbital haematoma, subconjunctival haemorrhage, diplopia, and restriction of eye movements superiorly (3rd nerve entrapment)
- Those with fractures involving the zygomatic arch may have restricted mouth opening due to the depressed arch impinging on the temporalis muscle, where it inserts on the mandibular coronoid process
- Occipitomental and sub-mentovertex facial X-rays will allow confirmation of a fracture and associated displacement
- Zygomatic fractures should be referred immediately to the maxillofacial surgeons for review and possible operative fixation.

Orbital (blow out) fractures

- Involve the orbital floor and the medial wall, and are usually associated with significant peri-orbital swelling and ecchymosis
- The infra-orbital nerve may be damaged causing paraesthesia over the infra-orbital area, and tethering of the muscles of the eye causing loss of upward movement of the eye and subsequent diplopia
- These signs may occur together or in isolation, and are individually suggestive of a fracture. Enopthalmos may be seen
- Facial X-rays may show the classic 'teardrop' sign, indicating the prolapse of the herniated orbital contents (peri-orbital fat and the inferior rectus muscle) through the orbital floor into the maxillary sinus
- However, if normal, but with persistent symptoms then CT scan of the orbital floor is a far more sensitive investigation.

⚠ A child presenting with signs of an inferior rectus muscle entrapment, such as diplopia on upwards gaze should have this surgically decompressed emergently by a facial specialist in theatre due to the risk of muscle necrosis. This pathology differs from the adult where there is no such trap-door effect and thus may be managed less urgently.

Mandibular fractures

- Due to the horseshoe structure of the mandible, fractures are generally bilateral and often occur at its weakest points—the condylar neck, the angle of the jaw, and the distal body
- The patient may present with malocclusion, pain, and swelling around the jaw, difficulty mouth opening, intra-oral bleeding and paraesthesia of the ipsilateral lower lip due to mandibular nerve damage
- The mandible may be deviated to one side, and intra-oral examination may reveal a palpable bony step of the dental margins
- Orthopantomogram (OPT) and mandibular X-rays will reveal the site of a mandibular fracture
- Bilateral or open fractures require IV antibiotic prophylaxis and referral to the maxillofacial surgeons for repair.

Mandibular dislocation

- This can occur uni- and bilaterally, and presents with the mouth hanging open and the patient drooling
- Palpating the temporomandibular joints may reveal swelling and tenderness
- In an athlete with recurrent dislocations, relocation can be performed pitchside by standing in front of the patient and applying slow, but firm manual pressure (protect your fingers by placing swabs on the teeth) bilaterally to the molars in an infero-posterior direction
- In an athlete presenting for the first time then this should not be attempted pitchside and referral to hospital for X-ray to ensure no associated fracture.

Maxillary fractures
- Are not commonly seen during sporting injuries
- They are commonly caused by high velocity blunt impact, and must be excluded when there is dental malocclusion present
- The patient may have associated airway disruption, and this must be secured before assessing the extent of these fractures by CT.

There are three main types of maxillary fracture according to the Le Fort classification system (Table 11.2).

Table 11.2 Le Fort classification of maxillary fractures

Le Fort Classification	Fracture and margins
I	Horizontal, extending from nasal septum to pterygoid plates
II	Pyramidal, extending from nasal bone down to pterygoid plates
III	Transverse, extending from nasal sinuses to pterygoid plates

Frontal bone fracture
- The supraorbital margins may be disrupted, and subcutaneous emphysema may be palpated
- Check the function of the superior orbital and trochlear nerves. Suspect a dural tear in extensive frontal injuries, which may involve fractures of the posterior wall of the frontal bone
- These fractures are often associated with polytrauma, and require physiological stability before CT imaging and definitive management.

Medical maxillofacial emergencies

The skin

Cellulitis
- Occurs around a site of trauma
- Causes erythema and swelling of the skin
- Oral antibiotics to treat common skin bacteria (*Staph. aureus* and *Staph. pyogenes*) are suitable for most cases
- However, peri-orbital cellulitis must be treated with high dose IV antibiotics to avoid spread into the orbital area so referral is required.

Spots and lesions
- If affecting the nasal area (the so-called 'danger area' of the face) can migrate posteriorly via the ophthalmic veins, causing haematological spread of infection into the cavernous sinus and can cause meningitis, or cerebral abscesses
- Patients will present with an obvious nasal region infection, and may have a pyrexia, confusion, and headache
- Treat with analgesia and antibiotics, and refer for specialist assessment.

Herpes zoster virus infection ('shingles')
A very painful skin infection, forming vesicles in the distribution of one dermatome. It results from reactivation of Varicella zoster in patients previously exposed. It is treated with analgesia and oral acyclovir.

Patients with ophthalmic shingles should be carefully monitored and referred to an ophthalmologist to avoid eye involvement.

Herpes gladiatorum ('scrumpox')
- A skin infection caused by the herpes simplex virus, and occurs following skin-to-skin (often stubble to face) contact, e.g. during a rugby scrum
- It is characterized by clusters of fluid filled blisters, which are painful
- Treatment consists of good hygiene, not sharing towels, excluding affected players until symptoms cease, analgesia, and acyclovir
- Scrumpox may be impetiginous and caused by *Staph. aureus* or *Staph. pyogenes*, and require antibiotic therapy
- Occasionally *Tinea barbae* may be the causative organism requiring treatment with anti-fungals.

Actinomycosis
- Caused by the bacterium *Actinomyces israelii*. It occurs in golfers who put golf tees in their mouth during play, and causes dental abscesses and sinusitis
- There is usually an underlying concurrent dental problem—poor dental hygiene or recent dental work
- Once in the tissues, it may also cause hard reddish purple skin lumps, that progress to form purulent discharging abscesses
- Treatment is long term, with up to 4 weeks of IV penicillin and several months of oral therapy. It may also be necessary to surgically drain abscesses and sinuses.

The eye

Conjunctivitis
- Viral or bacterial in origin, this can affect one or both eyes
- The patient will complain of red, gritty eyes with increased tearing
- Full eye examination must be performed to exclude foreign bodies or ulceration on the cornea
- Treatment should include analgesia, and topical chloramphenicol applied for 5 days.

Acanthoemoebic keratitis
- A water-borne infection, which can cause pain, keratitis, and ulceration in watersports participants
- Especially common in swimmers who wear contact lens in the pool
- Treatment is with analgesia and corneal debridement, followed by antimicrobial therapy.

The mouth

Toothache
- Caused by dental caries, broken fillings, and dental abscesses
- Symptoms include throbbing dental pain, headache, altered taste, and sensitivity to foods and temperature
- Treatment with anti-inflammatories is recommended, and if there is evidence of a swelling around a dental root then a 1-week course of antibiotics should be prescribed to treat dental abscess
- Such patients should be referred to their dentist for repair of caries or abscess incision and drainage.

Wisdom teeth (third molars) usually develop between the ages of 18–25 years old.
- They are normal teeth and do not need to be extracted unless they cause problems
- Impaction of the wisdom teeth occurs due to lack of space meaning they only partly come through the gums
- They can be associated with infection due to gum tissue that can sit on top of the teeth allowing food and bacteria to build up underneath and abscesses to subsequently develop
- Infections should be treated with antibiotics and dental review
- Certain types of impaction can cause weakness to the mandible and be associated with an increased incidence of mandibular fractures
- The problematic wisdom teeth can be extracted depending on a number of factors, such as the degree of impaction and the age of the patient
- Depending on how many need to be removed and their position they can be removed under local anaesthetic with or without sedation, or in hospital as part of a general anaesthetic
- If 'elective' then extraction should be undertaken during the off-season
- Return to light training can be between 7–10 days and return to contact sport usually 2–3 weeks depending on the complexity of the surgery.

Ulcers
- Breach in the oral mucosa exposing the underlying connective tissue
- Commonly caused by infection or trauma, these lesions are extremely painful, and should be treated with analgesia and chlorhexidine or salt mouthwashes
- Persistent oral ulceration should raise suspicion of underlying malignancy or systemic conditions, e.g. Aphthous ulceration in Crohn's disease, and refer to a specialist for investigation.

Herpes simplex virus
- Clinically manifests as 'cold sores' on the lips
- It initially presents with a burning tingling sensation before the appearance of crops of golden vesicles
- It can be treated with acyclovir, but the mainstay of treatment is good hygiene between players to avoid spread.

The sinuses
Sinusitis
- Results from infection (bacterial, viral, fungal, and allergic) or inflammation, and can cause excruciating pain
- It is associated with headaches and thick purulent nasal discharge, and can be very debilitating
- Treatment is supportive with analgesia and antibiotics if symptoms are prolonged
- Patients suffering from chronic (symptoms lasting beyond 12 weeks) or recurring sinusitis may benefit from maxillofacial referral for surgical drainage.

Chapter 12

Spinal injuries

Introduction *154*
Pitchside care of suspected spinal injury *156*
'Clearing' the cervical spine *158*
Recognizing neurological signs *159*
Complications of cord injury *160*
Cord injury and shock *161*
Back pain associated with acute disc prolapse *162*

Introduction

- Spinal injuries may consist of bony and/or ligamentous damage with or without neurological damage. Such injuries are uncommon in sport, but certain sports carry a higher inherent risk such as rugby or eventing.

For the purposes of this chapter:
- **Spinal injuries** will refer to injuries with or without neurological deficit
- **Spinal cord injuries** refer to those injuries which present with neurological deficit
- **Primary spinal cord injury** is the injury to the cord resulting in direct compressive forces from unstable bony architecture
- **Secondary spinal cord injury** is the result of changes at a cellular level caused by factors such as hypoxia or hypovolaemia.

Any medical professional who is pitchside must be able to:
- Recognize the potential for spinal injury with and without cord damage
- Recognize that there is the potential to cause worsening of the primary injury by failing to appropriately assess and immmobilize and secure the cervical spine
- This failure may lead to spinal cord injury in a previously undamaged spinal cord or further damage to a spinal cord that was damaged at the time of the original injury (e.g. a partial cord transection becoming complete)
- Close observation of the athlete may give the clinician vital clues as to the mechanism of injury and therefore the likelihood of spinal injury. This is especially useful when the athlete may have suffered concurrent head trauma and potentially not be capable of giving an (accurate) history.

If you do not clearly witness the incident, then:
- Consider the situation, e.g. was the injury sustained during the collapse of a rugby scrum or has a gymnast fallen from a piece of apparatus?
- Make your initial assessment whilst applying manual in-line stabilization to the cervical spine
- Obtain eye witness reports where possible
- Have a low threshold for suspecting spinal injury:
  - In some circumstances, it may quickly become obvious that you are not dealing with a spinal injury
  - At other times where there may be spinal pain but you do not suspect a spinal cord injury, then a formal procedure to clear the spine clinically may be attempted.

Essential equipment and training

To manage a spinal injury pitchside, the essential equipment consists of:
- Oxygen
- Spinal board, head blocks, and straps (along with application of a cervical collar this constitutes triple immobilization)
- Cervical collars (adjustable or various sizes, including paediatric if appropriate)
- IV access, drugs, fluids for neurogenic shock.

You will need to be confident in the following procedures:
- Primary survey assessment
- Manual in-line stabilization (MILS)
- Sizing and application of a cervical collar
- Log rolling
- Transfer and securing onto a spinal board
- Safely re-positioning the athlete from their position of injury to one where they may be transferred onto a spinal board (usually this means keeping their spine straight and placing them supine
- However, if their neurological symptoms worsen as you attempt to move them or pain/muscle spasm prevents movement, then you may have to stabilize them in the position in which you found them)
- Potentially directing untrained personnel to assist you in some of the above (only if the athlete must be transferred from the field of play before paramedics are in attendance).

Note: The above points assume that there are no other injuries requiring management. There is no substitute for practice and many courses are available locally and nationally to learn the practical techniques listed above.

Pitchside care of suspected spinal injury

It is important to treat all patients in a systematic fashion according to the principles of ABCDE, including a safe approach to the patient (see 📖 pp.13–14).

When you suspect a potential spinal injury, then assessment of the airway must be accompanied by manual in-line stabilization of the cervical spine. High flow oxygen should be applied immediately to help prevent secondary insult to the spinal cord.

Practical tips on airway assessment with cervical spine control

Athletes do not always fall helpfully into a supine position to enable easy assessment of their airway along with manual in-line stabilization.

- If they are not supine but you are still able to assess the airway, then stabilize them manually in the position in which you find them
- If there is any airway compromise which cannot be managed in their original position, then you will have to turn them
- Adapt the technique for log rolling, but remember the airway takes priority over potential spinal cord damage. If they are not breathing sufficiently to achieve adequate oxygenation, you may have to turn whilst maintaining what stabilizing forces around the spine possible
- If someone with airway compromise has a suspected cervical spine injury, a jaw thrust (not head tilt/chin lift) should be used to open the airway
- Manual in-line immobilization (MILS) may be adapted to provide jaw thrust concurrently should airway support be required (if persistent jaw thrust is required, you may want to consider an adjunct airway).

The following is a stepwise approach to the assessment and management of a suspected spinal injury pitchside:

- SAFE approach and call for assistance as the scene dictates
- Immediately apply manual in line immobilization and assess the airway.
  - Can the patient talk to you?
  - If possible, obtain a history from the athlete, especially regarding spinal pain and neurological symptoms. (Turning the athlete into a supine position may be required to assess and/or manage the airway adequately)
- Ask someone to call 999 for paramedic assistance (if they are not already in attendance)—ask them to tell the operator that you are dealing with a suspected spinal cord injury and get them to come back and confirm that they are on their way
- Continue with MILS, until triple immobilization is complete.
- This consists of:
  - Correctly-sized semi-rigid collar applied correctly
  - Head blocks or equivalent
  - Tape or straps placed over the forehead and blocks, attached to the extraction device, together with a second tape or strap over the chin
- Assessment of breathing and circulation (see 📖 pp.13–14 for details) and manage issues with ABC as they arise (see 📖 earlier chapters for details)

PITCHSIDE CARE OF SUSPECTED SPINAL INJURY

- Administer high flow oxygen
- Briefly assess disability:
  - AVPU or GCS (GCS; see p.116)
  - Active movement in all 4 limbs
  - Sensation to light touch in hands and feet
  - If there is any neurological deficit then assume a cord injury and manage accordingly
- Log roll onto the spinal board (see p.15 for details). Continue to apply manual in-line stabilization throughout this as the collar only reduces cervical movement by about 30%
- Put the head blocks in place and apply the straps or tape
- Continuously reassess ABC's and monitor for changes in neurology during the above
- Arrange transfer to the nearest Emergency Department (ED) capable of dealing with spinal injuries such as a major trauma centre. Depending on the condition of the athlete and your other responsibilities you may wish to accompany them.

Clinical practice tips regarding athlete extraction

- Whenever you are working in a new location or with a new team then aim to have a run through of how you would extract an athlete with a suspected cord injury before the competition starts.
- Make sure everyone (clinical and non-clinical) know their roles e.g. fetching equipment, assisting with log roll, calling the paramedics.

Note: The procedure is exactly the same for an athlete with a thoracic or lumbar spinal injury—the neck should still be immobilized as part of the triple immobilization.

'Clearing' the cervical spine

You may be called to see an athlete who has gone down and is complaining of neck pain, but in whom you think a spinal injury is unlikely. For example, a clash of heads on the football pitch and on assessment the athlete is fully alert, has no signs of a head injury, and is complaining of mild pain on one side of their neck.

- In such a scenario you may attempt to clear the cervical spine clinically.
- The starting point always remains the same, i.e. inline stabilization whilst assessing ABC.
- If ABCs are normal, then you may clear the spine clinically if ALL of the following criteria are met (based on NEXUS low risk criteria; Panacek et al. 2001):
  - (1) GCS 15/15 (and no evidence of intoxication)
  - (2) No distracting injury, e.g. ankle fracture dislocation
  - (3) No neurological deficit (moving all 4 limbs, normal sensation, not complaining of paraesthesia)
  - (4) No posterior midline cervical tenderness—ask someone else to stabilize the neck from the front whilst you palpate the spine
- If all the above are met then proceed to active movements as a final check (based on Canadian C-spine Rule; Stiell et al. 2003):
  - (5) Ask the athlete to gently rotate their head in a lateral direction, first one way then the next. Continue to support the head, but ensure the movements are active (i.e. the athlete is moving his neck not you!) and not passive. There should be 45° of lateral rotation in both directions without significant pain
  - (6) No concern over the mechanism of injury, i.e. after a fall from a horse you should have a very low thresh-hold of suspecting spinal injury even if steps 1–5 are clear
- If the athlete successfully progresses through the NEXUS criteria then release manual in-line stabilization and gently sit them up
- If they can take the weight of their head and move their neck reasonably comfortably then they can be managed as for a soft tissue injury
- If at any stage they fail a criterion or if the mechanism of injury is a concern then transfer to nearest appropriate ED.

Recognizing neurological signs

The conscious patient may complain of:
- Inability to move limbs
- Loss of sensation
- Altered sensation
- Burning pain in the limbs
- A mixture of all or some of the above.

A number of 'incomplete' cord syndromes have been described relating to the neurology signs that will be demonstrated depending on which aspect of the cord has been injured.

Central cord syndrome
- Usually results from falling directly onto the face resulting in a hyperextension injury
- Characterized by disproportionately greater motor loss in the upper extremities compared with the lower extremities—'able to walk but not move arms'
- Variable degree of sensory loss below the level of injury
- Incomplete cord injury.

Brown sequard
- Usually result of penetrating trauma
- Hemisection of the cord
- Motor loss and numbness to touch and vibration on the same side of the spinal injury
- Loss of pain and temperature sensation on the opposite side.

Anterior cord syndrome
- Partial spinal cord injury
- Often vascular in origin
- Complete muscle paralysis below the level of the injury with loss of pain and temperature sensation
- Proprioception and vibration sensation is not affected.

Complications of cord injury

The level of the injury may affect the patient's breathing.

C1–2
- Inability to breathe due to intercostal and diaphragmatic paralysis
- Requires immediate breathing support to survive.

C3–5
- Phrenic nerve may be involved leading to difficulty breathing
- Even if a patient is able to breathe, initially they will tire easily and need close monitoring.

C5–7
Seesaw respiratory pattern due to paralysis of intercostal muscles, but functioning diaphragm.

T1–L2
- Variable loss of intercostal muscle function and thus respiratory function
- The anatomical level of the primary injury may be falsely reassuring in that haematoma and swelling may be found 1–2 vertebral bodies more proximally than the level found on initial examination or imaging
- The pitchside doctor will need to treat all spinal injury patients with high flow oxygen and may need to provide respiratory support with a bag valve mask.

Cord injury and shock

▶▶ Initial management should include thorough and repeated assessment to ensure you do not miss an alternative cause for hypotension. (see Chapter 2).

Neurogenic shock/bradyarrhythmia

In those with cervical or upper thoracic cord injuries, the sympathetic chain may be damaged, leading to parasympathetic activity being unchecked.

- The patient will be 'warm and hypotensive' with bradyarrhythmia or even asystole
- Atropine can be used to treat bradycardia, (although this would not necessarily be expected as part of the standard pitchside drug bag)
- Ensure adequate oxygenation and enable rapid paramedic assistance and transfer to nearest ED if the athlete is showing signs of bradycardia
- IV fluids, e.g. normal saline may be administered to maintain a systolic blood pressure (BP) of 80–90 mmHg. There is a risk that chasing the BP with fluids will result in fluid overload and vasopressors may be required instead in the ED (It is, however, unlikely that fluid overload will be an issue in the pre-hospital setting)
- Beware of other causes of hypotension (e.g. from hypovolaemia, suggesting internal bleeding). If the shock is hypovolaemic, usually the pulse rate will be raised. Remember, however, the two forms of shock may co-exist and the key to managing these patients is regular repeated assessments.

Spinal shock

- This is not shock as classically defined in terms of a failure to perfuse vital organs
- It refers to the immediate loss of reflexes and flaccidity seen after cord injury with subsequent return of hyper-reflexia found weeks after the injury
- Spinal shock and neurogenic shock are not interchangeable terms.

⚠ Back pain associated with acute disc prolapse

Consider this in any sudden onset of acute back pain. The radiation of the pain will depend on the level of the disc affected. For example, cervical discs will radiate into the shoulders and arms, while lumbar discs will give pain radiating into the legs. The radiation of the pain occurs due to irritation of the nerve roots, rather than the cord and will give unilateral signs and symptoms.

- Initial treatment will be analgesia and, if associated with trauma, immobilization
- Neurological examination should identify the level of the disc affected.

Cauda equina syndrome

- Central disc herniation at L4–5 level below the end of the spinal cord (i.e. below L2/3)
- Severe pain
- Loss of peri-anal sensation due to involvement of S1–2 with saddle anaesthesia and decreased anal tone
- Loss of ability to control micturition with urinary retention
- This requires immediate referral for decompression.

▶▶ Remember that in patients over the age of 50 presenting with a traumatic back pain, the diagnosis of other conditions, such as an aortic aneurysm should be considered and abdominal examination carried out.

Further reading

Blackmore, C.C. (2003). Evidence-based imaging evaluation of the cervical spine in trauma. *Neuroimaging Clin N Am* **13**(2): 283–91.

Hoffman, J.R., Wolfson, A.B., Todd, K., Mower, W.R. (1998). Selective cervical spine radiography in blunt trauma: methodology of the National Emergency X-Radiography Utilization Study (NEXUS). *Ann Emerg Med* **32**(4): 461–9.

Panacek, E.A., Mower, W.R., Holmes, J.F., Hoffman, J.R. (2001). NEXUS group. Test performance of the individual NEXUS low-risk clinical screening criteria for cervical spine injury. *Ann Emerg Med* **38**(1): 22–5.

Stiell, I.G., Clement, C.M., McKnight, R.D., et al. (2003). The Canadian C-spine rule versus the NEXUS low-risk criteria in patients with trauma. *N Engl J Med* **349**(26): 2510–18.

Vinson, D.R. (2001). NEXUS cervical spine criteria. *Ann Emerg Med* **37**(2): 237–8.

Chapter 13

Thorax

Introduction *164*
Anatomy *165*
Preparation and risk management *166*
Trauma *168*

Introduction

Medical conditions or trauma involving the chest during sport and exercise are a rare but a potentially serious problem.

Although exercise itself, or the environment in which we exercise, can exacerbate underlying medical conditions such as asthma, the more common chest-related problems in sports are those involving trauma.

- Impairment can be as a result of blunt (such as a closed compression mechanism) or penetrating trauma
- The more severe injuries are usually as a consequence of a high velocity impact, such as is seen in motor racing
- However, chest injuries can occur in any contact sport or where there is a fall at speed or from a height, and these can ultimately be as potentially severe.

Anatomy

- The chest wall comprises of 12 pairs of ribs and the two layers of intercostal muscles that lie between them
- Beneath each rib lies the neurovascular bundle, containing an intercostal nerve, artery, and vein
- All the ribs are attached posteriorly to the 12 thoracic vertebrae. The first seven pairs of ribs articulate anteriorly with the sternum via the costochondral cartilages
- The following three pairs share a common cartilaginous connection to the sternum, whereas the last two pairs (eleventh and twelfth ribs) have no connection with the sternum and are termed *floating ribs*
- The sternum in turn articulates with the clavicles via synovial joints
- The chest cavity is separated from the abdomen by the muscular diaphragm, which can rise to the level of the fourth intercostal space during full expiration
- It is therefore essential that when assessing a chest injury, we are aware of the possibility of an underlying abdominal injury
- Abdominal viscera particularly at risk are the spleen, the liver, and the kidneys.

Preparation and risk management

It is essential that detailed preparation is undertaken prior to any sporting activity. Essential information required particularly relating to chest conditions would include:
- *Past medical history:* particularly any underlying lung or heart conditions
- *Relevant medications:* their requirements before, during, and after exercise and their relevance with the World Anti-Doping Agency
- *Any recent chest injuries:* as a graduated rehabilitation and return to contact sports may be required
- A concise knowledge of the environment in which the activity is to take place (see Chapter 6).

Standard medical equipment
- This should relate to the activity, potential injuries, and environment
- Appropriate protective equipment should be used depending on the sport, e.g. chest and spine protectors
- Appropriate sport-specific training and fitness testing, with adequate rest and staged return after injury and illness.

Trauma

Any assessment of the chest after trauma must first include an assessment of the airway and consideration of a cervical spine injury.

Assessment of patient

The patient's chest, back, and neck must be fully exposed. Injuries and respiratory or circulatory compromise can be identified by:

- *Looking*:
  - Respiratory rate
  - Quality and depth of breathing
  - Unequal or paradoxical chest movements
  - Use of accessory muscles
  - Central cyanosis
  - Distension of neck veins
  - Bruising and abrasions
- *Listening*:
  - Inspiratory stridor indicative of an upper airway compromise, e.g. foreign body
  - Expiratory wheeze indicative of a lower airway compromise, e.g. asthma
  - Reduced air entry
  - Abnormal chest percussion (dull or hyper-resonant)
- *Feeling*:
  - Position of trachea
  - Surgical emphysema
  - Unequal chest movements
  - Pain.

⚠ Significant internal injury to the chest can occur without an obvious external injury.

Rib fractures

- The protective framework of the upper part of the chest includes the scapula, the humerus, the clavicle, and all their muscular attachments
- Together these provide quite an extensive protective framework
- Any fracture to upper ribs (1–3) therefore suggests a magnitude of injury that places the head, spine, lungs, heart, and great vessels all at serious risk of injury
- The middle ribs (4–9) sustain the majority of blunt trauma
- Anteroposterior forces (such as a fall from a horse) generally force the ribs outwards resulting in a fracture of the midshaft of the rib
- Direct forces to the ribs, (such as elbows) generally drive them into the thorax with potential for injuries such as pneumothorax, haemothorax, or tension pneumothorax
- Fractures of the lower ribs (10–12) increase the suspicion of an associated intra-abdominal injury.

Because younger individuals have more flexible chest walls, their ribs are more likely to bend than to break.

⚠ There should therefore be a high level of suspicion of a serious associated injury in the presence of rib fractures in a child or young adult.
- Pain aggravated by deep breathing or coughing with localized tenderness or palpable crepitus over the affected rib would suggest a rib fracture
- In most cases the treatment is NSAID analgesia and rest for up to 6 weeks
- Breathing exercises are encouraged, as the pain can result in splinting of the thorax, which can impair ventilation and an effective cough
- This can lead to atelectasis and pneumonia, particularly in those who have underlying lung disease or who smoke
- Stress fractures of the ribs (most commonly the first rib) can also occur and are seen in athletes who compete in overhead sports, such as basketball or tennis
- There is no acute traumatic event, but due to the repeated contractions of the anterior scalene muscle the rib stresses and breaks
- Treatment is analgesia and rest with a graded return to full activity over 1–2 months.

Pneumothorax

A pneumothorax occurs when air accumulates in the pleural cavity, a potential space, which lies between the visceral and parietal pleura.
- This occurs either from the outside in the case of an open pneumothorax (which is rare in sport) or from the lung itself—a closed pneumothorax
- It can occur spontaneously in the absence of trauma, or as a result of a penetrating or crush injury.

Spontaneous pneumothoraces
- Can be primary or secondary:
  - Primary spontaneous pneumothoraces are more often seen in tall, thin young men without underlying lung disease. They are usually characterized by a rupture of an imperfection in the lining of the lung (bleb) causing the lung to deflate
  - Secondary pneumothoraces are as a result of underlying lung disease such as asthma, Marfan's syndrome, cystic fibrosis, infection, or carcinoma
- When a pneumothorax is present, the patient will complain of pleuritic pain, and they may be tachycardic and tachypnoic
  - Breath sounds are decreased on the affected side and the chest is hyper-resonant to percussion
  - There may be subcutaneous emphysema felt around the neck, axillae, or chest wall, but ultimately a chest X-ray is required to confirm the diagnosis
- In hospital, small traumatic pneumothoraces may be treated conservatively; however, most are safely treated with the insertion of a chest drain in the fourth or fifth intercostal space. Aspiration can be attempted, but is a more appropriate treatment for a primary spontaneous pneumothorax

⚠ A patient with a pneumothorax *should not* travel by air. Airlines currently arbitrarily advise that there should be a 6-week interval between X-ray confirmed resolution of a pneumothorax and travelling by air.

Pneumothorax and diving

Advice for return to diving is generally related to the nature of the pneumothorax. Because of the high risk of recurrence of a spontaneous pneumothorax (up to 50% in some studies) this is regarded as an absolute contra-indication to diving.

A pneumothorax secondary to trauma, however, is related to a specific injury that if fully healed should not predispose the pleura to risk of a further pneumothorax. In this situation, a normal clinical examination and CT scan is advised to show full healing of any rib fractures and full expansion of the lung prior to return to diving.

⚠ Tension pneumothorax

This is a life-threatening emergency and requires prompt recognition and treatment. As a result of a one-way valve leak, the air in the pleural cavity continues to accumulate. The resulting increase in the intrathoracic pressure gives rise to mediastinal shift and an increasing pressure on the interthoracic vessels. This leads to a reduction in venous return to the heart, and thus a decreased cardiac output resulting in profound hypotension and death if left untreated.

⚠ A tension pneumothorax is a clinical diagnosis based on the diagnosis of a pneumothorax associated with signs of shock.

Features include:
- Chest pain
- Hypotension
- Respiratory distress
- Tachycardia
- Distended neck veins
- A deviated trachea away from the affected side (although this is a rare finding)
- Hyper-resonant chest to percussion.

Treatment
- Treatment is high flow oxygen and immediate needle decompression—if appropriately trained:
  - This involves the insertion of a large bore cannula into the second intercostal space anteriorly in the mid-clavicular line
  - A loud hiss may be heard as the needle breaches the pleura and releases some of the intra-thoracic pressure (Fig. 13.1)
- This is a life-saving, but only temporary procedure as the cannula is at risk of kinking and blocking
- Regular assessment and the timely insertion of a chest drain is required.

Mid-clavicular line

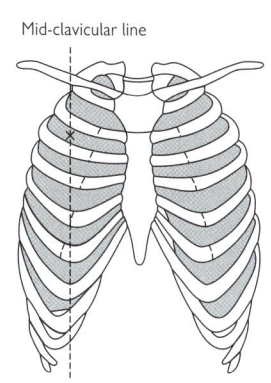

Fig. 13.1 Site for needle decompression of right tension pneumothorax. Reproduced from Wyatt et al., *Oxford Handbook of Emergency Medicine*, 2006, with permission from Oxford University Press.

Haemothorax

- A haemothorax is a condition that results from blood accumulating in the pleural cavity usually as a result of a lung laceration or a laceration to an intercostal or internal mammary vessels
- Its cause can be blunt or penetrating trauma and blood loss into the pleural cavity can be massive as each side of the thorax can hold 30–40% of the total circulating volume
- If left untreated it may progress to a point where the accumulating blood starts to put pressure on the mediastinum and great vessels in much the same way as a tension pneumothorax
- This together with the associated blood loss can quickly lead to profound hypotension, shock and subsequent death
- Diagnosis can be made clinically:
  - The patient will complain of pain with associated tachycardia and tachypnoea
  - Decreased or absent breath sounds on the affected side will be found in association with a chest that is dull to percussion
  - It is dullness to percussion that is one of the main clinical pointers to allow differentiation between massive haemothorax and tension pneumothorax where percussion is hyper-resonant
  - There may be additional signs of blood loss and shock depending on the size of the haemothorax
- A haemothorax is managed in the pre-hospital environment with high flow oxygen and judicious fluid replacement:
  - In the hospital setting treatment involves draining the blood already accumulated in the thoracic cavity
  - Blood in the cavity can be removed with the insertion of a chest drain and as the lung expands the bleeding will generally stop

- If the bleeding does not slow down or stop then urgent surgery will be required to temper the bleeding source.

⚠ If you have doubt about whether the athlete is suffering from tension pneumothorax or massive haemothorax, and they are peri-arrest with respiratory compromise, then there is much to be gained by decompressing the chest with a needle as described earlier. It will make little difference in the case of a massive haemothorax, but will be life-saving in tension.

Open pneumothorax
- Large defects of the chest wall, which remain open, result in an open pneumothorax
- A negative intrathoracic pressure is generated during inspiration so that air is entrained or sucked into the chest cavity through the hole in the chest wall
- If the opening in the chest wall is approximately two-thirds the diameter of the trachea, air passes preferentially through the chest defect with each breath
- The result is inadequate ventilation and a progressive buildup of air and, therefore, subsequent pressure in the pleural space
- Diagnosis should be made clinically during the primary survey
- Any wound in the chest wall that appears to be 'sucking air' into the chest or is visibly bubbling is diagnostic of an open pneumothorax
- Initial management is high flow oxygen and subsequent prompt closure of the defect with a sterile occlusive dressing taped on three sides. This produces a flutter-type valve, which allows air to pass out when the patient exhales, but gets sucked shut on inhalation preventing air from entering
- A chest drain is then required. Regular assessment is required as a dressing closed on all four sides can convert an open pneumothorax to a tension pneumothorax.

Flail segment
- A flail segment occurs as a result of multiple rib fractures, i.e. 3 or more rib fractures in 2 or more places
- The chest wall fails to move properly resulting in a paradoxical breathing pattern where the isolated area of chest wall moves inward with inspiration and outwards during expiration
- A flail chest is a high-energy injury and should prompt transfer to hospital for investigation of damage to underlying viscera (e.g. pulmonary contusion, pneumothorax, or haemothorax)
- Crepitus of rib fractures felt in an area, where the chest wall is seen to be moving paradoxically is diagnostic of a flail chest
- This is a potentially life-threatening injury and will frequently require a period of assisted ventilation. Initial treatment is to provide oxygen, analgesia, assess for other associated injuries and arrange immediate transfer to an appropriate emergency department that can continue to assess and if necessary further assist ventilation.

Cardiac tamponade

- Traumatic cardiac tamponade occurs when the pericardium fills with blood as a result of penetrating or blunt injury
- The pericardial sac is a fixed fibrous structure so only a relatively small amount of blood (~100 mL) is required to restrict cardiac contractility and reduce cardiac output
- The diagnosis can be difficult and the classic signs of hypotension, jugular venous distension, and muffled heart sounds (Beck's triad) are not always easy to elicit, especially in a noisy sporting arena
- If, however, a traumatic chest injury has occurred where there is a high index of suspicion for a cardiac tamponade and a patient is unresponsive to resuscitative efforts for hemorrhagic shock and/or a tension pneumothorax then a pericardiocentesis may be considered
- If you have been appropriately trained then this involves the removal of blood from the pericardium by a long 18G needle
- The needle is inserted 1–2 cm below the xiphisternum at 45° to the skin and advanced towards the left shoulder tip
- Aspiration of 20–30 mL of blood from the pericardium is diagnostic and may temporarily improve cardiac output until a more definitive treatment can be arranged.

Pulmonary contusion

- Pulmonary contusions are caused by a high energy, blunt trauma, and are the most common potentially lethal chest injury
- It is also commonly seen in patients with flail chest and multiple rib fractures
- The diagnosis is made radiologically in a patient who over a period of time becomes progressively short of breath and hypoxic
- Supportive measures before transfer to hospital include high flow oxygen, judicious fluids, analgesia, and appropriate monitoring.

Sternal fractures

These fractures occur as a result of direct high energy trauma. The primary significance is that it can indicate the presence of serious associated internal injuries, especially to the heart and lungs. Any athlete with a suspected fractured sternum must be assessed in hospital and will require a period of observation unless they have an isolated sternal fracture, a normal ECG and no associated injuries.

Signs and symptoms

- Crepitus
- Pain
- Tenderness
- Bruising
- Swelling over the fracture site.

The fracture may visibly move when the person breathes, and it may be bent or deformed, potentially forming a 'step' at the junction of the broken bone ends that is detectable by palpation. Associated injuries, such as those to the heart may cause symptoms, such as abnormalities seen on electrocardiograms.

Chapter 14

The abdomen

Introduction *176*
Anatomy *178*
Preparation and risk management *180*
Trauma *182*
Non-traumatic emergencies *188*
Minor injuries and conditions *192*

Introduction

- Assessment of the abdomen is a key part of the initial approach to an injured or unwell athlete and should be examined as part of the evaluation of circulation
- In sport the abdominal contents may be vulnerable to sudden deceleration, blunt impact, or penetrating injury
- Bleeding from vessels/solid organs or rupture of hollow viscera can lead to hypovolaemic shock or sepsis
- In-built protection comes from the lower ribs, tensed muscles, abdominal, and retroperitoneal fat, and can be augmented by protective equipment
- Even small and initially occult internal injuries can lead to devastating shock and in a fit athlete a considerable amount of blood can be sequestered in the abdominal cavity before external signs become evident
- Damaged viscera may be difficult to detect clinically and/or masked by other injuries. A high index of suspicion and repeated examinations by the same person are necessary, with a low threshold for transfer to hospital and imaging.

INTRODUCTION

CHAPTER 14 The abdomen

Anatomy

- The anterior abdomen extends from the trans-nipple line superiorly to the inguinal ligaments, and symphysis pubis inferiorly and laterally to the anterior axillary lines, with the flanks extending as far as the posterior axillary lines
- The upper abdominal cavity, bounded by the diaphragm, lies within the thoracic cage and rises as high as the fourth intercostal space in full expiration
- The lower part of the cavity lies between the alae of the iliac bones. The vertebral column and thick back muscles lie posteriorly with thinner musculature anteriorly and laterally
- These bony relations and contraction of the muscles offer a degree of protection from injury, but trauma to the lower thorax, back, and buttocks can impact on the contents of the abdomen
- It is helpful to divide the abdomen into four quadrants for descriptive purposes and to correlate areas of local tenderness with the underlying structures (Fig. 14.1 and Table 14.1).

Knowledge of patterns of referred pain can help identify the source in disease and injury:

Referred pain

- *Shoulder:* from undersurface of diaphragm
- *Tip of scapula:* from gallbladder
- *Left chest:* from spleen
- *Umbilicus:* from appendix or pancreas
- *Groin/testes:* from ureter.

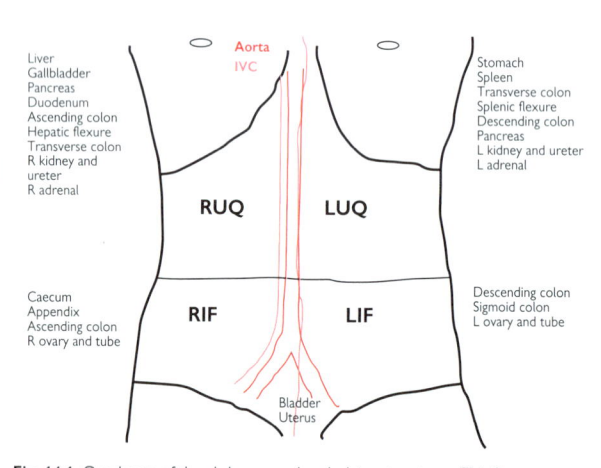

Fig. 14.1 Quadrants of the abdomen and underlying structures. This figure was published in *Sports Injury Assessment and Rehabilitation*, David C. Reid, p.716, figure 18.28, Copyright Elsevier (1991).

Table 14.1 Abdominal content

Solid organs	Hollow viscera
Liver	Stomach
Spleen	Small bowel
Pancreas	Large bowel
Kidneys	Gallbladder
Adrenals	Ureters
	Vasculature

Preparation and risk management

Reduce risks by ensuring:
- Appropriate protective equipment and adherence to rules
- Resting and using a staged return after injury and illness
- Relevant immunizations, especially if taking athletes abroad
- Especially when travelling observe good food hygiene and use clean water to avoid food poisoning/traveller's diarrhea.

Does an athlete require special protection or restriction of activities?
- *Previous liver laceration or trauma*: ↑ risk of further injury
- Congenital absence, loss of kidney, or testicle
- Bleeding disorders
- Sickle cell trait: ↑ risk of splenic infarction at moderate altitude
- Abdominal surgery: can usually return to training at 4 weeks, contact sports at 6–12 weeks or up to 6 months, depending on procedure
- *Glandular fever*: ↑ risk of splenic rupture.
  - Rest for duration of fever and return to contact sports only when back to full strength and FBC, LFTs, urinalysis and spleen size normal
  - The spleen normally takes up to 6–8 weeks to return to normal size and it is advisable to wait ~3 months before returning to contact sports unless an ultrasound can confirm normal size prior to this.

Know your athletes' Past medical history (PMHx)—ideally prior to any incidents. Underlying conditions may present with abdominal symptoms/signs:
- Diabetes mellitus
- Coeliac disease
- Inflammatory bowel disease
- Peptic ulcer disease
- Gallstones.

Trauma

Mechanism of injury

Blunt
Compression and crushing forces from direct blows can damage solid organs and rupture hollow viscera leading to bleeding and peritonitis.
- Kicks, punches, head-butting (especially with helmet), stamping in a ruck in rugby, trampling by a horse in equestrian events
- Collapse of a maul in rugby, pile-on in American football
- *Missiles:* balls (baseball, cricket), pucks
- *Equipment:* bats, sticks, gymnastic apparatus
- Deceleration forces can tear mobile structures at their points of fixed attachment (spleen, liver, small bowel):
  - *Fall from a height:* equestrian events, gymnastics, diving
  - Crashes in motor sport.

Penetrating
- Not commonly seen in sport.
- Stab or slash wounds cause cutting or lacerating injury
- Gunshot wounds may cause additional damage through cavitation, tumbling, and fragmentation
- Penetrating spleen or liver injuries from fractured ribs are sometimes seen.

Assessment
▶▶In the acutely-injured athlete the aim is a rapid focused assessment in the field, while summoning on-site help and arranging emergency transfer.
- **A**irway (with C-spine immobilization) and **B**reathing must be secured as per the initial assessment described in 📖 pp.13–14)
- In the assessment of **C**irculation obvious sources of bleeding should be controlled with direct pressure to any bleeding point, and splinting of fractures
- If possible large-bore IV access should be established and analgesia administered as needed
- There is no role for IM morphine in an acutely injured athlete due to unpredictable absorption rates
- Opiates should only be administered by the IV route
- Signs of shock should be sought—repeatedly
- Presence of tachycardia, narrowed pulse pressure, hypotension after abdominal trauma mandate emergent transfer to an appropriate hospital with appropriate fluid resuscitation (see 📖 Chapter 2)
- Imaging via computed tomography (CT) or focused assessment with sonography for trauma (FAST) scanning in the emergency department with subsequent surgical intervention will be required if a sustained response is not achieved

- In the haemodynamically normal athlete findings suggestive of significant injury again necessitate transfer for further management
- ▶Blunt abdominal trauma may be associated with delayed onset of haemorrhage and/or peritonitis and repeated assessment and adequate advice to the athlete are important.

Specific injuries

Diaphragm
- Traumatic rupture is usually associated with significant blunt abdominal trauma and commonest on the left (right protected by liver)
- Herniation of abdominal contents into the thorax can cause collapse of the left lung and respiratory embarrassment
- Chest X-ray (CXR) is usually abnormal and surgical repair required
- Small tears may be missed initially and present delayed or when herniated bowel becomes ischaemic.

Spleen
- The normal spleen lies under the diaphragm against the posterior 9th–11th ribs
- A solid, firm organ about the size of the palm of the hand and rarely damaged by direct blunt trauma in sport, it may be vulnerable to deceleration or trauma from fractured ribs
- Splenic enlargement occurs in a number of conditions (glandular fever, lymphoma, leukaemia, etc.) and, in this state, injury is much more likely
- Injuries are often missed—a slow leak of blood may be initially symptom-free followed by dull left flank and left shoulder tip pain (Kehr's sign)
- Subcapsular haematoma can lead to delayed rupture
- Most splenic injuries can be managed conservatively with careful observation
- Splenectomy may be required for significant bleeding or injury.

Liver
- Direct blows can cause subcapsular haematoma, usually associated with significant pain and tenderness
- Lacerations are rarely seen in sport, but may result from deceleration in falls from a height and in motor sport.

Stomach
Injury is unusual, but may be produced by epigastric spearing, e.g. by a hockey stick. Acidic stomach contents cause early peritoneal irritation, and there may be bloody gastric aspirate and free air on X-ray.

Pancreas
- May rarely be injured by direct trauma causing compression against the vertebral column (cycle handlebars) or by deceleration
- Clues are epigastric tenderness, pain radiating to the back, or an ileus (distention, absent bowel sounds)
- Amylase may be ↑, CT/endoscopic retrograde cholecystic pancreatogram (ERCP) are often required.

Duodenum and small bowel

Air trapped between a closed pylorus and duodeno-jejunal junction at the time of blunt trauma can result in rupture of the duodenum. Retroperitoneal position means signs of injury are difficult to detect. Bloody gastric aspirate or retroperitoneal air on X-ray suggests the diagnosis.

- Proximal jejunum and distal ileum are vulnerable to deceleration forces which produce tearing near fixed points of attachment
- There may be an associated lumbar spine fracture
- Persistent pain and progressive abdominal signs develop due to peritonitis, but signs may be subtle initially.

Large bowel

Significant rupture from blunt trauma results in massive peritoneal contamination and is often associated with other injuries. Onset of peritonitis may be delayed with small, isolated tears.

Genito-urinary

- Sporting injury is the commonest cause of renal trauma
- The kidneys are relatively protected by the lower ribs, fat, and psoas muscles, but remain vulnerable to direct blows to the back/flank. which result in crushing between the 12th rib and lumbar spine
- Renal contusion causes flank pain which may radiate to the costovertebral junction or lower abdomen with gross haematuria ± renal colic (clots)
- There are usually external signs of injury and tenderness over the loin with rigidity of the anterior abdominal wall
- Immediately refer to hospital any athlete with gross haematuria or signs of shock for further investigation—usually contrast CT
- Approximately 95% of such injuries can be managed expectantly and hypovolaemic shock is almost always due to other injuries (which will also almost all be picked up by CT)
- By contrast, disruption of the renal pedicle, injuries to the ureter, and renal vessels are rare in sport
- They are seen with deceleration, rarely cause haematuria, and are serious and potentially life-threatening, presenting with severe shock and requiring prompt surgical intervention
- Therefore, do not discount significant renal injury just because there is no gross bleeding when the patient passes urine (PU)
- Microscopic haematuria is unlikely to be detected pitchside
- If there is access to a urine dipstix and the result is positive for blood then as long as the athletes observations are normal and there is not a concerning mechanism of injury (such as high speed road traffic accident (RTA)) then the athlete can be managed conservatively and referral to hospital is unlikely to be required unless his clinical condition changes
- A repeat urine dip should be carried out in a further 2 weeks to ensure the microscopic bleeding has resolved
- If still present then referral to urology will be required to look for other causes of haematuria.

Rectus abdominis injury
- Paired rectus abdominis muscles run vertically either side of the linea alba from 5th–7th costal cartilages to pubic bone.
  - They are segmented by fibrous intersections adherent to the muscle sheath which becomes continuous with the aponeuroses of the lateral muscles
  - Superior and inferior epigastric arteries enter the sheath and run along the posterior surface of the rectus muscles
- The muscles can be damaged by direct blows or strained. Strain injuries can be classified as:
  - Grade 1 mild—no effect on exercise ability. Pain usually after activity
  - Grade 2 moderate—pain at the time of injury with pain reproduced contracting the muscle
  - Grade 3 severe—pain at time, debilitating
- Return to sport will clearly depend on the grade of injury from 2–3 weeks for grade 1, 4–6 for grade 2 and up to 3 months for grade 3
- A rectus abdominis haematoma occurs due to rupture of one of the epigastric arteries—usually the inferior epigastric. This is due to stretching of the vessel
- Most haematomas form below the umbilicus and are tamponaded by the sheath.
- Presentation is with sudden pain and a well-localized immobile mass, which does not cross the midline or lateral muscle border, and is present on sitting and lying
- Marked tenderness and guarding may make differentiation from an intra-abdominal problem difficult and necessitate imaging
- Athletes who are in extreme pain or with signs of shock should be immediately referred to hospital as occasionally surgical evacuation may be needed and very rarely bleeding from the damaged vessels continues leading to shock if not recognized.

⚠ Significant muscle/SC haematoma after minimal trauma may indicate an underlying blood disorder, such as leukaemia or Idiopathic thrombocytopenic purpura (ITP). Athletes with repeated bruising out of proportion to the mechanism of injury should have the above conditions considered, especially when associated with recurrent nosebleeds or anaemia. A full blood count (FBC) and coagulation should be performed by the athlete's general practitioner.

Investigation of traumatic abdominal injury

- ▶Haemodynamic instability, which does not show a sustained response to crystalloid/blood, is an indication for surgical intervention, not imaging
- This will always be carried out from the nearest appropriate Emergency Department (ED) and transfer should not be delayed if the athlete's condition is unstable
- A number of investigations can be performed (see Table 14.2 for comparisons):
  - Increasingly CT scan is the preferred option due to increased speed of the equipment and ready availability
  - In the ED a FAST scan may easily be performed at the bedside and is highly specific though less sensitive than CT.

Table 14.2 Comparison of diagnostic peritoneal lavage (DPL), FAST, and CT for evaluation of abdominal trauma

	DPL	FAST	CT
Type of patient	Haemodynamically abnormal	Haemodynamically abnormal	Haemodynamically normal and co-operative, sedated, or anaesthetized
Look for	Blood, GI contents, bile	Fluid	Organ injury, fluid, pneumoperitoneum
Advantages	Quick, bedside, high sensitivity (96–100%)	Quick, bedside, non-invasive, repeatable, high specificity (up to 99%) for injuries requiring surgery, can be used for other body areas	Anatomical detail, quantifies haemorrhage, identifies on-going bleeding, good for retroperitoneum, sensitivity ~97%, specificity ~95%
Disadvantages	Invasive, risk of perforation, misses diaphragm or retroperitoneal injury	Low –ive predictive value, operator dependant, bowel gas/subcutaneous emphysema = distortion, misses clotted blood, diaphragm, bowel, some pancreatic injuries	Expensive, time-consuming, requires transfer, conventional scan may miss bowel, diaphragm and some pancreatic injuries, contrast and radiation exposure

Non-traumatic emergencies

Athletes may present with the full spectrum of abdominal and gastrointestinal (GI) complaints seen in the general population.

▶▶As for any acutely unwell athlete, assessment and management is guided by ABCDs with urgent transfer to hospital.

Acute cholecystitis
- Gallstone impaction in the biliary tree causes acute RUQ pain, which may radiate to back or shoulders
- There may be fever, sweating, nausea, and vomiting ± jaundice. Right upper quadrant (RUQ) tenderness/peritonism is maximal on inspiration (Murphy's sign)
- Rigors imply progression to cholangitis (infection)
- Admission to hospital will be required with IV fluids, anti-emetics, analgesia, and antibiotics the mainstay of treatment
- If cholecystectomy is required then this can be done either as an open procedure or laparascopically
- Return to sport will depend on the procedure and the sport performed, but may be as early as 2 weeks.

Acute liver failure
- Relevant causes in athletes include:
  - Exertional heatstroke
  - Paracetamol excess
  - Viral hepatitis, rarely as a side effect of anabolic steroids or creatine
- *Presentation:* jaundice, fever, nausea, vomiting, hepato(spleno)megaly, and/or complications such as hypoglycemia, bleeding, encephalopathy, sepsis, hepatorenal syndrome
- ▶Check and correct using blood glucose monitor (BM).

Appendicitis
- Commonest cause of acute abdomen in the UK, mainly in young adults and teenagers
- Presents with colicky peri-umbilical pain localizing to the right iliac fossa (RIF), anorexia, nausea, or diarrhoea
- There may be fever, flushed appearance, tachycardia, tenderness (rebound), and guarding in RIF maximal over McBurney's point with pain there on pressing in the left iliac fossa (LIF) (Rovsing's sign)
- Peritonitis, sepsis, and shock occur with perforation
- Return to play will again depend on whether there was associated perforation and the nature of the operation whether an open or laparoscopic procedure
- A graded return to activity starting with gentle exercise 2–4 weeks after operation should be expected in uncomplicated cases.

Inflammatory bowel disease
- Ulcerative colitis is commoner in ♀ and non-smokers
- Commoner than Crohn's and the commonest cause of prolonged bloody diarrhoea in the UK
- Suspect if 'infective gastroenteritis' fails to resolve
- Initial treatment is with fluid and electrolyte replacement. This has particular importance in athletes with a history of inflammatory bowel disease (IBD) and concomitant gastroenteritis/traveller's diarrhoea
- Acute complications include dehydration, haemorrhage, toxic dilatation, intestinal obstruction (Crohn's), perforation, and sepsis.

Indicators of a severe attack
- Abdominal pain
- >6 bloody stools, day, pus
- Systemically unwell
- Signs of hypoproteinaemia/anaemia
- Abdominal distention, tenderness, rebound
- Shock

Intestinal obstruction
- Presents with colicky abdominal pain, anorexia, nausea, vomiting (early if small bowel), abdominal distention (less if small bowel), constipation—not always absolute, 'tinkling' bowel sounds
- Fever and peritonism imply strangulation
- Commonly due to adhesions or herniae, more rarely tumour, ingested foreign body, gallstone ileus, intussusception, volvulus, or Crohn's
- Athletes in sports where intra-abdominal pressure is raised (e.g. weight-lifting) maybe more at risk of hernia formation including at unusual sites such as Spigelian (lateral border of rectus muscles, most often below the umbilicus, and difficult to palpate).

Paralytic ileus
This adynamic form of obstruction occurs more commonly in children with various causes including—gastroenteritis, hypokalaemia, narcotics.

Strangulated hernia
Athletes involved in heavy lifting are at risk of hernias and this may become strangulated. Always check the hernial orifices and femoral orifice for irreducible masses in patients with non-specific abdominal pain.

Pancreatitis
- Presents with severe epigastric pain, which may radiate to the back and is often better when leaning forward (pancreatic position)
- Often accompanied by vomiting
- Chief causes are gallstones and alcohol
- Drugs may be relevant in athletes and many have been implicated, both prescribed (sulphonamides, metronidazole, tetracyclines, sodium valproate, etc.) and those used for 'performance enhancement', e.g. steroids or diuretics in sports with weight limits or where low body weight is advantageous, such as boxing and gymnastics
- Third spacing of fluid can be substantial leading to shock

- Necrosis and bleeding may produce periumbilical (Cullen's sign) or flank discolouration (Grey Turner's sign).

Upper gastrointestinal bleed
- Presents with haematemesis and/or melaena
- Fit athletes can remain haemodynamically normal despite significant blood loss, i.e. postural dizziness or hypotension may be an early sign of incipient collapse
- Peptic ulcer disease and oesophagitis/gastritis account for 80%
- Non-steroidal anti-inflammatory drug (NSAID) use may be associated
- Rarer causes:
  - Mallory–Weiss tear (commonly after excess alcohol)
  - Crohn's
  - Meckel's diverticulum (fresher per rectum (pr) blood, ♂>♀)
  - Vascular malformations
  - Malignancy
  - Coagulopathy/platelet disorder.

⚠ Minor injuries and conditions

Stitch
- Sharp pain (usually around right lower ribs)
- Commonly seen in less fit individuals and when exercising too soon after eating
- Actual aetiology is unknown, but various conditions have been proposed, such as the diaphragm being pulled when the solid organs stretch as you exercise
- Can 'run through' by leaning over to that side, pressing with fingers or stretching up the arm on the affected side, breathing out through pursed lips. May need to lie with arms above head/legs bent
- Specific breathing exercises may help to prevent it occurring, such as timing of respiration relating to running stride.

Winding
- A blow to the abdomen when muscles are relaxed can lead to the athlete feeling unable to breathe freely (diaphragmatic spasm). This can therefore cause great distress
- Check **A**irway and **B**reathing, loosen clothing, encourage the athlete to relax, and sit leaning forward over flexed knees
- Normal breathing usually returns quickly
- Ensure there is no serious underlying injury by monitoring pulse and BP
- Symptoms should settle quickly, but if they persist or worsen then intra-abdominal injury should be considered and referral to hospital made.

Skin wounds
- Irrigate and cover with an occlusive, non-adherent dressing
- Any suggestion that depth extends to muscle or beyond, apply pressure if necessary and transfer to hospital.

Skin irritation
- Torso skin may be affected by contact dermatitis, e.g. from nickel in clothing/equipment or from plants—poison ivy, primula, etc.
- Treatment is with cold compresses, steroid cream, and avoidance of irritants.
- Intertrigo is an irritant dermatitis in skin folds (submammary, groin) due to the combination of sweat and friction
- Treatment is as before, plus attention to secondary fungal or bacterial infection.

Gastrointestinal complaints
- Heartburn, nausea, vomiting, and loss of appetite are all common ♀ > ♂ particularly with intense activity and in less experienced athletes
- Importance lies in excluding serious underlying causes (peptic ulcer disease, ischaemic heart disease (IHD)), symptoms may respond to dietary and/or activity modification
- Faecal occult blood loss is very common in endurance athletes

- Again, importance lies in excluding underlying causes. Proper hydration and prophylactic H_2 blocker may help.
- Nausea, stomach cramps, and diarrhoea may be seen with creatine use
- *Traveller's diarrhoea* (nausea, watery diarrhoea, cramps) is most often due to *E. coli* and lasts 3–5 days
- Oral fluid and electrolyte rehydration is usually sufficient. Loperamide (not with fever or dysentery) or bismuth may help, antibiotics (co-trimoxazole) are reserved for protracted illness.

Athletic pseudonephritis

- Abnormal urinalysis is common after strenuous aerobic activity particularly in long-distance runners
- Red blood cell count (RBC), white blood cell count (WBC), haemoglobin (Hb), myoglobin, protein, and casts may all be seen and on occasion gross haematuria
- The condition is benign, usually causes at most mild discomfort and settles with rest from strenuous activity for 24–48 h
- Persistent symptoms warrant investigation.

Chapter 15

Pelvic trauma

Introduction *196*
Anatomy *197*
Assessment *198*
Fractures and dislocations *200*
Soft tissue injuries *204*
Other causes of acute pelvic pain *206*

Chapter 15 Pelvic trauma

Introduction

- Pelvic trauma is common in the world of sport. It is a spectrum ranging from a simple strain to a devastating, life-threatening pelvic ring fracture
- Despite being common it can be notoriously difficult to diagnose accurately with many injuries presenting in a similar fashion
- It also has to be remembered that there are many non-muscular structures in this area that may be the cause of pain and pain is often referred to the knee
- An accurate diagnosis is key to allowing appropriate treatment and rehabilitation.

Anatomy

- The hip and pelvis are two distinct, but interrelated parts of the human body:
  - The bony pelvis connects the trunk and legs, supporting the trunk and containing intestine, urinary bladder, and the internal sex organs
  - The bony pelvis comprises 3 bones on either side—the ilium, ischium, and pubis
- Anteriorly the pubic bones are united by a cartilaginous joint known as the pubic symphisis
- Posteriorly the bony sacrum connects with both ilia at the sacroiliac joints and its upper portion provides connection with the vertebral column
- The acetabulum is the concave surface of the pelvis formed by the fusion of the 3 pelvic bones
- It meets with the head of the femur and together they form the hip joint
- The hip joint is a ball and socket joint capable of an extensive range of movement (see Table 15.1).

Table 15.1 Muscles of the hip

Movement	Muscle
Flexion	Sartorius, rectus femoris, iliopsoas (iliacus and psoas)
Extension	Gluteus maximus, hamstrings
Adduction	Gracilis, pectineus, adductor longus, adductor brevis, adductor magnus
Abduction	Gluteus medius, gluteus minimus, tensor fascia lata
External rotation	Gluteus minimus, piriformis, obturator internus, quadratus femoris
Internal rotation	Gluteus medius, adductor magnus, semimebranosus, semitendinosus

Assessment

History
- At the pitchside the most important part of the initial assessment is to secure the airway, breathing, and circulation (ABC)
- The pelvis is included as part of the circulation assessment as a significant volume of blood that can be lost due to a fracture in this area
- Obtain details of the mechanism of injury
- This may come from direct observation of the injury at the pitchside, from the athlete or team-mates
- A history of allergy, medications, past medical history, last eaten, events preceding (AMPLE) history is appropriate in initial assessment:
  - Injury mechanism—was the trauma direct, e.g. fall from horse, or indirect, e.g. sprinting or jumping? Was the trauma a high or low impact/velocity, e.g. motor vehicle crash at speed? Was there any associated twisting/rotational component either of the back or of the hip (especially with the foot planted)?
  - Mobility—has the athlete been able to weight-bear since, i.e. could he carry on and continue to compete or has he not been able to stand since? Is the pain localized to one specific area, e.g. muscle insertion? Is the pain there constantly or only when actively moving?
  - Were there any preceding problems that make the clinical assessment more difficult, e.g. is there a history of osteitis pubis, previous surgery, or injuries to the pelvis, groin, hip, or lower back?
- From the AMPLE history make a plan about how best to analgese the athlete, i.e. contra-indications to non-steroid anti-inflammatory drugs (NSAIDs)
- ♀ *Last menstrual period*: worth noting in females of child-bearing age as conditions such as ectopic pregnancy may be missed or initially attributed to problems such as groin strain:
  - X-rays of the pelvis may need to be taken in hospital as part of the initial 'primary' assessment in a significant injury
  - Being aware of the pregnancy status can prove helpful in determining specific films taken and minimizing radiation doses.

Examination
Look
- For any swelling, bruising, or deformity
- Previous scars
- Observe gait if the athlete is able to walk
- Do not force them to their feet until you are have made a full assessment of their active then passive movements to ensure that no further harm will result from them weight-bearing.

Feel
- For any tenderness, warmth, crepitations, etc.
- Check pulses and assess the neurovascular status of the lower limbs.

Move
- Assess the active range of movement before the passive
- Perform any specific tests appropriate for the affected area.

Fractures and dislocations

Fractures

Pelvic ring fractures
- Fractures to the pelvis are a result of high energy blunt trauma
- They are associated with a high morbidity and mortality secondary to complications from the fracture itself and associated injuries
- As with all major injuries the ABCD assessment must be followed and associated cervical spine injury considered
- Pelvic fractures are commonly seen in the equestrian, motorsport, and cycling environments
- Pelvic fractures occur as a result of one of three loading forces, lateral compression, anterior posterior (AP) compression (open book), and vertical shear (Table 15.2).

Table 15.2 Loading forces causing pelvic fractures

Force	Example of force
Lateral compression	Side impact in motor vehicle accident
AP compression	Head on collision in vehicle accident
Vertical shear	Fall from height

Treatment
- Resuscitate ABCD (Chapter 2)
- Obtain IV access as soon as possible. Give analgesia with morphine and start IV fluids if available
- ⚠ Do not attempt to 'spring' the pelvis as it is unreliable and may cause further damage
- Use pelvic splint if available to tamponade and stop bleeding. A number of these are commercially available, but a sheet tied around the pelvis may be a useful temporizing measure
- Continue to monitor pulse and blood pressure (BP)
- Transfer urgently to definitive centre.

Complications
- Haemorrhage is the most serious immediate complication of pelvic fracture
- Massive retroperitoneal haemorrhage may occur from bony fragments and lacerated blood vessels
- The retroperitoneal space can hold up to 4 L of blood before tamponade occurs
- Continued bleeding may therefore result in shock
- Associated injuries are extremely common owing to the huge forces involved. The most common are:
  - Head injury
  - Long bone fracture
  - Nerve injury (sacral plexus, sciatic)

- Thoracic injury
- Urethra
- Bladder
- Intra-abdominal solid and hollow viscus organs
- Diaphragm.

Sacral fractures

- May occur in isolation or as part of a pelvic fracture with or without sacro-iliac joint disruption. 30% present late, and delay in presentation is associated with an increased incidence of chronic pain and neurological dysfunction
- Again equestrian sports are particularly linked to this type of injury
- Fractures may be transverse or vertical, and due to the possibility of neurological involvement around the sacral foramina it is vital that a full neurological assessment is made
- Note the athlete may still be able to mobilize after the injury with the only finding being tenderness elicited by palpating the sacrum
- Return to sport will usually be a minimum of 6–8 weeks, but may be longer depending on the sport.

Initial management

- In the initial stages of assessment it may be very difficult to distinguish the athlete suffering from an uncomplicated sacral fracture from someone suffering a complicated pelvic injury and so initial treatment as per ABCD should be carried out
- Unless the athlete is mobile, transfer to hospital is likely to be required and imaging initially with plain film X-rays will be necessary
- Further imaging with computed tomography (CT) may be required along with magnetic resonance imaging (MRI) should there be any evidence of neurological involvement.

Avulsion fractures

- These fractures are most commonly seen in the adolescent age group
- They are due to the sudden forceful contraction of a muscle pulling a piece of the bone off
- There are 3 main sites involved (Table 15.3).

Table 15.3 Location of avulsion fracture

Site	Muscle	Action
Anterior superior iliac spine (ASIS)	Sartorius	Jumping
Anterior inferior iliac spine (AIIS)	Rectus femoris	Kicking, e.g. football
Ischial tuberosity	Hamstrings	Sprinting, hurdling

- Athletes may describe a sudden pop followed by pain in the hip or groin
- Tenderness is elicited by palpating the affected site and bruising may be noted
- Distinction between injuries with associated avulsion fractures and those without, i.e. musculotendinous strains may be very difficult

- If the history is suggestive and there is specific insertion tenderness then X-rays should be obtained
- Generally, these injuries will settle with rest and conservative management, but sometimes they may not heal or the fragment may be too large
- Referral to orthopaedic services is recommended for follow-up as soon as a bony avulsion has been identified to allow a decision regarding operative treatment to be made
- In general, if the X-ray demonstrates more than 2 cm displacement of the bony fragment from the pelvis then operative management will be preferred to allow a quicker return to play.

Stress fractures
- Stress fractures are the result of overuse injuries
- Fatigued muscles transfer the stress to the bone causing a fracture
- In the pelvic region they are most commonly seen in either the pubic rami or neck of femur
- Runners, especially long distance, are the group most likely to be affected
- Military trainees are also a high risk group
- Females suffer more than males: this is probably related to hormone-induced osteoporosis
- Palpation of the ramus will prove tender if a fracture is present, but neck of femur fractures are more difficult to diagnose
- In femoral neck stress fractures a high degree of suspicion is required in those most at risk
- Patients will complain of a pain in the anterior groin that worsens with activity and resolves with rest
- It may then progress to being constant
- Pain may radiate to the knee and may be described as a deep-seated ache
- X-rays should be undertaken, but often the fracture is not visible. CT or MRI may be needed to allow diagnosis
- Operative fixation will be required in the vast majority of cases and urgent orthopaedic referral will be required
- Complications include avascular necrosis and non-union (if conservative management is used.)

Acetabular fractures
- Rarely occur in isolation as they too are a result of high energy forces
- They are commonly associated with pelvic ring fractures and hip dislocations
- Complications, associated injuries, and assessment are the same as for pelvic ring fractures.

Dislocation of the hip
- Dislocations of the hip can be posterior, anterior, or central
- Dislocation of the hip requires a significant force and other injuries are common
- Posterior dislocations account for approx 90% of hip dislocations in sports

- They occur when great force strikes the flexed knee with the hip flexed, adducted, and internally rotated
- They are most commonly seen in contact sports like American football and rugby, where players are tackled and land with other players piling on top of them. They have also been documented in motor sports, skiing, and snowboarding.

Examination

In a posterior dislocation typically the leg is shortened, internally rotated, with flexion and adduction at the hip.

Initial management

- Resuscitate per ABCD
- Obtain IV access and give analgesia (with opiate if possible)
- Assess neurovascular status of the affected limb. The sciatic nerve and its common peroneal branch are most commonly involved in posterior dislocations:
  - Look for foot drop, and decreased power and sensation
  - Ensure you assess the knee joint as well for associated fractures
- Arrange urgent transfer to hospital
- There is a significant increase in long term hip joint damage if the hip is not reduced within 6 h
- There are reports of this being managed at the pitchside in the first few minutes after dislocation before muscle spasm intervenes
- This can only be advised if the operator has experience in the techniques used to achieve this, and it would be expected that this procedure is usually carried out in a hospital environment.

Return to play

- Imaging will usually be carried out at 6 weeks to ensure no signs of avascular necrosis
- Gentle jogging may then be undertaken with a full return to sport between 4–6 months post-injury.

Soft tissue injuries

Soft tissue injuries are common in athletes. The incidence of these may be reduced by an adequate warm up and stretching programme prior to the activity. Evidence for this, however, is still controversial.

Strains

Strains occur when the muscle fibres tear as a result of overstretching. They can be graded into three severities, but it can be difficult to grade them accurately (Table 15.4).

Table 15.4 Grades of strain

Grade	Description
I (mild)	Stretching or minor tearing of a ligament or muscle
II (moderate)	Ligament or muscle partially torn, but still intact
III (severe)	Ligament or muscle is completely torn and joint is unstable

Adductor strain
- Occur where there is a violent external rotation with the leg in a widely abducted position
- Changing direction suddenly in sports such as tennis, basketball, and tackles in football can all be responsible
- Injuries are often acute on chronic
- Many perceive this to be an overuse injury
- A number of factors may contribute to development of an adductor strain including imbalances between the strength of the adductors and the gluteal muscles
- Acute injuries will present with the athlete often describing a sudden, sharp, ripping pain in the affected groin
- There may be previous experience of niggling groin pain in this area
- They may be swelling and tenderness over the origin of the adductor and there will be pain on resisted adduction
- Initial treatment of the acute injury involves withdrawal from play, rest, and ice
- Compression bandages may be symptomatically helpful
- Mainstay of treatment of these injuries is identifying those with chronic strains and rehabilitating them before a superimposed acute injury occurs
- Once identified, strengthening the adductors, and core exercises is crucial in these cases prior to return to full activity
- Length of time away from play is dependent on a number of factors, such as the grade of strain, and the response to a controlled, supervised rehabilitation programme
- MRI or ultrasound (US) scanning may be very useful in determining the extent of the injury and assessing for other differential diagnoses
- Chronic injuries may take up to 6 months to fully settle.

SOFT TISSUE INJURIES

Hip flexor strain
- The hip flexors are the rectus femoris (which is also involved in knee extension) iliacus and psoas
- Any or all three muscles may be affected though iliopsoas is most commonly affected
- Hip flexor strains tend to occur either as a result of an explosive movement such as a burst of speed when running or when striking an object with your foot—such as a ball
- Pain is present over the anterior upper thigh and is associated with movements involving the flexors
- This can be assessed by asking the athlete to bring his knee towards his chest—the pain may be reproduced on resisted extension of the hip
- It may be confused with an adductor strain, but can be differentiated by the absence of pain with lateral movements
- Treatment is usually symptomatic with rest and ice progressing to ultrasound and massage under the direction of the physiotherapists
- Return to play will again depend on the grade of strain but may take up to 6 weeks.

Hamstring strain
- Account for approximately 1/3 of all sports-related lower limb injuries, and are recurrent in about 1/3
- Injuries tend to occur in sports such as football that require explosive extension of the knee, as when sprinting
- Symptoms may be insidious, but are more likely to be dramatic with the athlete pulling up 4 or 5 strides into a sprint
- An audible pop may be heard. There will be point tenderness over the injured muscle and possibly extending to the ischial tuberosity
- A palpable defect may be present and muscle spasm evident
- MRI will define the extent of the injury as well as excluding associated avulsion fracture of the ischium
- Plain films may be useful if there is a question of associated fracture and MRI is unavailable
- Initial treatment involves withdrawal from play, ice, and compressive bandages. Analgesia and the use crutches is recommended until able to mobilize without pain
- A graded return to full activities will be required using a supervised rehabilitation programme. As a rough guide:
  - Grade 1 strains—2–3 weeks
  - Grade 2 strains—3–6 weeks
  - Grade 3 strains—6–8 weeks

! Other causes of acute pelvic pain

Slipped upper femoral epiphysis
- Seen in the 10–17-years age group, ♂>♀(3:1). Occurs in left leg more than right
- May present as sudden onset groin pain following trauma, or insidiously over weeks as gradually increasing groin pain or worsening limp
- Pain may be felt in the groin, medial thigh, or the knee. Up to 40% of patients will develop bilateral involvement
- The patient may hold their hip in external rotation, with pain reproducible on passive internal rotation
- Both AP and 'frog leg' views of the pelvis should be taken
- Operative fixation will be required so urgent orthopaedic review is necessary
- Prophylactic fixation of the contralateral limb remains controversial
- Supported weight bearing using crutches will usually be required for up to 8 weeks post-surgery with a return to play not advocated by some until the physis has closed.

Ectopic pregnancy
For any female of child-bearing age who presents with acute pelvic pain this must be kept in mind. Occurs in approximately 1% of pregnancies with 95% of ectopic pregnancies occurring in the fallopian tubes. Symptoms usually occur between weeks 4 and 10 of the pregnancy.

Symptoms may include:
- Unilateral groin pain
- Vaginal bleeding
- Postural hypotension
- Shock with tachycardia and decreased BP
- Shoulder tip pain.

Treatment will depend on the initial presentation, but if the patient is unstable then immediate surgery is warranted. Even if the patient has normal observations then bear in mind that deterioration can occur quickly and catastrophically if rupture occurs.
- Manage the patient by addressing the ABCs
- Cannulate and start IV fluid, as well as opiate for the pain
- Immediately transfer to the nearest Emergency Department (ED).

Return to sport is unlikely to be on the athletes mind, but will vary depending on the extent of the surgery required.

Testicular torsion
- Is a true urological emergency and can present with groin pain. It is most common in the men <30-years-old with most between the ages of 12 and 18 years
- The majority of patients will usually complain of acute onset of unilateral scrotal pain
- Torsion results in disruption of the blood supply to the teste and the teste itself will become non-viable if the torsion is not reversed. A success rate approaching 100% for retaining viability of the teste occurs if the procedure is done within 6 h of the onset of symptoms.

Symptoms
- Unilateral pain usually acute onset
- Lower abdominal pain
- Scrotal swelling
- Vomiting.

Signs
- *Swollen scrotum:* may be warm and red
- Markedly tender to palpation
- Teste lying horizontal (bell-clapper)
- Loss of cremasteric reflex on the affected side (not seen in epidiymitis)
- High temperature is unusual.

Diagnostic tests are usually not required as this is a clinical diagnosis.
Blood tests have little value, but ultrasound may be useful as long as it does not delay the surgical procedure.

Treatment
Administer analgesia and immediately refer to the nearest ED—ideally one with on-site urology cover.
Return to play can usually be around a month post-fixation.

Sports hernia (Gilmore's groin)
Commonly associated with kicking sports, such as football, rugby, and American football. It is caused by weakening of the posterior inguinal wall.
- Patients will complain of a gradual onset of deep groin pain
- The pain will increase with manoeuvres, which increase intra-abdominal pressure and may radiate to the testicles
- On examination there will be no palpable hernia as it is only the posterior abdominal wall that is involved
- Diagnosis is difficult and often by exclusion
- Patients should be referred for surgical assessment on an outpatient basis.

Osteitis pubis
- Is inflammation at the pubic symphysis caused by repetitive contraction of the muscles that attach to the pubic bones and pubic symphysis
- Pain has a gradual onset and tenderness is elicited when palpating the pubic symphysis
- It is most commonly seen in footballers and long distance runners though can be seen in dancers, ice skaters, and weight lifters
- It is more prevalent in ♂ aged 30–50 years
- It is not commonly encountered in the paediatric population.

Bursitis

Iliopsoas bursitis
- Is commonly associated with iliopsoas tendonitis due to their close proximity
- Together they are known as the iliopsoas syndrome
- Patients will describe anterior thigh pain and sometimes a snapping sensation in the hip
- There may be a palpable mass owing to the increasing size of the bursa.

Trochanteric bursitis
The trochanteric bursa has a superficial and deep component. Patients will normally describe lateral thigh pain. Pain can be reproduced by hip adduction (superficial) or resisted active abduction (deep).

Apophysitis
- An apophysis is a growth plate that provides a point for a muscle to attach to
- If the muscle attached is excessively tight it can put increased tension on the apophysis, which results in inflammation and apophysitis
- There are several at the pelvis that can be affected
- It most commonly affects adolescents who participate in running, dancing, and football
- They will complain of pain in the area of the associated apophysis, but it may be more diffuse and will worsen with activity
- X-rays are important to exclude avulsion fractures.

Chapter 16

Upper limb injury

Introduction *210*
Clavicular injuries *212*
Shoulder injuries *214*
Elbow injuries *218*
Forearm injuries *220*
Wrist injuries *222*
Hand injuries *224*
Thumb injuries *226*

Chapter 16 Upper limb injury

Introduction

Limb injuries, whilst unlikely to cause mortality, are the biggest cause of morbidity faced by athletes.

Upper limb sporting injuries are a common presentation to emergency departments. One of the most common mechanisms of injury occurs as a result of falling onto an outstretched hand (FOOSH) as a reflex reaction to a fall. Direct blows to the upper limb are also a common mechanism of injury, as are injuries secondary to ball-games resulting in hyperextension to the wrist.

Often injuries occur in individual sports in a manner that is predictable in both the mechanism of injury and presentation.

⊙ Clavicular injuries

Assessment
- As with all orthopaedic trauma, assessment begins with 'look, feel, move' before assessment of distal neurovascular deficit
- There will be tenderness over the fracture site, and there may be obvious deformity and swelling at the fracture site acutely
- The patient will usually support the injured limb by holding the forearm
- Most clavicular injuries will severely limit movement at the gleno-humeral joint
- Acromio-clavicular injuries will cause pain on adduction of the arm across the chest with the elbow flexed.

Claviclular fractures
- Most clavicular injuries occur as a result of direct force to the shoulder, either as a direct fall or blow
- Clavicular injuries may also occur as a result of a FOOSH
- The commonest site of fracture is at the junction of the middle and outer thirds
- Middle third fractures are also common. Fractures of the outer third are less common and those of the medial third rarer still
- Adolescents and young adults will often fracture in a 'greenstick' pattern
- No manipulation or reduction of clavicle fractures is required acutely
- Approximately 3% of clavicle fractures will be associated with a pneumothorax so assessment of the chest is mandatory.

Acromio-clavicular injury
These often occur after a fall onto the shoulder. They are graded radiologically, although deformity at the acromio-clavicular (AC) joint may be noted pitchside, with the distal tip of the clavicle sitting superiorly to the acromion.

Sterno-clavicular injury
- These are relatively rare and result from a blow to the front of the shoulder resulting in the clavicle 'popping' out anteriorly
- Asymmetry, swelling, and local tenderness of the medial end of the clavicle is noted compared with the other side
- ⚠ Rarely the dislocation occurs posteriorly and can cause compressive symptoms on the mediastinal structures
- This will require surgical decompression with elevation of the dislocated clavicle
- CT is usually required to confirm this diagnosis as it is commonly not picked up on plain imaging.

Treatment
- Acute treatment entails supporting the arm in a broad arm or polysling, usually with the elbow at 90° of flexion. However, do not force the arm into this position—the patient is likely to present in their own 'position of comfort'
- Definitive treatment for clavicle fractures can either be conservative with operative fixation a consideration in displaced fractures
- Return to play is variable depending on factors such as the age of the athlete the displacement of the fracture fragments and the sport
- An adult returning to contact sports is likely to require up to 3 months or so of rehabilitation.

ⓘ Shoulder injuries

Dislocations

The gleno-humeral joint may dislocate anteriorly, posteriorly, or inferiorly. The vast majority of dislocations are anterior.

Anterior dislocation

- These usually occur from a FOOSH when the shoulder is externally rotated or where the trunk rotates internally after a FOOSH
- The patient will be in immediate pain and will support the upper limb with the opposite hand, at the elbow, or forearm
- The shoulder will often look 'squared off' in less muscular subjects
- Palpation under the acromion will reveal a palpable gap
- If the axillary nerve is damaged then there may be paraesthesia in a 'badge' distribution over the deltoid.

Treatment

- Reduction should not be carried out pitchside unless
  - This is a recurrent injury that the sportsman has had before or
  - There is neurovascular compromise or
  - There will be a significant delay to hospital assessment
- The arm should be supported in a broad arm sling in a position of comfort to the patient.

Methods of reduction

- Analgesia will be required—Entonox® is ideal
- There are numerous methods of reduction of anterior dislocations, most of which involve a degree of abduction and external rotation of the shoulder
- All 3 techniques should be performed gently and gradually
  - Lie the athlete supine—support the affected arm and gently lift the arm in an upwards direction trying to achieve 90° flexion at the shoulder. If you continue to support the arm and gently pull skywards the athletes body weight will act as traction and the dislocation can reduce
  - Lie the athlete semi-recumbent—extend the elbow and apply gentle traction to pull the arm in a downwards direction. The operator should lean backwards whilst holding the athletes arm. *No other force is required*
  - Lie the athlete prone—with their arm hanging over the side of the treatment table. Ask them to hold onto a weight such as a heavy water bottle. Gravity will allow the dislocation to reduce
- A balance needs to be struck as to where and when to reduce
- There is always the possibility of an associated fracture and also the potential of medico-legal issues if this is found on imaging carried out in hospital after a pitchside reduction
- In athletes with significant swelling or any doubt as to the diagnosis then splint the arm in a sling and transfer for imaging.

Posterior dislocation
- The mechanism of injury is usually a fall onto an internally rotated hand or a direct blow to the front of the shoulder
- Classically, this occurs as a result of either a seizure or electric shock where the shoulder is forced into hyper internal rotation
- Clinically, there is usually no deformity
- The athlete will have pain on active and passive movement out of proportion to the clinical findings
- Administer analgesia, apply sling, and refer to hospital.

Inferior dislocation (luxio erecta)
- This injury is very rare (approximately 0.5% of shoulder dislocations)
- Usually seen in high impact motorsport accidents and occasionally in falls from height, such as in gymnastics
- The arm is usually fully abducted with the elbow held flexed and resting on or above the head
- Administer analgesia and refer to hospital.

Shoulder fractures

These can mimic dislocations with the patient presenting holding the injured arm supported with the other hand.

Neck of humerus fractures
These are relatively uncommon injuries in sport
- Commoner in the young and the elderly
- Usually the result of a FOOSH with or without a further load landing on top of the limb, i.e. another athlete
- The normal contour of the shoulder is unlikely to be lost, thus helping to distinguish it from an anterior dislocation
- X-ray will allow distinction of the type of injury and whether it involves the surgical or anatomical necks
- Fractures of the surgical neck may involve the brachial plexus, notably the axillary nerve and this should be looked for with paraesthesia in a badge distribution overlying the deltoid
- Administer analgesia, apply sling, and transfer to hospital
- Definitive treatment may be conservative or operative, but early rehabilitation is key in assisting a return to sport with contact sport usually taking about 3 months.

Scapula fracture
- Usually the result of a direct blow to the posterior chest wall
- Typically, affects the blade of the scapula with obvious bruising and swelling found on assessment
- Complications are related to the associated injuries that are sustained at the same time such as pneumothorax, haemothorax, and rib fractures
- A full ABC assessment must be carried out
- The vast majority of scapula fractures are treated conservatively with splinting using a sling, which can be fully discarded by about 6 weeks.

Shaft of humerus fractures
- These may result from a direct blow to the side of the arm or a FOOSH
- The diagnosis is rarely in doubt, with localized tenderness, swelling +/− bruising
- Complications include associated vascular injuries and radial nerve palsy resulting in wrist drop
- Check distal pulses and neurology
- Administer analgesia, provide a sling or collar and cuff, and refer to hospital
- Definitive treatment is usually conservative.

Rotator cuff injuries

The rotator cuff muscles serve to stabilize the glenohumeral joint.
- Supraspinatus initiates abduction
- Infraspinatus and teres minor are responsible for external rotation
- Subscapularis provides internal rotation.

Rotator cuff injuries are diagnoses of exclusion in terms of pitchside assessment. They are almost impossible to diagnose pitchside or indeed acutely as the hallmark of these injuries is weakness in function and pain. Since pain will limit the ability to move, these are most commonly diagnosed on MRI, US, or at subsequent examination once the acute pain has settled.

ⓘ Elbow injuries

Dislocation
- Dislocated elbow may occur in isolation or with associated fracture. It may be closed or compound
- Clinical appearances will show a loss of the normal anatomical triangle formed between the olecranon and the medial and lateral epicondyles on either side
- A visible deformity will be present. There is usually considerable soft tissue swelling
- An immediate check must be made for the presence or loss of brachial and distal pulses, as well as the median and ulnar nerves, which can also be injured
- If there are absent pulses and no immediate nearby ED facility then consideration should be given to reducing the dislocation
- Most dislocations occur in a postero-lateral direction and reduction is usually achieved using 2 operators
  - The first operator stabilizes the upper arm with the elbow flexed
  - With a second person applying traction distally, the first operator uses their thumbs to push the olecranon in a distal direction
  - This should allow the dislocation to reduce and the normal 'triangle' appearance of the elbow to be restored
  - A check should be made of the neurovascular status and the patient immediately referred to hospital for imaging and definitive treatment.

Fractures

Supracondylar fractures
- These usually are as a result of a FOOSH and are commonest in childhood. They can cause vascular compromise by impinging on the brachial artery and neurological compromise by impinging on the ulnar nerve
- There will be significant swelling and tenderness but the triangular anatomical relationship between the olecranon and epicondyles will be intact
- Treatment involves analgesia, applying a sling and referral to hospital
- Operative management will be dictated by the age of the patient, the degree of angulation and displacement, as well as neurovascular status.

Radial head/neck fractures
- Usually caused by FOOSH
- Occasionally caused by direct blow to elbow
- Patient usually unable to fully extend and supinate elbow
- There will usually be point tenderness over the radial head or neck as well as a haemarthosis of the elbow joint
- Plain imaging is required and treatment is usually conservative in a sling, or collar and cuff.

Olecranon fracture
- The olecranon tends to fracture as the result of landing on the point of the elbow
- Localized bruising, tenderness, and swelling result
- Management depends on the displacement of the olecranon fragment caused by the pull of triceps with displaced fractures requiring operative fixation
- Administer analgesia, apply sling, and refer to hospital.

⚠ Forearm injuries

Fractures

Isolated ulnar shaft fracture
- A direct blow to the forearm or a fall against a hard surface may result in an isolated fracture to the ulna
- This may also be seen in sports where 'defensive' injuries occur as a result of bringing the hands and forearms upwards to protect the face
- Localized tenderness and swelling may be apparent
- It is vital to check for the presence of an associated radial dislocation as these injuries can occur together
- Imaging will be required of the entire forearm in a suspected ulnar shaft fracture
- For this reason administer analgesia, apply sling, and refer to hospital
- Undisplaced fractures may be treated in a cast with displaced fractures requiring operative fixation.

Isolated radial shaft fracture
- Unusual injury to have an isolated fracture to the proximal 2/3rds of the radius
- Usually the result of a fall or direct blow
- Always assess and X-ray for associated dislocations
- Non operative treatment is rare.

Fractures to both radial and ulna shafts
- Usually the result of significant force
- Highly unstable as no ability for either bone to be splinted by the other
- Clinically apparent due to pain, swelling +/− deformity
- Assessment of neurovascular status is mandatory
- Internal fixation is almost always required.

Dislocations

Monteggia fracture dislocation
- Fractured shaft of ulna
- Dislocation of the radial head.

The elbow and wrist joints must be examined closely in any suspected forearm fracture in order to look for an associated dislocation of the radial head in an ulnar shaft fracture. X-ray will reveal both problems with operative fixation required to reduce the dislocation.

Galeazzi fracture dislocation
- Fractured shaft of radius between middle and distal thirds
- Dislocation of the distal radio-ulnar joint (wrist joint).

Mechanism is usually direct blows to the forearm or a fall. X-ray is again required to confirm the extent of the injuries and operative fixation is required.

⚠ Wrist injuries

Fractures

Distal radius and ulnar fractures
- These injuries are usually caused by a FOOSH or a hyperextension injury, e.g. being struck by a ball
- Distal radius fractures are the most common of the radius fractures
- They can occur in isolation or in conjunction with an ulnar fracture
- The majority of displaced fractures displace dorsally, resulting in a 'dinner fork' appearance
- Assessment of the median nerve is required, as well as palpation of the distal pulses
- These injuries may require manipulation, open reduction, and internal fixation or conservative management
- Any clinically obvious deformity will invariably mean that the patient will require manipulation of the fracture so splint, analgese, and refer to hospital
- Depending on the type of fracture it may be possible to return to sport relatively quickly wearing a custom fit splint in the case of an undisplaced radial styloid fracture for example. More commonly, it will take about 6 weeks.

Colle's fracture
Fracture of the radius within 2.5cm of the wrist joint with dorsal angulation. Classically-associated with an ulnar styloid fracture and causes a 'dinner-fork' type deformity.

Smith's fracture
Fracture of the radius with volar angulation. Usually as a result of falling onto a flexed wrist.

Barton's fracture
Unstable intra-articular fracture of the volar aspect of the distal radius extending into the wrist joint.

Scaphoid fractures
- Usually caused by a FOOSH, causing swelling and tenderness in the anatomical snuffbox and tenderness on axial loading of the thumb or index finger
- Also assess for tenderness of the volar aspect of the scaphoid tubercle
- Due to the intricate blood supply, avascular necrosis can occur and so treatment of the 'clinical' diagnosis with splintage or casting is mandatory even in the presence of normal X-rays
- MRI if available will provide a definitive diagnosis. If unavailable immediately then follow up is required in 10–14 days after injury even in the presence of a normal X-ray
- Return to sport is usually in the order of 6–12 weeks.

Dislocation

Lunate dislocation
- Usually the result of FOOSH
- Whilst there will be pain and swelling, the symptoms will usually be out of keeping with the signs
- Paraesthesia in the median nerve distribution may be apparent and is a pointer to the diagnosis
- X-ray is required to confirm although the appearance is only truly appreciated on the lateral view
- Reduction is required so administer analgesia and refer.

Peri-lunate dislocation
- Uncommon in sport
- The result of high velocity forces
- Usually associated with significant swelling, but occasionally this is not the case
- There is significant soft tissue disruption including ligamentous rupture. The lunate maintains its alignment with the radius (in comparison with a lunate dislocation), whilst the capitate is displaced dorsally relative to the lunate
- Again operative reduction is required so analgese, and refer.

⚠ Hand injuries

Fractures

Metacarpal fractures
- Most commonly fractured is the neck of the 5th metacarpal as a result of a punch injury or 'boxer's fracture'
- Deformity, extensor lag, or rotational deformity may be present, although rotational deformity is much more common in proximal or middle phalangeal fractures
- Occasionally, there may be carpo-metacarpal subluxation, which may be subtle both clinically and radiologically. (These can cause significant morbidity and should be referred for specialist opinion)
- Any wound overlying any knuckle should prompt specific questions regarding the aetiology
- A fight bite should be considered as the cause. This will require a thorough examination to ensure no foreign body contaminants, such as fractured teeth
- Irrigation and cleaning of these wounds should take place and referral for X-ray as determined by clinical exam
- Consideration for hepatitis B and C and human immunodeficiency virus (HIV) should be made
- Prophylactic antibiotics should be commenced if a human bite is the cause of the wound, although this is no substitute for thorough cleaning of the wound
- Treatment of uncomplicated wounds rarely requires operative correction and can be managed with a variety of treatments form simple neighbour strapping to a volar slab for 10 days.

Proximal and middle phalangeal fractures
- A common injury in ball games
- Patterns of injury can often be predicted by the mechanism of injury
- Most isolated transverse fractures are stable, but fractures that are oblique or intra-articular are more likely to be unstable
- Clinical examination should help to elicit concerning features such as rotational deformity, which will require correction
- Pitchside treatment involves analgesia and neighbour strapping with referral for X-ray.

Distal phalangeal fractures
- Usually, the result of crush injuries to the tip of the finger such as another player standing on the patient's finger
- Very painful injuries that require splinting to assist pain
- If compound then ensure thorough cleaning and remove the nail if necessary
- Antibiotics prophylactically have been historically given, but are of no proven benefit.

Volar plate injuries
- Occur secondary to hyperextension to the proximal interphalangeal joint
- Common in basketball players and goalkeepers
- Examination reveals a fusiform swelling around the proximal interphalangeal joint (PIPJ) with maximal tenderness over the volar aspect of the joint
- There may be an associated fracture involving the base of the middle phalanx
- These injuries require splinting and reassessment of function after about 10–14 days.

Dislocations

Proximal and distal interphalangeal joint dislocation
- These tend to dislocate with the distal bone dislocated dorsally
- Whilst sportsmen occasionally self-reduce these injuries, there is a risk that the cause of the deformity is due to a displaced fracture rather than dislocation and as such an X-ray is usually advised prior to any reduction
- Volar dislocations are much rarer and are often irreducible and unstable
- Once reduced the PIPJ should be kept in full extension, but the distal interphalangeal joint (DIPJ) left free to minimize the risk of boutonniere deformity.

Flexor tendon rupture
- There are two flexor tendons in each finger
  - Flexor digitorum superficialis (FDS), which flexes the proximal interphalangeal joint
  - Flexor digitorum profundus (FDP), which flexes the distal interphalngeal joint
- Any loss of flexion at either necessitates X-ray and in the case of a wound, surgical exploration
- Due consideration should also be given to exploration to any wound found on the volar aspect of either the palm or fingers even in the absence of loss of function as injury to these areas may result in occult injuries with delayed rupture if not treated.

Mallet injuries
- Common injury—exterior tendon rupture to digital phalanx
- May be innocuous, such as when tying shoelaces or after direct trauma causing forced flexion on an extended finger
- Injuries can be associated with no bony injury on X-ray or associated intra-articular fracture of the base of the distal phalanx
- They require splinting in a mallet splint for a minimum of 6 weeks.

⚠ Thumb injuries

Bennett's fracture dislocation
- Mechanism of injury is usually forced abduction or direct force along the long axis of the thumb
- It is common in skiers, ballgames, and cyclists
- Results in an intra-articular fracture to the base of the thumb carpometacarpal joint, which is inherently unstable and will require operative fixation.

Ulnar collateral ligament rupture
- Caused by forced abduction of the thumb
- Common is skiers, especially on dry slopes
- Untreated this injury will cause permanent disability by causing interference of grasp
- There will be tenderness and swelling over the ulnar aspect of the metacarpophalangeal joint of the thumb
- Complete rupture paradoxically may not be particularly painful and present with obvious laxity on stressing the joint
- All injuries should be referred for X-ray and definitive treatment—ranging from cast or splint through to operative correction.

Chapter 17

Lower limb injury

Lower limb injury 228
The thigh 230
Knee injuries 232
Leg injuries 238
Ankle injuries 240
Foot injuries 246
Ottawa Foot and Ankle Guidelines 249

Lower limb injury

- It is calculated that approximately 40–60% of sport injuries seen in EDs in the UK affect the lower limb.

⚠ The thigh

Femoral fractures

- Large forces are required to break an adult femoral shaft and these injuries are often associated with violent or multisystem trauma
- It is extremely important to exclude other serious injuries, including those to pelvis, hip, and knee
- Pre-existing conditions increasing risks of fracture also need to be considered (e.g. osteoporosis/athletic female triad, metastatic, or other metabolic disease)
- There is usually a shortened externally rotated/abducted hip, severe pain and inability to weight bear. In distal (supracondylar) fractures the gastrocnemius will pull the more distal fragment away from the proximal end.

▶▶ Fractures of the femoral shaft can cause a very fast and life-threatening haemorrhage. This is more pronounced in compound injuries.

- Apply principles of airway, breathing, circulation (ABC) assessment
- Obtain IV access immediately with two large bore cannulae
- Blood should be cross-matched as soon as possible
- Start fluid resuscitation, as this could be a life-threatening haemorrhage
- Give opioid analgesia
- Splinting with Thomas or other traction splints will reduce complications of haemorrhage/fat embolus and will help pain control.

Femoral stress fractures

- Femoral stress fractures are not common, but should be suspected in an athlete who has undergone a sudden increase in their training schedule. The athlete may complain of poorly localized pain in the anterior thigh, which may refer proximally or distally into the knee
- MRI or bone scan may be more sensitive than radiographs in detecting this fracture
- Treatment involves relative offload with conservative management preferred for compression-side fractures and surgical fixation for some tension-side fractures
- Depending on the nature of the fracture, correction of predisposing factors may need to be considered
  - Smoking
  - Athletic female triad
  - Hormonal disturbances and lower limb mechanics have all been associated with stress fractures in the lower limb.

Hamstring origin avulsion

- This is a relatively common injury in adolescents and should be suspected in any athlete in this age group presenting with a hamstring strain. The larger avulsions of the ischial apophysis may be identified by X-ray
- MRI will demonstrate injured bony contours and muscle status with no radiation exposure
- Only displacements of greater than 3 cm are thought to require surgical fixation

- However, if avulsion is detected early referral to orthopaedic specialist is required. Surgical reattachment is becoming increasingly popular and is associated with better outcomes in recent literature
- Avulsion of ischial origin is also seen in adult power lifters and is the result of an award sudden forced hip flexion on an extended knee
- Early surgical intervention has a good prognosis.

Muscle injuries

Although not life-threatening muscle injuries are common and cause considerable time away from sport. They can be classified into grades I–III:
- Grade I is a minor strain with pain on active resisted contraction of the muscle, where the athlete may complete his participation before reporting the injury
- Grade II pain on active unopposed contraction and stretch
- Grade III which is a full thickness tear.

This will be important to the sportsman because it will determine his time to return to sport from anything up to 2 weeks.
- Grade I: 2 weeks
- Grade II: 2–8 weeks.
- Grade III: 8+ weeks for full thickness tears. The rectus femoris (kicking, jumping, sprinting) and hamstring muscles (sprinting, football) are commonly injured.

Emergency treatment of an injured muscle should include ice and compression as soon as possible.
- This minimizes bleeding into the muscle and is thought to reduce scar formation and therefore return to sport or active work time, as well as making a recurrence less likely.
- Referral to a physiotherapist will ensure active graduated return to activity using a progressive functional rehabilitation programme optimizing muscle health and healing.
- Imaging with MRI and ultrasound may be appropriate in the higher-level sportsman.

Quadriceps contusion
- The quadriceps contusion ('dead leg') follows direct impact into the anterior thigh usually by a knee, shoulder, or foot
- The athlete is usually able to continue activity until bleeding increases pressure within the thigh and a dull ache inhibits the affected quadriceps
- There is a diffuse tenderness to palpation over the affected area and range of movement is affected. Vastus intermedius is crushed against the femur and is more commonly affected
- Immediate treatment should be ice and compression to minimize bleeding and time out from sport. This can be days to weeks depending on the force of impact and immediate management of the lesion
- Gentle mobility and range of movement exercises should be encouraged. No imaging is usually required unless a significant muscle tear is suspected.

Knee injuries

Fractures

Tibial plateau fractures
- Tibial plateau fractures may be seen in high velocity injuries, such as skiing or in low-energy knee twisting mechanisms
- The patient will complain of difficulty in weight bearing and pain
- These fractures need to be excluded in all higher grade collateral ligament injuries
- Radiographs may show obvious fracture or it may be harder to detect if the fracture is undisplaced
- If mechanisms alert the clinician to possibility of fracture a horizontal lateral radiograph may show presence of fat–fluid level (lipohaemathrosis)
- Magnetic resonance imaging (MRI) will show any associated meniscal or anterior cruciate ligament (ACL) injury
- Emergency management involves analgesing and splinting the knee in extension and non-weight bearing crutches
- Conservative treatment is occasionally possible in minimally displaced fractures but arthroscopy may allow direct visualization of articular surfaces and menisci and undetected detached osteochondral fragmentation.

Patellar fractures
- A fracture of the patella usually follows a direct impact onto this sesamoid bone from a fall or from direct contact
- Occasionally, it follows forced and sudden contraction of the quadriceps muscle
- A congenital bipartite patellar can be confused with a fracture and can occur in the lateral upper pole, lateral margin, or inferior pole and can mimic a fracture symptomatically as the impact can disrupt and inflame the synchondrosis
- Anteroposterior (AP) and lateral X-rays will be required and give idea of degree of displacement of fragments
- X-ray of the contralateral side may help exclude bipartite patella as these are rarely unilateral
- Emergency management involves analgesia and splinting the knee
- Patellar fractures should be referred for surgical opinion
- Fractures with minimal displacement, well preserved articular surfaces and intact extensor mechanism can be managed conservatively
- Patellar fractures with overlying skin wounds can undergo delayed fixation and should be covered with antibiotic prophylaxis.

Dislocations

Knee
- The knee joint is a very stable joint and as such dislocations are rare
- When they occur they are usually the results of significant forces such as the tibia being forced backwards in a road traffic accident (RTA) or a fall from height

- Associated injuries should always be sought and the ABC approach followed
- The knee will appear clinically deformed, the athlete in extreme pain
- Neurovascular examination should be carried out to ascertain the associated injuries to both the popliteal artery and the peroneal nerve
- If a vascular deficit is found pitchside then consideration must be given to reducing the dislocation pre hospital. This is usually performed by carrying out longitudinal traction
- This decision will be multifactorial, i.e. having an appropriate medical facility minutes away it may be more appropriate to split the limb as best possible, analgese and immediately transfer
- Imaging both plain film and computed tomography (CT) will be required, and serial vascular assessments should be performed with the patient being required to be admitted for these serial observations
- It should be remembered that significant vascular injury can occur with normal examination of pulses and so vascular assessment will involve some form of investigation whether that be angiography, ankle brachial index, or ultrasonography
- Associated fractures and ligament disruption is almost invariable and surgical management will be dictated by the presence of these findings.

Patellar dislocations/subluxations

- Patellar dislocations most commonly occur laterally and can be atraumatic or traumatic
- Traumatic dislocations will follow a history of significant traumatic force following jumps or rotational movements and are accompanied by haemathrosis and severe pain
- The patients describe popping or 'knee dislocation' and until closer inspection may mimic ACL rupture. The patella may spontaneously reduce, or require analgesia and manipulation
- Examination reveals significant effusion, a tender medial border, tenderness, and apprehension on gentle lateral pressure on the patella
- Athlete may be unable to raise straight leg as active contraction of the quadriceps will be very painful. (Exclude patella tendon rupture or quads tendon rupture by palpation of defects proximal and distal to patella)
- To reduce a patellar dislocation analgese the athlete (Entonox® is ideal) extend the knee, whilst applying gentle pressure to the patella in a medial direction
- Risk factors include generalized ligamentous laxity (hypermobility), genu valgum, patella alta (where the patella sits much more superiorly than normal) and compromise to static stability of the knee. (e.g. dysplastic patella or hypoplastic lateral condyle)
- X-rays should include skyline as well as antero-posterior (AP) lateral and intercondylar views to look for associated osteochondral injuries/medial patellar facet injuries and resultant loose bodies. MRI will show bone bruising on the lateral femoral condyle and medial patella and it may show a degree of insult to the chondral surfaces or demonstrate loose fragment not detected by radiographs

- First episodes of traumatic patellar dislocations may be treated conservatively. A period of immobilization is a necessity to allow healing of the medial stabilizing structures
- Arthroscopy is indicated in recurrent dislocators (approx 50% of first time dislocators)
- It is also indicated in first patella dislocation for detection/excision or reattachment of osteochondral fragments and detailed inspection of chondral surfaces where a high degree of injury is suspected on MRI
- Additionally allows repair of medial patello-femoral ligament to aid stability.

Tendon ruptures

Patellar tendon ruptures

- Sudden unexpected eccentric contraction of powerful quadriceps muscle, e.g. landing awkwardly, can cause patellar tendon to rupture
- Athletes are usually under the age of 40 and the rupture is more commonly closer to the inferior patella pole
- The athlete will experience localized pain and inability to maintain leg extension and the patellar will be visibly retracted proximally if rupture is complete
- Straight leg raise may be inhibited with pain and effusion in a partial tear.
- Radiographs will demonstrate any bony avulsion and a high riding patella. Ultrasound (US) will show degree of tear if not clinically obvious
- Partial tears may be treated conservatively with 3–6 weeks immobilization, but experienced surgical opinion may be warranted to determine whether remaining tendon will cope with functional load in an athletic population
- Tears need early surgical reconstruction as repair less successful if late.

Quadriceps tendon ruptures

- Quadriceps tendon ruptures will usually happen in the older athletes or those with associated systemic conditions such as gout, diabetes, hyperthyroidism, or renal failure
- It is more common in males and may be partial or full thickness
- The athlete is unable to walk or extend his leg
- Knee flexion may be intact if pain permits
- Quadriceps rupture is usually extremely painful
- A haemathrosis will develop and a defect may be palpable usually just proximal to the patellar
- The defect may not be immediately obvious with a tense haemathrosis Surgical correction is required within 48 h to obtain a good result
- Radiographs will show a low lying patella and MRI will demonstrate extent of tear.

Meniscal injuries

- Usually, the result of a twisting knee injury with a foot anchored on the ground. Classically, the effusion develops over 24 h, although no effusion may develop
- The athlete may feel a significant amount of pain and hear a snap, tear, or may feel nothing

KNEE INJURIES

- This injury is usually associated with joint line tenderness
- A positive McMurray test with reproduction of pain or 'a clunk' on combined flexion and rotation of the tibia makes menisceal injury more likely
- The older athlete may have a greater predisposition following degenerative change with a relatively small trauma
- More severe menisceal injuries with pain and restriction of range/fixed flexion may occur in bucket handle tears as displaced menisceal fragments may prevent normal articular movement. This should prompt rapid arthroscopy
- Look for chondral involvement +/– ACL involvement in the more traumatic injuries.

Ligament injuries

Anterior cruciate ligament injuries
- ACL injury can happen as a result of a sudden deceleration, rotation, jump, or by any fall on the athletes flexed knee
- Typically occurs in football, basketball, or skiing, but can happen in any sport reproducing the injury mechanism described
- More commonly there will be a tense haemathrosis developing over a couple of hours, but there may be little swelling especially if previous insult to the ligament may have rendered few fibres intact by the time of the complete disruption
- The athlete will normally be unable to continue participation in the activity due to the pain:
  - They may describe a snapping or crack and occasionally describe the knee 'going out of its normal position'
  - You may have a window to examine effectively if pain permits immediately after injury
  - Examination is more difficult and less accurate for several days once haemathrosis, pain, and muscle spasm take hold
- Lachmans test is both more sensitive and specific than anterior drawer test:
  - Remember to compare to contralateral side, as different degrees of laxity may be normal to any individual athlete
  - Pivot shift is very effective in demonstrating torn ACL in a very relaxed athlete
- ACL can be accompanied by meniscal injuries, collateral ligament rupture, or a Segond fracture where there is an avulsion just distal to the lateral tibial plateau
- The pivot shift may be absent in the presence of tear of the medial collateral ligament and beware of capsular tears where effusions may leak out of the torn capsule confusing the clinician away from serious internal derangement of the knee
- Good history taking is important.

Lachmans test
- Lie the athlete supine
- Flex the injured knee to 20–30°

- Place one hand behind the tibia with the thumb coming round the front of the lower leg to rest on the tibial tuberosity
- Place the other hand above the knee and attempt to pull the lower leg anteriorly
- A definite end point should be felt and this should be compared with the unaffected knee.

Posterior cruciate ligament (PCL) injuries
- This classically occurs as an RTA injury where the tibia is translated posteriorly under force
- In sport it will usually happen in a hyperextension injury
- Unless posterolateral corner structures are involved the degree of posterior translation is usually minimal and therefore most noticeable at 90° flexion (compare with contralateral side) with a relaxed quadriceps muscle
- Examination would reveal tibial posterior sag/reverse Lachmans and posterior drawer
- Thorough examination of the posterolateral corner is important
- X-rays can aid bony avulsion or other associated fractures that may need urgent surgical intervention
- MRI will help confirm diagnosis
- Isolated posterior collateral ligament (PCL) injuries tend to do well conservatively, but follow-up needs to be done to exclude associated posterolateral corner injuries when patient is pain free
- Rehabilitation will be essential in order to compensate for the posterior instability.

Medial collateral ligament injuries.
Usually sustained after a valgus strain to the knee. They can be classified in terms of severity into three grades:
- Grade 1 (tenderness, pain on valgus stress but no laxity at 30° flexion)
- Grade 2 (tenderness over the ligament, pain, and laxity at 30° flexion but a solid end feel, usually accompanied by swelling)
- Grade 3 (laxity at 30° flexion with no end feel. There may be a sensation of instability, but less pain following the injury since all fibres are in theory disrupted)
- The higher the severity the longer the healing time (approx 2 weeks for grade 1 to >8 weeks for grade 3)
- MRI will confirm diagnosis and will aid the clinician in excluding associated cruciate ligament injuries if clinically difficult due to pain
- Most of these injuries will do well conservatively if given time and the resulting laxity is controlled by the use of a splint. Surgical intervention is required for persistent laxity beyond the prescribed healing period.

Lateral collateral ligament injuries
These injuries are less common than medial collateral ligament (MCL) injuries. Posterolateral corner injuries/instability should be considered for all lateral collateral ligament injuries, as these will require surgical intervention.

ⓘ Leg injuries

Fractures

Tibia and fibular fractures
Rotational injuries in most lower limb dominant sports can result in comminuted (usually spiral) fractures of the tibia and fibula. Direct trauma may also result in fractures.
- The athlete will be in pain
- Swelling and deformity are usually obvious
- Do not be distracted by the lower limb injury, and exclude other life-threatening injuries first using the ABC approach
- Open fractures need immediate cover with sterile, moist swabs soaked in saline/water and splintage. A photograph of the wound is useful to stop repeated removal of the dressing.
- Check tetanus cover and arrange immediate hospital referral.
- Immobilization will help pain, and opioid analgesia may be required.

The popliteal artery can be injured following proximal tibial fractures, and the common peroneal nerve can complicate a proximal fibula fracture so lateral foot sensation and foot dorsiflexion should be documented during assessment. All tibial and fibula fractures can further be complicated by emergent compartment syndromes so careful neurovascular observation should follow in the hours and days following these fractures. The deep peroneal nerve can be assessed by testing sensation between the first and second toes.

Maisonneuve fracture
- This is an ascending fracture of the shaft or proximal fibula
- It follows a severe ankle ligament injury where the ankle syndesmosis is disrupted and therefore unstable
- There may be an associated medial malleolus fracture
- Fibular examination should follow all severe ankle injuries
- Syndesmosis injuries are discussed under ankle injuries.

Stress fracture of the tibia
- Tibial stress fracture can present with gradual or sudden shin pain and are located on the tibial medial border.
- Posterior cortex fractures can present with calf pain and history can be confused with a gastro-soleus muscle injury.
- A palpable lump may be felt around the area of the fracture if anterior and chronic.
- Radiographs may miss subtle stress fractures unless they are more chronic in nature. MRI or bone scan and CT will be more sensitive.
- Biomechanics (rigid pes cavus, over-pronated foot), sudden increase in training schedule or change of surface, athletic female triad, hormonal or metabolic disorders should be screened for and addressed.
- Longitudinal stress fractures occur in the distal third of the tibia and have a better prognosis. Stress fractures of the anterior cortex have

a poorer prognosis and can be career ending due to non-union and progression to fracture.
- The athlete should be removed from aggravating activity and risks explained since symptoms will quickly settle.
- The athlete can be offloaded with crutches and an orthotic boot.
- Referral to a specialist with experience in dealing with stress fractures in athletes should be sought early.

Fibular stress fractures
- Usually associated with abnormal foot biomechanics increasing the tractional load of the peroneal muscles.
- Athlete is locally tender at the site of injury but will usually be able to weight bear.
- Relative offload in orthotic boot and referral for biomechanics assessment will usually allow adequate healing.

Muscle injury

Gastrocnemius/soleus
- The gastrocnemius muscle can be injured when landing forward or during a sudden start to a run or jump
- The medial belly is most commonly injured
- Plantar flexion may be painful and the athlete may require crutches
- A heel raise may help alleviate symptoms and allow earlier weight bearing.

Soleus injuries may happen insidiously during a run or landing after a jump.
- They can be differentiated from a gastrocnemius injury when stretching of the calf with the knee in flexion reproduces pain.
- Emergency treatment of calf muscles should involve early ice and compression as previously described for the muscles of the thigh.

CHAPTER 17 Lower limb injury

⊙ Ankle injuries

Ankle fractures

Lateral malleolus
- Very common injury in sport resulting usually from an inversion injury
- Depending on the type of fracture, the athlete may be able to carry on playing and only complain of pain after ceasing activity
- Examination should be based on the Ottawa ankle guidelines, which have a high sensitivity in excluding bony injury (see 📖 p.249)
- Examination will identify bony tenderness over the lateral malleolus. The medial malleolus should also be palpated as should the entire lower leg paying particular attention to the head and neck of fibula
- Bruising and swelling may be apparent immediately, but may take time to develop
- X-ray will usually reveal the fracture with treatment depending on a number of factors including association of medial malleolar or posterior malleolar fractures
- The fracture can be classified using the Weber classification where:
  - Type A—usually stable injuries with the fracture below the mortice line
  - Type B—spiral fracture starting at the level of the mortice. Potentially unstable depending on associated medial ligamentous or bony injury
  - Type C—fracture above the level of the mortice with associated instability
- Stable fractures may require very little treatment other than symptomatic support whether in a cast or rigid boot. Unstable fractures may require open reduction and internal fixation.

Medial malleolus
- Less common than lateral fractures
- May occur in isolation, but are more commonly associated with lateral malleolar fractures
- Again, examination using the Ottawa guidelines will detect these fractures
- If a medial malleolar fracture is suspected, examination should proceed to look for an associated injury that would render the ankle complex unstable, such as a proximal fibula fracture or injury to the syndesmosis
- Immediate management is as for lateral malleolar fracture, including ice, analgesia as required, and immobilization prior to X-ray.

Talar dome osteochondral injuries
- Ankle ligament injuries can often be associated with talar dome lesions
- Unless considerable in size and, therefore, higher in grade these may be undetected in plain X-ray
- The mechanism usually involves compression to the medial or lateral talus by the tibial plafond
- Talar dome osteochondral injuries can be graded on a scale of I–IV depending on severity

- MRI and CT scanning will allow grading of an osteochondral injury of the ankle. Grade I–II can usually be treated conservatively with a period of offload
- Arthroscopy is warranted for higher grades, which may warrant microfracture and/or removal of loose bodies depending on the degree of severity.

Lateral and posterior talar process fractures
- Posterior talar process fractures can occur in forced plantar flexion and may require 6-week cast immobilization or excision
- Lateral talar process fractures occur in forced dorsiflexion and inversion producing shearing forces into the talus by the calcaneus
- Often confused with lateral ligament sprain. Athlete will present with pain and tenderness anterior and inferior to tip of lateral malleolus, and difficulty with persistent weight-bearing
- The athletes may experience difficulty with prolonged weight-bearing, particularly if fracture extends into posterior facet of subtalar joint
- Mortise view will demonstrate the fracture especially in 20–25° of plantar flexion
- Radiographs can underestimate fragment size
- Further investigation by CT is recommended for accurate sizing and extension of fracture
- Fractures with more than 2 mm displacement or larger than 1 cm are treated surgically as risk of non-union is high
- Conservative treatment involves immobilization in non-weight bearing cast for 4–6 weeks.

Talar stress fractures
- Stress fractures of the talus usually involve the posterolateral aspect
- They are most commonly seen in track, field athletes, and footballers
- Swelling and pain may vary from inability to weight bear to asymptomatic MRI appearances
- CT is required to establish extent of fracture
- Treatment involves cast immobilization and correction of predisposing factors, e.g. over-pronation, athletic triad.

Ankle dislocation
⚠ A potentially catastrophic injury for an athlete, and should be considered as an orthopaedic emergency.
- Usually associated with a fracture of the ankle, but not always
- The ankle can dislocate in a number of different directions, but posteriorly is the most common with the talus forced backwards in relation to the tibia
- Immediate management as always should exclude more significant injuries via the ABC approach
- The athlete will require analgesia—Entonox® is ideal until IV access is gained to allow administration of opioids if available
- Assessment should focus on diagnosis and identification of an associated neurovascular compromise and/or possible compromise to the overlying skin from displaced bone causing tethering

- If these issues are found, then pitchside reduction will be required unless there is a very short transport time to the nearest ED
- Reduction involves manual traction to the ankle usually best achieved by holding the heel in one hand with the other hand on the dorsum of the foot and pulling in a distal direction. Counter traction should be applied proximally, ideally with the athlete's knee flexed to reduce hamstring resistance
- Once reduced splint and transfer
- Cover any compound injury with saline soaks and splint. A photograph avoids repeated removal of the dressing
- Further management will be directed on the associated injuries found post-reduction.

▶ X-ray should confirm the reduction and are not required to be taken prior to the reduction taking place in the ED.

Tendon injuries

Achilles tendon rupture
- Complete or incomplete ruptures are more likely in athletes after the age of 30
- It may occur in a tendon with previous painful tendinopathy or may occur in a tendon previously asymptomatic
- The acute rupture is not always painful
- There may be an audible snap as the tendon tears and athlete may describe 'being struck on the back of the leg'
- There is usually a reduction in function
- On examination the acute swelling may vary.
- Squeezing of the calf may still plantar flex the foot (Simmonds's test) in a partial rupture but the degree of plantar flexion may be diminished on comparison to the contralateral side
- Complete tears will usually leave a palpable defect unless haematoma fills in the gap
- MRI and US will aid the clinician in establishing the degree of tear, but surgical exploration may be warranted even in partially torn tendons to establish the percentage of torn segment
- Longitudinal tears of the tendon may be more easily missed on imaging
- A surgical opinion is warranted early in an athlete. It is generally accepted that surgical repair is advisable for active individuals performing at a higher functional level.

Tibialis posterior ruptures
- An athlete with tibialis posterior rupture will present with a flattened foot arch (compare to contralateral foot) and pain in the navicular tubercle, often extending posteriorly and proximally behind the tibia
- Absence or defect in the tendon may be palpated and will be detected by US and MRI
- Surgical reconstruction is required to restore normal foot arch and power/control in lower limb dominant sports.

Tibialis posterior dislocation
- Dislocation of the tibialis posterior tendon can occur in a forceful dorsiflexion and inversion of the foot
- There is some pain and swelling in the area as the aponeurosis is torn
- The subluxed tendon can be palpated anterior to the medial malleolus
- MRI will demonstrate oedema around the injured area and dynamic ultrasound can demonstrate the subluxing tendon
- Early surgical reconstruction is required in the elite athlete (typically a ballet dancer).

Ligament injuries

Lateral ligament injuries
- Usually caused by a forced inversion lateral ligament. Injuries are very common in a numerous number of sports
- Mechanism can involve a degree of plantar flexion and, therefore, the anterior talo-fibular ligament is usually torn before the calcaneofibular ligament
- Clinical picture depends on severity of the injury and the athlete may be able to finish their event or need assistance in leaving the field
- Swelling may develop immediately or over several hours and compression and ice will reduce degree of swelling and may therefore assist rehabilitation
- Ottawa ankle rules offer the physician a guide as to when to image is required and have a sensitivity of approximately 98%
- Once fracture is excluded, grading can give a guide to prognosis and return to sport:
  - *Grade I:* no ligament laxity
  - *Grade II:* some laxity (compare to contralateral side) but solid endpoint
  - *Grade III:* laxity without endpoint
- More severe grades may benefit from MRI/follow-up to exclude missed osteochondral lesions or fractures.

Deltoid injuries
- The deltoid ligament is better thought of as a complex of ligaments stronger than lateral ligaments in combination. It is probably more commonly injured than previously thought
- The more commonly described injury follows a forced high-energy eversion of the ankle and the athlete is usually unable to weight bear
- There will be immediate emerging swelling and the ankle may be dislocated
- Radiographs can show associated fractures of fibular syndesmosis and talar dome. Occasionally associated with lateral ligament injuries
- MRI and US may show oedema and ligament disruption
- Disruption of the anterior deltoid part of the complex in dancers and footballers following a combined dorsiflexion external rotation insult may cause instability in the anteromedial ankle causing ongoing pain when injury mechanism is reproduced
- They will be varying degrees of tenderness and swelling over the anterior deltoid area
- Surgical exploration may be warranted with continuing pain around the medial ankle as imaging may be deceiving and surgical correction may be required.

Syndesmosis injuries

- Tears of the anterior inferior tibio-fibular ligament can occur within sports involving repeated rotation of the ankle joint (e.g. football, rugby). History of 'tackle from behind' or direct impact to the distal fibula will often precede this injury
- The athlete will generally be unable to continue participation
- There will be some difficulty weight bearing although they can usually progress to walking once the initial pain subsides
- Minor sprains will generally be able to continue playing
- The athlete will describe high ankle pain. High ankle swelling will develop after several hours but may not be marked or may travel distally confusing the clinician onto thinking there is lateral ankle ligament injury
- Pain will be reproduced by combination of ankle dorsiflexion and external rotation
- Palpation of the ligament will usually be painful. Mortise and lateral view will be normal
- Stress diastases views will reveal a separation of the tibia and fibula
- MRI is good at detecting the extent of syndesmosis injury and instability
- Instability should be surgically repaired because of the danger of future arthritis
- Additionally, athletes requiring high rotational stability will be unable to progress to normal functional levels
- Traditional methods of syndesmosis repair by screw fixation are slowly being replaced by tightrope repair
- This is favoured in an athletic population due to earlier return to sport secondary to decreased ankle stiffness during rehabilitation and less morbidity associated with metalwork in the area
- Syndesmosis injuries can be associated with medial malleolar fractures.

Foot injuries

Fractures

Base of fifth metatarsal fractures
Two types of fractures are commonly described at the base of fifth metatarsal.
- The peroneus brevis tendon attaches to the base of the fifth metatarsal and may avulse a fragment in inversion injuries:
  - This fracture may be associated with a lateral ankle ligament injury
  - There can be involvement of the metatarso-cuboid articular surface
  - This fracture has a good prognosis when treated conservatively by offload and immobilization (3–6 weeks) followed by graduated return to loading
  - This fracture is not to be confused with the normal apophysis of the 9–14 age-group (Apophyseal line runs parallel to metatarsal shaft)
- A fracture seen more distally, 1.5 cm distal to the metatarsal tubercle, at the diaphyses (Jones fracture) disrupts blood supply to the displaced fragment
- This is associated with a poorer prognosis and will often require internal fixation especially in the athletic population where quick return to sport can be associated with non-union.

Calcaneal fractures
- These usually occur after a fall from height. The majority are intra-articular as a result of axial loading, whilst 30% are extra-articular and can be associated with rotational forces being applied to the hindfoot
- Axial load type fractures are associated with spinal fractures in up to 15% so these injuries need to be excluded and should be assumed until proven otherwise
- Clinical examination will reveal tenderness on squeezing the heel, with likely swelling and bruising (though these may be delayed signs)
- Immediate management will involve splinting the ankle with analgesia appropriate to manage the patient's symptoms
- Compartment syndrome due to swelling should be regularly assessed for, and the foot elevated and iced
- Orthopaedic management will be directed by the findings on plain film, with reconstructed CT images playing a more frequent role in determining treatment.

Anterior calcaneal process fracture
- The anterior calcaneal process can be injured in avulsion (more commonly) and compression
- Avulsion fractures occur after combined adduction and plantar flexion that results in avulsion of the anterior process by the bifurcate ligament
- Compression fractures follow forced forefoot abduction where calcaneus and cuboid are compressed against each other
- There is resulting tenderness just anterior to the sinus tarsi opening, anterior and inferior to the anterior tibio-fibular ligament, distinguishing this injury from lateral ankle ligament sprains

- Lateral hindfoot and, lateral oblique views of the ankle will best demonstrate this fracture but MRI may be necessary
- These fractures require immobilization in below knee cast for 4 weeks if picked up early and conservative treatment is possible depending on the size of the fragment. Refer for orthopaedic opinion.

Calcaneal stress fractures
- More commonly seen in those walking unaccustomed to the load or marching this is usually an insidious onset injury. The athlete complains of heel pain and is tender on calcaneal squeeze test
- Radiographs may show sclerotic appearances if the injury has been present for some time. Prognosis is generally good following a period of relative offload.

Navicular stress fractures
- Navicular stress fractures can present with midfoot pain and swelling
- The athlete may report 'aching' present for some time, but worse after a particular activity
- Since this condition can be associated with a poor outcome for the future career of the athlete, tenderness over the navicular should be treated and investigated as a stress fracture until this condition is excluded
- Radiographs are not sensitive, so CT and MRI are recommended for diagnosis and evaluation
- Non-weight-bearing immobilization is required, after which tenderness is re-assessed
- This provides the clinician with a good opportunity to attempt to correct risk factors, which include reduced range of motion in the ankle, athletic female triad, and over-pronation
- CT may additionally provide more accurate evaluation of a co-existing tarsal coalition.

Lisfranc fracture dislocation

The tarsometatarsal joint (Lisfranc joint) may be dislocated dorsally when a high-energy impact is sustained on a plantar flexed foot through an axial plane. Even without associated fractures this injury is career-ending if untreated due to complications of mid-foot collapse and post-traumatic arthritis.

- Compartment syndrome of the foot is also associated with this condition
- There will be a history of significant traumatic episode and the athlete will complain of midfoot pain, and may or may not be able to weight bear
- Swelling will develop over the midfoot and the Lisfranc joint will be tender to palpation
- Pain can be reproduced by abduction and pronation of the forefoot over a fixed hindfoot
- Blood supply may be compromised in severe injuries as dorsalis pedis may be injured or compressed
- The Lisfranc injury may not be immediately obvious on X-rays, as spontaneous reduction of the joint may have taken place. Fractures at

the base of second metatarsal and anterior cuboid may be evident, and should suggest a Lisfranc dislocation
- Weight-bearing views may help in demonstrating relationship between first and second metatarsal, but may not be well tolerated by the individual
- MRI and CT may be required
- If no gross instability remains in a less severe injury 6 weeks of below knee immobilization is required
- Observation of neurovascular supply should be maintained for several weeks
- Precise anatomical reduction required and this often involves open reduction internal fixation (ORIF)
- Note that dislocations without a fracture often have a poorer outcome despite ORIF.

Sesamoid injuries

Fractures
- Located within the flexor hallucis brevis the sesamoid bones confer mechanical advantage to this tendon, and assist weight bearing across the 1st metatarso-phalangeal (MTP)
- Fractures usually involve the medial sesamoid
- The onset may be sudden or more insidious in nature and may follow forefoot weight bearing activities or sudden landing
- Swelling is limited but direct palpation over the affected bone is excruciatingly tender
- AP lateral and oblique, as well as axial sesamoid views will identify the fracture
- Bipartatite medial sesamoids could be confused with fracture where edges are usually irregular in the latter
- MRI can be helpful
- Treatment includes immobilization in non-weight-bearing cast
- Loading should be returned gradually and the sesamoid should be offloaded with orthotics, as this is a fatigue fracture
- Excision of the sesamoid is used when conservative approaches fail, but is not recommended in the athlete. It is associated with development of hallux valgus (if medial sesamoid resected) or halux varus (if lateral resected)
- Excision has also been associated with cock-up/claw toe deformity and first MTP stiffness.

Sesamoiditis
- Trauma, infection vascular, necrosis, and systemic inflammatory conditions can all cause inflammation of the sesamoids
- Sesamoid shape may also influence the amount of soft tissue micro-trauma that they cause in surrounding tissues when loading
- Radiograph sesamoid views and MRI will help distinguish from other conditions affecting the sesamoids
- Treatment requires offload and orthotic prescription
- Infiltration with corticosteroid may help accelerate the recovery from symptoms as mechanical causes are corrected
- Excision should be avoided for reasons listed above.

ⓘ Ottawa Foot and Ankle Guidelines

These validated guidelines have a sensitivity of about 98% in excluding a fracture to the ankle or foot after injury.

Ankle

X-rays are only required if there is any pain in the ankle region (between the malleoli) and any one of the following:
- Bone tenderness along the distal 6 cm of the posterior edge of the tibia or tip of the medial, malleolus *or*
- Bone tenderness along the distal 6 cm of the posterior edge of the fibula or tip of the lateral malleolus *or*
- An inability to bear weight both immediately and in the ED for four steps.

Foot

X-rays are only required if there is any pain in the area of the midfoot and any one of the following:
- Bone tenderness at the base of the fifth metatarsal (for foot injuries), *or*
- Bone tenderness at the navicular bone (for foot injuries), *or*
- An inability to bear weight both immediately and in the ED for four steps.

Further reading

Stiell IG, Greenberg GH, McKnight RD, et al. (1993). Decision rules for the use of radiography in acute ankle injuries. Refinement and prospective validation. *J Am Med Ass* **269**: 1127–32.

Chapter 18

Paediatrics

Introduction *252*
Physical (anatomical) *253*
Physiological *254*
Pathological *255*
Psychological *256*
Protection *257*
Choking child *258*
Asthma *260*
Seizures *262*
Limping child *264*
Head injury *267*
Useful drug doses in children *269*

Introduction

The United Nations Convention on the Rights of a Child states that a child is considered 'every human being below the age of eighteen years'. This definition has been accepted by all 4 UK governments.

We all have a social responsibility to encourage children to participate in sport, whether that be in our roles as doctors, physiotherapists, teachers, or most importantly parents. The benefits of regular exercise in the long-term health of a population should be built on a foundation that promotes that regular exercise should be undertaken at as young an age as possible.

Children should not, however, be viewed simply as small adults. There are many differences that should be considered in ensuring that children are enabled to exercise in a safe environment.
- Physical (anatomical)
- Physiological
- Pathological
- Psychological
- Protection.

We shall look at these different areas to highlight the kind of problems that may be encountered.

⚠ Note in the presentation of cardiac arrest please refer to 📖 p.82.

⚠ Note in the presentation of anaphylaxis please refer to 📖 p.96.

Physical (anatomical)

All children develop and grow at different rates and these weights and heights are charted on plots giving centile measurements. These charts demonstrate the great differences in weight and height between children at the same age or in the same class at school. Growth spurts tend to occur around puberty—with girls usually commencing puberty slightly earlier than boys. These changing physical characteristics can play a part in affecting the psychological development of a child, especially if a child develops particularly early or late in comparison with their peers.

Physical differences play an important part in the injury rates of children. Rugby is a sport that recognizes the potential difference in physical size between children at different ages and the problems that can arise as a result of this. As such, there is a graded introduction into this game using smaller pitches and 'touch', rather than tackle-based games.

Analgesia is prescribed usually on a weight basis. Most over the counter medications such as paracetamol or ibuprofen will have a dosage regime on the side of the bottle, but for more precise dosing, it is important to measure or calculate the child's weight to prevent under- or over-dosing. This is highly important in the prescription and administration of any drug and not just analgesia.

In situations of critical illness, such as epilepsy or cardiac arrest where time is especially pressing, knowledge of the child's weight will allow accurate calculation, and aid administration of medications timeously and safely.

Various formulae have been used to calculate a child's weight, based on age. As long as the child is between the ages of 1 and 13 years old the following formula can be used:

$$\text{Weight (kg)} = (\text{Age} \times 3) + 7$$

For example, a 6-year-old would be estimated to weigh 25 kg.

⚠ Remember this is a rough estimate.

Physiological

Children's physiology changes remarkably as they grow. Respiratory rate, heart rate, blood pressure (BP) will continue to change until adult levels are reached. This is important when trying to assess an injured child and interpret their clinical condition. Realizing that it can be normal for a child to have a resting pulse rate of 120 bpm and a respiratory rate of 20 bpm can have a major impact on how you proceed in your management.

Paediatric brain physiology is similar to that of adults in terms of cerebral autoregulation and perfusion pressures. Children tend to have a lower cerebral perfusion pressure than adults but this is offset by their lower BP.

Different to adults, however, children can become much more easily hypovolaemic and this can occur due to blood loss from scalp wounds—much less common in adults.

⚠ Children usually have a marked physiological reserve and can appear to be coping up until the point where they decompensate dramatically.

See Table 18.1 for a range of normal findings (Wyatt et al., 2006, p. 629).

Table 18.1 Normal (expected) physiological values at different ages*

Age (years)	Respiratory rate	Heart rate	Systolic BP
<1	30–40	110–160	70–90
1–2	25–35	100–150	80–95
2–5	25–30	95–140	80–100
5–12	20–25	80–120	90–110
>12	15–20	60–100	100–120

Expected systolic BP = 80 + (age in years x 2) mmHg.

Adapted from the American Academy of Pediatrics and the American College of Emergency Physicians, 2004, 2007. Used with permission.

Pathological

As a result of the physical differences between the immature and adult skeleton, different types of pathologies and fractures can arise. The following fractures are specific to children for example:
- *Torus (Buckle):* typically stable injuries that can be treated usually by a wrist splint. May be very little to find clinically
- *Greenstick:* a break in one cortex and a bend in the other. May be unstable and change position. Manipulation may be required. Cast minimum treatment
- *Epiphyseal:* the Salter Harris classification describes the 5 different fractures that can affect the growth plates. Management depends on the extent of the injury, but these can cause considerable morbidity
- *Plastic bowing:* an uncommon injury that usually occurs in association with a second fracture that is the cause of the shortening, i.e. distal radius fracturing and resulting bowing of the ulna.

Fractures are just one example of the differences in pathology that will be suffered by a child. There are many others that should be borne in mind, including childhood illnesses, such as chickenpox, which may affect both the child athlete and potentially his classmates too if undetected.

Psychological

- Children need to be allowed to develop both physically and psychologically
- Care needs to be taken to provide an appropriate environment for exercise to take place
- This includes appropriate areas both for training, playing, and changing
- Adequate supervision needs to take place at all times, whilst balancing the issues of privacy.

Bullying can take many forms, but at its most basic, it is either physical or non-physical, where either may be absolutely intolerable and devastating for the child. It may originate from other children, but occasionally from adults as well. Pressure to succeed felt by the touchline parent may be directed towards a child who they see as underperforming. This is clearly unacceptable, and may inhibit the child and hinder them from wanting to participate in any form of exercise in the future.

Children must be treated as individuals. They must be encouraged foremost to participate in exercise and, thereafter, to maximize their potential. This takes a great deal of skill and patience to get the best out of each child. Whatever problems that may prevent or delay a child from participating in sport, such as extreme self-consciousness should be sought for and addressed.

Protection

Child protection is an area that should never be compromised when dealing with children and sport. It is encumbant on any health professional to consider issues relating to child protection when presented with a child seeking medical attention. Any injury sustained by a child should have an adequate explanation to accompany it. Sport can be used as a convenient excuse to explain away an injury and whilst in the overwhelming majority of patients this will be an appropriate explanation, other factors should always be in the back of the clinicians mind.
- Delay in presentation
- Recurrent unexplained injury
- Unusual patterns of injury
- Withdrawn child
- Multiple attendances to Emergency Department (EDs)
- Unusual time of attendance to EDs.

These factors are just some of the many red flags that may present to the team physician. It should be remembered that the difficulty in identifying a child with child protection issues lies in that a child may present with all the red flags and have absolutely no issues, or present with none of the red flags and be at risk. Herein lies the problem. In order to mitigate risk it is vital that any adult dealing with children has undertaken adequate training in child protection issues and had an adequate assessment made of themselves according to local policies and procedures.

Help, advice, and information may be sought from the child's GP, health visitor, school nurse, or social work team.

Statutory guidance is available in England via *Working Together to Safeguard children 2010*, whilst in Scotland the Protection of Children (Scotland) Act 2003 also provides guidance.

⚠ 'If you don't consider it, you will miss it.'—is an adage that holds true in all medical disciplines, but is never more important than in the assessment of child protection.

Choking child

- Children may choke at any age, although it is more common in younger children.
- If the presentation has been witnessed then the diagnosis is usually clearly apparent and the algorithm below can be followed.
- In cases where the event is not witnessed, a high index of suspicion should be given in any child who suddenly develops:
  - Cyanosis
  - Drooling
  - Stridor
  - Clutching throat
  - Dyspnoea
  - Wheeze
  - Intractable coughing
  - Silent chest.

Differential diagnoses of this presentation therefore includes anaphylaxis, asthma, and epiglottitis. The sudden nature of the onset of the airway obstruction, however, is key in making the diagnosis.

Management

The initial management follows the flow diagram in Fig. 18.1.

- Assessment is made as to whether the child has an effective cough or not
- If they are able to cough and shift air into the lungs then leave them in a position of comfort. They should be encouraged to cough and regularly checked to ensure no deterioration
- If the cough is ineffective then check the child's consciousness level. If they are unconscious then open the airway, perform 5 rescue breaths and start cardiopulmonary resuscitation (CPR). If they are conscious then perform 5 back blows followed by 5 abdominal thrusts (or 5 chest thrusts if the child is under 1-year-old)
- Back blows are performed by striking the child between the scapula. After each blow, check to see if the foreign body has become dislodged
- Abdominal thrusts are performed by standing behind the child. Make a fist and place this hand between the child's umbilicus and xiphisternum. Place the other hand on-top of the closed fist, and pull sharply inwards and upwards
- Chest thrusts are performed with the hands in the same position as for CPR, but with a rate in the region of 1 s per thrust.

CHOKING CHILD

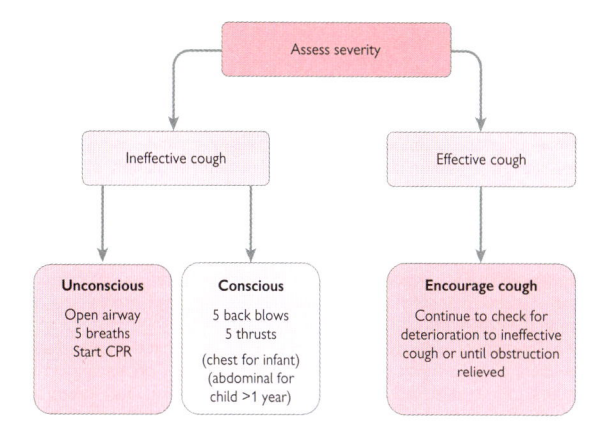

```
                    Assess severity
                    /            \
         Ineffective cough    Effective cough
           /        \                |
   Unconscious    Conscious      Encourage cough
   Open airway   5 back blows   Continue to check for
   5 breaths     5 thrusts      deterioration to ineffective
   Start CPR     (chest for infant)  cough or until obstruction
                 (abdominal for  relieved
                 child >1 year)
```

Fig. 18.1 Choking child algorithm. Reproduced with the kind permission of the Resuscitation Council (UK).

Asthma

The incidence of asthma is on the increase especially in the paediatric population.

The classic presentation is wheeze, breathlessness, and cough. There may be a history of atopy or nocturnal coughing. Acute asthma attacks are relatively common and usually resolve with inhalation of a short-acting beta-2 agonist. In situations where the child deteriorates, treatment should be carried out as detailed below.

The differential diagnosis differs slightly in children compared with adults where children are more prone to choking, and this should be remembered and considered. Other potential causes of shortness of breath, such as anaphylaxis, pneumothorax, and pneumonia are also potential differentials.

Management of asthma is similar to that of adults in that the exacerbation should be classified into one of the categories below depending on the features found on assessment. The age of the child is also taken into account. The remainder of this chapter refers to the management of a child over 5 years old. (As per Scottish Intercollegiate Guidelines Network (SIGN) guidelines 101).

Initial pre-hospital treatment involves administration of a beta-agonist such as salbutamol. 2 puffs should be given every 2 min (preferably via a spacer).

Criteria for referring to hospital
- More than 10 puffs of salbutamol required
- Any features of acute severe or life-threatening as detailed in Box 18.1.

Treatment of acute asthma
- Sit the child up to aid lung expansion and reassure
- Assess and classify into one of the 3 categories in Box 18.1. Note that peak exploratory flow rate (PEFR) is vital
- Note past medical history; risk of severity increases with past history of hospital admission for asthma, ventilation, >3 types of asthma drugs and repeated presentations to the Emergency Department (ED)
- Initial management is with inhaled bronchodilators (e.g. salbutamol) 2 puffs every 2 min then reassess, including PEFR
- If there are any features of a severe or life-threatening exacerbation, or SaO_2 <94% then commence oxygen at as high a flow rate as possible—ideally 15 L/min via non-rebreathable facemask (CO_2 retention is never an issue at this stage)
- In all cases of acute asthma give po prednisolone 30–40 mg, usually for 3 days
- A nebulizer should be used, if available, in any child with an acute severe or life-threatening exacerbation. If there is a poor response to beta agonist add ipratropium bromide to the nebulized beta agonist

Box 18.1 Acute severe and life-threatening features

Moderate exacerbation
- Increasing symptoms
- PEF between 50 and 75% of best or predicted
- No features of acute severe asthma

Acute severe exacerbation
Any ONE of:
- PEF between 33 and 50%
- SaO_2 <92%
- Cannot complete sentences in one breath or too breathless to feed/talk
- Pulse >125 bpm
- Respiration >30 bpm

Life-threatening exacerbation
Any ONE of:
- PEF <33% or unable to carry out
- SaO_2 <92%
- Silent chest
- Poor respiratory effort
- Cyanosed
- Hypotensive
- Exhausted
- Coma

⚠ Bradycardia is a pre-terminal event.

Seizures

See p.38 and 98.

Seizures can occur in children for many reasons. Some of these such as febrile convulsions are unique to children and do not occur in adults.

Causes of seizures in children
- Epilepsy
- Trauma—head injury
- Infection
- Hypoglycaemia
- Febrile convulsions
- Cerebral palsy
- Congenital.

This list is not exhaustive. Best management is based on prevention so ensure you are up to date with each athlete's medication if they are known to fit. Focus of management of epilepsy or seizures of any aetiology is clearly prevention. When a seizure occurs, the management is prescriptive. Being prepared is vital—ensure you have access to the correct equipment including a mobile phone.

Status epilepticus is defined as seizure activity, ongoing for more than 30 min, or repeated seizures without consciousness being regained. It is a life-threatening condition with a high mortality, the rate of which increases with the increasing duration of the seizure.

Management aims
- Maintain an airway
- Terminate the seizure if not self-terminated within 2 min
- Identify potential reversible causes namely hypoglycaemia.

⚠ Remember that cardiac arrest caused by ventricular fibrillation may present as a short-lived seizure. Check for a pulse in all patients suffering from a seizure.

When to phone an ambulance
- Status epilepticus
- Seizure lasting longer than 5 min
- Athletes first seizure
- Seizure as a result of injury
- Injury resulting from seizure
- Multiple seizures.

Medications
There are a number of medications belonging to the benzodiazepine family that can be used to terminate seizures.

All members of the benzodiazepine family have a similar side-effect profile, such as respiratory depression and hypotension. The extent of these effects varies between drugs, but being familiar with these effects is paramount, as is having the correct equipment to deal with them when they arise.

Management of seizures

- Maintain airway as able—use a naso- or oropharyngeal airway if tolerated (an oropharyngeal airway may prove impossible to insert in a fitting athlete due to teeth clenching)
- Administer 15 L of oxygen as available
- Check for a pulse
- If fitting for more than 2 min
- Obtain IV access if possible and check using a blood glucose monitor (BM)
  - If IV access is obtained then administer 0.1 mg/kg lorazepam
  - If no IV access then use 0.5 mg/kg diazepam pr or 0.5 mg buccal midazolam and try again for IV access
- Phone an ambulance if fitting for more than 5 min
- If still fitting after 10 min
  - If IV access is obtained then administer 0.1mg/kg lorazepam
  - If still no IV access then use a further 0.5mg/kg diazepam PR or 0.5mg/kg buccal midazolam and try again for IV access
- ENSURE AMBULANCE HAS BEEN CALLED.
(Adapted from APLS)

ⓘ Limping child

The differential diagnosis for a child presenting with a limp is exceptionally varied and causes originating anywhere from the spine to the toe nails should be sought. Pain from the hip is often felt in the knee so hip pathology should always be considered in a child with knee pain.

Different causes will occur at different ages such as transient synovitis being more common in the under 10-year-olds and a slipped femoral epiphysis in the over 10-year-olds. The child may or may not complain of pain—indeed, the limp may be detected by the clinician or a concerned parent without the child even being aware of it. Fever is a most concerning symptom and septic arthritis should always be considered in such presentations.

Management will depend on the likely cause found via a thorough history and examination. In many cases, radiological and blood tests will not be required, and a wait and see plan may be put in place, as long as the child is reassessed regularly. In more complex cases or where there is any doubt as to the pathology then specialist referral for imaging and further investigation will be required.

Potential causes of a limping child

▶ In *all* age groups *always* consider the possibility of non-accidental injury (NAI).

- *Age 0–4:*
  - Trauma—toddlers fracture (#)
  - soft tissue injury (STI) to foot
  - Septic arthritis/Osteomyelitis
  - Transient synovitis
  - Hair tourniquet
  - Juvenile rheumatoid arthritis
  - Rarely—malignancy.
- *Age 4–10:*
  - Trauma—fracture or STI to lower limb including epiphyseal injuries
  - Septic arthritis/osteomyelitis
  - Transient synovitis
  - Perthes disease
  - Leukaemia
  - Juvenile rheumatoid arthritis.
- *Age 10–18:*
  - Trauma—fracture or STI to lower limb including epiphyseal injuries, and avulsion fractures
  - Slipped upper femoral capital epiphysis (SUFE)
  - Septic arthritis/osteomyelitis
  - Leukaemia and malignancies
  - Juvenile ankylosing spondylitis.

History
Important factors in the history include:
- Trauma: If so then what was the mechanism
- Associated fever: should raise concern over infective cause such as septic arthritis. Mandates referral for blood and imaging work-up
- Associated night pain
- Associated systemic upset or weight loss
- Multiple joints affected
- Previous history: perthes is bilateral in approximately 15%
- Family history of joint diseases/HLA B27.

▶▶ Remember to be careful to allow the parent or child to answer without direct questioning initially. It is all too easy to be distracted by an 'injury' where the parents or child tries to help you by attributing the symptoms to a possible trauma when, in fact, this is a red herring.

▶▶ Night pain and weight loss are vague symptoms, but should raise concerns of a potentially significant aetiology, such as malignancy.

Examination
The examination made will be directed depending on whether there has been a history of trauma or not.
- In any case of a traumatic injury the athlete should be assessed using the ABC approach and a focused assessment made thereafter of the injured limb including the joints above and below the injured area.
- In atraumatic limping, examination should include a general examination of the athlete to include pulse and temperature.
- The child's weight should also be taken.
- Assessment of the child's gait should be made followed by an examination, starting with the lumbar spine and working down to assess the pelvis, hips femur, knee, lower limb then the ankle, foot, and finally the toes if a cause for the limp has not been found by this point.
- Each joint should be assessed using the standard joint examination principles of *look*, *feel*, and *move*.
- Symmetry should be assessed by examining the unaffected leg as this will help to clarify the normal range of movement and also allow you to assess for polyarthropathy too.

Investigations
- Will depend on the clinical findings and the working diagnosis.
- In any child with a fever and a restricted range of hip movement, referral should be made for a work-up of laboratory tests to include full blood count (FBC), c-reactive protein (CRP), X-ray and possible ultrasound (US) with a view to hip joint aspiration depending on local policies.

Septic arthritis
⚠ Septic arthritis is an orthopaedic emergency.
- Suspect in any child with a fever and a painful/inability to weight bear (Note: there may be no fever)
- Usually *Staph. aureus*

- Can occur in any age, but the majority of patients are around 3 years old
- May be little in the way of clinical findings of erythema, warm joint, or swelling. Child may hold the hip flexed abducted and rotate externally
- Immediately refer for blood tests and imaging followed by antibiotics and joint washout.

Perthes' disease
- Aseptic (avascular) necrosis of the femoral head
- The classic cause of a 'painless' limp. Aetiology unknown
- Also known as (Legg–Calve–Perthes' disease)
- Boys are affected more than girls by a factor of about ×4
- Peak age is usually in the 4–10-year-old group
- Occurs bilaterally in about 10–15% so ask about previous history
- Pain may be referred to the anterior thigh or the knee
- Pain may be found maximally on internal rotation and abduction
- Diagnosis is confirmed with X-ray
- Treatment may either be conservative with splinting and traction or be surgical via an osteotomy. Either way the aim is to maximize the femoral head regaining its correct anatomical shape
- Long-term outcomes vary depending on the extent of necrosis and age the condition develops with best outcomes in the younger population
- Return to sport can be considered once the child is pain free and X-ray appearances confirm healing of the femoral head.

Slipped upper femoral capital epiphysis
- Boys affected more than girls by a factor of about ×3
- Increased incidence in obese children and some medical conditions, such as metabolic disorders of growth, hypogonadism, and hypothyroidism. Peak age is usually in the 10–17-year-old group
- May occur bilaterally in about 40% (usually within 2 years of the first hip) resulting in some athletes opting for prophylactic fixation of an unaffected hip
- Progressive pain in hip/groin. Pain on internal rotation and abduction
- Treatment is invariably surgical after X-ray diagnosis
- Crutches and graded weight-bearing for at least 2 months
- Return to play once pain free. Some advocate X-ray confirmation of the physis closing prior to return to contact sport.

Transient synovitis of the hip
- This is a particularly common cause of a limp in children (especially under the age of 10 years old)
- It is best considered a diagnosis of exclusion, i.e. there is absolutely nothing to suggest a septic arthritis as discussed before
- Aetiology is thought to be secondary to a viral infection and, as such, there may be a history of a recent or ongoing coryzal illness
- Investigations are non-specific with only mild if any elevation in inflammatory markers. X-ray will be normal and is not routinely required
- US will diagnose the effusion, but there is no distinction between the causes for the effusion, i.e. septic arthritis
- Management is symptomatic with rest simple analgesia and anti-inflammatories.

Head injury

Paediatric head injuries are common. Over 500,000 children present to EDs across the UK each year as a result of head injury. The majority of these will be 'minor' implying that there is no serious intracranial pathology.

⚠ However, 1:500 children initially classified as having a 'minor head injury' will actually ultimately have serious intracranial pathology.

Initial assessment of the head injured child

▶▶ The initial assessment of a child with a head injury is no different to that of an adult with a head injury (see 📖 also p.116)

History is again key.
- What was the mechanism of injury?
- Was the child unconscious? If so for how long?
- Has the child vomited?
- Did they suffer a seizure (pre- or) post-injury?
- Have they been amnesic and is so, for how long?

These questions form the basic framework for the decision-making criteria about whether the child needs to go to hospital and needs imaging.

Examination is again primarily used to both assess and treat injuries as they are found.
- Protect the cervical spine and assess the airway
- Reassurance will be required so talk calmly to the child
- Involve the parents if present (*Do not*, however, allow them to move the child until you have completed your assessment.)
- Ensure assistance has been called for
- Proceed to assessing breathing and circulation (bear in mind the differences in normal values in differing age groups)
- Over the age of 5 years, the adult GCS assessment scoring system (see 📖 p.116) or alternatively, the AVPU system can be used when assessing disability. Under the age of 5 an adjusted Glasgow Coma Score (GCS) system is used, although this is a rare sporting event and, as such, AVPU is recommended in this age group
- Log roll should be carried out as per the guidance detailed on 📖 p.15:
  - If the child is small it may be more appropriate to use 2 persons to log roll the child rather than 3
  - This will depend on the length of the child and is really a judgment call
  - Best advice is that if the 3 persons standing to roll the child cannot place their hands appropriately because they are in each others way then only 2 will be required.

Head injury management

The way children with head injuries are managed has changed in recent years after the publication of guidelines such as NICE and SIGN 110, and CHALICE.

These papers have focused on the best methods of investigating these injuries—who to image and when. This guidance is invaluable to the pitchside clinician who can much more readily decide who to refer to hospital.

Indications for referral to the ED
- GCS <15 at initial assessment
- Post-traumatic seizure (generalized or focal)
- Focal neurological signs
- Signs of a skull fracture
- Loss of consciousness
- Sever and persistent headache
- Repeated vomiting (two or more occasions)
- Post-traumatic amnesia >5 min
- Retrograde amnesia >30 min
- High risk mechanism of injury
- Coagulopathy
- Clinical suspicion of NAI.

Indications for CT scan immediate
- GCS 13 or less in ED
- GCS 14 or 15/15, but witnessed the loss of consciousness (LOC) >5 min
- GCS 14 or 15/15, but suspicion of open or depressed skull #
- GCS 14 or 15/15, but focal neurology
- GCS 14 or 15/15, but basal skull #.

Indications to consider CT scan within 8 h
- GCS 14 or 15, but presence of bruise, swelling, or lac >5 cm
- GCS 14 or 15, and post-traumatic seizure (no history of epilepsy)
- GCS 14 or 15, and any amnesia lasting >5 min
- GCS 14 or 15, and a history of significant fall
- GCS 14 or 15, and 3 or more discrete episodes of vomiting
- GCS 14 or 15, and abnormal drowsiness (slow to respond).

Return to sport guidelines

The guidance detailed in p.124 is applicable to children aged 10 and above. Further research is being undertaken to provide evidence on the safest way to return a child to sport in the ages below this. At present the guidance as laid out in p.124, i.e. rest followed by a graded return to full activities is the suggested advice.

Useful drug doses in children

See Table 18.2.

Table 18.2 Useful drugs dosages to consider

Paracetamol po	loading dose 20 mg/kg then 10–15 mg/kg
Ibuprofen po	loading dose of 10 mg/kg then 7 mg/kg
Lorazepam IV	0.1 mg/kg
Diazepam pr	0.5 mg/kg
Morphine IV	0.1 mg/kg
Adrenaline in cardiac arrest	0.1 mL/kg of 1:10,000

Further reading

British Thoracic Guidelines/Scottish Intercollegiate Guidelines Network (2008, revised 2011). Available at: www.sign.ac.uk/pdf/qrg101.pdf.

Wyatt JP, Illingworth RN, Graham CA, et al. (2006). *Oxford Handbook of Emergency Medicine*. Oxford: Oxford University Press.

Chapter 19

Athletes with a disability

Introduction 272
Principles of treatment 272
Special considerations 273
Autonomic dysreflexia 274

Introduction

Disability sport is the term used for any sport undertaken by someone with a disability (Table 19.1). It therefore covers a wide range of sports and athletes with 20 summer and 5 winter sports at Paralympic games.

Table 19.1 Sports undertaken by people with disabilities

Summer Paralympic sports				Winter sports
Archery	Football 5-a-side	Rowing	Volleyball (sitting)	Alpine skiing
Athletics	Football 7-a-side	Sailing	Wheelchair basketball	Biathlon
Boccia	Goalball	Shooting	Wheelchair fencing	Cross-country skiing
Cycling	Judo	Swimming	Wheelchair rugby	Ice sledge hockey
Equestrian	Powerlifting	Table tennis	Wheelchair tennis	Wheelchair curling

Five major impairment groups are recognized for the elite athletes in the Paralympics.
- Visual impairment
- Spinal-cord-related disability (congenital or acquired)
- Limb deficiencies (congenital or acquired)
- Cerebral palsy
- Les Autres (for athletes who do not fit into other categories).

Athletes with intellectual impairment will be reintroduced at the 2012 Paralympics in a limited number of sports following issues relating to classification systems, but are involved in a number of sports at the community level.

Athletes with disabilities can compete in a wide range of sports as part of the Paralympics, and a wider range of sports and activities within communities.

Principles of treatment

The principles of treatment for injuries are identical to those in able-bodied athletes. See Chapter 2 for all injuries that follow the ABCDE approach.

Special considerations

- Knowledge of the regulations covering the sport is important, although outside the scope of this book (see www.paralympic.org for further information)
- Each individual sport will potentially use specialist equipment and a working knowledge of this equipment will be vital. For example, when working with athletes using wheelchairs, it is vital to know how to release the athletes quickly from their chairs in event of significant trauma
- Field of play recovery also needs consideration for each sport and should be practiced by the team prior to the commencement of events—e.g. in wheelchair events a crash involving a number of wheelchair athletes on a track will pose a significant challenge to most field-of-play medical response teams unless adequately rehearsed
- The nature of the injuries likely to be experienced depend on the nature of the sport—e.g. alpine skiing or sledge hockey with high impact collisions as compared with archery. However, it is important to note that a high index of suspicion is required, for fractures with minimal trauma in athletes with paralysis and consequent osteoporosis/osteopenia. For example, a sideways fall onto the lateral hip in a chair can result in hip fractures, although the forces involved do not appear significant
- Knowing the athletes you are caring for is always important, but not always possible. So understanding the different impairment groups involved in each sport will give an indication of the type of medical issues likely to be faced. However, in the Les Autres groups this can be challenging and, in athletes with rare conditions, the use of a textbook is important!
- Sometimes a condition will not only have physical limitations, but may have intellectual and emotional components, which need to be considered in the treatment of the athlete
- In athletes with intellectual impairment, consent to treatment can be an issue, which should be considered prior to participation
- There is often a higher incidence of epilepsy in these athletes and provision for this should be considered in the planning of an event
- The co-existence of other diseases and use of medications is more frequent in this group of athletes and these may affect response to injury. For example, tetraplegic athletes with limited respiratory reserve will deteriorate quicker with chest trauma than an able bodied athlete
- Skin care of the stump in amputee athletes needs careful consideration and repeated observation, to ensure that breakdown of the tissue does not occur
- There is also the potential for penetrating injuries if prosthesis breaks suddenly during an event.

Autonomic dysreflexia

- This occurs in patients with a chronic or acute spinal cord lesion above T5–6
- It is an exaggerated increase in blood pressure (BP) as a result of a noxious stimulus below the level of the lesion
- The autonomic nervous system depends on a balance between the parasympthatic and sympathetic nervous systems
- The sympathetic system is associated with the fight or flight response, which includes:
  - Dilation of the pupil
  - Increase in heart rate
  - Vasoconstriction
  - Release of catecholamine hormones (adrenalin)
- The parasympathetic system produces opposite responses, which includes:
  - Constriction of the pupil
  - Decrease in heart rate
- The sympathetic and parasympathetic nerves have different pathways in the body with the sympathetic system having a major output between the 5th thoracic and 2nd lumbar segments of the spinal cord
- In a patient with a spinal cord lesion above the level of the 5th and 6th thoracic vertebrae, a painful stimulus below the level of the lesion will produce a response by the sympathetic system, which may result in:
  - Vasoconstriction
  - High BP
  - Pounding headache
  - Anxiety
  - Pallor
  - Goosebumps
- The skin changes will occur below the level of the lesion only
- The parasympathetic system is unable to counteract these effects below the level of the lesion and so produces bradycardia and flushing of the neck and face by vasodilation.

Symptoms of autonomic dysreflexia
- Anxiety
- Pounding headache
- Sweating
- Chest pain.

Signs of autonomic dysreflexia
- Flushing of face and neck
- Hypertension with bradycardia
- Possible cardiac arrythmias
- Dilated pupils
- Goosebumps below the level of the lesion
- Cold peripheries.

AUTONOMIC DYSREFLEXIA

The baseline BP in a spinal cord patient is often relatively low and so a significant rise may not be appreciated—it is important to know the baseline BPs for all athletes at risk of this complication.

The increase in BP is a medical emergency, and prompt recognition and treatment is essential.

Causes
Any noxious stimuli below the level of the lesion can cause the condition. These may be painful, uncomfortable, or physically irritating. The most common cause is overfilling of the bladder followed by gas- or stool-filled bowel.

Causes in the bladder
- Retention
- Infection
- Over-filled collection system
- Calculi.

Causes in the bowel
- Constipation
- Digital stimulation
- Haemorrhoids and fissures
- Infection.

Causes in the skin
- Pressure sores
- In-growing toenail
- Burns
- Restrictive clothing below the level of the lesion
- Wrinkled clothing or pressure from a foreign body.

Other causes
Include:
- Sexual activity
- Menstrual cramps
- Injuries such as fractures.

Treatment
The most important treatment is the identification and removal of the stimulus. Sometimes this will be obvious, but it is recommended to ensure a thorough examination for the cause using a step approach. Always complete all steps.

Therefore:
- *Step 1:* check bladder
- *Step 2:* check bowel
- *Step 3:* check skin
- *Step 4:* check other.

Treatment is required to lower BP. This can be achieved with either:
- Nifedepine 10 mg (capsules that can be chewed or split into the mouth)
- Glyceryl trinitrate (GTN) spray.

During the initial management, arrangements should be made for transfer to hospital unless rapid resolution of the symptoms and signs are achieved.

Chapter 20

Aggressive patients

Introduction *278*
Explaining aggression and violence *279*
Preventing aggression or violence in athletes *280*
Dealing with aggressive or violent athletes *281*
Summary *282*

CHAPTER 20 Aggressive patients

Introduction

Aggressive or violent acts are often associated with sport. When people are brought together in competition, they demonstrate their physical and tactical supremacy within pre-established rules or laws of the game, but a strong desire to win may lead them to overlook these rules. This can lead to actions that endanger their opponents' well-being.

In professional sport, these acts tend to be highlighted by the media and sometimes appear to provoke violent acts by supporters who may be incensed or inappropriately inspired by the on-pitch activities.

Within a sporting environment, aggressive behaviour might not just be between competitors, but athletes might be aggressive to staff (including doctors) or even spectators

Effective communication with aggressive or violent patients, whether in a sporting environment or not, is obviously challenging. It is essential to bear in mind one's own safety and to proceed cautiously when engaging such patients.

Explaining aggression and violence

Aggression and violence in a sporting environment has a number of possible causes or precipitating factors (see Box 20.1 for relevant definitions).

- *Misunderstanding or misinterpretation:*
  - Lack of language skills
  - Cultural differences
  - Misinterpretation of body language
- *Personality types involved:*
  - Competitive, fearless
  - Accustomed to violence (on the field of play), but unable to make a distinction when they cross over the boundary where such behaviour is unacceptable
- *Emotions:*
  - Disappointment
  - Frustration
  - Anger—loss, failure, blaming others
- *Confusion:* consider medical causes especially hypoglycaemia:
  - Pain (e.g. From sports injuries)
  - Brain injury
  - Metabolic (e.g. dehydration, heat exhaustion)
  - Infective
  - Neoplastic causes (e.g. brain tumour)
  - Drugs—stimulants, alcohol, or anabolic steroids
- *Mental illness:*
  - Psychosis (e.g. due to schizophrenia or bipolar illness)
  - Depression
  - Anxiety state or panic attack.

Box 20.1 Definitions

- *Aggression:* behaviour in which there is intent to harm or cause damage, though this may not be a conscious decision
- *Violence:* physically harmful or damaging behaviour, where there is pre-meditation or planning
- *Assertive:* behaviour associated with trying to control a situation, but with no intent to cause harm or damage

Preventing aggression or violence in athletes

It is often possible to prevent potential acts of aggression or violence from escalating. Engendering mutual trust and respect is important to building a good doctor–patient relationship. It is advisable to:
- Consult out of the media spotlight and 'public eye' as much as possible
- Consult in a room suitable for medical purposes where possible
- Explore the needs and expectations of the athlete sensitively
- Explain the reasons for carrying out any action or procedure and ensure agreement or consent so that actions may not be misconstrued (e.g. as an assault.)
- Remain impartial—do not appear to take sides with management, coach, other players, or the opposition
- Arrange a chaperone.

Facilities
- Sports physicians should impress upon management that it is essential to provide a suitable medical room, the layout of which should be planned bearing in mind dealing with aggressive or violent patients
- An easy route of escape for the doctor and a panic alarm facility should be available with other staff aware of the expectations if the alarm is sounded.

Early warning signs

Changes in character or behaviour
- The player's on- or off-pitch behaviour may change before their actions turn aggressive. These changes may be subtle or obvious
- Typically, dehydrated or heat-affected players lose position or role sense in their team, and the sports physician should assess and manage their condition appropriately
- There may be a character change in a sportsman suffering the delayed effects of a head injury
- Appropriate, urgent assessment, investigation, and management can prevent an even more catastrophic outcome.

Education
- The governing bodies of sports have a duty to educate players about the dangers of aggressive behaviour in their sport and to encourage the ethics of fair play
- The doctors involved in sports must play their part by upholding the laws of the sport and spirit of the game. They must also adhere rigidly to the professional ethics and regulations that govern their medical profession.

Dealing with aggressive or violent athletes

Situations can arise rapidly and unexpectedly in which a doctor will feel threatened by an athlete. It is important that the doctor's own behaviour remain non-aggressive and does not lead to the situation escalating with significant injury to doctor, athlete, anyone else, or damage to property.

The following tips may be helpful:
- Use calm tones
- Use reassuring words
- Body language:
  - The doctor should let his arms hanging down
  - Have the palms turned into an open position
- Move towards an exit and away from aggressor
- Express empathy—e.g. 'I'm sorry you feel like this' or 'I want to understand why you feel like that.'
- Express willingness to help—'Tell me how I can make the situation better.'
- Avoid pointing, confrontation, staring, arguing, or raising one's voice.

Help and restraint

- The doctor must use their discretion as to when to summon help with a panic alarm, phone, or by shouting
- Having sufficient other bodies available will be essential to bring the situation under control if the athlete is intent on violent acts
- Those trained in restraint and crowd control (e.g. the police) would be valuable, although the familiar faces of other squad members or support staff might be more calming to the athlete.

Record keeping

When the doctor has achieved control of the situation, they should make comprehensive notes and involve appropriate other parties, such as:
- Psychiatrist
- Police
- Sports club or governing body officials
- Athlete's family.

There may be situations whereby the confidentiality of the doctor–patient relationship has to be breached. Each case will be unique and the merits and drawbacks of breaking confidentiality must be considered. If there is ethical uncertainty, it is advisable to obtain professional advice (e.g. from one's professional registration body) before deciding how best to proceed.

Summary

- Aggressive and violent behaviour may be present in a sports environment
- Some aggressive acts result from circumstance due to the sport, but others may originate in a mental or physical illness of the athlete
- Sports doctor must prepare themselves to deal with situations where their own well-being is threatened by an aggressive athlete
- Sports doctors must be vigilant for early signs in athletes that might lead to aggressive or violent behaviour.

Chapter 21

Breaking bad news

Introduction *284*
General principles *286*

Chapter 21 Breaking bad news

Introduction

A sports doctor will occasionally be responsible for imparting bad news to an athlete or participant within the sporting arena.

This information can have a significant impact on a patient's fitness to play, general health, or career earnings.

Selected examples include:
- Informing an athlete that they cannot compete in a major competition due to injury
- That their injury is so severe that it may threaten their future involvement in competitive sport.

Although the environment a sports doctor works in may be different from that of a hospital, hospice, or community clinic, the principles of 'breaking bad news' remain the same. The importance of doing this fundamental task well cannot be overstated.

General principles

Prepare ('before')
- Bad news should ideally be communicated in person. Traditionally, this is done by a senior and experienced medical doctor, but that may not always be possible
- It is never a pleasant task, but do not avoid meeting the patient or leave them 'stranded' without any news. Anticipation can be worse than the actual news itself!
- If it is your responsibility to tell the patient and they are not immediately present, ask a receptionist or colleague to contact the patient and make an appointment to see you. (Asking a third person to arrange this appointment ensures that the news does not get 'leaked' if the patient quizzes you, and gives you the opportunity to create an ideal environment beforehand in which to convey the news.)
- Alternatively, it may sometimes be appropriate to call the patient yourself if they already have an inkling of what the problem is and are expecting a telephone call from you
- Follow this up by arranging a subsequent face-to-face discussion to talk about their problems in greater detail
- The patient may like to be accompanied by their coach or family member. Allow them to do so
- If dealing with a child or teenager, it is ideal if you can have the parent/s present when you convey the information. This may not always be possible, e.g. when a child or teenager has travelled to a training camp or competition in a foreign country
- Remember that if you are asked to discuss the medical condition with a concerned third party, e.g. relatives or carers other than the parent or guardian of a child, you must have the patient's consent if he/she is in a position to give it
- Familiarize yourself with the facts as far as possible. If discussing imaging results, consider discussing the imaging investigations in detail with a radiologist beforehand. It can also be valuable to have the images available to show the athlete
- Try to anticipate the types of questions you may be asked and consider how you might answer them. Have a clear plan for dealing with the problem—this may involve a specialist opinion, detailed rehabilitation plans or structured advice for the future
- Ensure a private, quiet environment where possible
- Create 'protected time'
- Turn off your mobile phone or pager
- Do not appear to be in a hurry
- Allow time for the patient and others present to ask questions.

Communicate ('during')

- Establish previous knowledge
  - What does the patient know already?
  - What were they expecting?
- A 'warning shot across the bow' to prepare them may be helpful. This can include phrases such as 'I'm sorry to say it is rather bad news'. Allow a moment for this to sink in
- Establish how much detail the patient wants to know
- Be aware of subtle visual and verbal cues. This is helpful in establishing a rapport and trust if this is the first time the sports doctor is meeting the patient
- Use language that the patient will understand. The level of comprehension will depend upon the age and educational background of the patient, but in general, avoid jargon, technical terms, and abbreviations
- If appropriate, structure the discussion into stages, such as diagnosis, implications, management (and prognosis in the case of patients with a terminal illness. This situation will be rare within a sporting context)
- Be aware that patients often take in only a fraction of the information conveyed to them initially and repetition may be necessary
- It is not essential to cover all aspects in great detail immediately
- Attempt to convey optimism, but still be honest and realistic, especially when dealing with a patient's expectations
- Expect the unexpected:
  - Patients can react in all sorts of ways to receiving bad news
  - Be empathic and do not be judgmental
- Observe to see how the patient is coping, but resist the urge to 'make everything better immediately'. Patients need time to let the news sink in
- Listen to your patient for their thoughts, ideas, and any immediate questions they may have
- Do not expect to deal with everything in one session
- Know when to conclude the consultation. 'Would you like to leave it for now and we can discuss it again when you are feeling ready?' Bear in mind they may wish you to speak to someone else or have someone with them for the next meeting
- Agree the short-term plan and further follow-up.

Conclude ('after')

- Finish with a brief summary and try to conclude on an optimistic note where possible. No matter how bad the news is, it is important that you do not rob the patient of all hope!
- Give appropriate written material or patient information leaflets if you have some available
- Inter-professional communication may be very helpful to ensure the patient is well supported. In the sporting arena, this will usually include coaches, managers, and relevant team staff:
  - Inform other colleagues involved in the patient's care if appropriate, but ensure the athlete's consent is obtained beforehand

- The input of a sports psychologist can be very helpful for aiding the elite athlete in coping with disappointment, injury, and the often arduous process of rehabilitation
- Respect the patient's right to confidentiality at all times
- Some athletes will cope with bad news by 'externalizing' blame—for example, blaming a physiotherapist or other doctor for a delay in diagnosis or what they perceive to be substandard care. Be careful not to 'add fuel to the fire' with careless remarks!
- Record clear and contemporaneous notes of the discussion. You or your colleagues may need to refer to it in future
- Imparting bad news can be an emotional (and often difficult) experience for the doctor, as well as the patient, so take a moment to recognize this and collect your thoughts before moving on to the next task.

Further reading

Knott, L. (2008). *Breaking Bad News.* www.patient.co.uk.

Midgley, S.J., Heather, N., Davis, J.B. (2001). Levels of aggression among a group of anabolic-androgenic steroid users. *Med Sci Law* **41**(4): 309–14.

Pope, H.G.J., Katz, D.L. (1990). Homicide and near-homicide by anabolic steroid users. *J Clin Psychiat* **51**(1): 28–31.

Simpson, C. (2004). When hope makes us vulnerable: a discussion of patient-healthcare provider in-teractions in the context of hope. *Bioethics* **18**(5): 428–47.

Tenenbaum, G.E., Singer R.N, Duda J. (1997). Aggression and violence in sport: an ISSP position stand. *J Sports Med Phys Fitness* **37**(2): 146–50.

VandeKieft, G.K. (2001). Breaking bad news. *Am Fam Physician* **64**(12): 1975–8.

Websites

(2009). Useful resources for UK Health Professionals. *Breaking Bad News.* www.breakingbadnews.co.uk website. 2009.

Chapter 22

Communication

Introduction *292*
Communication: athlete confidentiality *293*
Communication: defining roles *294*
Communication: external opinions *295*
Communication when travelling abroad or to major championships *296*
Communication with the media: press releases *298*
Media interviews *300*

Introduction

Excellent communication skills and the ability to work alongside colleagues are essential qualities for all clinical doctors, particularly those working within the sporting team. Both these skills are specifically mentioned in the General Medical Council (GMC) guidance for doctors *Good Medical Practice*.

The nature of the multidisciplinary team in performance sport necessitates clear strategic direction and definition of individual's roles. Within the sporting environment, the medical team is one part of the overall performance team.

The performance team is the ultimate multidisciplinary team and is often composed of individuals with very different professional, educational, social, and sporting backgrounds. The knowledge and skills of these individuals, all of which are critical to team or athlete success, are not always aligned in fundamental approach. There is also the potential for significant overlap of roles and responsibilities.

Composition of multidisciplinary team in sporting environment

- Athlete
- Coach, manager, selectors
- Strength and conditioning coach
- Administrators
- Sport and exercise medicine physician
- *Therapists:* physiotherapist, chiropractors, osteopaths, soft tissue therapists, others
- Nutritionist
- Physiologist
- Psychologist
- Biomechanist
- Podiatrist
- *External consultants:* radiologists, orthopaedic surgeons, others.

Challenges to effective communication in this environment

- Athlete medical confidentiality
- Lack of defined roles and responsibilities
- Essential requirement for strong relationships of trust between team members
- Ability to travel abroad and spend prolonged periods of time with other team members
- Different medical opinions given to athlete/coach from members within the multidisciplinary team
- Different medical information given to athlete/coach from external medical opinions (solicited or unsolicited)
- Time pressures
- Media requests
- Electronic notes databases.

Communication: athlete confidentiality

As stated in *Good Medical Practice*, patients have 'a right to expect that information about them will be held in confidence by their doctors'. This is fundamental to all medical practice and is essential to maintain the professional integrity and trust of all athletes in the physician's care.

However, disclosure of medical information to non-medical personnel in the multi-disciplinary team is necessary for the performance team to function effectively. There are some practical suggestions for dealing with this issue in the sporting team.

Athlete contracts and consent
- These should state that medical information that impacts on the athlete's ability to perform will be disclosed to the head coach/manager
- The physician should still request consent after each consultation before disclosing medical information to coaches
- Athletes may withdraw consent at any time and for any particular condition. In this case, the doctor should inform the head coach that consent for disclosure has been withdrawn.

Transfer of information
- The relevant medical information should be passed in a secure format to only the individuals that need to know for purposes of team selection or rehabilitation planning
- These individuals should be made aware that information is not to be passed on without further athlete consent and must be stored securely
- Any transfer of information to the media should be done with athlete consent.

Meetings
- Attendance of both the coach and athlete at clinical reviews or at team meetings can be a useful way of involving coaches in receiving medical information
- Regular team meetings between the head coach and lead medical officer are invaluable.

Other athletes
- The medical team must have a private room facility for reviewing patients if desired
- Members of the medical team should never discuss an athlete's medical issues with other athletes or in the patient's absence in communal training or rehabilitation areas
- Professionalism should be maintained at all times.

Communication: defining roles

Multidisciplinary teams in elite sport are usually composed of individuals with enthusiasm and intelligence, diverse skill sets, a passion for the sport and a willingness to perform duties not specifically recognized as part of their job description.

Indeed, this is usually encouraged as part of being an excellent team member. Such energy, passion, and intelligence can, however, lead to individuals offering advice and information regarding another team member's area of expertise.

Although useful and appropriate if channelled skillfully, there are a number of possible –ive consequences. First, the athlete can receive mixed messages, which can be both detrimental to their understanding or their rehabilitation goals. This type of communication can also undermine practitioners in their area of expertise and lead to sub-standard overall care.

Recommendations for good practice can include:
- *Clearly define roles and responsibilities of team members:*
  - With regards to athletes' sustaining a new injury, the role and responsibility of the team doctor might be defined primarily as diagnosis, investigation, and early intervention, or management
  - The physiotherapist's primary role and responsibility may be defined as the rehabilitation or exercise prescription through to return to sport
  - As the team relationships and dynamics evolve and become more sophisticated, both the doctor and the physiotherapist will communicate appropriately with each other to influence each practitioner's primary responsibility
- *Encourage and facilitate discussion within the multidisciplinary team:*
  - Facilitate and support communication within the team with both formal meetings and informal conversations
  - Do not comment directly to athletes regarding issues that come under other team members (coaches or medical practitioners) areas of expertise
  - Individual disagreements should be discussed by the practitioners concerned and within the team, never with the athlete directly.

Communication: external opinions

Effective referral to external consultants is an essential requirement for a medical physician to be successful in an elite sporting environment. It is important to establish excellent communication and relationships.

Two examples are provided; although it is recognized that expertise from other specialties may also be warranted.

Radiologists

- It is useful for the athlete's physician to have an excellent relationship with a small number of local radiologists
- The sports physician should be aware of the individual nuances in reporting
- The sports physician's expectation of the nature of communication from the radiologist should be clearly defined
- To ensure good record keeping, written reports should always be produced and filed in the patient's notes, even if a verbal report has been discussed beforehand with the athlete or athlete's physician
- It is usually inappropriate for the radiologist to communicate with the athlete regarding diagnosis, rehabilitation plans, or healing time frames.

Surgeons

The choice of surgical referral should be made by the athlete's sports physician after discussion with the athlete.

The decision to refer should be based on a number of considerations including:

- Detailed awareness of the procedures the surgeon can offer
- Expertise of the surgeon
- The surgeon's understanding of elite sport and experience with elite athletes
- Accessibility
- The surgeon's ability to communicate appropriately with the athlete and coach, and to involve the managing medical team in decision-making
- It is usually helpful to discuss the referral verbally with the surgeon prior to the consultation. This should be followed with a professional written correspondence. It is ideal that the managing sports physician attends the surgical consultation.

Communication when travelling abroad or to major championships

Major championships and travelling abroad provide many additional pressures that require effective communication within the multidisciplinary team.
- Provision should be made for appropriate written documentation regarding athlete's medical presentations. A database with an on- and offline facility is particularly useful to maintain athlete's medical notes
- Daily clinical meetings are particularly to be recommended:
  - The timing of these will depend on the competition schedule and the timing of the team management meeting
  - If possible, the clinical meeting should directly precede the team management meeting so that the medical representative is fully updated for the team management meeting
- Individual practitioners should communicate their own needs to the leader of the medical team
- Travelling abroad with a team can be an exhausting activity and individuals should be mindful of keeping their productivity and effectiveness high by taking appropriate nutrition, rest, and recovery.

Communication with the media: press releases

Sports physicians working as elite team doctors or governing body medical officers will often come under pressure to divulge medical information about their patients to the media.

An awareness of the requirement for confidentiality and professional obligation to respect it is essential at all times.

If you are asked to provide information about patients, you must:
- Inform patients about the disclosure, or check that they have already received information about it
- Anonymize data where unidentifiable data will serve the purpose
- Be satisfied that patients know about disclosures necessary to provide their care, or for local clinical audit of that care, that they can object to these disclosures, but have not done so
- Seek patients' express consent to disclosure of information, where identifiable data is needed for any purpose other than the provision of care or for clinical audit—save in the exceptional circumstances
- Keep disclosures to the minimum necessary
- Keep up to date with and observe the requirements of statute and common law, including data protection legislation

Sporting organizations vary in their approach to informing the public of the injuries and illnesses that afflict their players. Most appoint media relations officers who will often communicate messages to interested journalists by e-mail.
- The media officer will be tasked to gauge the public perceptions of the organization by reading the newspapers, and listening to interviews and comment on radio and television
- They will also be best placed to advise the medical officer about possible misconceptions.

Doctors may have the opportunity to influence the content of such press releases.
- A proactive approach is recommended for the club doctor who should check the content is accurate and that the wording has the full consent of the player before submitting it
- The doctor should try to anticipate what will happen as a consequence of releasing this information and the press release should be written in a language that is readily understood by the non-medical public
- There is no benefit to the doctor being quoted in the press release
- It is generally better that the statement comes from the organization, club, or governing body.

Consider that club officials (e.g. coach, captain, performance manager, chief executive) and other parties with vested interests (e.g. agents, sponsors) may need to be briefed (with the patient's full consent) before the statement goes public.

The press release should be as complete as possible, because any omissions will attract further questions from curious and usually persistent journalists.

When preparing a press release, consider providing the following information:
- What happened? (circumstances, problem, diagnosis)
- What is happening? (current management)
- What is going to happen? (future management plan)
- How bad is it? (severity/prognosis, i.e. predict missed matches, key events).

Media interviews

Occasionally, the media may want to interview the medical professional looking after an elite sports-person who has become injured or unwell. Should an interview be agreed, the doctor should prepare carefully.

When preparing for interviews with media:
- Request recorded live interviews
- Rehearse and know your intended message well
- Agree with the athlete the information they consent for you to impart in the interview
- Prepare a response to questions that are not anticipated or covered by the athlete's consent, e.g. 'I am not in a position to be able to comment on that at this time'
- Ask the interviewer to brief you on intended questions in advance
- Rehearse with the interviewer, if possible
- Tidy up your appearance
- Consider the proposed interview environment—minimize loud background sounds and sights that may give an unprofessional image.

In the interview (or press conference):
- Look and sound confident
- Repeat your prepared message
- Anticipate potential pitfalls
- Do not breach confidentiality providing information beyond that which is covered by the athlete's consent
- Avoid commenting on unprepared issues. You may need to state and restate, 'I am not in a position to be able to comment on that at this time'.

Further reading

Gregory, P.L., Seah, R., Pollock, N. (2008). What to tell the media—or not: consensus guide-lines for sports physicians. *Br J Sports Med* **42**(10): 485–8.

General Medical Council. (2006). *Good Medical Practice*. London: GMC.

BOA statement. (2000). The British Olympic Association's position statement on athlete confidentiality. *Br J Sports Med* **34**: 71–2.

Index

A

abdomen 175
  anatomy 178-9
  assessment 176
  bleeding, and hypovolaemic shock/sepsis 176
  minor injuries and conditions 192
  non-traumatic emergencies 188
  preparation and risk management 180
  quadrants structure 178
  referred pain 178
  trauma 182
    assessment 182
    investigations 186
    mechanism of injury 182
    specific injuries 183
    surgical intervention 186
  viscera, detecting damaged 176
abductor strain 204
ABLS see adult basic life support (ABLS)
acanthoemoebic keratitis 151
acetabular fractures 202
acetazolamide (Diamox®) 73
actinomycosis 150
acute coronary syndrome see myocardial infarction/acute coronary syndrome (MI/ACS)
acute mountain sickness (AMS) 66, 68
  management 69-70
  symptoms 68
  typical onset 68
adrenaline 29, 97
  cardiac arrest 269
  topical local anaesthetic (LAT) 142
adrenals 179
adult advanced life support (ALS) 28
  advanced airway management 29
  algorithm 28, 30
  arrests, prolonged/non-shockable 29
  automated external defibrillator (AED) 28
  collapsed athlete, assessment of 53
  drugs, IV administration of 28

key points/changes 29
rhythms
  abnormal 28
  shockable versus non-shockable 28, 30
adult basic life support (ABLS) 18, 20
  algorithm 20-1
  cardiac compressions 23-4
  cardiopulmonary resuscitation (CPR) 18
  defibrillation 18, 24
  drowning 24
  head tilt, chin lift 22
  jaw thrust 23
  manual in-line immobilization (MILS) 18
  mouth to mouth resuscitation, risks to rescuer 24
  outcome 1: patient responds 20
  outcome 2: no response 20
  outcome 1: patient breathing normally 20
  outcome 2: not breathing normally 20
  rescue breaths 24
  sudden cardiac death 18
  see also paediatric basic life support (PBLS)
advanced airway management 29, 134
AED see automated external defibrillator (AED)
aggression 277
  competition, and sport 278
  dealing with 281
    confidentiality 281
    help and restraint 281
    record keeping 281
  definition of 279
  explanations for 279
    assertive behaviour, definition of 279
    confusion 279
    emotions 279
    mental illness 279
    misunderstanding 279
    personality types 279
  prevention of 280
    early warning signs 280
    education 280
    facilities, suitable 280
airway injuries 129

advanced airway management 134
  endo-tracheal (ET) intubation 134
  laryngeal mask airway (LMA) 134
  surgical airway techniques 135
face injuries 131
incidence of 130
management of 134
  ABC assessment 134
  airway adjuncts 134
  basic manoeuvres 134
neck injuries 131
presentation of 132
  agitation/respiratory distress 132
  facial soft tissue trauma 132
airway management see advanced airway management
allergens, common 96
allergy, versus anaphylaxis 96
ALS see adult advanced life support (ALS)
altitude sickness 66
  acute mountain sickness (AMS) 66, 68
  altitude, definition of 66
  barometric pressure 66
  differential diagnosis 67
  high altitude cerebral oedema (HACE) 66, 71
  high altitude pulmonary oedema (HAPE) 66, 72
  key learning points 74
  normal physiology, and altitude 67
  prevention 67
  risk factors 74
amenorrhoea 49
amiodarone 29, 110
AMS see acute mountain sickness (AMS)
anaemia, and arthritis 48
anaphylactoid reaction, versus anaphylaxis 96
anaphylaxis 94, 96, 258
  allergens, common 96
  versus allergy 96
  versus anaphylactoid reaction 96

clinical manifestations 96
management of 97
  adrenaline 97
  chlorphenamine 97
  hydrocortisone 97
  IV fluid challenge 97
ankle injuries 240
  ankle dislocation 241
  ankle fractures 240
    lateral and posterior talar process fractures 241
    lateral malleolus 240
    medial malleolus 240
    talar dome osteochondral injuries 240
    talar stress fractures 241
  ligament injuries 243
    deltoid injuries 243
    lateral ligament injuries 243
  Ottawa foot and ankle guidelines 249
  syndesmosis injuries 244
  tendon injuries 242
    Achilles tendon rupture 242
    tibialis posterior dislocation 243
    tibialis posterior ruptures 242
anomalous coronary artery origins 80, 87
anterior cord syndrome 159
aortic dissection 104
aortic rupture 81
apophysitis 208
appendicitis 188
arrhythmnogenic right ventricular dysplasia 81
arrythmias 42
arthritis 48
  and anaemia 48
  ankylosing spondylitis 48
  rheumatoid arthritis 48
assertive behaviour, definition of 279
assessment, of athlete 11
  evaluation, continuing 15
  extremity trauma 16
  initial assessment 12–16
  log roll 15
  preparation 12
  rapid assessment, and synchronous resuscitation 12
    A: assess the airway 13
    B: assess the breathing 13
    C: assess the circulation 14

D: assess neurological disability 14
E: expose the patient 14
asthma
  acute exacerbations of 94
    acute asthma, treatment of 95
    differential diagnosis 94
    life-threatening exacerbation 95
    moderate exacerbation 94
    severe exacerbation 94
    triggers, common 94
  in children 260
    acute asthma, treatment of 260
    acute severe and life-threatening features 261
    differential diagnosis 260
    hospital referral, criteria for 260
    incidence of 260
    management 260
    presentation 260
  exercise-induced asthma (EIA) 36, 94
  pre-existing 36
asystole 28
athletic pseudonephritis 193
atropine 28
automated external defibrillator (AED) 7, 26, 28
autonomic dysreflexia 274–5
  causes of 275
    in bladder 275
    in bowel 275
    other causes 275
    in skin 275
  signs of 274
  symptoms of 274
  treatment 275
avulsion fractures, pelvic 208

B

back pain, acute disk prolapse 162
bad news, breaking 283, 287
  communication 287
  conclusion 287
  importance of 284
  preparation 286
Barton's fracture 222
basic life support see adult basic life support (ABLS); paediatric basic life support (PBLS)
Bennett's fracture dislocation 226

benzodiazepine 98, 262
bladder, autonomic dysreflexia in 275
blood disorders 185
blood pressure
  children, and systolic BP 254
  pulse, and systolic BP 14
  see also hypertension; hypotension
bowel
  autonomic dysreflexia in 275
  trauma 179, 184
bradyarrhythmia 161
breath, shortness of see shortness of breath (SOB), acute onset
Brown sequard 159
bullying 256
bursitis 208
  iliopsoas bursitis 208
  trochanteric bursitis 208

C

CAD see coronary artery disease (CAD)
calcaneal fractures 246
cardiac compressions 23–4
cardiac death, sudden 77
  acquired 81
    ischaemic heart disease 81
    post-viral cardiomyopathy 81
  aetiology 80
  congenital 80
    anomalous coronary artery origins 80
    aortic rupture 81
    arrhythmnogenic right ventricular dysplasia 81
    hypertrophic cardiomyopathy (HOCM) 80
    idiopathic concentric left ventricle (LV) hyptertrophy 80
    long QT 80
    valvular disease 81
    Wolff–Parkinson–White 80
  epidemiology 78
    hypertrophic cardiomyopathy 78
    ischaemic heart disease 78
    screening 78
  management 86
    anticipation 86
    defibrillator access 86

INDEX

equipment requirements 86
presentation 82
  under 35-year-olds 82
  over 35-year-olds 82
prevention 87
  exercising, and viral illness 87
  pathology and treatments 87
screening 84
  electrocardiogram (ECG) 85
  screening tools 84
  team screening 84
  Veneto experience, northern Italy 84
cardiac tamponade 173
cardiopulmonary resuscitation (CPR) 18, 26
  see also pitch side resuscitation bag
cardiorespiratory arrest 17
  adult advanced life support (ALS) 28
  adult basic life support (ABLS) 18, 20
  critical care incidents, planning for 31
  paediatric basic life support 26
cardiovascular disease 42
  conduction disturbances (arrythmias) 42
  coronary artery disease (CAD) 42
caudia equina syndrome 162
cauliflower ear 142
cellulitis 150
central cord syndrome 159
cerebral hyperthermia 56
cerebral oedema 62
cerebral palsy 39
  classification of 39, 39
  considerations 39
  management 39
cerebral swelling, diffuse 125
cervical spine clearance, NEXUS criteria 117, 158
cheekbone fractures 146
chest pain emergencies 102
  non-pleuritic causes 103
    aortic dissection 104
    myocardial infarction/acute coronary syndrome (MI/ACS) 103
  pleuritic causes, potential 102
    musculoskeletal 103
    pericarditis 102
child protection 257

children see paediatrics
chlorphenamine 97
choking child 258
  differential diagnosis 258
  management 258–9
cholecystitis, acute 188
clavicular injuries 212
  acromio-clavicular injury 212
  assessment 212
  clavicular fractures 212
  sterno-clavicular injury 212
  treatment 213
collapse, during exercise 5, 51, 54
  altitude sickness 66
  assessment principles 53–4
    blood sodium 53
    early symptoms and signs 53
    hydration status 53
    loss of consciousness 53
    rectal temperature 53
    site of collapse 53
  collapsed athlete, assessment of 53
  exercise-associated hyponatraemia (EAH) 62
  heatstroke 56
  hypothermia 58
  specific causes 52
  treatment 54
Colle's fracture 222
communication 291
  abroad/major championships, travelling to 296
  aggression, explanations for 279
  bad news, breaking 287
  confidentiality 293, 298
  effective communication, challenges to 292
  external opinions 295
  importance of 292
  media, communication with 298
  multidisciplinary teams 292, 294
  planning and preparation 6
  roles, defining 294
compartment syndrome, of the foot 247
competition, and sport 278
concussion 122
  definition of 122
  diagnosis of 122
  features of 122
  history 123
  return to play (RTP) protocol 123–4

see also head injuries
confidentiality 293
  aggression, dealing with 281
  athlete contracts, and consent 293
  media, communication with 298
  meetings 293
  other athletes 293
  transfer of information 293
conjunctivitis 151
consciousness see loss of consciousness
consent
  confidentiality 293
  disability, athletes with 273
coronary artery disease (CAD) 42
CPR see cardiopulmonary resuscitation (CPR)
cricothyroidotomy 135
critical care incidents, planning for 31
  courses 31
  defibrillator, availability of 31

D

deep vein thrombosis (DVT) 100
defibrillators 18, 31, 86
  see also automated external defibrillator (AED)
dental injuries 144
  avulsed teeth 144
  dentoalveolar injuries 144
  displaced teeth 144
  fractured teeth 144
dexamethasone 73
diabetes mellitus 34
  description and incidence of 34
  diabetes management 35
  and exercise 35
  glucose regulation, impaired 34
  hyperglycaemia 92
  hypoglycaemia 90
  and infection 35
  insulin 34
diabetic ketoacidosis (DKA) 92
diagnostic peritoneal lavage (DPL) 186
diaphragm trauma 183
diazepam 269
disability, athletes with 271
  autonomic dysreflexia 274

disability, athletes with (cont.)
  comorbidity 273
  consent 273
  field of play recovery 273
  impairment groups, understanding 272–3
  injuries, nature of 273
  prosthesis, injury from 273
  regulations 273
  special considerations 273
  specialist equipment 273
  sport types 272
  stump skin care 273
  treatment principles 272
disc prolapse, acute 162
DKA see diabetic ketoacidosis (DKA)
drowning 24
drugs
  controlled, problematic nature of 9
  doses, in children 269
  hypertension treatments 44
  world antidoping agency 36
duodenum/small bowel trauma 179
duty of care 2
DVT see deep vein thrombosis (DVT)
dysreflexia see autonomic dysreflexia

E

EAH see exercise-associated hyponatraemia (EAH)
eating disorders 49
ECG see electrocardiogram (ECG)
ectopic pregnancy 206
elbow injuries 218
  dislocation 218
  fractures 218
    olecranon fracture 219
    radial head/neck fractures 218
    supracondylar fractures 218
electrocardiogram (ECG) 84–5
encephalitis 107
endo-tracheal (ET) intubation 134
endurance events 4–5
Entonox® 16
environmental conditions 4
epilepsy 38
  generalized 38
  grand mal 38

  partial 38
  petit mal 38
  status epilepticus, definition of 262
  see also seizures
epiphyseal fracture 255
equipment 6
  kit, assembling own 9
  pitch side resuscitation bag 6–7
  sudden cardiac death 86
  world antidoping agency (WADA) code 6–7
ethical responsibilities 2
European Resuscitation Control Guidelines (2010) 18, 20
exercise-associated collapse (EAC) see collapse, during exercise
exercise-associated hyponatraemia (EAH) 62
  assessment 62
  notes 63
  prevention 63
  pulmonary and cerebral oedema 62
  risk factors 62
  treatment 63
exercise-induced asthma (EIA) 94
extradural haematomas 125
eye injuries 143, 151
  acanthoemoebic keratitis 151
  conjunctivitis 151

F

face injuries 131
  see also maxillofacial injuries
falling onto an outstretched hand (FOOSH), reflex reaction 210
  clavicular fractures 212
  elbow injuries 220
  shoulder fractures 215
  shoulder injuries 214
  wrist injuries 222–3
female athlete triad 49
  amenorrhoea 49
  eating disorders 49
  osteopenia 49
femoral fractures 230
fibular fractures 238
flail segment 172
focused assessment with tomography for trauma (FAST) 186
FOOSH see falling onto an outstretched hand (FOOSH), reflex reaction

foot care, and diabetes mellitus 35
foot injuries 246
  fractures 246
    anterior calcaneal process fracture 246
    base of fifth metatarsal fractures 246
    calcaneal fractures 246
    calcaneal stress fractures 247
    navicular stress fractures 247
    Lisfranc fracture dislocation (tarsometatarsal joint) 247
  Ottawa foot and ankle guidelines 249
  sesamoid injuries 248
    fractures 248
    sasamoiditis 248
forearm injuries 220
  dislocations 220
    Galeazzi fracture dislocation 220
    Monteggia fracture dislocation 220
  fractures 220
    both radial and ulnar shaft fractures 220
    isolated radial shaft fracture 220
    isolated ulnar shaft fracture 220
  thumb injuries 226
    Bennett's fracture dislocation 226
    ulnar collateral ligament rupture 226
frontal bone fracture (maxillofacial) 148

G

Galeazzi fracture dislocation 220
gallbladder 179
gastrocnemius injury 239
gastrointestinal complaints 192
general medical emergencies 89
  anaphylaxis 96
  asthma, acute exacerbations of 94
  chest pain emergencies 102
  diabetes mellitus 90
  headache, emergency causes of 106
    non-traumatic causes 106
    traumatic causes 106

metabolic acidosis 101
palpitations 108
seizures 98
shortness of breath (SOB), acute onset 100
genitourinary trauma 184
Gilmore's groin 207
Glasgow Coma Scale 116, 157, 267
best motor response 116
best verbal response 116
eye opening 116

H

HACE see high altitude cerebral oedema (HACE)
haematomas
extradural 125
intracerebral 126
muscle/SC haematoma, significance of 185
septal 146
subdural 125
subperichondral to the ear (cauliflower ear) 142
haemothorax 171
hamstring strain 205
hand injuries 224
dislocations 225
flexor tendon rupture 225
fractures 224
treatment 224
distal phalangeal fractures 224
metacarpal fractures 224
proximal and middle phalangeal fractures 224
volar plate injuries 225
mallet injuries 225
HAPE see high altitude pulmonary oedema (HAPE)
HCM see hypertrophic cardiomyopathy (HCM)
head injuries 113
background 114
hypotension, avoiding 114
incidence 114
outcomes 114
children 267
incidence of 267
initial assessment 267
management 267
concussion 122
diffuse cerebral swelling 125
extradural haematomas 125
intracerebral haematomas 126
minor head injury 118

advice 119
assessment 118
classification 118
Modified Maddock's questions 118–19
significant head injury 119
pitchside assessment 116
pitchside equipment 115
pre-event preparation 115
scalp injuries 126
significant head injury 120
subdural haematomas 125
headache, emergency causes of 106
non-traumatic causes 106
history red flags 106
hypertensive crisis 107
meningitis/encephalitis 107
subarachnoid haemorrhage 106
temporal arteritis 107
traumatic causes 106
heart failure 45
see also cardiac death, sudden
heatstroke 4, 56
assessment 56
cerebral hyperthermia 56
heat gain and loss, causes of 56–7
treatment 56
hernia, sports 207
herpes gladiatorum ('scrumpox') 150
herpes simplex virus 152
herpes zoster virus infection ('shingles') 150
high altitude cerebral oedema (HACE) 66, 71
management 70–1
symptoms and signs 71
typical onset 71
high altitude pulmonary oedema (HAPE) 66, 72
drugs 73
management 70, 72
pathophysiology 73
symptoms/signs 68, 72
typical onset 72
Hillsborough disaster 4
hip
anatomy 197
dislocation 202
examination 203
initial management 203
return to play 203
see also pelvic trauma
hip flexor strain 205
HOCM see hypertrophic obstructive cardiomyopathy (HOCM)

hydrocortisone 97
hyperglycaemia 92
diabetic ketoacidosis (DKA) 92
doctor, considerations for 92
hyperosmolar complications 92
metabolic acidosis 92
hypertension 43
assessment 43
blood pressure levels, classification of 43
drug treatments 44
management 44
hypertensive crisis 107
hyperthermia 56
hypertrophic cardiomyopathy (HCM) 78, 80, 84, 87
hypertrophic obstructive cardiomyopathy (HOCM) 46
hypoglycaemia 90
blood glucose measurement 90
doctor, considerations for 91
insulin-dependent athlete, considerations for 91
loss of consciousness 90
symptoms and signs 90
hyponatraemia see exercise-associated hyponatraemia (EAH)
hypotension, avoiding in head injuries 114
hypothermia 5, 58
assessment of 58–9
further notes 60
neurological changes 58
physiological effects 58
risk factors 58
treatment of 59
mild 59
moderate 59
severe 60
hypovolaemic shock
bleeding 176
children 254
see also shock

I

ibuprofen 269
idiopathic concentric left ventricle (LV) hypertrophy 80
inflammatory bowel disease (IBD) 189
insulin 34
intestinal obstruction 189
paralytic ileus 189
strangulated hernia 189

INDEX **307**

intracerebral haematomas 126
ion channelopathies 87
  long QT syndrome 87
  Wolff–Parkinson–White syndrome 87
ischaemic heart disease 78, 81

K

kidneys 179
knee injuries 232
  dislocations 232
    knee 232
    patellar dislocations/subluxations 233
  fractures 232
    patellar fractures 232
    tibial plateau fractures 232
  ligament injuries 235
    anterior cruciate ligament injuries 235
    Lachman's test 235
    lateral collateral ligament injuries 236
    medial collateral ligament injuries 236
    posterior cruciate ligament injuries 236
  meniscal injuries 234
  tendon ruptures 234
    patellar tendon ruptures 234
    quadriceps tendon ruptures 234

L

Lachman's test 235
laryngeal mask airway (LMA) 134
larynx, injuries to 131
LAT see topical local anaesthetic (LAT)
leg injuries 238
  fractures 238
    fibular stress fractures 239
    Maisonneurve fracture 238
    stress fracture of the tibia 238
    tibular and fibular fractures 238
  muscle injury 239
    gastrocnemius 239
    soleus 239
lignocaine 142
limping, child 251
  causes 264
    by age 264
  examination 265
  history 265
  investigations 265
  management 264
  Perthes' disease 266
  septic arthritis 265
  slipped upper femoral capital epiphysis 266
  transient synovitis of the hip 266
Lisfranc fracture dislocation 247
liver 179
  failure, acute 188
  trauma 183
long QT syndrome 80, 87
lorazepam 269
loss of consciousness
  collapse, during exercise 53
  consciousness, checking for 12
  head injuries, pitchside assessment of 117
  hypoglycaemia 90
  see also Glasgow Coma Scale; head injuries
lower limb injury 227
  ankle injuries 240
  foot injuries 246
  incidence of 228
  knee injuries 232
  leg injuries 238
  thigh injuries 230

M

magnetic resonance imaging (MRI) 84
Maisonneurve fracture 238
mallet injuries 225
mandibular dislocation 147
mandibular fractures 147
manual in-line immobilization (MILS) 18, 156
marathons 4
maxillary fractures 148
  Le Fort classification of 148
maxillofacial injuries 137
  ABC with cervical spine control assessment 138
  anatomy, facial 139
  dental injuries 144
  incidence of 138
  management
    principles 140
    examination 140
    facial nerve assessment 140–1
    history 140
  maxillofacial fractures 146
    frontal bone fracture 148
    mandibular dislocation 147
    mandibular fractures 147
    maxillary fractures 148
    nasal fractures 146
    orbital fractures 147
    zygomatic fractures 146
  medical maxillofacial emergencies 150
    eye 151
    mouth 151
    sinuses 152
    skin 150
  soft tissue injuries 142
    abrasions 142
    eye injuries 143
    haematomas 142
    lacerations 142
    mouth injuries 143
    tetanus prone wounds 138
    wound cleaning 138
MD see muscular dystrophy (MD)
media officers 298
Medical Defence Union (MDU) 2
meningitis 107
meniscal injuries 234
mental illness, and aggression 279
metabolic acidosis 92, 101
metacarpal fractures 224
metatarsal fractures 246
MI/ACS see myocardial infarction/acute coronary syndrome (MI/ACS)
MILS see manual in-line immobilization (MILS)
Monteggia fracture dislocation 220
morphine IV 269
mountain sickness see acute mountain sickness (AMS)
mouth emergencies 151
  herpes simplex virus 152
  toothache 151
  ulcers 152
  wisdom teeth 151
mouth injuries 143
mouth to mouth resuscitation, risks to rescuer 24
MRI see magnetic resonance imaging (MRI)
multidisciplinary teams
  communication 292, 294

INDEX

composition of 5, 292, 294
muscle/SC haematoma, significance of 185
muscular dystrophy (MD) 41
myocardial infarction/acute coronary syndrome (MI/ACS) 103

N

nasal cavities, injury to 130
nasal fractures 146
neck injuries 131
neurogenic shock 161
neurological/neuromuscular disorders 38
  cerebral palsy 39
  epilepsy 38
  muscular dystrophy (MD) 41
  Parkinson's disease 39
NEXUS clinical criteria, for c-spine clearance 117, 158
nifedipine 73

O

olecranon fracture 219
open pneumothorax 172
opiates 16
oral cavities, injury to 131
orbital fractures 147
osteitis pubis 207
osteopenia 49
Ottowa foot and ankle guidelines 249

P

paediatric basic life support (PBLS) 26
  ABC approach 26–7
  outcome 1: patient responds 26
  outcome 2: no response 26
paediatrics 251
  asthma 260
  child protection 257
  choking child 258
  drug doses, in children 269
  head injury 267
  limping child 251
  pathological features, of children 255
  physical (anatomical) features, of children 253
    growth rates 253
    injury rates 253
    medication, and body weight 253
  physiological features, of children 254
    brain physiology 254
    heart rate 254
    respiratory rate 254
    systolic BP 254
  psychological features, of children 256
  seizures 262
  see also asthma, in children
palpitations 108
  examination 108
  history 108
  investigation 108
  management of 109–10
  recurrent supraventricular tachycardias (SVT) 108
pancreas, trauma to 179, 183
pancreatitis 189
paracetamol 269
paralytic ileus 189
Parkinson's disease 39
patellar dislocations/ subluxations 233
patellar fractures 232
peak expiratory flow rate (PEFR) 95
pelvic trauma 195
  acute pelvic pain, causes of 206
  anatomy 197
    hip, muscles of 197
    hip and pelvis 197
  assessment 198
    examination 198
    history 198
  diagnosis of 196
  dislocation of hip 202
    examination 203
    initial management 203
    return to play 203
  fractures 204
    acetabular fractures 202
    avulsion fractures 201–2
    complications 205
    initial management 203
    loading forces causing 200
    pelvic ring fractures 204
    sacral fractures 201
    stress fractures 202
    treatment 205
  incidence of 196
  soft tissue injuries 204

contusions 230
strains 204
percutaneous needle cricothyroidotomy 135
pericarditis 102
peripheral vascular disease 44
Perthes' disease 266
phalangeal fractures 224
pitch side resuscitation bag 6–7
planning and preparation 1
  communication 6
  documentation 9
  duty of care 2
  environmental conditions 4
  equipment and medication 6
  ethical responsibilities 2
  indemnity 10
  medical personnel required 5
  participants 2
  preparation 2
  responsibilities 3
  security/identification 10
  sports type 2
  transportation 6
  venue 4
plastic bowing 255
pneumonia 94, 101
pneumothorax 94, 169
  and diving 170
  spontaneous 169
  tension pneumothorax 170
  treatment 170
    needle decompression, right tension pneumothorax 170–1
post-viral cardiomyopathy 81
pre-existing conditions, athletes with 33
  arthritis 48
  cardiovascular conditions 42
  diabetes mellitus 34
  female athlete triad 49
  neurological and neuromuscular disorders 38
  respiratory conditions 36
pseudonephritis, athletic 193
pulmonary contusion 173
pulmonary embolism 94, 100
pulmonary oedema 62, 94, 100
pulse, and systolic BP 14

pulseless electrical activity (PEA) 28

R

radial fractures 220
radial head/neck fractures (elbow) 220
record keeping
  aggression, dealing with 281
  documentation 9
rectus abdominis injury 185
renal trauma 184
rescue breaths 24
respiratory conditions, pre-existing 36
resuscitation see cardiopulmonary resuscitation (CPR)
return to play (RTP) protocol
  concussion 123–4
  head injury, children 268
  pelvic trauma 203
rib fractures 168
rotator cuff injuries 216

S

sacral fractures 201
salbutamol 36
salmeterol 36
scaphoid fractures 222
screening, cardiac 84
  electrocardiogram (ECG) 84–5
  family history 84
  magnetic resonance imaging (MRI) 84
  screening tools 84
  symptoms and signs 84
  team screening 84
  Veneto experience, northern Italy 84
'scrumpox' (herpes gladiatorum) 150
seizures 98
  ambulance, when to call 98
  children 262
    ambulance, when to call 262
    causes of in children 262
    management 262–3
    medications 262
  management 38, 98
  medications 98
  status epilepticus 98
septal haematomas 146
septic arthritis 265
sesamoid injuries 248

'shingles' (herpes zoster virus infection) 150
shock 14
  children 254
  cord injury 161
  hypovolaemic 176
shortness of breath (SOB), acute onset 100
  pneumonia 101
  pulmonary embolism 100
  pulmonary oedema 100
shoulder injuries 214
  dislocations 214
    anterior dislocation 214
    inferior dislocation 215
    methods of reduction 214
    posterior dislocation 215
    treatment 214
  rotator cuff injuries 216
  shoulder fractures 215
    neck of humerus fractures 215
    scapula fracture 215
    shaft of humerus fractures 216
sinuses 152
  sinusitis 152
skin emergencies 150
  actinomycosis 150
  autonomic dysreflexia 275
  cellulitis 150
  herpes gladiatorum ('scrumpox') 150
  herpes zoster virus infection ('shingles') 150
  spots and lesions 150
  wounds 192
skin irritation 192
slipped upper femoral epiphysis 206, 266
Smith's fracture 222
soleus injury 239
spectator first aid cover 3
spinal injuries 153
  back pain, acute disk prolapse 162
  cervical spine, 'clearing' 158
  cord injury 161
    neurogenic shock/ bradyarrhythmia 161
    spinal shock 161
  cord injury complications 160
  definitions 154
  equipment and training, essential 155
  neurological signs, recognising 159
  pitchside care 156
    airway assessment, with cervical spine control 156

athlete extraction 157
manual in-line stabilisation (MILS) 156
primary spinal cord injury 154
recognition of 154
secondary spinal cord injury 154
spleen, trauma to 179, 183
sports hernia (Gilmore's groin) 207
spots and lesions, skin 150
St John's Ambulance volunteers 3
sternal fractures 173
stitch 192
stomach, trauma to 179, 183
strangulated hernia 189
subarachnoid haemorrhage 106
subdural haematomas 125
subperichondral haematomas to the ear (cauliflower ear) 142
supracondylar fractures 220
supraventricular tachycardias (SVT) 108
syndesmosis injuries 244

T

tachycardia
  abdomen trauma 182
  palpitations, management of 109–10
  recurrent supraventricular tachycardias (SVT) 108
talar fractures 240
tatracaine 142
temporal arteritis 107
tension pneumothorax 170
testicular torsion 206
  signs 207
  symptoms 207
  treatment 207
tetanus prone wounds 138
thigh injuries 230
  femoral fractures 230
  hamstring origin avulsion 230
  muscle injuries 231
    classification of 231
    emergency treatment 231
    quadriceps contusion 231
thirst mechanism 63
thorax 163
  anatomy 165
  preparation and risk management 166
  history 166

standard medical equipment 166
trauma 164, 168
  assessment 168
  cardiac tamponade 173
  flail segment 172
  haemothorax 171
  open pneumothorax 172
  pneumothorax 169
  pulmonary contusion 173
  rib fractures 168
  sternal fractures 173
thumb injuries 226
tibial plateau fractures 232
tibialis posterior dislocation 243
tibialis posterior ruptures 242
tibular fractures 238
toothache 151
topical local anaesthetic (LAT) 142
Torus (Buckle) fracture 255
trachea, injuries to 131
transient synovitis of the hip 266

U

ulcers 152
ulnar fractures 220

United Nations Convention on the Rights of a Child 252
upper gastrointestinal bleed 190
upper limb injury 209
  clavicular injuries 212
  elbow injuries 220
  FOOSH, reflex reaction 210
  forearm injuries 220
  hand injuries 224
  shoulder injuries 214
  upper limb, direct blows to 210
  wrist injuries 222
ureters 179

V

valvular cardiac disease 81
vasculature 179
ventricular fibrillation (VF) 28
ventricular tachycardia (VT) 28
violence see aggression
volar plate injuries 225

W

wet bulb globe temperature index (WBGT) 4, 57

winding 192
wisdom teeth 151
Wolff–Parkinson–White syndrome 80, 87
world antidoping agency (WADA)
  code, and equipment 6–7
  insulin 34
  salbutamol 36
  salmeterol 36
wound cleaning 138
wrist injuries 222
  dislocation 223
    lunate dislocation 223
    peri-lunate dislocation 223
  fractures 222
    Barton's fracture 222
    Colle's fracture 222
    distal radius and ulna fractures 222
    scaphoid fractures 222
    Smith's fracture 222

Z

zygomatic fractures 146

OXFORD MEDICAL PUBLICATIONS

Oxford Handbook of Sport and Exercise Medicine

Published and forthcoming Oxford Handbooks

Oxford Handbook of Midwifery 2e
Edited by Janet Medforth, Susan Battersby, Maggie Evans, Beverley Marsh, and Angela Walker

Oxford Handbook of Adult Nursing
Edited by George Castledine and Ann Close

Oxford Handbook of Cancer Nursing
Edited by Mike Tadman and Dave Roberts

Oxford Handbook of Cardiac Nursing
Edited by Kate Johnson and Karen Rawlings-Anderson

Oxford Handbook of Children's and Young People's Nursing
Edited by Edward Alan Glasper, Gillian McEwing, and Jim Richardson

Oxford Handbook of Clinical Skills for Children's and Young People's Nursing
Edited by Paula Dawson, Louise Cook, Laura-Jane Holliday, and Helen Reddy

Oxford Handbook of Clinical Skills in Adult Nursing
Edited by Jacqueline Randle, Frank Coffey, and Martyn Bradbury

Oxford Handbook of Critical Care Nursing
Sheila K Adam and Sue Osborne

Oxford Handbook of Dental Nursing
Edited by Elizabeth Boon, Rebecca Parr, Dayananda Samarawickrama, and Kevin Seymour

Oxford Handbook of Diabetes Nursing
Edited by Lorraine Avery and Sue Beckwith

Oxford Handbook of Emergency Nursing
Edited by Robert Crouch, Alan Charters, Mary Dawood, and Paula Bennett

Oxford Handbook of Gastrointestinal Nursing
Edited by Christine Norton, Julia Williams, Claire Taylor, Annmarie Nunwa, and Kathy Whayman

Oxford Handbook of Learning and Intellectual Disability Nursing
Edited by Bob Gates and Owen Barr

Oxford Handbook of Mental Health Nursing
Edited by Patrick Callaghan and Helen Waldock

Oxford Handbook of Musculoskeletal Nursing
Edited by Susan Oliver

Oxford Handbook of Neuroscience Nursing
Edited by Sue Woodward and Catheryne Waterhouse

Oxford Handbook of Nursing Older People
Edited by Beverley Tabernacle, Marie Honey, and Annette Jinks

Oxford Handbook of Orthopaedic and Trauma Nursing
Rebecca Jester, Julie Santy, and Jean Rogers

Oxford Handbook of Perioperative Practice
Edited by Suzanne Hughes and Andy Mardell

Oxford Handbook of Prescribing for Nurses and Allied Health Professionals 2e
Edited by Sue Beckwith and Penny Franklin

Oxford Handbook of Primary Care and Community Nursing
Edited by Vari Drennan and Claire Goodman

Oxford Handbook of Respiratory Nursing
Edited by Terry Robinson and Jane Scullion

Oxford Handbook of Women's Health Nursing
Edited by Sunanda Gupta, Debra Holloway, and Ali Kubba

Oxford Handbook of Sport and Exercise Medicine

Second edition

Edited by

Domhnall MacAuley
Specialist in Sport and Exercise Medicine and visiting Professor at the University of Ulster. Editor (Primary Care) at the BMJ

OXFORD
UNIVERSITY PRESS

OXFORD
UNIVERSITY PRESS

Great Clarendon Street, Oxford, OX2 6DP,
United Kingdom

Oxford University Press is a department of the University of Oxford.
It furthers the University's objective of excellence in research, scholarship,
and education by publishing worldwide. Oxford is a registered trade mark of
Oxford University Press in the UK and in certain other countries

© Oxford University Press 2013

The moral rights of the authors have been asserted

First Edition published in 2007

Second Edition published in 2013

Impression: 1

All rights reserved. No part of this publication may be reproduced, stored in
a retrieval system, or transmitted, in any form or by any means, without the
prior permission in writing of Oxford University Press, or as expressly permitted
by law, by licence or under terms agreed with the appropriate reprographics
rights organization. Enquiries concerning reproduction outside the scope of the
above should be sent to the Rights Department, Oxford University Press, at the
address above

You must not circulate this work in any other form
and you must impose this same condition on any acquirer

British Library Cataloguing in Publication Data

Data available

Library of Congress Cataloging in Publication Data

Library of Congress Control Number: 2012940770

ISBN 978-0-19-966015-5

Printed in China by
C&C Offset Printing Co., Ltd.

Oxford University Press makes no representation, express or implied, that the
drug dosages in this book are correct. Readers must therefore always check
the product information and clinical procedures with the most up-to-date
published product information and data sheets provided by the manufacturers
and the most recent codes of conduct and safety regulations. The authors and
the publishers do not accept responsibility or legal liability for any errors in the
text or for the misuse or misapplication of material in this work. Except where
otherwise stated, drug dosages and recommendations are for the non-pregnant
adult who is not breast-feeding

Links to third party websites are provided by Oxford in good faith and
for information only. Oxford disclaims any responsibility for the materials
contained in any third party website referenced in this work.

Contents

Foreword to first edition *vii*
Foreword to second edition *ix*
Preface to first edition *xi*
Acknowledgements *xii*
Contributors *xiii*
Symbols and Abbreviations *xvii*

1	Immediate care	**1**
2	Sports injury	**35**
3	Physiotherapy and rehabilitation	**65**
4	Benefits of exercise	**95**
5	Exercise physiology	**123**
6	Metabolic	**171**
7	Aids to performance	**197**
8	Disability	**213**
9	Arthritis	**227**
10	Cardiorespiratory	**259**
11	Infectious disease	**311**
12	Dermatology	**323**
13	Women	**351**
14	Older people	**371**
15	Head and face	**383**
16	Spine	**423**
17	Shoulder	**455**
18	Elbow and forearm	**503**
19	Wrist and hand	**529**
20	Abdomen	**547**

21	Hip and pelvis	559
22	Knee	619
23	Ankle and lower leg	649
24	Foot	685
25	The team physician	711

Index *741*

Foreword to first edition

The excellent authoritative *Oxford Handbook of Sport and Exercise Medicine* is published at a singularly appropriate time. The Government has just, belatedly many think, recognized an NHS Faculty of Sport and Exercise Medicine. The new Faculty was launched at the Royal College of Physicians by HRH Princess Royal, herself an Olympic equestrian medallist now having a daughter with equal equestrian achievements.

It is fortunate that Professor Domhnall MacAuley has agreed to edit this remarkable volume. To his credit he has been one of the leaders of the campaign for the Faculty as well as advancing sports medicine practice and teaching (and is now a Senior Editor with the *BMJ*). He is to be congratulated on this book, which although rather modestly described as a handbook, is in fact a comprehensive encyclopaedia of sport and exercise medicine. Its layout and indexing make it a quickly accessible practical guide to all sports injuries both common and rare. It will be welcomed by all sports medicine practitioners, both doctors and all the others in allied professions like physiotherapy. It is a worthy successor to the *Oxford Textbook of Sports Medicine*, first published by Oxford University Press in 1994 under the editorship of Mark Harries, then physician to the British Olympic Medical Centre, with his colleagues Clyde Williams, William Stanish, and Lyle Michaeli.

You may ask why official recognition of sport and exercise medicine is so important. The reason is that, by its very nature, sports medicine is a polymorphous animal comprising an unusually large number of disparate and loosely-linked subspecialties: respiratory and cardiac physiology and medicine, physical medicine, physiotherapy, and orthopaedics to name but a few. For the past 50 years it has not been possible to create an overall umbrella body within which all can co-operate and work together. The faculty will now do just this. Though the success of joining the pantheon of 70 recognized specialties is a triumph in itself, it is only the beginning: more NHS posts are needed, more skilled accident and emergency (A&E) sports medicine trained staff. Also recognized is the inclusion of sports medicine in qualifying and advanced examinations. A significant victory has been advanced, but many more battles lie ahead before sport and exercise medicine finds a proper place in British medicine.

The government may have been persuaded that this was the right moment for recognition with the realization that in 2012 some 10,000 athletes from around the globe will converge on London for the Olympic Games. Britain can be a showcase for sports medicine as the sports men and women will need and rightly expect the highest quality of care for injuries they sustain, which inevitably occur when bodies are strained to the limit and beyond. It should never be overlooked too that prompt and effective treatment of sports injuries brings benefits to the health service as a whole by encouraging better management of comparable traumatic injuries in civilian life.

A further factor the government has recognized is that with average television viewing of 9h a week for our children, coupled with bad diets, we face an obesity epidemic more serious than almost any country. The habit of exercise must be gained in childhood. Exercise for exercise's sake alone rarely appeals to the young, but almost all will respond with enthusiasm to some kind of sport well taught and supervised. This is badly neglected in many schools, with playing fields sold off and sports teaching a minor part of teacher training and curriculum time. Such a programme including competitive sport needs alongside it a better sports injury service.

So, the future is bright for the *Oxford Handbook of Sport and Exercise Medicine* and for sports medicine in Britain. The success of both is fully deserved and I wish both well.

Sir Roger Bannister
October 2006

Foreword to second edition

This new edition of the *Oxford Handbook of Sport and Exercise Medicine* reflects the rapid development of the specialty in the last six years, since Sport and Exercise Medicine (SEM) was recognized as a full specialty within the National Health Service in Great Britain in 2005. Following four years as a junior doctor there are now four years of specialist training in the recognized SEM curriculum. With the creation of consultant specialists in SEM there is the opportunity to deliver an effective SEM service within the NHS. This Handbook can be used in the clinic by specialists and generalists; by team doctors preparing to care for their groups of athletes or actually delivering that care on the touchline; by GPs seeing anyone who cannot or should be exercising; and by other members of the multidisciplinary team interested in any aspects of SEM. The format of the Oxford Handbook enables concise yet comprehensive coverage of the broad SEM curriculum from musculoskeletal injury, to cardiorespiratory illness, to infectious disease, to exercising with a disability, to doping in sport. In daily practice, it is useful for anyone interested in the field of sport and exercise medicine to have a quick reference guide and also to be confident that it is authoritative and accurate.

One of the reasons that SEM was recognized as a specialty was because of the challenge of sedentary behaviour and lifestyles. Whether care of athletes is delivered on the playing field, in the changing room, in primary care, or in an out-patient department, the main aim is to keep athletes and patients exercising, get them back to their sport and exercise as quickly as possible, and maintain fitness while injured or ill. The ability to plan rehabilitation with an accurate diagnosis and prognosis is hugely important to success and adherence of anybody trying to stick to a long term exercise and sport programme. The clear and well-presented information in this Handbook will thus play an important part in keeping people active. There are many factors needed to start individuals and athletes on their path to an exercise habit and SEM will play an important part by empowering clinicians to contribute to the onset as well as, crucially, the continuation of exercise. Both athlete/patient and physician can approach the diagnosis, rehabilitation, treatment, and graded return to exercise following illness or injury with confidence if they have an accurate diagnosis and prognosis. Access to a book that is authoritative, clear, easy to reference, and immediately to hand will make a real difference to this. The Olympic and Paralympic Games in London in 2012 have been a catalyst for many legacy initiatives and this new edition published in Olympic year can be considered one of those legacies as a quality reference practitioners can trust. Most users will not read the Handbook from cover to cover in one sitting, but like any good reference or dictionary you will find yourself following trails and picking up interesting topics beyond what you were initially looking for. I hope you will use this Handbook to improve your

Practice and care of athletes and all patients who exercise, as well as enjoying discovering the wealth of knowledge and information so clearly laid out inside.

Dr Richard Budgett OBE FSEM FISM FRCP
2012

Preface to first edition

Sport medicine is fast and reactive. You need an immediate answer to most problems, but you may not need the breadth of a major textbook or the detail of the specialist work. What is needed is a quick and accessible overview—and one you can easily carry around. This book is designed as your companion in everyday sport and exercise medicine. All you need in one source.

From ankles to altitude, blood doping to bursitis—everything you ever wanted to know about sport and exercise medicine—in your pocket. Arranged by systems, focused on the patient, it offers an immediate guide to all aspects of diagnosis and treatment, exercise benefits, and epidemiology.

Sports medicine is an evolving discipline. The science and research base is expanding and there are changing views on the value of many treatment modalities, the utility of preventive strategies, and the optimal exercise prescription. Clinicians are looking for evidence and patients are increasingly aware of the need for a scientific approach. This book brings together the common problems and diagnoses in sport and exercise medicine with a focused summary of the latest strategies, management plans, and evidence-based protocols.

The aim is to provide a rapid access overview of sport and exercise medicine. The objective is to produce a comprehensive text that is filled with essential information presented in a user-friendly, easily accessible format. It has all the essential information, with blank pages for the readers' own updates, local procedures, or personal notes. We set out to provide a comprehensive basic text. It is directed at the increasing numbers of students of physiotherapy, sport therapy, sports science, and exercise and rehabilitation who are searching for a suitable textbook. It is particularly relevant to postgraduate students on Masters courses in sport medicine and undergraduate medical students, many of whom undertake electives, special study modules, and intercalated degrees in sport and exercise medicine. It should also be the first line reference handbook for general practitioners with a special interest, and the foundation text for career professionals in the emerging specialty of sport and exercise medicine. It has been compiled by expert educators in the field, all of whom have been involved in teaching at undergraduate, masters, and specialist level and it has an international flavour, in keeping with worldwide development of the discipline.

Acknowledgements

Like sport, if it looks easy, it probably means thorough preparation, hard work, talent, and teamwork. If you enjoy this book, then the credit must go to the great team of people involved in putting it together. Each contributor wrote a number of sections that were moved around and finally placed together to build the chapter structure. It is essentially a huge jigsaw where some chapters have up to four authors. We had a team of reviewers who worked hard to ensure that chapters were up-to-date and comprehensive. They were excellent. We must also give credit to those pioneers of academic sport and exercise medicine who defined the boundaries of this new discipline, sought specialist recognition, formed colleges, and created the examination structure. We are only following in their wake. Thank you to the friends, partners, and families who keep the show on the road, while we follow our love of SEM.

I would particularly like to thank Sir Roger Bannister. He has been such a wonderful inspiration to all of us in sport and exercise medicine, not only though his personal sporting achievements, but through his leadership, guidance, and stewardship of our emerging discipline. I will always cherish his quiet words of wisdom and advice and I feel very privileged to include his Foreword, written for the first edition. It is also a pleasure to include the words of Richard Budgett, a friend and colleague for many years. We share a passion for excellence in sport and sports medicine and I have great admiration for his huge contribution to the specialty, leading to his most recent role as Chief Medical Officer to the Olympic Games.

DM
2012

Contributors

Dr Chris Bleakley
Lecturer
Ulster Sports Academy
Faculty of Life and Health Sciences
University of Ulster, Ulster, UK

Dr Carolyn Broderick
Staff Specialist, Paediatric Sports Medicine, The Children's Hospital at Westmead, Westmead, Australia; and Senior Lecturer, Exercise Physiology, Faculty of Medicine, University of New South Wales, Sydney, Australia

Stefano Campi
Department of Orthopaedic and Trauma Surgery
Campus Bio-Medico University
Rome, Italy

Professor Michael Cullen
Consultant in Sport and Exercise Medicine, Musgrave Park Hospital, Belfast, UK

Mr Bernard Donne
Director of Human Performance Laboratory, Departments of Anatomy and Physiology,
Trinity College,
Dublin, Ireland

Dr Philip Glasgow
Head of Sports Medicine, Sports Institute Northern Ireland, University of Ulster, Ulster, UK

Dr Peter L. Gregory
The New Dispensary, Warwick; formerly Course Director Masters Programme in Sport and Exercise Medicine, University of Nottingham, UK

Scott H. Grindell
Sports Medicine and Orthopedic Physician, Spectrum Health, Reed City Campus, Reed City, Michigan, USA

Professor W. Stewart Hillis
Emeritus Professor and Senior Research Fellow, Glasgow University, Glasgow, UK

Zoe Hudson
Editor, *Physical Therapy in Sport*, Elsevier; and Honorary Senior Clinical Lecturer, Centre for Sports and Exercise Medicine, Barts and the London School of Medicine and Dentistry, Queen Mary University of London, London, UK

Dr Tim Jenkinson
Consultant in Rheumatology, Sports and Exercise Medicine, Royal National Hospital for Rheumatic Diseases, Bath, UK

Dr Constance Lebrun
Associate Professor, Faculty of Medicine & Dentistry, Department of Family Medicine, Consultant Sports Medicine Physician, Glen Sather Sports Medicine Clinic, University of Alberta, Canada

Dr Umile Giuseppe Longo
Department of Trauma and Orthopaedic Surgery
Campus Biomedico University
Rome, Italy

Dr John A. MacLean
Medical Director, National Stadium Sports Medicine Centre, Hampden Park, Glasgow; and International Team doctor, Scottish Football Association; Course Director, MSc Sport & Exercise Medicine, University of Glasgow, Glasgow, UK

CONTRIBUTORS

Professor Nicola Maffulli

Centre Lead and Professor of Sports and Exercise Medicine; Consultant Trauma and Orthopaedic Surgeon, Queen Mary University of London, Barts and The London School of Medicine and Dentistry; and William Harvey Research Institute Centre for Sports and Exercise Medicine, Mile End Hospital, London, UK

Dr Nick Mahony

Assistant Professor of Anatomy and Course Coordinator MSc in Sports and Exercise Medicine, Trinity College, Dublin, Ireland

Dr Paul McCrory

Associate Professor, Centre for Health, Exercise and Sports Medicine, University of Melbourne; Brain Research Institute, Florey Neurosciences Institutes, University of Melbourne; and Australian Centre for Research into Injury in Sport and its Prevention, International Research Centres for Prevention of Injury and Protection of Athlete Health supported by the International Olympic Committee (IOC), Australia

Professor Niall Moyna

School of Health and Human Performance, Dublin City University, Dublin, Ireland

Professor T.D. Noakes

Discovery Health Professor of Exercise & Sports Science at the University of Cape Town, Department of Human Biology, Sports Science Institute of South Africa, Cape Town, South Africa

Professor Moira O'Brien

Emeritus Professor of Anatomy, Trinity College, University of Dublin; Hon Medical Director of the Masters in Sports and Exercise Medicine, Trinity College Dublin; President of the Irish Osteoporosis Society; and Consultant in Osteoporosis and Sports Medicine, Euromedic, Dundrum, Ireland

Professor Robert J. Petrella

Professor, Department of Family Medicine, Faculty of Medicine and Dentistry, Schulich School of Medicine and School of Kinesiology, Faculty of Health Sciences, University of Western Ontario; and Beryl and Richard Ivey Research Chair, Lawson Health Research Institute, London, Ontario, Canada

Dr Mark Ridgewell

Programme Director, Masters in Sport and Exercise Medicine, Metropolitan University, Cardiff, UK

Dr Ian Shrier

FACSM Centre for Clinical Epidemiology and Community Studies, Lady Davis Institute for Medical Research, Jewish General Hospital, Montreal, Quebec, Canada

Professor Cathy Speed

Consultant in Rheumatology, Sports and Exercise Medicine Addenbrooke's Hospital Cambridge, UK

Dr Simon Till

Consultant Rheumatologist & Sports Physician, Royal Hallamshire Hospital, Sheffield, UK

Professor Denaro Vincezo
Department of Trauma and
Orthopaedic Surgery
Campus Bio-medico University
Rome, Italy

Dr Nick Webborn
Medical Director, Sussex Centre
for Sport and Exercise Medicine,
University of Brighton; Research
Fellow of the Chelsea School,
University of Brighton; and
Honorary Clinical Senior Lecturer
in Sport & Exercise Medicine,
Queen Mary, University of
London, London, UK

Dr Catherine Woods
Head of School, School of Health
and Human Performance, Faculty
of Science and Health, Dublin City
University, Ireland, UK

Symbols and abbreviations

↑	increased
↓	decreased
≈	approximately
η	blood viscosity
AAF	adverse analytical finding
ABC	airway, breathing, and circulation
ABCD	airway, breathing, circulation, and disability
ACE	angiotensin converting enzyme
ACEI	angiotensin-converting enzyme inhibitors
ACL	anterior cruciate ligament
ACR	agonist–contract–relax
ACSM	American College of Sports Medicine
ACTH	adrenocorticotrophic hormone
ADAMS	Anti-Doping Administration and Management System
ADH	antidiuretic hormone
ADL	activities of daily living
ADO	anti-doping organization
ADP	adenosine diphosphate
AED	automated external defibrillator
AF	atrial fibrillation
AHA	American Heart Association
AHR	airway hyper-responsiveness
AIDS	acquired immune deficiency syndrome
AITFL	antero-inferior tibio-fibular ligament
ALS	advanced life support
ANA	antinuclear antibody
ANS	autonomic nervous system
AP	antero-posterior
APL	abductor pollicis longus
AS	ankylosing spondylitis
ASIS	anterior superior iliac crest
ATA	atmosphere absolute
ATFL	anterior talofibular ligament
ATLS	advanced trauma life support
ATP	adenosine triphosphate
ATP-PC	adenosine triphosphate-phosphocreatine

AV	atrioventricular
AVN	avascular necrosis
a-vO$_2$ diff	arteriovenous difference in oxygen concentration
AVPU	alertness, verbal, pain, unresponsive
bd	twice daily
BEH	benign exertional headache
BLa	blood lactate
BLS	basic life support
BMC	bone mineral content
BMD	bone mineral density
BMI	body mass index
BMR	basal metabolic rate
BNF	*British National Formulary*
BP	blood pressure
CABG	coronary artery bypass graft
CAD	coronary artery disease
CA-MRSA	community acquired methicillin-resistant *Staph. aureus*
CCP	citrullinated protein
CDC	Center for Disease Control
CFL	calcaneofibular ligament
CFO	common flexor origin
CHD	coronary heart disease
CHF	cardiac failure
CHO	carbohydrate
CJD	Creutzfeld Jakob Disease
CMC	carpo-metacarpal
CMO	chief medical officer
CMV	cytomegalovirus
CNS	central nervous system
CO	cardiac output
CON	concentric
COPD	chronic obstructive pulmonary disease
CeP	cerebral palsy
CP	creatine phosphate
CPK	creatine phosphokinase
CPR	cardiopulmonary resuscitation
CR	contract–relax
CRAC	contract–relax–antagonist–contract
CRP	C-reactive protein
CRT	cardiac resynchronization therapy
CSF	cerebrospinal fluid

SYMBOLS AND ABBREVIATIONS

CT	computed tomography
CTD	connective tissue disease
CVA	cerebrovascular accident
CVD	cardiovascular disease
CVS	cardiovascular system
CTE	chronic traumatic encephalopathy
CWI	cold water immersion
DB	dry bulb
DBP	diastolic blood pressure
DCO	doping control officer
DCS	diffuse cerebral swelling
DEXA	dual energy X-ray absorptiometry
DIP	distal interphalangeal
D_{max}	maximum displacement
DMARD	disease modifying agents
DOMS	delayed onset muscle soreness
DSD	disorders of sex development
DVT	deep vein thrombosis
EAH	exercise associated hyponatraemia
ECC	eccentric
ECF	extracellular fluid
ECG	electrocardiogram
ECRB	extensor carpi radialis brevis
ECRL	extensor carpi radialis longus
ECU	extensor carpi ulnaris
EDC	extensor digitorum communis
EDV	end diastolic volume
EEA	energy expenditure for activity
EEG	electroencephalogram
EIA	exercise-induced asthma
EIB	exercise-induced bronchospasm
EMD	electromechanical dissociation
EMG	electromyography
ENMG	electoneuromyography
ENT	ear, nose, and throat
EPB	extensor polaris brevis
EPO	erythropoetin
ER	external rotation
ESR	erythrocyte sedimentation rate
ESV	end systolic volume
ESWT	extra-corporeal shock wave therapy

SYMBOLS AND ABBREVIATIONS

ETC	electron transport chain
EVH	eucapnoeic voluntary hyperpnoea
FABER	flexion abduction external rotation
FAD	flavin adenine dinucleotide
FAI	femoroacetabular impingement
FBC	full blood count
FCR	flexor carpi radialis
FCU	flexor carpi ulnaris
FDS	flexor digitorum superficialis
FEV	forced expiratory volume
FFA	free fatty acids
FH	family history
FG	fast twitch glycolytic fibres
FOG	fast twitch oxidative-glycolytic fibres
FPL	flexor policis longus
FPT	functional performance tests
FRAST	Free Running Asthma Screening Test
FSEM UK	UK Faculty of Sport and Exercise Medicine
FSH	follicle stimulating hormone
FT_b	fast twitch fibres
FVC	forced vital capacity
GAPA	Global Advocacy for Physical Activity
GCS	Glasgow Coma Scale
GERD	gastroesophageal reflux disease
GFR	glomerular filtration rate
GH	growth hormone
GI	gastrointestinal
GMC	General Medical Council
GnRH	gonadotrophin-releasing hormone
GT	globe temperature
GTN	glyceryl trinitrate
GU	genito-urinary
GXT	graded incremental tests to volitional exhaustion
HBOT	hyperbaric oxygen therapy
Hb	haemoglobin
Hct	haematocrit
HDL	high density lipoprotein
HGH	human growth hormone
HIV	human immunodeficiency virus
HK	hexokinase
HMB	beta-hydroxy-beta-methylbutyrate

HPV	human papilloma virus
HR	heart rate
H-R	hold–relax
HRR	heart rate reserve
HRT	hormone replacement therapy
HSE	Health & Safety Executive
HSV	herpes simplex virus
IA	intra-articular
IBD	inflammatory bowel disease
ICP	intracranial pressure
ICD	implantable cardioverter defibrillator
ICP	intracranial pressure
ICS	inhaled corticosteroids
IDET	intradiscal electrothermal annuloplasty
IGF-1	insulin-like growth factor 1
IHD	ischaemic heart disease
IHS	International Headache Society
IM	intramuscular
InfM	infectious mononucleosis
IntA	intrinsic asthma
IO	intraosseous
IOC	International Olympic Committee
IPC	International Paralympic Committee
IR	internal rotation
ITB	ilio-tibial band
IV	intravenous
IVC	interior vena cava
IVP	intravenous pyelogram
IZ	injury zone
JVP	jugular venous pressure
JIA	juvenile idiopathic arthritis
LABA	long-acting beta2 agonists
LCL	lateral collateral ligament
LDL	low density lipoprotein
LFT	liver function test
LH	luteinizing hormone
LMA	laryngeal mask airway
LOC	loss of consciousness
LSD	long slow distance
LV	left ventricle
LVH	left ventricular hypertrophy

M	mass
MAP	mean blood pressure
MCL	medial collateral ligament
MCP	metacarpophalangeal
MCV	mean corpuscular volume
MCS	microscopy and culture
MDI	measured dose inhaler
MET	metabolic equivalent
MFC	medial femoral condyle
MJL	medial joint line
MK	myokinase
MPHR	maximum predicted heart rate
MRA	magnetic resonance angiography
MRI	magnetic resonance imaging
MRSA	methicillin-resistant *Staphylococcus aureus*
MST	metre shuttle test
MSU	mid-stream urine sample
MT	metatarsal
MTPJ	metatarsophalangeal joint
NAD	nicotinamide adenine dinucleotide
NCAA	National Collegiate Athletic Association
N	maximum force
NIDDM	non-insulin dependent diabetes mellitus
NFL	National Football League
NGB	national governing body
Nm	maximum moment
NP	neuropsychological
NSAIDs	non-steroidal anti-inflammatory drugs
OA	osteoarthritis
OCD	osteochondritis dissicans
OCP	oral contraceptive pill
OPG	osteoprogerin
ORIF	open reduction internal fixation
OTC	over-the-counter
PA	physical activity
P-A	postero-anterior
PABA	para-aminobenzoic acid
PaO_2	partial pressure of oxygen in the arterial blood
$PaCO_2$	partial pressure of carbon dioxide in the arterial blood
PC	provocative concentration
PCI	percutaneous coronary intervention

PCL	posterior cruciate ligament
PCOS	polycystic ovary syndrome
PCR	phosphocreatine (energy system)
PCS	post-concussion syndrome
PEA	pulseless electrical activity
PEF	peak expiratory flow
PEFR	peak expiratory flow rate
PFJ	patello-femoral joint
PFT	pulmonary (lung) function test
PFK	phosphofructokinase
PFPS	patellofemoral pain syndrome
Pi	inorganic phosphate
PIN	posterior interosseous nerve
PIP	proximal interphalangeal
PM	particulate matter
PMS	premenstrual syndrome
PMH	past medical history
PNF	proprioceptive neuromuscular facilitation
PNS	parasympathetic nervous system
pO_2	partial pressure of oxygen
POMS	profile of mood states
POP	plaster of Paris
PPI	proton pump inhibitor
PRICE	protect, rest, ice, compression, elevation
PRICES	protect, rest, ice, compression, elevation, and support
PRP	platelet-rich plasma
PSIS	posterior superior iliac crest
PTFL	posterior talofibular ligament
PTH	parathyroid hormone
PV	plasma volume
PVL	Panton-Valentine leukocidin
PUVA	psoralen with UVA
PWC	physical work capacity
Q	cardiac output
qid	4 times a day (quarter in die)
QSART	quantitative sudomotor axon reflex tests
r	arteriolar radius
RA	rheumatoid arthritis
RBC	red blood cells
RCC	red cell count
RDA	recommended daily allowance

RER	respiratory exchange ratio
Rf	respiratory frequency
RF	rheumatoid factor
rg-CT	reverse gantry computerized tomography
RH	relative humidity
RICES	rest, ice, compression, elevation, stabilization
RM	repetition maximum
ROM	range of movement
RPE	rate of perceived exertion
RPM	revolution per minute
RR	respiratory rate
RSO	resting sweat output
RT	resistance training
RTA	road traffic accident
RTP	return to play
RV	residual volume
SA	surface area
SABA	short-acting beta2 agonist
SAC	Standardized Assessment of Concussion
SAH	subarachnoid haemorrhage
SAID	specific adaptations to imposed demand
SAR	sit and reach test
SARA	sexually-acquired reactive arthritis
SBP	systolic blood pressure
SC	subcutaneous
SCAT	Standardized Concussion Assessment Tool
SEM	sports and exercise medicine
SF	skin-fold
SIA	sinoatrial
SIJ	sacro-iliac joint
SLAP	superior labrum anterior to posterior
SLE	systemic lupus erythematosus
SLR	straight leg raise
SNS	sympathetic nervous system
SO	slow oxidative
SOC	stage of change
SPECT	single photon emission computer tomography
ST	slow twitch fibres
STEMI	ST elevation myocardial infarction
STPD	standard temperature and pressure for a dry gas

SYMBOLS AND ABBREVIATIONS

SUCFE	slipped upper capital femoral epiphysis
SV	stroke volume
SVR	stroke volume resistance
SVT	supraventricular tachycardia
TB	tuberculosis
TBI	traumatic brain injury
TCA	tricarboxylic acid cycle
TFCC	triangular fibrocartilage complex
TGA	transposition of great arteries
TGF-β	transforming growth factor beta
TIA	transient ischaemic attack
tid	three times a day
TLac	lactate threshold (aerobic/anaerobic threshold)
TNF	tumour necrosis factor
TOE	transoesophageal echocardiography
TPR	total peripheral resistance
TT	time trial
TTE	transthoracic echocardiography
TUE	therapeutic use exemption
TV	tidal volume
UCL	ulnar collateral ligament
U&E	urea and electrolytes
UKAD	UK Anti-doping
ULTT	upper limb tension test
URTI	upper respiratory tract infection
UTI	urinary tract infection
US	ultrasound
UVA	ultraviolet A
Uvb	ultraviolet B
V_A	alveolar ventilation
VC	vital capacity
V_E	pulmonary ventilation
V_m	minute ventilation
VF	ventricular fibrillation
VI	visually impaired
VJH	vertical jump height
VMO	vastus medialis obliquus
VO_2	oxygen uptake
VT	ventricular tachycardia
VZV	Varicella zoster virus

WADA	World Anti-Doping Agency
WB	wet bulb
WBV	whole body vibration
WBGT	wet bulb globe temperature
WCC	white cell count
WHO	World Health Organization

Chapter 1

Immediate care

Sports first aid 2
First aid facilities at venues 3
Approach to the acutely ill or injured athlete 3
Crisis management: the primary survey 4
Basic life support 6
Resuscitation of children 12
Advanced adult life support 14
Automated external defibrillators 18
Secondary survey 22
Major emergencies in sport 23
The unconscious athlete 23
Choking 24
Bleeding and shock 26
Anaphylaxis 30
Drowning 32
Ongoing assessment, documentation, and transfer to definitive care 33

Sports first aid

- Assess the airway, breathing, and circulation (ABC).
- Assess and monitor level of consciousness.
- Direct the casualty on to the appropriate agency.
- Keep within recognized first aid guidelines.
- We all have a 'Duty of Care' (Good Samaritan), but will have a different standard of care, whether doctor, nurse, physiotherapist, etc.
- In children, there is an additional responsibility. Contact parents immediately—you are '*locum parentis*'—responsible for their care and management and must have written consent to 'administer' medication.

Roles and responsibilities of first aider

- *Assess*: what has occurred.
- *Protect*: self and others.
- *Identify*: nature of illness/injury.
- *Treat*: by severity and safety.
- *Transport*: remove to care.
- *Accompany*: remain with casualty.
- *Report*: to doctor or paramedic.
- *Isolate*: to prevent cross-infection.
- *Secure*: valuables and clothing.
- *Inform*: family.

Recording incidents

Health & Safety Executives (HSE) have a form to record.
- Name and address of casualty.
- Date and time of incident.
- Details.
- Witnesses.
- Injury.
- Treatment.
- Disposal.
- Include your name and contact details.

First aid facilities at venues

It is important to know the venue and the key staff, including the location of the first aid room, medical help, and the particular emergency procedures for the venue. Remember when telephoning for help to give the exact location and try to meet the ambulance where possible. This is especially important at a large venue.

The Taylor Report has set criteria for safety at sports grounds with specific advice regarding doctors, ambulances, etc., depending on the expected crowd size.

Make sure that the first aid room is open and has the following:
- *Telephone:* with emergency contact numbers.
- Large, clean room with good lighting.
- Stretcher.
- Couch, pillows, and blankets.
- Hot and cold running water with soap and towels.
- Ice and bags.
- First aid kit.

Approach to the acutely ill or injured athlete

Best achieved by a pre-planned (and trained) team approach, with each team member aware of their individual roles and responsibilities. However, in many sporting situations the first aider will be the only suitably trained individual.

Prioritize if there is more than one casualty. Multiple casualties are common especially in contact sports. A quiet casualty is a potentially dead casualty. Remember the possibility of injury to or illness in the spectators.

Direct visualization of the injury mechanism will help to prioritize or give a clue as to diagnosis.

The general approach can be summarized as:
- Establish scene safety.
- Rapid primary survey with resuscitation and immediate treatment of life- and limb-threatening injuries.
- A detailed secondary survey.
- Initiation of definitive care based on the above.

Crisis management: the primary survey

DRS ABC
- D = Danger.
- R = Response.
- S = Shout or Send for help.
- ABC = Assess and treat as required.

Danger could include hazards such as electricity, water, and height. Remember that in a sporting situation the most common danger is the game and its participants so always:

STOP THE GAME!

For ABC see 📖 Basic Life Support, p. 6

Disability

Some authors consider Disability within the primary survey (ABCD). This consists of a brief neurological assessment to assess the level of consciousness of the casualty. This best achieved and noted by using the AVPU scale (**see** Box 1.1), rather than the more detailed, but complicated Glasgow Coma Scale (GCS; may be used by health professionals). This assessment allows a decision regarding urgent transfer to hospital for a more detailed assessment, especially when the neurological signs are deteriorating.

Possible spinal injury

Any unconscious casualty or one who complains of neck pain, numbness, weakness, or paralysis should be assumed to have a neck injury until proved otherwise. This is particularly important where the mechanism of injury is suggestive of potential cervical damage. Such situations include a fall from height (diving, horse riding, climbing, etc.), injuries at speed (motor racing, etc.) or where the cervical spine is seen to hyperextend, flex, or rotate (rugby, American football, etc.).

Exposure during the primary survey

Remove enough clothing to allow detailed examination (remember not to remove headgear in suspected spinal injury except for resuscitation). Preserve casualty dignity as much as possible and avoid hypothermia by covering with a blanket/clothing.

There is a delicate balance between the time required for an extensive primary survey and the 'load and go' approach of early transport for more definitive care. This decision will be based on the nature of the injuries, experience of those present, the need for more definitive care, such as need for surgery, advanced airway management, vascular access, distance to secondary care, and mode of transport available. The casualty should be constantly monitored during this assessment and ongoing care including ABC and AVPU.

CRISIS MANAGEMENT: THE PRIMARY SURVEY

Basic life support

Introduction

The publication of the 2010 UK Resuscitation Council Guidelines 2010 marks the 50th anniversary of modern cardiopulmonary resuscitation (CPR). In 1960 the first paper on survival of cardiac arrest by 14 patients by application of closed chest cardiac massage was published, and later that year the combination of chest compressions and rescue breathing was introduced.

Following an initial assessment of the possible *danger* to the casualty and those carrying out the resuscitation and the *response* of the casualty, basic life support (BLS) comprises:
- Airway maintenance.
- Rescue breathing.
- Chest compression.

BLS guidelines are for out-of-hospital, single rescuer, adult BLS, and imply no equipment is employed—a simple airway or facemask should be used if available.

Chain of survival

A cardiac arrest is the ultimate medical emergency with the chances of survival considerably improved if appropriate steps are taken to deal with the emergency. It is now recognized that a chain of interventions contribute to a potentially successful outcome of a cardiac arrest—the 'Chain of survival' (Fig. 1.1).

The 4 steps of the chain are:
- Early recognition and call for help to prevent cardiac arrest
- Early CPR
- Early defibrillation
- Early advanced life support (ALS)

Fig. 1.1 Chain of survival diagram. Reproduced from Nolan J, et al. *Resuscitation* 2006; **71:** 270–1 with kind permission from Elsevier.

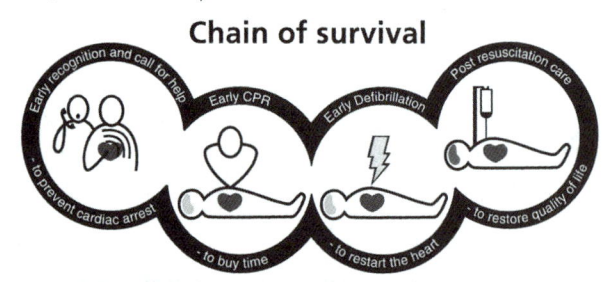

International consensus

Resuscitation guidelines in the UK are set by the Resuscitation Council (UK), which is itself a member of the European Resuscitation Council. There is now a desire to seek consensus among all areas of the world and as a result the International Liaison Committee on Resuscitation (ILCOR) was formed in an attempt to ensure that guidelines for resuscitation are uniform in all countries.

Purpose of BLS

- Maintain adequate ventilation and circulation until means can be obtained to reverse the underlying cause of the arrest—in practice by defibrillation.
- BLS is a 'holding operation'. On occasions, particularly when the primary pathology is respiratory failure, it may itself reverse the cause and allow full recovery.
- Failure of the circulation for 3–4 min (less if the victim is initially hypoxic) will lead to irreversible cerebral damage.
- Assessment of the carotid pulse is time-consuming and leads to an incorrect conclusion (present or absent) in up to 50% of cases. For this reason, training in detection of the carotid pulse as a sign of cardiac arrest is no longer recommended for non-healthcare persons.
- The safety of both rescuer and casualty are paramount, but the risk to the rescuer during CPR is minimal. While there have been isolated reports of transmission of infections such as tuberculosis, transmission of human immunodeficiency virus (HIV) during CPR has never been reported.
- Barrier devices with one-way valves have been shown in laboratory studies to prevent transmission of oral bacteria from the victim. Rescuers should therefore take all appropriate safety precautions if the casualty is known to have a serious infection. Compression-only CPR may be appropriate in this instance.
- In non-asphyxial cardiac arrest as blood oxygen remains high initially, ventilation is less important than compressions. Thus, the priority is to start with compressions.
- Jaw thrust is not recommended for lay rescuers as it is difficult to learn and perform, and best left for more experienced personnel in cases of suspected neck injury.

2010 Guideline changes

The Resuscitation Council recently updated the BLS Guidelines to reflect the fact that an interruption in chest compressions is common and associated with a reduced chance of survival for the victim. Ideally, compressions should be given continuously, while giving ventilations independently—possible only in ALS with an advanced airway in place. Compression-only CPR will increase the number of compressions and eliminate pauses, but at the expense of any ventilation. New guidelines emphasize the importance of the correct depth and rate of compressions.

Guideline changes
- When obtaining help ask for an automated external defibrillator (AED) if available.
- Compress the chest to a depth of 5–6cm at a rate of 100–120/min (previously 100/min).
- Give each rescue breath over 1s, rather than 2s.
- Do not stop to check the victim or discontinue CPR unless the victim starts to show signs of regaining consciousness, such as coughing, opening his eyes, speaking or moving purposefully *and* starts to breathe normally.
- Teach CPR to laypeople with an emphasis on chest compression, but include ventilation as the standard, particularly for those with a duty of care.

Sequence of events for BLS (Fig. 1.2)
- Check for danger (rescuer and victim).
- Check for response—squeeze and shout ask 'Are you all right?'
- If response, leave in position in which found or place casualty in the recovery position. Try to find out any information about the casualty, send for help if required, and reassess regularly.
- *If no response*:
  - Shout for help.
  - Turn casualty on his back.
  - *Open the airway*—head tilt, chin lift, and remove any visible loose objects from mouth. Leave well-fitting dentures and gum-shields.
  - If cervical spine injury suspected then use jaw lift instead of head tilt.
- Keeping the airway open Look, listen, and feel for normal breathing for *no more than 10s*. If in doubt, act as if the casualty is not breathing.
  - Look for chest movement.
  - Listen at the casualty's mouth for breath sounds.
  - Feel for air on your cheek.
- If breathing, place casualty in the recovery position, send for help if required, and reassess regularly.
- *If not breathing*:
  - Send for help and ask them to bring an AED if available. If on your own use your mobile or nearby phone to call for an ambulance or when no other option exists go for help at this stage and return to continue BLS. In some circumstances it is recommended that 1 min of CPR is given before a lone rescuer goes for help (see 📖 p. 9). If the casualty is not breathing do not check for signs of circulation but proceed immediately to commence chest compressions.
  - Kneel by the side of the casualty.
  - Place the heel of one hand in the centre of the casualty's chest and place the heel of the other hand on top of the first. Less emphasis on exact hand placement is encouraged in the revised guidelines to prevent further time being lost prior to commencing compressions.
  - Interlock fingers of both hands, extend arms vertically above the sternum, and depress the sternum 5–6cm × 100–120/min without losing contact between your hands and the sternum. Pressure should be on the centre of the sternum, not the lower sternum,

ribs, or upper abdomen. Compression and release should take an equal amount of time.
- Combine chest compressions with rescue breaths:
  - After 30 compressions open the airway again (head tilt/chin lift)
  - Pinch the soft part of the nose with thumb and index finger, allow casualty's mouth to open, but maintain chin lift, take a normal breath, place your lips around the casualty's mouth ensuring a good seal, and blow steadily into the mouth watching for the casualty's chest rise—the breath should take 1s—this is an effective *rescue breath*. Repeat for a second rescue breath – the 2 breaths should take no more than 5s.
  - Return hands to the correct position on the sternum and give a further 30 compressions.
  - Continue with chest compressions and rescue breaths in a ratio of 30:2.
- *Do not interrupt resuscitation.* Do not stop to recheck the casualty unless he shows signs of life (as described above).
- If the rescue breaths do not result in the chest rising as in normal breathing then:
  - Check the casualty's mouth and remove any visible obstruction.
  - Recheck there is adequate head tilt and chin lift.
  - Check adequate seal around the casualty's mouth.
  - Do not attempt more than 2 breaths each time before returning to chest compressions.
- Continue resuscitation until:
  - More qualified help arrives and takes over.
  - The victim shows signs of life
  - Exhaustion.

Compression-only CPR
- Use if untrained or unwilling to give rescue breaths.
- Give at a continuous rate of 100–120/min.
- Do not stop unless casualty shows signs of regaining consciousness (as above).

When to go for help
When there is more than one rescuer, then one should go for help immediately. With a single rescuer and if the casualty is an adult, then assume the cause is cardiac and go for help before commencing cardiac compressions when no other option exists, e.g. using nearby or mobile phone.

It may be worthwhile performing resuscitation for 1min before going for help if:
- The cause is respiratory.
- Trauma.
- Choking.
- Drug or alcohol intoxication or poison.
- Drowning or extreme cold.
- The casualty is a child.

Two-person resuscitation
- Send one person for help as the second commences resuscitation.
- Work as a coordinated team on opposite sides of the casualty.
- Maintain airway at all times.
- Ensure a smooth and quick transition between ventilation and compressions. In particular, ensure the minimum of delay without interruption of chest compressions.

Further points re BLS
- *Use of oxygen:* no evidence of benefit except in drowning and will interrupt chest compressions.
- *Mouth to nose ventilation:* effective alternative if casualty's mouth seriously injured or cannot be opened.
- *Bag-mask ventilation:* requires considerable skill and particularly difficult for single rescuer. Reserve for experienced rescuer or where risk of poisoning.
- *Importance of chest compressions:* when teaching BLS it is important to emphasize the importance of the compression element of resuscitation, particularly the new rate of 100–120/min, the increased depth of 5–6cm and minimizing the interruptions in compressions.
- If the casualty vomits during resuscitation (seen particularly in drowning), turn the casualty on their side ensuring the head is towards the floor and the mouth open to allow the vomit to drain away. Ensure the mouth is clear of debris before turning onto back, ensuring a clear airway and recommencing CPR.

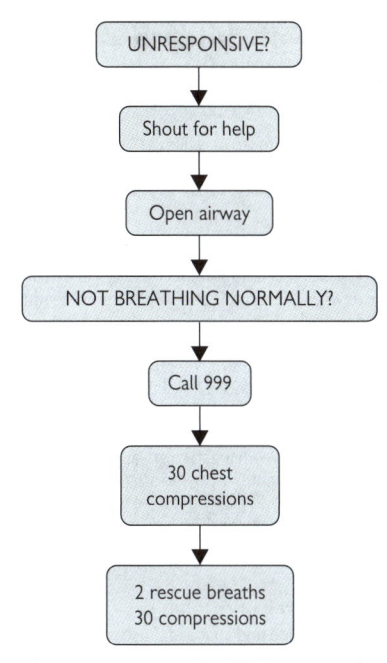

Fig. 1.2 Adult BLS algorithm. Reproduced with kind permission from the Resuscitation Council UK (Resuscitation Council Guidelines 2010).

Resuscitation of children

Changes in resuscitation of children have resulted from both new scientific evidence (limited) and the need to maintain simplicity to assist teaching and retention.

The fear of causing harm to a child as a result of resuscitation is unfounded. For ease of teaching and retention, laypeople should be taught that the adult sequence should be used for children who are not responsive and not breathing.

Guideline changes
- While ventilation is a vital component of asphyxial arrest rescuers who are unable or unwilling to do this should be encouraged to perform compression-only CPR.
- Pulse palpation for 10s is unreliable for determining effective circulation even when performed by health professionals and should not be the sole determinant of the need for CPR. Pulse checks are not part of layperson CPR.
- It has been shown that chest compression is frequently too shallow. As a result the guidelines have changed from 'approximately one-third' to 'at least one-third' of the antero-posterior (AP) diameter of the chest. The guidelines encourage advising 'don't be afraid to push too hard'. Use 2 fingers for an infant under 1 yr.
- To maintain consistency, the rate of compression is as in adults—100–120/min.

Use of AEDs in children
- More evidence of the safe and successful use of AEDs in children less than 8 years has become available since the last guideline change in 2005.
- AED manufacturers now supply purpose-made pads and programmes which limit the output to 50–75J.
- If no paediatric adjusted machine is available, an adult AED may be used.

BLS sequence (Fig. 1.3)
- For laypeople and those health professionals who have no experience of paediatric resuscitation the adult 30:2 sequence should be used with the following modifications:
  - Give 5 initial rescue breaths before starting chest compression.
  - If the responder is alone, perform 1min of CPR before going for help.
- For 2 or more health professionals performing CPR, who have experience of paediatric resuscitation a ratio of 15:2 should be used, i.e. which utilizes more rescue breaths.

RESUSCITATION OF CHILDREN   13

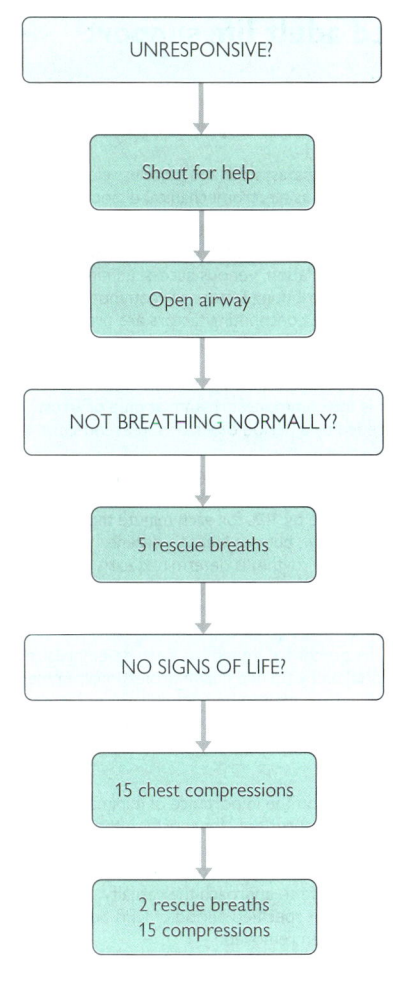

```
UNRESPONSIVE?
    ↓
Shout for help
    ↓
Open airway
    ↓
NOT BREATHING NORMALLY?
    ↓
5 rescue breaths
    ↓
NO SIGNS OF LIFE?
    ↓
15 chest compressions
    ↓
2 rescue breaths
15 compressions
```

Call resuscitation team

Fig. 1.3 Paediatric BLS algorithm. Reproduced with permission from the Resuscitation Council UK. (Resuscitation Council Guidelines, 2010).

Advanced adult life support

Introduction
Heart rhythms associated with cardiac arrest can be divided into two groups:
- *Shockable rhythms:* ventricular fibrillation (VF)/pulseless ventricular tachycardia (VT); and
- *Non-shockable rhythms:* asystole and pulseless electrical activity (PEA), which is also known as electromechanical dissociation (EMD).

The main difference between the two is the need for defibrillation in those with VF/VT. All other actions including chest compressions, airway management and ventilation, venous access, administration of adrenaline, and correction of contributing factors are common to both.

Where any of these contributing factors are present, resuscitation will require specific intervention to treat/reverse the cause.

Shockable rhythms (VF/VT)
- In adults, VF is the commonest rhythm at time of arrest.
- May be preceded by a period of VT or supraventricular tachycardia (SVT).
- Best survival rates in this group, especially when shock delivered promptly.
- Survival rates decline by 10% for each minute that the arrhythmia persists. BLS can slow, but not halt this decline.
- It is vital that patient rhythm is determined early via monitoring electrodes, or defibrillator paddles.
- Start BLS if any delay in defibrillation, but this should not delay shock delivery.
- The role of the precordial thump has been de-emphasized and should only be undertaken by trained health professionals immediately in monitored/witnessed arrest when defibrillator not immediately to hand. Greater success with pulseless VT than in VF.

Treatment
- See Algorithm.
- Increased emphasis on the importance of minimal interruption in chest compressions with pauses only for specific interventions.
- Remember to remove oxygen delivery equipment during defibrillation.
- CPR should be restarted immediately once the shock has been delivered and it is safe to approach the casualty – ideally <5 seconds.
- Recommendation for specified period of CPR before out-of-hospital defibrillation has been removed.
- Manual defibrillators should be charged to 150-200J for the first shock and 150-360J for subsequent shocks.
- Following the third shock, resume chest compressions immediately and then administer adrenaline 1mg IV and amiodarone 300mg IV while performing a further 2 minutes of CPR.
- Give further adrenaline 1mg I/V every 3-5 min (during alternate cycles of CRP).
- If organized electrical activity compatible with a cardiac output is observed during a rhythm check, confirm by checking a central pulse and if present, commence usual post-resuscitation care.

ADVANCED ADULT LIFE SUPPORT

- If asystole observed, switch to the non-shockable side of the algorithm.
- The single shock strategy has replaced the previous three-shock strategy in an attempt to minimize the interruption to compressions during defibrillation.
- Despite the lack of positive long-term survival data in humans, the use of adrenaline is still recommended based on animal and short-term survival data in humans. The basis of this is the resultant vasoconstriction which increases cerebral and myocardial perfusion pressure. The higher coronary blood flow increases the frequency and amplitude of the VF waveform and should improve the chance of successful defibrillation. On the down side animal work has suggested that adrenaline may cause post-arrest cardiac dysfunction.

Non-shockable rhythms (PEA and asystole)

- PEA is the absence of a palpable pulse in the presence of cardiac electrical activity which would normally result in a cardiac output. Survival in asystole or PEA is unlikely unless a reversible cause can be identified and treated — see 📖 Potential reversible causes or contributory factors for reversible causes.

Treatment
- See Fig. 1.4.
- Start CPR 30:2
- In asystole always check leads are attached correctly.
- Give adrenaline 1mg IV
- When airway established continue CPR 30:2 but without interruption for ventilation
- Consider possible reversible causes and correct as appropriate
- Recheck rhythm after 2 min. If VF/VT proceed as shockable algorithm.
- Give further adrenaline every 3-5 min.

Atropine
- Atropine antagonizes the effect of acetylcholine at parasympathetic muscarinic receptors, blocking the effect of the vagus nerve on both SA and AV nodes, increasing sinus rate and AV node conduction. 2005 guidelines suggested the use of atropine but this has been removed from the 2010 guidelines due to lack of benefit in available studies. It has been suggested that atropine is less likely to be of use as the cause of the arrest is more likely to be due to primary myocardial damage than excessive vagal tone.

Potential reversible causes or contributory factors

During any cardiac arrest, potential causes or aggravating factors for which specific treatment exists should be considered. For ease of memory, these are divided into two groups of four based upon their initial letter—either H or T:

The four 'Hs'
- Hypoxia.
- Hypovolaemia.
- Hyperkalaemia, hypokalaemia, hypocalcaemia, acidaemia, or other metabolic disorders.
- Hypothermia.

The four 'Ts'
- Tension pneumothorax.
- Cardiac tamponade.
- Toxic substances or therapeutic substances in overdose.
- Thrombo-embolic or mechanical obstruction (e.g. pulmonary embolus).
- The use of ultrasound (US) in experienced hands during cardiac arrest may assist in the detection of reversible causes, but it's use should not interrupt chest compressions

Airway management and ventilation

Assess the airway
Patients requiring resuscitation often have an obstructed airway. Utilize a simple airway adjunct initially.

Provide artificial ventilation as soon as possible if spontaneous breathing absent or inadequate. As expired air has only 17% oxygen, replace with oxygen enriched air as soon as possible via a pocket mask, bag-mask device, laryngeal mask airway (LMA) or by intubation.

Deliver a volume sufficient to observe the chest rising over 1s with 1s allowed for expiration at a rate of 2 ventilations after 30 compressions.

When a tracheal tube is *in situ* continue ventilation independent of chest compressions at a rate of about 10 breaths/min.

The 2010 guidelines suggest increased emphasis on the use of capnography (the monitoring of CO_2 concentration in respiratory gases) to confirm and monitor tracheal tube placement and quality of CPR.

Intravenous access and drugs
- Intravenous (IV) access should be established if this has not been achieved already.
- The central veins provide the optimal route as they allow drugs to be delivered rapidly into the central circulation.
- Peripheral venous cannulation is quicker, easier to perform, and safer in inexperienced hands.
- Drugs administered by the peripheral route must be followed by a flush of at least 20mL of fluid to assist their delivery into the central circulation.
- Delivery of drugs via an endotracheal tube is no longer recommended as drug concentrations are variable compared to intravenous use. In addition the large volumes of intratracheal fluid impair gas exchange. Where IV access cannot be established the use of the intraosseous (IO) route is suggested. This involves injection directly into the bone marrow—the tibial and humeral sites are recommended.

Drugs
- The use of adrenaline, amiodarone, and atropine has been discussed above.
- No anti-arrhythmic drug given during a human cardiac arrest has been shown to improve survival. However, there remains a case for the use of other agents during a cardiac arrest despite the poor evidence. These agents are outside discussion in this section, but include magnesium, bicarbonate, and calcium.

Post-resuscitation care
- There is increasing interest in post-resuscitation care as a means of improving the rate of successful hospital discharge. Although not for further discussion, areas of interest include:

- Post-arrest hyperoxaemia.
- Prevention of further cerebral and myocardial damage, in particular the prevention of hypoxia, hypercarbia, seizure activity, pyrexia, and hyperglycemia.
- Post-arrest cardiac intervention including angiography and angioplasty.
- Therapeutic hypothermia.
- Vasoactive agents for myocardial dysfunction

```
Unresponsive?
Not breathing or
only occasional gasps
        │
        └──> Call resuscitation team
        │
CPR 30:2
Attach defibrillator/monitor
Minimise interruptions
        │
   Assess rhythm
   ┌────┴────┐
Shockable    Non-shockable
(VF/Pulseless VT)  (PEA/Asystole)
   │                  │
 1 Shock     Return of spontaneous circulation
   │                  │                  │
Immediately      Immediate post      Immediately
resume CPR       cardiac arrest       resume CPR
for 2 min        treatment            for 2 min
Minimise         • Use ABCDE          Minimise
interruptions     approach           interruptions
                 • Controlled
                  oxygenation
                  and ventilation
                 • 12-lead ECG
                 • Treat precipitating
                  cause
                 • Temperature control/
                  therapeutic hypothermia
```

During CPR
- Ensure high-quality CPR: rate, depth, recoil
- Plan actions before interrupting CPR
- Give oxygen
- Consider advanced airway and capnography
- Continuous chest compressions when advanced airway in place
- Vascular access (intravenous, intraosseous)
- Give adrenaline every 3–5 min
- Correct reversible causes

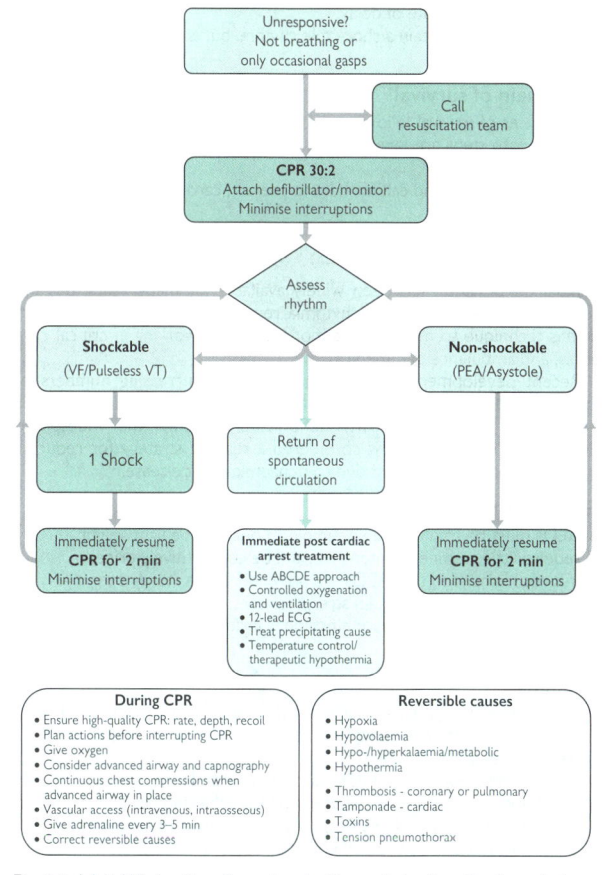

Reversible causes
- Hypoxia
- Hypovolaemia
- Hypo-/hyperkalaemia/metabolic
- Hypothermia

- Thrombosis - coronary or pulmonary
- Tamponade - cardiac
- Toxins
- Tension pneumothorax

Fig. 1.4 Adult ALS algorithm. Reproduced with permission from the Resuscitation Council UK (Resuscitation Council Guidelines 2010).

Automated external defibrillators

- Electrical defibrillation is well established as the only effective therapy for cardiac arrest due to VF or pulseless VT.
- The scientific evidence to support early defibrillation is overwhelming, the single most important determinant of survival being the delay from collapse to delivery of the first shock.
- Every year in the UK approximately 30,000 people sustain a cardiac arrest outside hospital and are treated by the emergency medical services. The chances of successful defibrillation decline at a rate of 10% with each minute of delay.
- BLS will help to sustain a shockable rhythm, but is not a definitive treatment.

The 'chain of survival'
The chances of survival following cardiac arrest are considerably improved if appropriate steps are taken to deal with the emergency. The four steps of the train are:
- Early recognition and call for help to prevent cardiac arrest
- Early CPR
- Early defibrillation
- Early advanced life supports (ALS).

Manual defibrillation has been widely available for many years, but the requirement for training in arrhythmia recognition limits the application of this technique to medical practitioners, nurses working in critical care areas, and ambulance paramedics.

Recent developments in AEDs have enabled increasing numbers of individuals to perform defibrillation safely and effectively.

Increased provision of early defibrillation through the widespread deployment of AEDs is now considered a realistic strategy for reducing mortality from cardiac arrest due to ischaemic heart disease.

Equipment
- AEDs must be totally reliable, simple to operate, be lightweight, require little routine maintenance, and be competitively priced.
- It is recommended that AEDs are provided with a sturdy carrying pouch, which should contain strong scissors, and a disposable safety razor, as well as spare electrodes including specialized paediatric pads.

Training
- Any individual with responsibility for the management of cardiac arrest in the hospital or community should be trained in, and authorized to perform defibrillation using an AED.
- The Resuscitation Council (UK) also recommends the provision of AEDs and training in early defibrillation for other individuals who may be called upon to provide emergency cardiac arrest management. These might include police officers, fire fighters, security personnel, airline cabin crew, and others.

- AEDs should be deployed within a medically controlled system under the direction of a medical adviser who should ensure adequate training of AED users, with periodic refresher training.
- General practitioners should be proficient in BLS and, certainly when responding to a patient with symptoms of chest pain, should bring an AED with them. There is substantial research to show that general practitioners are capable of performing successful early defibrillation.
- There may be occasions when it is appropriate for staff other than nurses and doctors to defibrillate. These may include physiotherapists supervising cardiac rehabilitation exercise classes, and physiological measurement technicians supervising exercise tests. In the community it may be appropriate to train dental surgeons and pharmacists. These individuals should be trained in defibrillation using an AED.
- AEDs have been used successfully in the community by lay first responders, including police officers, fire fighters, security staff, airline cabin crew, and members of first aid and rescue organizations. The Resuscitation Council (UK) recommends that AEDs be made available wherever large crowds gather, e.g. at sports stadiums, pop concerts, theatres, cinemas, and shopping complexes.

2010 Guideline changes

There are no major changes to the sequence for AED use. It is emphasized that an AED can be used safely and effectively without previous training. Lay-people can even be instructed in their use by video self-instruction, rather than instructor-led courses, thus minimizing cost and time for training. The guidelines emphasize the importance of minimizing interruptions in chest compressions during AED use.

Sequence of actions for AED (Fig. 1.5)

- Follow adult BLS sequence as described above. Do not delay commencing CPR unless an AED is available immediately.
- *As soon as the AED arrives*, continue CPR (if more than 1 rescuer present), switch on the AED, follow the voice prompt and attach the electrodes to the casualty's bare chest. Ensure no one touches the casualty during the analysis of the casualty's rhythm.
- *If a shock is advised*, ensure no one touches the casualty, push the shock button—usually indicated by a flashing light. Fully automated AEDs will deliver the shock automatically. Continue as instructed and ensuring minimal interruption in chest compressions.
- *If no shock is advised*, resume CPR (30:2 ratio). Follow voice prompts.
- *Continue to follow the AED voice prompts* until qualified help arrives, the casualty regains consciousness and starts to breathe normally, or the rescuer becomes exhausted.

Use of AEDs in children

- More evidence of the safe and successful use of AEDs in children less than 8 yrs has become available since the last guideline change in 2005.
- AED manufacturers now supply purpose-made pads and programmes which limit the output to 50–75J.
- If no paediatric adjusted machine is available, an adult AED may be used.

Placement of AED pads

Place as shown on the diagram with each pad positioned vertically, one to the right of the sternum, the other on the left mid-axillary line—ensure this pad is sufficiently lateral and clear of breast tissue.

Although labelled left and right it does not matter if the pad placement is reversed and the rescuer should not lose time in changing the pads.

Ensure the chest is sufficiently exposed with removal of enough chest hair to achieve electrical contact and minimize the risk of a shock to the casualty, but do not delay defibrillation if a razor is not immediately available.

If the casualty is wet, e.g. victim of drowning, dry as best as able, especially to allow the pads to adhere to the chest. Avoid direct contact (of anyone present) with the casualty when the shock is delivered.

If supplemental oxygen is being used remove the mask and place it at least 1m away.

The key is to provide good quality CPR while awaiting the AED and minimize interruptions during the process of using the AED. The use of a period of CPR before AED use, when it is available, is no longer recommended.

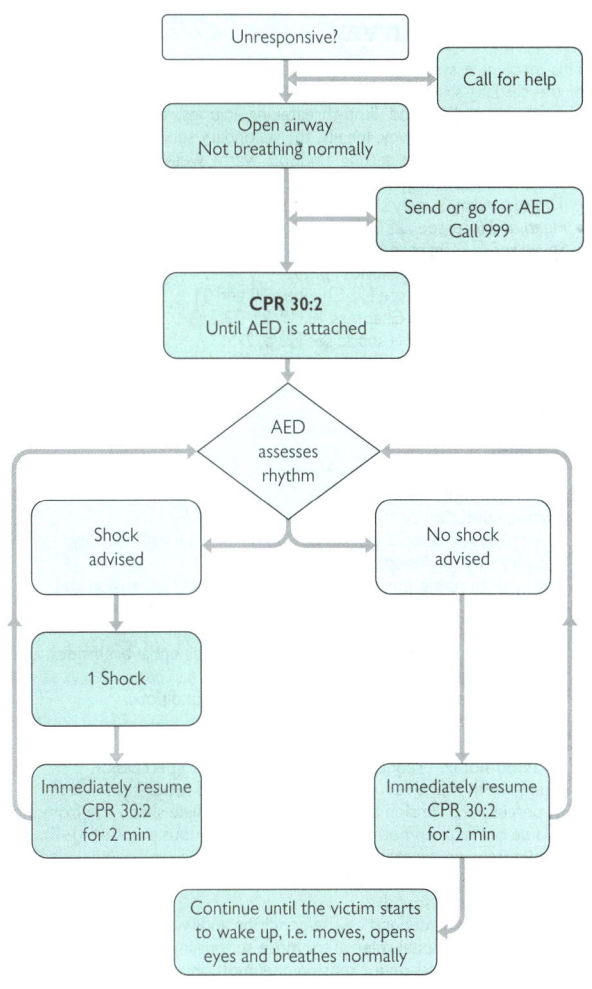

Fig. 1.5 AED algorithm. Reproduced with permission from the Resuscitation Council UK (Resuscitation Council Guidelines, 2010).

Secondary survey

This involves a systematic examination of the entire body from the top of the casualty's head to their feet. This should be carried out following assessment of life- and limb-threatening injuries, and their treatment during the primary survey. Ideally, the secondary survey should be carried out in an appropriate setting (indoor, warm well-lit environment), by experienced medical staff with appropriate equipment available.

The secondary survey should include:
- *Head and face:* see Chapter 15.
- *Spine:* see Chapter 16.
- *Chest:* see 'Chest injuries', p. 22.
- *Abdomen and pelvis:* see Chapters 20 and 21
- *Limb injuries:* see Chapters 18, 19, 21–23.
- *Assessment for possible shock:* see p. 27.

Chest injuries

Trauma to the chest can result in:
- Rib fractures.
- Flail chest.
- Pneumothorax and/or haemothorax.
- Diaphragm rupture.
- Cardiac contusion or tamponade.
- Injury to major vessels, e.g. aorta. Can result from high velocity, deceleration injuries as in skiing, motor sport.
- Extensive circumferential burns may restrict chest expansion and ventilation.
- Chest examination should include:
  - Inspection for chest movement—is it normal, equal both sides, and signs of injury.
  - Assess breathing rate—increased in most conditions.
  - Palpation for tenderness, e.g. rib injury.
- Auscultation and percussion:
  - haemothorax—reduced breath sounds, dull to percussion
  - pneumothorax—reduced breath sounds and hyper-resonant to percussion. Tension pneumothorax has midline shift away from the side of the pneumothorax, raised jugular venous pressure (JVP), hypotension, tachycardia, shock
- Cardiac tamponade: raised JVP, hypotension, tachycardia, shock, diminished heart sounds.
- Management will depend on the condition and will include analgesia for rib injury, hospital referral for more serious injury and emergency needle decompression for tension pneumothorax. Tamponade will require urgent pericardiocentesis under echocardiography guidance.

Major emergencies in sport

- Bleeding and shock.
- Head injuries.
- Cervical spine injuries.
- Choking.
- The unconscious casualty.
- Severe facial injuries.
- Hypothermia, heat stroke, and altitude sickness.
- Abdominal trauma.
- Cardiac and pulmonary emergencies.
- Major limb injuries:
  - Fractures and dislocations.
  - Major ligament injuries.
- Medical emergencies:
  - Diabetes.
  - Seizures.
  - Acute asthma attack.
  - Severe allergic reaction.
  - Poisoning.

The unconscious athlete

Lack of *oxygen* or *nutrient* to the *brain*

Causes of unconsciousness

- *Lungs*: respiratory problem, injury, or poison.
- *Heart*: lack of adequate circulation to brain.
- *Metabolism*: diabetes, drugs, alcohol, infection, too hot, too cold.
- *Brain*: lack of oxygen, head injury, epilepsy.

Management

- DRS ABC + recovery position if no C-spine suspected.
- Look for clues as to cause.
- Treat if possible.
- Monitor casualty continuously.
- Call for help.

Monitoring the unconscious casualty

Glasgow Coma Scale most widely used worldwide, but difficult for first-aider to understand and use. Simpler versions are available including AVPU (Box 1.1).

Box 1.1 AVPU scale

A	=	Alertness	Avpu	=	Alert
V	=	Verbal	aVpu	=	Responsive to speech
P	=	Pain	avPu	=	Responsive to pain
U	=	Unresponsive	avpU	=	Unresponsive

Choking

Recognition
Choking is the obstruction of the airway by a foreign body. Recognition is key. Do not confuse with fainting, heart attack, seizure, etc.

Choking is serious. It may lead to partial or complete airway obstruction. It may lead to the casualty becoming unconscious, and is potentially fatal if the obstruction is not removed.

Treatment
Ask the question 'Are you choking?'

Signs of severe airways obstruction include:
- Casualty unable to speak or only nods when asked if chocking.
- Casualty unable to breath.
- Breathing sounds wheezy.
- Silent cough.
- Unconscious casualty.

If blockage is partial and the casualty is conscious and breathing, support the casualty, and *encourage patient to cough*.

- If coughing does not remove the object then try carefully to remove any obvious objects from the mouth. Take care not to push anything further down the airway.
- Call 999.
- If casualty shows signs of exhaustion but is conscious, then ensure someone has called 999.
- Carry out *back blows* up to ×5. Stand to the side and slightly behind the casualty Support the chest with one hand and lean him forward to allow gravity to assist the expulsion of the object. The back blows are done with the heel of the hand between the scapulae, checking with each blow to see if the object has been expelled.
- If the back blows fail, carry out up to 5 *abdominal thrusts* (casualty bending forwards, both hands in clenched fist placed just below lower edge of sternum, and pull inwards and upwards).
- Alternate 5 back blows and 5 abdominal thrusts until the obstruction has been relieved (Fig. 1.6).
- If the casualty becomes unconscious support them carefully to the ground, call an ambulance immediately if not already done and proceed to BLS.
- If the casualty successfully expels the object it is advisable to advise an immediate medical opinion in all but the mildest cases in case further foreign material remains in the airway, causing later complications. This is particularly important if the casualty has a persistent cough, difficulty swallowing, or a sensation of something still stuck in the throat.

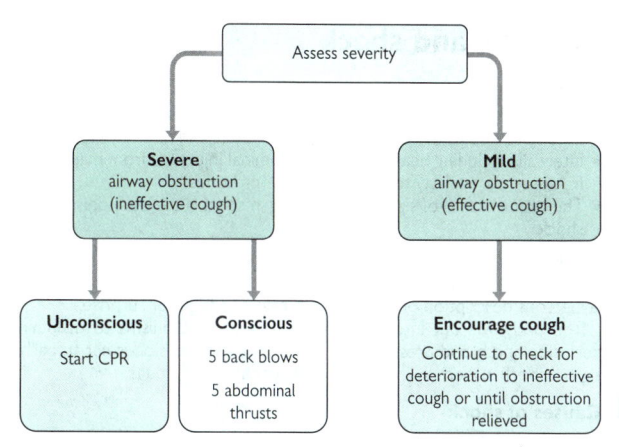

```
                    ┌─────────────────┐
                    │ Assess severity │
                    └─────────────────┘
                    ╱                 ╲
        ┌──────────────────┐   ┌──────────────────┐
        │     Severe       │   │      Mild        │
        │ airway obstruction│   │ airway obstruction│
        │ (ineffective cough)│  │ (effective cough) │
        └──────────────────┘   └──────────────────┘
          ╱           ╲                  │
┌──────────────┐ ┌──────────────┐ ┌────────────────────┐
│ Unconscious  │ │  Conscious   │ │  Encourage cough   │
│              │ │              │ │ Continue to check  │
│  Start CPR   │ │ 5 back blows │ │ for deterioration  │
│              │ │ 5 abdominal  │ │ to ineffective     │
│              │ │   thrusts    │ │ cough or until     │
│              │ │              │ │ obstruction        │
│              │ │              │ │    relieved        │
└──────────────┘ └──────────────┘ └────────────────────┘
```

Fig. 1.6 Adult choking algorithm. Reproduced with permission from the Resuscitation Council UK (Resuscitation Council Guidelines, 2010).

Choking child

Recognition
- As in adults the immediate reaction is to cough in an attempt to expel the foreign body. Active intervention required when coughing becomes ineffective and then must be commenced rapidly as asphyxia occurs more rapidly in children.
- Majority of chocking events in children occur during eating and are therefore often witnessed by an adult—as a result intervention more likely when child still conscious.

Treatment
Largely as in adults, but note:
- Only clear superficial debris—danger of moving objects further down airway and increasing obstruction.
- Substitute chest thrusts for abdominal thrusts in infants.
- Support infants and small children in a head-down prone position to allow gravity to assist expulsion.

Bleeding and shock

Introduction
In sport, bleeding most commonly arises as a result of trauma:
- Externally due to direct trauma: wounds, facial, and nasal injuries etc.
- Internally including head, chest, or abdominal injury, or from major fractures: particularly to the pelvis and long bones.
- The major hazard of significant bleeding in sport is the development of shock.

Shock is defined as an inadequate perfusion of the body's vital organs.

Clinical shock is very different and much more serious that the laypersons description of 'shock' which refers to fright or surprise.

The body will put into place compensatory mechanisms to maintain perfusion and blood pressure (BP) initially, so hypotension is *not* an early sign of shock, especially in children and healthy young adults.

Causes of shock
- *Cardiogenic = pump failure:*
  - Myocardial infarction/myocarditis.
  - Thoracic aortic dissection/acute valvular regurgitation.
  - Cardiac arrhythmias.
  - Cardiac depressant drug overdose.
- *Hypovolaemia:*
  - Blood loss—external or internal haemorrhage.
  - Other fluid loss such as diarrhoea, vomiting, burns etc.
- *Anaphylaxis:*
  - Food allergy especially peanuts.
  - Insect stings especially bees and wasps.
- *Spinal:* neurogenic shock may occur in a cervical spine injury.
- *Systemic:*
  - Sepsis.
  - Liver or adrenal failure.
  - Drug overdose, e.g. vasodilators, paracetamol.

Management of bleeding
Use gloves to provide a barrier and prevent infection (2-way).
- Minor cuts and abrasions can often be managed at the pitchside and the casualty allowed to continue their sporting activity. The wound should be irrigated with clean water. (Sterile water if possible, but not essential.)
- Dirt and embedded foreign bodies can be removed by the gentle force of the water in the cleaning process, but significant foreign objects, such as glass, should be left in place. Cover with a non-adhesive dressing and allow to return to play if appropriate.

Note that some sports have rules determining return to play in bleeding injuries, e.g. boxing, while other sports allow temporary substitution of a player 'blood substitution' e.g. rugby.
- All dirty wounds, where the bleeding is more severe or complicated (possible infection, foreign object, close to an important structure)

should be referred to hospital for adequate cleaning and tetanus immunization.
- First aid management of bleeding wounds includes application of pressure over the bleeding point and elevation above the level of the heart where possible and without aggravating the injury, e.g. bleeding in open leg fracture.

Internal bleeding in sport most commonly results from a fracture (especially pelvis and femur), chest injury (haemothorax), or abdominal injury (ruptured spleen, liver or kidneys). There will be no initial external signs of bleeding—a significant volume of blood can be lost into a body cavity with little external signs.

Assessment and management of shock

Assessment

The patient's airway should be secured:
- Initial 'First Aid' history and assessment may give clues as to the cause, e.g. bleeding wound, chest pain, bee sting, etc.
- If BP is so low that it is unrecordable then treat as a medical emergency and call for an ambulance and any available medical assistance immediately.
- Assess danger and response.
- *Assess/open airway:* look for obstruction, vomit, or blood and clear if possible.
- *Check breathing:* classically rapid and laboured.
- *Check cardiac rhythm:* pulse weak and thready ? arrhythmia.
- Check BP.
- *Check skin:* cold and clammy in pump failure and hypovolaemia. May be fevered in sepsis, but beware peripheral shutdown in severe sepsis with cold skin.
- *Check for signs of blood loss:* open wound, evidence of fracture, abdominal trauma, etc.
- *Check for any evidence of allergic reaction:* wheeze, stridor, soft tissue swelling, etc.
- Assess conscious level.

Management

- Danger, response, ABC and send for help.
- Give oxygen if available.
- Try to stabilize cause if possible, e.g. stop bleeding.
- Lie casualty flat with head down and feet up: those with asthma or cardiac aetiology may feel uncomfortable in this position.
- Maintain temperature.
- Reassure.
- Monitor ABC and conscious level.
- Do not give anything to eat or drink.
- Insert large bore cannula ×2 if available and trained to do so and commence IV fluids if available. Though blood or colloid may be more appropriate the SFAE study (2004)[1] found saline to be equally effective.

1 SFAE study (2004). A Comparison of Albumin and Saline for Fluid Resuscitation in the Intensive Care Unit. N Engl Med J 350: 2247–56. Available at: M http://www.nejm.org/doi/full/10.1056/NEJMoa040232.

In-hospital management includes aggressive intravenous fluid support, insertion of a central line, urinary catheterization, assessment and treatment of the underlying condition including appropriate drugs, and investigations such as CXR, ECG, bloods (U&E, FBC, LFTs, cross-match, septic screen, cardiac screen, etc.).

Anaphylaxis

Anaphylaxis is defined as a "severe life-threatening generalized or systemic hypersensitivity reaction". It is characterized by a rapidly developing life-threatening airway and/or breathing, and/or circulation problems usually associated with skin and mucosal changes (Fig. 1.7). Atopic individuals are particularly at risk but it can occur in those without any past history.

Common precipitants include:
- *Insect bites, and especially bee and wasp stings:* cause shock in ≈10–15min.
- *Food and food additives (e.g. peanuts, fish and eggs):* cause shock in ≈30–35min.
- *Drugs (e.g. aspirin, non-steroidal anti-inflammatory drugs (NSAIDs), iron injections, vaccines etc.):* IV drugs—cause shock in ≈10–15min.

Presentation

Casualty looks and feels unwell with a feeling of 'impending doom'.
- *Airway problems:* airway swelling, stridor, hoarse voice.
- *Breathing problems:* shortness of breath, wheeze, confusion (hypoxia) and cyanosis (late sign). Finally respiratory arrest.
- *Circulation problems:* signs of shock (see 📖 Shock, p. 27)
- *Skin/mucosal problems:* often the first feature and present in 80% of cases. Rash, erythema, urticaria, angioedema.

Management

Treat as a medical emergency and call for help:
- Secure the airway.
- Give 100% oxygen.
- Lie patient flat with head down (left lateral tilt if pregnant).
- Establish IV access.
- If possible measure BP, respiratory rate (RR), heart rate (HR), oxygen saturation, skin colour, capillary refill time.

Administer

- *Adrenaline:* intramuscular (IM) not IV, adult 500micrograms, child 6–12 years 300 micrograms, child <6 yrs 150 micrograms.
- IV fluids: colloid if available.
- IM/slow IV chlorampheniramine, 10mg in adults.
- IM/slow IV hydrocortisone, 200 mg in adults.
- Consider nebulized salbutamol if persistent bronchospasm.

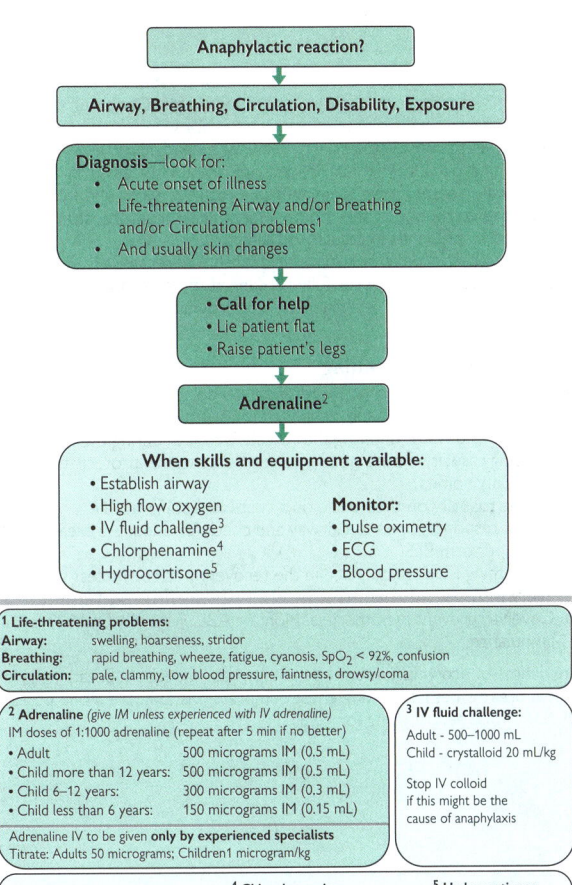

ANAPHYLAXIS

Anaphylactic reaction?

Airway, Breathing, Circulation, Disability, Exposure

Diagnosis—look for:
- Acute onset of illness
- Life-threatening Airway and/or Breathing and/or Circulation problems[1]
- And usually skin changes

- Call for help
- Lie patient flat
- Raise patient's legs

Adrenaline[2]

When skills and equipment available:
- Establish airway
- High flow oxygen
- IV fluid challenge[3]
- Chlorphenamine[4]
- Hydrocortisone[5]

Monitor:
- Pulse oximetry
- ECG
- Blood pressure

---

[1] **Life-threatening problems:**
Airway: swelling, hoarseness, stridor
Breathing: rapid breathing, wheeze, fatigue, cyanosis, SpO_2 < 92%, confusion
Circulation: pale, clammy, low blood pressure, faintness, drowsy/coma

[2] **Adrenaline** (give IM unless experienced with IV adrenaline)
IM doses of 1:1000 adrenaline (repeat after 5 min if no better)
- Adult: 500 micrograms IM (0.5 mL)
- Child more than 12 years: 500 micrograms IM (0.5 mL)
- Child 6–12 years: 300 micrograms IM (0.3 mL)
- Child less than 6 years: 150 micrograms IM (0.15 mL)

Adrenaline IV to be given **only by experienced specialists**
Titrate: Adults 50 micrograms; Children 1 microgram/kg

[3] **IV fluid challenge:**
Adult - 500–1000 mL
Child - crystalloid 20 mL/kg

Stop IV colloid
if this might be the
cause of anaphylaxis

	[4] Chlorphenamine (IM or slow IV)	[5] Hydrocortisone (IM or slow IV)
Adult or child more than 12 years	10 mg	200 mg
Child 6–12 years	5 mg	100 mg
Child 6 months to 6 years	2.5 mg	50 mg
Child less than 6 months	250 micrograms/kg	25 mg

Fig. 1.7 Anaphylaxis algorithm. Reproduced with permission from the Resuscitation Council UK (Resuscitation Council Guidelines, 2010).

Drowning

Potential drowning may occur in a variety of sporting environments including swimming pools, rivers, and open water. Drowning can occur in a surprisingly small volume of water especially when the casualty has an altered level of consciousness, e.g. following a head injury.

Drowning occurs when an inadequate amount of air is in the lungs due to water entering the lungs. When a casualty is rescued from water, water may come out of the mouth—most likely from the stomach. It is important to prevent the casualty inhaling this.

Every casualty from a drowning incident should receive prompt medical attention, even if they appear fully recovered, as there is the possibility of later swelling of the airway. All victims of drowning should be treated for potential hypothermia.

Management of drowning

- Remove the casualty from water if safe to do so. The rescuer should not put himself at risk, e.g. deep water, fast-flowing river.
- Try to avoid water entering the casualty's mouth during the rescue. If carrying casualty ensure head is lower than chest to protect the airway if casualty vomits.
- Lie the casualty on their back, on a coat/blanket if available.
- Check response, open the airway and check for adequate breathing. If none, perform BLS.
- If breathing is adequate place in the recovery position, unless spinal injury is suspected, e.g. diving.
- Cover to prevent hypothermia. Monitor ABC + AVPU. Dial 999 for an ambulance.

In victims of drowning when the casualty has inadequate breathing give 5 initial breaths before starting chest compressions (30:2). If alone perform BLS for 1min before going for help.

Ongoing assessment, documentation, and transfer to definitive care

Ongoing assessment

Continued reassessment and evaluation of response to treatment is vital. Try to obtain additional information from witnesses, friends, and family members as to the exact mechanism of presentation and any underlying medical conditions, medication taken, etc. Continued observation and monitoring of ABC and AVPU may allow early identification of deterioration.

Documentation

Remember to pass on all relevant medical information to secondary care and any appropriate individuals.

Patient confidentiality remains paramount and no information should be given to other that the casualty's relatives and health professionals involved in ongoing care. Never give any medical information to the media without the casualty's consent. Best practice suggests the casualty speaks directly to the media.

Accurate medical notes should be written as soon as practicable after transfer or other 'disposal', e.g. casualty goes home with an accompanying adult. It is rarely possible to make notes during the assessment and treatment unless another individual is present to note down information. If more than one health professional is involved in the care of the casualty, it is advisable for all to agree and sign the documentation. There are a variety of accident report forms available for this purpose.

Transfer to definitive care

In minor injury or illness the casualty can be allowed home with an accompanying adult. As mentioned before there is a delicate balance between the time required for assessment and treatment and the 'load and go' approach of early transport for more definitive care. This decision will be based on the nature of the injuries, experience of those present, need for more definitive care such as for surgery, advanced airway management, vascular access, distance to secondary care and mode of transport available

Chapter 2

Sports injury

Injury management *36*
General management plan for acute sports injuries *38*
Management of acute soft tissue injury *40*
Care of wounds, cuts, and grazes *44*
Non-steroidal anti-inflammatory drugs *48*
Strain and sprain *52*
Ligaments *54*
Bone *58*
Sports injury in children *62*

Injury management

The initial management of an acute sporting injury is vital as optimal treatment will shorten the recovery time, protect the athlete from further injury, and enable the athlete to return to training and competition as soon as possible. Delayed or inappropriate treatment has the opposite effect and may adversely affect an athlete's career.

Good initial management requires on-site recognition of the injury and prompt initiation of treatment. It requires a team approach with experienced medical and physiotherapy staff working with coaches, referees, and administrators.

Sports injuries may be as a result of trauma or overuse and can involve any of the tissues of the body. The most commonly involved are muscles, ligaments, and tendons, (soft tissue injury) or the bony skeleton. Some serious joint injuries may involve a combination of bone and soft tissue.

Injuries to the head and cervical spine or the thoracic and abdominal organs are potentially life threatening.

Acute injury
- Bleeding occurs with tissue damage.
- Immediate swelling and the resultant pressure on surrounding structures causes secondary effects.
- Response follows the classical inflammatory pattern—see 'Non-steroidal anti-inflammatory drugs', p. 48 for an explanation.
- Local oedema increases tissue pressure, further delays healing, and lengthens rehabilitation.
- In immediate treatment of acute injury, the objective is to interrupt this cycle, limit bleeding, and swelling, reduce inflammation, and reduce the size and extent of the injury.

Overuse injuries
This type of injury leads to the same cycle of response, without local bleeding. Continued activity causes repetitive micro-trauma, tissue inflammation, and damage. The treatment of overuse injury follows the same plan.

Soft tissue inflammation
This follows the classic pattern of:
- Swelling.
- Heat.
- Erythema.
- Pain and loss of function.

The treatment plan is based on this process and cycle as described above.

General management plan for acute sports injuries

Preparation and planning
The management of sports injury requires preparation and planning. Factors include:
- Equipment and facilities.
- First aid kit and doctors bag.
- Liaison with officials, administrators, and coaches.
- Membership of 'The Medical Team', which includes a variety of health professionals.

On-site availability
On-site availability allows:
- Initiation of the appropriate management immediately.
- Direct observation of the mechanism of injury—this aids accurate diagnosis.

This, ideally, includes presence at both training and matches or competition. This helps to build trust with the coaching staff and the athletes. It also allows further input into the athlete's preparation in areas such as:
- Pre-season screening and assessment.
- Fitness assessment.
- Planning of training schedules.
- Monitoring rehabilitation, arranging surgical opinions/operations, etc.

Event management
Medical input may be needed in planning of events, and may include advice on playing surface, equipment, adequate time for warm-up and rest, training facilities, and first aid equipment. Good event management will not only limit injury risk (e.g. by not playing on dangerous surfaces), but will also ensure prompt and appropriate management at the time of the injury.

Observation
This includes:
- Observation of training and warm-up, etc., to ensure good technique.
- Observation of exact injury mechanism will result in prompt and appropriate treatment.
- Observation of the sport so that the doctor is familiar with the rules and likely injuries which will result.

History
An appropriate history is vital to ensure correct diagnosis and treatment. In acute sports injury the athlete may be distressed both by the pain and the implications of serious injury.

The exact nature and location of the pain will give a guide as to the structures injured. In Achilles tendon or anterior cruciate ligament rupture, for example, the athlete may describe an audible 'pop'.

Clinical examination

Early examination, before swelling and the inflammatory response ensues, may give clues as to the diagnosis, which are more difficult to elicit at a later time. Initial pitch side assessment is usually helpful but at times it may be more appropriate to carry out a clinical examination at a better location, e.g. first aid room. Protective equipment should be removed to allow full examination, unless this will worsen the injury, e.g. fractured tibia. Sporting headgear should not be removed unless to enable Basic Life Support to be performed especially where spinal injury is suspected.

The initial examination should:
- Establish a preliminary diagnosis.
- Determine whether the athlete can continue.
- Determine whether further treatment is required, e.g. at hospital.

Treatment

- *Emergency care:* injuries to the head, cervical spine, and chest, and those to major joints or bones should be considered as an emergency and managed appropriately.
- *Triage:* this includes transport from the field and, if required, onwards to hospital for X-ray, further examination, etc. Good communication with the hospital and the athlete/coach to ensure appropriate after care. Arrangements for review as soon as practical.
- *Immediate injury care:* if standard care is appropriate it should follow the PRICES/POLICE regimen—see 📖 Management of acute soft tissue injury, p. 40.

Return to play

Return to training and competition is determined by whether:
- Return will not worsen the injury.
- Return will not increase the risk of further injury.
- The athlete will be able to perform at pre-injury level.
- The athlete's return will not place other competitors at risk.

This decision should take into account factors such as the importance of the event, time left in the event, future schedule, and playing conditions.

The medical team should observe the athlete closely on their return to ensure rehabilitation is complete and no further damage is taking place.

Judgement on return to play should be based solely on the health of the athlete and should take precedence over the wishes of the coach, relatives, club, supporters, and sometimes, the wishes of the athlete him/herself.

Management of acute soft tissue injury

The 'PRICES' mnemonic incorporates the various treatment modalities for acute soft tissue injuries:
- P = Protect
- R = Rest
- I = Ice
- C = Compression
- E = Elevation
- S = Support

POLICE substitutes Optimal Loading for Rest.

Protect

This refers to a number of types of protection such as:
- Protect the athlete so they do not make the injury worse.
- Protect and support surrounding structures.
- Protect other competitors.
- Protection of the injured part may include crutches, splints, slings, braces, taping, strapping, etc.

Rest

True rest is difficult to enforce—and in practice usually unnecessary.

Absolute rest

Severe soft tissue injuries may require a short period of bed rest or immobilization in plaster or brace to limit movement to a minimum. Absolute rest will also be required initially after an operation.

Relative or active rest

An athlete can often maintain some activity. This will usually be part of the treatment programme and is important psychologically. Relative activity ensures:
- Maintenance of muscle strength.
- Maintenance of general cardiovascular conditioning and aerobic fitness, e.g. hydrotherapy.

Exercise is a recognized part of the treatment programme for soft tissue injury. Damaged ligaments benefit from the 'stress' of weight-bearing and movement. Excessive rest will prolong the inflammatory phase and lengthen the time to return to play.

A recent (2010) UK consensus conference on the PRICES regime recommended that the duration of the unloading (Protection/Rest) and speed of progression of rehabilitation depends on the severity of the injury, the injury mechanism, and the type of soft tissue injured (ligament v tendon v muscle).

More recently, a modification of the acronym substitutes **O**ptimal Loading for Rest and the acronym becomes POLICE. Optimal loading is more appropriate in facilitating early rehabilitation. Available at: http://bjsm.bmj.com/content/early/2011/09/07/bjsports-2011-090297.full.pdf

Ice

The application of cold (cryotherapy) has been advocated since the classical description of inflammation by Celsus in the 1st century AD (redness, swelling, heat, and pain) to which Virchow, in 1858, added loss of function.

Theoretical benefits of cryotherapy

- Limitation of bleeding via vasoconstriction. The theory of reflex vasodilatation remains controversial.
- Limitation of swelling.
- Limitation of inflammation and further tissue damage. This may be due to the effect of histamine on vascular membranes and on neutrophils and leucocytes.
- Reduction in metabolism in local tissues. This reduces enzyme function, inhibits pain and decreases swelling and oxygen consumption.
- Assists with pain control—however, beware the athlete who becomes 'pain free' with ice and wishes to resume playing. Ice inhibits pain in 2 ways:
  - Relief of surrounding muscle spasm.
  - Slowing of sensory pain impulses.

How to apply ice

Ice comes in a variety of forms including crushed ice (better than ice cubes as the contact is better), chemical ice packs, reusable gel cold packs, and those combined with compression, e.g. cryocuff. Be careful as only melting iced water is at 0°C. Ice taken directly from a freezer may be at a much lower temperature.

Coolant sprays work by evaporation thus reducing skin temperature. They do not achieve sufficient depth of cooling to be effective in reducing muscle temperature.

Debate continues as to the optimum frequency and time of application. An intermittent protocol is more effective than continued application.

The primary clinical effect of the application of ice is a reduction in pain. Ice, preferably crushed, should be applied for 10–20min every 2h initially. Ice should not be used continuously for longer than 20–30min. There is no agreed scientific consensus re the duration of the use of ice though it would appear to most beneficial in the first 48–72h.

Ice works via conduction. As adipose tissue is an excellent insulator, ice application may have to be extended in those areas with greater body fat.

A thin damp barrier should be used at the cooling interface to avoid reduction of the clinical effectiveness.

Contraindications to using ice

- Broken or damaged skin.
- Where nerve damage is suspected and sensation altered.
- Altered circulation is suspected.
- When ice application increases pain.

Compression

The early use of compression will:
- Support the injured area.
- Decrease swelling.
- Ice can be combined with compression. Later, compression can be replaced by a supportive bandage or strapping. Taping is best done by an experienced sports physiotherapist to achieve maximum benefit.

It is recommended that the compressive modality configures to the shape of the body part and provides a gradual compressive force. Compression provides additional benefits in terms of biomechanical support, control of the range of movement and reassurance to the injured athlete. It also corroborates the severity of the injury.

Elevation

- Contributes to the reduction in blood flow and as a result, swelling. The lower tissue pressure will contribute to the reduction in pain.
- Must be at a significant angle, i.e. greater than 45° for a lower limb.
- Should be combined with support of the elevated part, e.g. pillows.
- While there is no optimal duration of the elevation it should be maintained at least over the first 24h. Distal body parts will require longer periods of elevation.

Support

Support aims to help to stabilize the injured tissue and prevent further injury. Under controlled conditions it may allow the athlete to return to competition earlier.

Support also allows an early commencement of controlled and monitored activity such as weight bearing, which will shorten the rehabilitation period and facilitate an earlier return to sport.

Care of wounds, cuts, and grazes

A wound is defined as a 'disruption of the tissues produced by an external mechanical force'. Wounds include:
- Contusions.
- Abrasions.
- Lacerations.
- Incised and puncture wounds.

Open wounds are very common in contact sports such as football, rugby, hockey and ice hockey, American football, etc. They are also common in sports where falls often occur such as cycling and riding. Wounds account for 25–30% of the workload in emergency departments.

Prognosis is dependent on the type of trauma and the extent of the damage.
- Severe bleeding and clinical shock.
- Infection.
- Complications secondary to the extent of the damage, e.g. blood vessel, nerve, and tissue damage.

Abrasions

An abrasion (Latin *abradere*–to scrape) is a superficial injury. Damage is only to the epidermis so it should not actively bleed (though in practice abrasions may extend into the dermis). A scratch is linear, while a graze suggests a broader impact.

The cause is normally a glancing contact with a rough surface. Tangential impact produces a moving abrasion, which indicates direction by the pattern of damage to the epidermis and may leave trace material such as grit. This type is most common in sport on artificial surfaces, such as Astroturf.

Direct impact produces an imprint abrasion with the pattern of the causative object.

All abrasions reflect the site of impact (contrast contusions).

Contusions (bruises)

A contusion involves bleeding into the soft tissue due to the rupture of a small blood vessel resulting from a direct, blunt force, e.g. a punch. A haematoma is a contusion where a larger amount of bleeding results in a pool of blood.

Contusions and strains comprise 60–70% of all sports injuries and are of variable severity from simple skin damage to contusions of internal organs. Most go unreported and untreated. Typically caused by blunt trauma, such as a blow or a fall. Uncomplicated contusions do not breach skin surface and there is no external bleeding.

It is important to exclude other causes of bleeding including abnormalities of the clotting system in diseases such as leukaemia, thrombocytopenia, liver disease, and vitamin deficiencies (Vitamin C).

Pathology

Trauma causes rupture of capillaries and possible venules (arterial damage rare). After impact, bleeding may continue for some time due to circulatory pressure. If the volume of bleeding is sufficient, swelling occurs. If extravastrated blood collects in a pool it is known as a haematoma. Local inflammatory reaction occurs at a site with necrotic tissue, caused by macrophage infiltration.

Site of bruising does not always indicate the exact site of injury, as blood will track through tissues under influence of gravity and body movement. (e.g. bruising along lower border of foot in ankle ligament and thigh bruising in fractured hip)

Deeper bruising will result in a slower appearance of surface skin discolouration. Changes in colour will give an inaccurate estimate of the time of the initial impact.

Signs and symptoms
- Soreness and pain with active movement.
- Visible trauma and swelling.
- Residual function is unaffected compared to injuries such as a muscle rupture.
- Will require formal assessment before return to play.

Differential diagnosis
Soft tissue injury including muscle rupture, ligament sprain, etc.

Wound healing
- Most wounds are treated by primary closure with a close approximation of the wound edges—primary intention. This may involve suturing or items such as Steristrips or wound glue.
- Secondary wound healing occurs when the wound is initially left open. This may occur when there is infection or in the case of a crush injury with extensive tissue damage.
- Wound healing may also be affected by:
  - *Anatomical site*: poor over tibia.
  - *Vascular supply*: poor in peripheral vascular disease.
  - *Movement:* e.g. over a joint.
  - *Wound configuration:* e.g. jagged edges.
  - *Mechanism of injury*: incised wounds heal quickly.
  - *General health and nutrition of the casualty*: older patients, those on steroids, etc.

Assessment of wounds

It is important to obtain an accurate history (with accurate note taking) including:
- Time of injury.
- Mechanism of injury.
- First aid treatment—if any.
- Tetanus immunization status—if any.
- Allergies or hypersensitivities (esp. tapes, dressings, etc.).
- Medication—if any.

A formal examination and assessment of the wound is then made, which should include:
- Anatomical site.
- Size: width and length.
- Depth.
- Configuration: straight, jagged edge, etc.
- Tissue loss.
- Deformity.
- Loss of function including motor and/or sensory loss.
- Pain.
- Bleeding: actual and estimated.

Management

First aid
- Elevation with support.
- Direct pressure: with sterile dressing if available.
- Pressure dressing: not tourniquet.
- Apply closure strips if appropriate triage measure until hospital transfer is possible.

Cleaning
- Essential to prevent infection and remove foreign body fragments.
- Protective barrier effect of skin is broken in wounds allowing micro-organisms to enter deeper tissues.
- Wounds that 'look' clean are not necessarily sterile—consider all traumatic wounds as contaminated.
- May require pain relief (including entonox) and/or anaesthetic to ensure adequate cleansing.

Which cleansing agent?
- Irrigate to remove contaminants with water—sterile if available. No evidence of increased infection with drinking-quality tap water.
- There are a variety of antiseptic solutions, which will assist wound cleansing. For an anti-bacterial action has been suggested that 20 min contact time is required.

Wound closure
- A variety of methods are available depending on nature of wound, time since injury, etc. Some wounds may be best treated by delayed closure.
  - Sutures.
  - Steristrips.
  - Staples.
  - Adhesive.

Dressings
Many now commercially available. Choice depends on factors such as:
- Nature and location of wound.
- Presence and risk of infection.
- Amount of exudates.

Tetanus
All casualties should have current tetanus status established and be immunized as per current Department of Health guidelines.

Return to sport
This will depend on a number of factors including:
- Nature of wound—size, method of closure, edges, etc.
- Site of wound especially if over a joint.
- Nature of sport.

Non-steroidal anti-inflammatory drugs

As the level of competition increases and greater competitive performance is required, there is a point where the 'strain' on the skeletal framework exceeds that which body can withstand, resulting in damage to connective tissues and joints.

The inflammatory response (Box 2.1)
- Enables the body's defensive and regenerative resources to be channelled into tissues which have suffered damage or are contaminated with abnormal material (e.g. invading micro-organisms).
- The term inflammation is derived from the Latin *inflammare*—to set on fire. It is used to describe the pathological process that occurs at the site of tissue damage. Classical description by Celsus 1st century AD.
- Four signs of inflammation are redness, swelling, heat, and pain. Cold application (cryotherapy) has traditionally been used in managing inflammation.
- Prior to the 20th century *phagocytosis* was considered the primary movement of inflammatory reaction with specialized cells able to move 'amoeba-like' to the site of the noxious agent, to ingest and destroy foreign material such as bacteria. The importance of a vascular system was later recognized—without this there would be no redness or heat associated with the inflammatory response.
- Inflammation is a dynamic process that may, at times, cause more harm to the organism than the initiating noxious stimulus itself. Hay fever, for example, can be incapacitating but occurs as a consequence of the reaction of our defence system to harmless airborne pollen.
- Not all inflammatory reactions are useful—there are no benefits from the inflammatory reactions that occur in diseases such as rheumatic fever or rheumatoid arthritis.

Vascular changes
- The immediate reaction of skin is redness due to increased blood flow through the inflamed area. Its duration depends on the severity of the stimulus.
- Skin temperature rises and approaches that of the deep body temperature.
- The whole capillary bed at the damaged site becomes suffused with blood at an increased pressure as capillaries dilate and closed ones open up. Venules open up with increased venous flow.
- Thus two of the cardinal signs of inflammation *heat* and *redness* are caused by this increase in blood flow to the affected area.

Swelling
- Results from changes in the permeability of the blood vessel wall to protein. Normally the tissue fluid is composed of water with some low-molecular-weight solutes. The very low protein content compared to the blood is because of the impermeability of the blood vessel wall, which inhibits protein movement from blood vessel to the surrounding tissues.

- Normally the vascular pressure generated from the heart forces water out of the blood at the arteriolar end, while the colloid osmotic pressure exerted by the protein in the blood draws water back at the venous end. Without the presence of the plasma protein, blood volume would rapidly diminish due to net movement of water from the blood to the tissues.

Pain
- May also be due to release of pain-inducing chemicals at the site of the reaction.
- Due in part to the increased pressure on sensory nerves caused by the accumulation of the oedematous fluid.

Mediators
- Lewis first proposed the *mediator* concept in 1927: he called this the H-substance. The first class discovered were *prostaglandins*—formed by the action of cyclo-oxygenase on arachidonic acid.
- Abundant in body: stored in granules in mast cells—found in high levels in lungs, GI system, and skin.
- Produce vasodilatation: redness and temperature and increased blood vessel permeability to protein—swelling.
- At high concentration can also produce pain.

Leucocytes in inflammation
- More persistent inflammatory reactions involve the influx of leucocytes, of which the most important in inflammation is the polymorph/neutrophil. Normal extra vascular tissue contains few polymorphs but, in inflammation, these cells pass from the blood into damaged tissue.
- Polymorphs are the first inflammatory cells to accumulate at the site of injury—they are *phagocytic* and ingest and digest invading micro-organisms and tissue debris.

Acute inflammation will gradually resolve in time with no damage or, if more severe, synthesis of connective tissue to form a scar.

Box 2.1 The inflammatory response

- An influx of blood giving rise to the characteristic *heat* and *redness*.
- A movement of plasma protein and associated water into the tissue, causing *swelling*.
- An influx of phagocytic cells that have the potential to cause tissue destruction.
- *Pain*, perhaps due to pressure on the nerve endings caused by the swelling or to the effect of chemical mediators of pain being released.
- Finally, and perhaps most importantly to the sportsman, *loss of function*—Virchow's fifth sign.

The use of anti-inflammatory drugs to treat inflammatory conditions

- Hippocrates mentions chewing of willow bark and the first synthetic analogue was produced in the 19th century, called acetylsalacilic acid and given the trade name aspirine.
- Now 20 or so aspirin-like drugs are available—aspirin and ibuprofen are on general sale.
- No clear evidence of any single agent being more effective than others—or indeed more effective than aspirin!

Mechanism of action

- In 1971, John Vane and his colleagues published 3 papers in *Nature* which outlined their ability to suppress the synthesis of prostaglandins. Their activity is to:
  - Reduce the symptoms of heat and redness as prostaglandin normally promotes an increased blood flow.
  - Reduce pain as there will be no hyperalgesia without prostaglandin.
  - Reduce oedema and swelling as the permeability increasing effect of chemical agents on blood vessel walls would not be subject to the normal exaggerating action of prostglandin.
- The use of NSAIDs in inflammatory conditions is well-established and they are a simple and relatively safe means of reducing the inflammatory response to injury and assist return to competitive fitness more rapidly.
- There is no unequivocal evidence that newer agents have more efficacy, but fewer gastric side-effects.
- Advantages in the early treatment of inflammatory responses to injury, in early post-injury stage.
- Effectiveness of treatment over longer periods is less apparent. In self-limiting injuries the differences between treatment and placebo groups diminish with time.
- Early NSAIDs were all based on aspirin but now there are more than 20 individual drugs. Ibuprofen is most widely used and available for purchase over the counter.
- Newer drugs were developed to lessen the gastric side effects, and in particular GI bleeding, which is especially important in the elderly. The most recent drugs which selectively inhibited cyclo-oxygenase 2 (COX 2), appeared to have an excellent initial side-effect profile. Recent reports suggest an increased risk of cardiovascular events.
- The current scientific evidence suggests that the use of NSAIDs can result in a modest inhibition of the initial inflammatory response and its symptoms, particularly pain. There use is most beneficial in soft-tissue injury associated with definite inflammatory conditions such as bursitis or synovitis. However, this may be associated with a negative effect later in the healing phase. It should be noted that corticosteroids have generally been shown to adversely affect the healing of acute injuries.

Topical NSAID agents
- Their concept is to maximize level of drug at site of injury while minimizing systemic, especially gastrointestinal, adverse effects.
- There is evidence that they achieve high levels of the active drug in the underlying tissues.
- Clinical trials demonstrate the active drug to be more effective than placebo but the differences slight.
- The effectiveness was greater in the first 2 weeks of treatment. Especially in acutely painful musculoskeletal conditions.
- *British National Formulary* concludes that they '…may provide some slight relief of pain…'

Strain and sprain

A strain is a partial or complete tear of a muscle or tendon. The most commonly strained muscles are those that cross two joints during an eccentric, rather than concentric, contraction. Lower limb muscles like rectus femoris, biceps femoris, semitendinosus, adductors, hamstrings, and medial head of the gastrocnemius are more frequently injured. Muscle strain more commonly occurs at the myotendinous junction, the weakest link in the muscle. Ligament injury is very common in sports medicine. Knee, ankle, elbow, shoulder, and fingers are the most common joints affected.

- *Grade 1 injury:* small number of fibres damaged, resulting in some pain and swelling, with minimal loss of strength, function, or stability.
- *Grade 2 injury:* more fibres damaged, with moderate pain, swelling, and loss of function, strength, or stability.
- *Grade 3 injury:* complete tear of the tissue. May result in instability of a joint or a gap in the muscle fibres.

Diagnosis is by clinical examination. An ultrasound scan or an MR scan may be helpful.

STRAIN AND SPRAIN

Ligaments

Anatomy and physiology
- Ligaments are of variable shapes and sizes with fibres running parallel between two bony points of insertion. Some appear as less distinct sheets of connective tissue.
- Most are extra-articular (though cruciates are intra-articular).
- Variable blood supply, e.g. poor for cruciates, good for medial collateral of knee.
- Most research on the cruciate ligaments because of their vital role in knee stability.
- Ligament tensile strength is lost with immobility—plaster cast immobilization for 8 weeks required 9 months rehabilitation to recover tensile strength.
- Conversely, there may be increased ligament strength with a formal training programme.

Histology
- Parallel collagen fibres running in a wave pattern to allow a spring-like stretch and lengthening. This allows an adjustment of tension and reduces the risk of injury.
- At the ligament insertion into the bone there is a transition from fibrous tissue to fibrocartilage, which becomes mineralized as it attaches to bone.

Composition
- Mainly type I collagen (some type III), elastin and proteoglycans. 65% by weight is water.
- The stiffness of the ligament increases with loading, which allows limited movement, but resists excessive load.

Function of ligaments
- Maintenance of joint alignment and the gliding motion of joint surfaces. Ligament disruption will result in mal-alignment and subsequent early joint degeneration.
- Proprioception around the joint.
- Support the skeleton, e.g. spinal ligaments.
- Maintain pressure on articular cartilage.

Classification of ligament injuries
- *Grade I*: mild sprain with no instability and firm end-point on stressing.
- *Grade II*: moderate sprain with mild instability and softer end-point on stressing.
- *Grade III*: severe sprain with significant instability.

Mechanism of injury
Injury may occur as a result of direct trauma, or indirectly when there is a sudden mechanical stress to the joint. One of the most common ligament injuries is to the medial collateral ligament of the knee when there is a forced valgus injury. This may occur, even when the point of contact is distal, due to the long levers of the lower leg. If, for example,

the sportsman is struck on the lateral side of the lower leg when the foot is fixed, the knee joint is forced medially. This tends to open up the medial side of the joint and, unfortunately, may also damage the meniscus and cruciate ligament(s).

Ligament healing

Classically, ligament healing is divided into 3 phases:

Inflammatory or substrate phase
This begins immediately after the acute injury with the classical inflammatory response of bleeding, swelling, cellular infiltrate of inflammatory cells, and white blood cells with later fibroblast aggregation.

Cellular proliferation phase
From 4 days until 2–3 weeks after injury. Fibroblasts proliferate and collagen is produced. Macrophages and mast calls are abundant. A new capillary network is established.

Remodelling phase
Ongoing and probably continuous. Fibroblast infiltration and collagen production peak and diminish. Collagen scar forms, which gradually remodels from the healing type III to type I collagen fibres.

Factors affecting ligament healing

The degree of injury
The injury itself is the initial stimulus for repair. Traumatically torn tissue usually disrupts the length of the ligament and incomplete tears repair more easily.

Wound stress
A topic of much debate and research. Initial protection of the site (for about 2 weeks) allows some strength to be regained. Later, however, mobilization and a degree of stress is essential if maximal repair is to be achieved.

Adequate blood supply and nutrition
Adequate blood supply is important for:
- Transport of inflammatory cells that initiate wound healing.
- Ensure optimum wound healing.
- Decrease the risk of infection.
- Improve wound healing if infection ensues.

It has also been suggested that vitamin C, protein, and cystine will facilitate tissue healing.

Prevention of ligament injury

Factors that may help to prevent or limit damage and consequently time lost from sport include:
- *Understanding the risk:* high-risk sports are those played at high velocity where direct trauma is more likely. These result in a higher risk of ligament injury.
- *Rules of the sport:* modification of the rules in contact sports may reduce the injury risk.

- *Sporting environment:* certain climatic conditions, such as heavy rain or ice, will alter the surface on which sport is played and thus the injury risk.
- *Use of protective equipment and devices:* these include both protection to prevent injury, such as protective padding, and also the use of protective braces and supports to minimize repeated injury to an already damaged, incompletely healed ligament.
- *'Prehabilitation':* while the immediate goal of training programmes is to optimize performance, it will also have the additional benefit of reducing the incidence of injury. This can be achieved by:
  - High standard of coaching and training.
  - Warm-up and stretching programmes.
  - Endurance and strength training.
  - Proprioceptive, flexibility, and agility training.
- *Medical screening of the athletes:* assessment of:
  - Previous injury and degree of rehabilitation achieved.
  - Excessive ligamentous laxity may be picked up on screening examination.
  - Incompetence of other supporting ligaments.
  - Poor muscle strength.
  - Other factors such as the use of alcohol or drugs may increase injury risk.
- As with all febrile illness, athletes should not return to sport until fever subsides.

Bone

The human body comprises a variety of different materials, which can be divided into 2 groups based on function:
- Active structures that produce force: muscles.
- Passive structures that do not produce force: bones, cartilage, ligaments, and tendons.

Functions of bone

The adult human skeleton consists of 206 individual bones. These:
- Provide support.
- Act with muscles as levers to transfer force.
- Protect the internal organs.
- Metabolic: calcium storage and metabolism.

Types of bone

Cortical

(Latin meaning bark.) Also known as compact bone.
- Predominant in limbs—appendicular skeleton.
- Surrounds trabecular bone as a protective covering.
- Main role is to provide skeletal strength.
- 3 layers: outer periosteum, middle intracortical layer, and inner endostium, next to the marrow cavity.
- Contain neurovascular 'haversian canals' with capillaries and nerve fibres.

Trabecular

(Latin *trabs* means timber.) Also known as cancellous or spongy bone.
- Forms bones of axial skeleton, e.g. skull, rib cage, and spine.
- Minimal part of skeletal strength.
- Major metabolic role.
- Made up of strands or trabeculae of bone whose pattern is determined by the forces applied to the bone.

Classes of bones

- *Long bones*: hollow shaft and two extremities, e.g. humerus and tibia. Found in limbs and act as levers to transmit force generated by muscles.
- *Short bones*: cubical in shape, cortical cover, and spongy core. Include carpal and tarsal bones.
- *Flat bones*: layers of cortical bones with spongy centre. Include sternum, skull bones, ribs, and scapula. Provide large area for tendon attachment and protective function.
- *Irregular bones*: adapted shape for particular function. Include pubis, maxilla, and vertebrae.

Bone metabolism

Bone composition
- *Bone cells:* osteoclasts and osteoblasts.
- *Bone matrix:*

- 40% organic—type 1 collagen, proteoglycans, and growth factors.
- 60% inorganic—calcium hydroxyapatite.

Calcium metabolism
- Regulated by parathyroid hormone (PTH) and vitamin D.
- Recommended daily intake = 1000mg.
- Excreted by kidneys.

Bone turnover
- Balance of osteoblast and osteoclast activity.
- Affected by hormones such as oestrogen, glucocorticoids, and thyroxine.
- Bone 'stress' is important.

Normal bone metabolim
- Peak bone mass in early adulthood.
- Plateau until 35–40 years.
- Rapid annual decline (1–2%/year) in women after the menopause.
- Male bone loss begins later (45 yrs) and at a slower rate.
- Osteoporosis is the decrease in bone mass (per unit volume). Primary osteoporosis is normally post-menopausal and is determined by reduced oestrogen. Other risk factors include:
  - Race.
  - Heredity.
  - Early menopause/hysterectomy.
  - Smoking/alcohol/drug abuse.
  - Calcium intake.

Standard investigations include measurement of bone density (DEXA scan) and calcium metabolism. Treatments include dietary measures, calcium, and vitamin D, hormone replacement therapy, and bisphosphonates. Screen for osteoporosis in those with a fracture, or 2 or more risk factors.

Secondary osteoporosis can result from a variety of causes such as:
- Poor diet.
- Endocrine causes.
- Drug induced, e.g. steroids.
- Chronic disease, e.g. rheumatoid arthritis and chronic renal disease.
- Malignancy.

Bone biomechanics

Wolff's law (1892) stated that 'The shape of bone is determined only by the static stressing …' While in general terms this is largely true, the effect of stress on bone is not as simple. Stress can have a variety of effects; as seen in a healing fracture or in bone atrophy. Wolff did not take into account the effect of heredity, where stress will not influence an inherited bone deformity.

When loaded, bone becomes increasingly 'stiff', thus less likely to fracture under load (spine). Fracture will occur, however, when the load exceeds the ultimate strength of the bone.

Stress fractures are clinical manifestations of bone fatigue. This occurs due to increased load repetitions which, individually, are within the normal acceptable load. Animal studies, for example, show a 5-fold increase in stress fractures from walking to jogging. The bones of the lower limb are more highly loaded and react with less strain at a given level of stress.

Fracture, which is the pathological result of load, may result from:
- Excessive force.
- Weakened bone.
- Small bone diameter.
- Excess frequency of load.
- Reduced recovery time between repeated loadings.

Bone remodelling is a slow process. A gradual progression in training intensity allows bone response which prevents stress fractures.

Bone shape is optimal for a normal load pattern so that bone deformity or an excessive load both contribute to the risk of skeletal injury.

Bones in children and adolescents deform at a lower load than in adults. The bone is weaker than the attached ligaments or tendons and is thus more likely to suffer avulsion fractures.

Bone and physical activity
- *Effect of gravity*: bone mass has a positive correlation to body mass. Astronauts suffer an increased excretion of calcium and decreased bone mineralization that is not reversed by exercise in non-weight-bearing conditions.
- *Effect of inactivity*: bed rest induces a weekly loss of bone mass with a mineral loss of up to 30%. The effects of prolonged bed rest may not be reversible.
- *Effects of muscular activity*: muscular activity has a positive loading effect on the skeleton. Less activity and deteriorating muscle mass in the elderly increases fracture risk.
- *Effects of physical activity*: multiple studies show a positive correlation between bone mass and physical activity with benefits at any age.
- *The female athletic triad*: is a combination of excessive athletic activity, negative effects on bone metabolism, amenorrhoea, and eating disorder.

Sports injury in children

Epidemiology
- Acute sports injuries occur 1.8–2.5 times more commonly in boys than girls.
- The incidence of sports injury increases with chronological age and pubertal stage.
- Peak rate of injury is at 12 yrs in girls and 14 yrs in boys.
- In contact sports, injuries occur more commonly in post-pubertal than pre-pubertal children.
- Peak fracture incidence coincides with the adolescent growth spurt.
- Winter sports appear more injurious than summer sports for children.

Mechanisms of injury
How children differ from adults
- The immature skeleton requires special consideration.
- Identical mechanisms of injury produce different pathologies in children compared with adults.
- Existence of growth plates and apophyses (insertion of muscle-tendon units into immature bone) largely account for the different injury profile observed in children.
- Growth cartilage is thicker and more fragile during adolescence.
- Immature articular cartilage appears to be weaker and more vulnerable to compressive loading.
- Increases in limb length and muscle mass result in greater moments of inertia around joints at a time of relative weakness in the growth plates and articular cartilage.
- In children growth plate injuries and avulsion fractures are more common than ligament and tendon tears.

Osteochondroses
Pathology
- Group of conditions affecting the growing skeleton and articular cartilage.
- May be intra-articular (e.g. osteochondritis dissecans), physeal (e.g. Scheuermann's disease) or extra-articular (e.g. traction apophysitis).

Cause and prognosis
- Vary in aetiology and frequency of occurrence.
- More common in boys than girls.
- Causative factors are not fully understood.
- Stress, ischaemia and genetics are all implicated to varying degrees.
- Differ in treatment and prognosis: some resolve spontaneously, others require surgical intervention.

Traction apophysitis
Commonest type of osteochondrosis
Cause
Repetitive traction forces at the vulnerable tendon-growth plate interface as a result of growth and loading.

Treatment
- Local anti-inflammatory measures including ice.
- Unloading the inflamed tendon-bone interface by avoiding or reducing provocative activities (usually running and jumping in lower limb traction apophysitis).
- Improving flexibility of the involved muscle-tendon unit.
- Graduated strengthening program.
- Gradual reintroduction of activity.

The specifics of these conditions will be discussed later under the region they affect.

Chapter 3

Physiotherapy and rehabilitation

Stretching 66
Balance and proprioception 68
Plyometrics 70
Proprioneurofacilitation (PNF) 71
Taping and strapping 72
Principles of rehabilitation 74
Sports-specific fitness tests 76
Types of skeletal muscle fibre 77
Features of skeletal muscle 77
Muscle training (isokinetic/isometric/isotonic) 78
Principles of strength training 79
Biomechanical assessment 80
Orthotics 81
Physiotherapy 82
Electrophysical agents 84
Gait analysis 85
Injury prevention, screening, and prehab 86
Cold therapy (cryotherapy) 92

Stretching

Many people confuse stretching, flexibility, and mobility. Stretching is an intervention, flexibility is the limits of range of motion (ROM) due to muscle-tendon, and mobility is the limits of ROM due to capsule-ligaments. The effects of stretching depend on whether one is trying to affect the muscle-tendon, or the capsule-ligament. This topic focuses only on muscle-tendon.

Pre-activity stretching
- ROM is increased. Increases in ROM are superior if warm-up is done prior to stretching.
- The increase in ROM is partly due to decreased stiffness of the tissue, and partly due to a decrease in the sensation of pain associated with the stretch.
- A single bout of stretching decreases the strength of tissue in animal studies in the immediate post-stretch period.
- The results below are unchanged whether or not warm-up is done prior to stretching:
  - Decreases tests of performance for strength and jump height in every study (over 20). Running speed changes are conflicting across different studies, but different methodologies prevent definitive conclusions.
  - No effect on overall injury rate when performed regularly. Some authors suggest the risk for some injuries are reduced with stretching before exercise. If so, then other injuries must be increased as the total number of injuries is unchanged.

Daily stretching (not pre-activity)
- ROM is increased with daily stretching.
- The results below are unchanged whether or not warm-up is done prior to stretching:
  - Daily stretching increases strength of tissue in animal studies.
  - Three studies have shown an approximate 20% reduction in injuries with daily stretching, but 2 of these had small sample sizes and did not achieve statistical significance.
  - Tests of performance for strength, jump height, and running speed are improved with daily stretching.

Dynamic stretching

Dynamic stretching is usually described as moving the joint through its *functional* ROM expected during activity, first slowly, and then more quickly; forcing a muscle into a lengthened condition when it is being contracted and relaxed is usually called ballistic stretching. Commonly described, 'dynamic stretching' activities include squats, push-ups, skipping, and hopping. With this definition, dynamic stretching is really just a form of warm-up and would be expected to have the same effects. There are no studies comparing the effects of *dynamic stretching* to traditional *dynamic warm-up*.

Additional comments

If daily stretching outside periods of exercise is protective against injury, but stretching immediately prior to activity is not associated with a reduction in injuries, it must mean that stretching immediately prior to activity removes the protective effect of daily stretching, i.e. it is harmful. However, because the overall effect of importance to the subject is whether the risk is increased when they stretch vs. when they don't stretch, this point is purely academic.

Balance and proprioception

Over the last 40yrs, we have recognized that balance and proprioception are important in the prevention and rehabilitation of injuries.

Definitions
- *Balance*: ability to maintain a given posture.
- *Proprioception:* (used interchangeably with kinaesthesia) control of movement and posture. There are 4 contributing sensations:
  - Limb position and movement.
  - Muscle effort, tension, heaviness, and stiffness.
  - Timing muscle contractions.
  - Body posture and size representation across more than one joint.

Many different physiological processes contribute to proprioception. These include afferent nerve fibres from:
- *Musculoskeletal*: muscle spindles, tendon organs, joints (ligaments, disks, and menisci).
- *Other*: cutaneous, pain fibres.

Biomechanics
The body sways to-and-fro in all directions. When the body's centre of pressure is not immediately under its centre of mass, the body moves. Resting muscle tone provides stiffness that prevents some motion. Muscles dynamically contract to restore position following perturbations.

Clinical research
Patient relevant outcomes include:
- Falls, and/or fall causing injury.
- *Fear of falling:* someone with poor balance may alter behaviour to avoid falls. This can have a dramatic impact on quality of life.

Measuring proprioception
Because proprioception is a composite of 4 different sensations, a true measure of proprioception is complex and requires sophisticated laboratory equipment. Most clinical studies that evaluate 'proprioception' are actually measuring balance. Some simple ways people measure balance in healthy subjects for sport medicine studies include (in order of difficulty):
- Standing on one leg
- Standing on one leg with eyes closed.
- Standing on one leg on a foam pad.

Although none of these methods actually has very good reliability, balance still seems to be a very important predictor of injury. How? Reliability is a measure of 'noise'. Injuries are a measure of 'signal'. As long as the signal-to-noise ratio is high, it is irrelevant how large the absolute value of the noise is.

Role for primary prevention
Exercises designed to improve proprioception have been successful in the primary prevention of:
- Falls in the elderly.
- Anterior cruciate ligament tears in girls.
- In a recent study, proprioceptive exercises for the ankle reduced ankle injuries by 20%, but the results were not statistically significant.

Role for secondary prevention
Many studies show proprioceptive exercises are effective in reducing re-injury rate following an ankle sprain. They may also be effective following anterior cruciate ligament reconstruction.

Other benefits
Proprioceptive exercises are effective in the elderly, frail elderly, those with Parkinson's disease, and patients post-hip fracture. Despite the lack of research on other musculoskeletal topics, the basic science and theoretical evidence suggest that it is a promising intervention with very low risk.

Plyometrics

Purpose
Plyometrics train power. Power is the ability to generate force in a very short period of time (e.g. jumping, sprinting). One study suggested that plyometrics are used by 90% of USA Division I strength and conditioning coaches and another suggested they are used by 94% of National Football League coaches.

Definition
Plyometrics is a very specific type of exercise. Some basic terms:
- *Concentric exercise*: the muscle shortens as it generates force.
- *Eccentric exercise*: the muscle lengthens as it generates force because it is unable to overcome a greater force being applied to it.

Plyometrics refers to any exercise where the muscle goes through an eccentric contraction-concentric contraction cycle repeatedly at a fast rate. In physiological studies, it is also called the stretch-shortening cycle, but those studies often limit themselves to one cycle—plyometrics requires repetitions.

Plyometric examples
- Jumping up and down.
- Push-ups and clap hands when body is high.

Theoretical reasoning
- Plyometrics is based on the specific adaptations to imposed demand (SAID) principle.
- If one trains strength, strength is increased, but there are very small gains in power and endurance. Weightlifters are not marathon runners and marathon runners cannot lift heavy weights.
- Plyometrics should be used for jumping sports or when acceleration is essential (sprint start).
- There are no meta-analyses or systematic reviews comparing plyometrics with other types of training. Some studies show it to be superior while others show no difference. The opposing results may be due to differences in populations and/or required power output.

Safety
- Plyometrics represent a high intensity workout.
- As exercise intensity increases, the stress applied to muscles, tendons, and ligaments increases.
- If the stress applied to a tissue is greater than it can absorb, an injury occurs.
- As with all exercises, the best way to prevent injury is to start slowly and increase gradually.
- Some reviews now suggest that plyometrics should be an important part of injury prevention programs.

Proprioneurofacilitation (PNF)

Definition
There are both PNF stretching and strengthening exercises. The common use of the term is for stretching.

Theory
The theory behind PNF stretching is that an antagonist muscle contraction causes reflex inhibition of the agonist muscle (e.g. quadriceps inhibits hamstring), which would lead to greater increases in ROM. Some forms use a contraction of the agonist muscle as well.

Types of PNF stretching
For each of the examples, the hamstring muscle is being stretched. Different authors use different nomenclature for the same procedures. I have chosen the one that seems reasonable if one considers the hamstring as the agonist muscle and the quadriceps is the antagonist muscle. The subject is lying on the floor on their back.
- *Contract–relax (CR)*: the leg is lifted passively by a partner. The subject contracts the hamstring muscle for a short period (2–10s) and then relaxes the muscle. As the muscle is relaxed, the partner passively raises the leg higher to increase the stretch on the agonist.
- *Contract–relax–antagonist–contract (CRAC)*: this is the same as the CR method, but following the passive stretch, the quadriceps is actively contracted by the subject.
- *Agonist–contract–relax (ACR)*: this is a confusing name. In fact, the subject contracts the antagonist (quadriceps/hip flexors) to stretch the agonist (hamstring), and the muscle is supported during the rest phase. A variation termed hold–relax (H-R) is to contract the hamstring before resting.

Experimental evidence
Since being widely promoted in the mid-1970s, there have been several studies examining the effectiveness of PNF stretching. The results are:
- With respect to ROM, studies suggest ACR and CRAC (these two have not been directly compared) superior to CR, which is superior are H-R, which is superior to static stretching.
- There is no inhibition of muscle reflex activity. In fact, the EMG of the stretched muscle is increased with PNF compared with static stretching. The mechanism for the increase in ROM remains to be determined.
- There is a change in the muscle visco-elasticity with PNF stretching for the immediate period following the stretch, but there are no long-term changes in visco-elasticity even though ROM increases. These changes are similar to those seen with static stretching.
- Taken together, the above suggests that PNF stretching has a greater analgesic effect than static stretching and this may be the reason for the increased ROM.

Taping and strapping

Taping and strapping refer to the use of bandage material wrapped around a joint with the objective of improving stability of that joint. Taping refers to the use of an adhesive tape and strapping refers to the use of non-adhesive wrap.

Background
There is both static and dynamic stability of a joint:
- *Static stability* (or mechanical instability) refers to passive mobility of a joint. Typically, this is tested by a second person while the subject's muscles are relaxed. Mainly ligaments provide stability.
- *Dynamic stability* (or functional instability) refers to the mobility of a joint during active motion. Mainly muscles provide stability.
- *Example*: The normal AP movement observed in the knee with the Lachman's or Anterior Drawer test, tests static stability. This movement does not occur during walking or running (i.e. dynamic stability).
- *Dynamic stability* is more clinically relevant than static stability and measured by joint displacement following a sudden force (e.g. trap-door). Injury or re-injury rate is even more clinically relevant.

Effectiveness
- Most of our knowledge comes from ankle studies or anecdotal experience.
- For large joints, taping and strapping have lost 20–50% of their effect on static stability within 15–20min. Whether this is true for small joints exposed to lesser forces remains to be determined.
- Taping and strapping appear to improve dynamic stability in most studies. This is associated with an increase in resting electromyography (EMG). Improved muscle activity results in increased stiffness of the joint (should protect against injury).
- Clinical trials suggest taping and strapping are effective in preventing ankle injuries.
- Anecdotal evidence suggests that they are useful to limit motion for injured small joints, such as wrists, fingers, toes.
- Some clinicians will also tape acromio-clavicular joints, knees, and shoulders. The effectiveness for these joints is controversial and should be evaluated on an individual basis, i.e. tape the joint and if the patient feels it allows them to compete with less pain it is effective for that patient.
- Taping is also used to limit joint movement to reduce stress on tendons in patients with symptoms (e.g. Achilles tendonopathy, anti-pronation taping). The effectiveness of these methods in general has not been well studied. That said, these types of taping should be evaluated using n-of-1 trials. Simply put, make decisions about a particular individual by measuring pain with and without tape repeatedly in that individual.

Potential deleterious effects

There are no studies on long-term effects. Probable potential deleterious effects include:
- Allergic reaction to the adhesive used in tape. Pre-wrap and hypoallergenic tape may reduce this problem.
- Tenosynovitis if tendon is superficial. Small foam pads placed over the tendons may reduce this problem (e.g. anterior tibialis and Achilles tendons for the ankle).

Principles of rehabilitation

The principles of rehabilitation following any injury can be broadly classified into three phases—early, middle, and late. These stages are not mutually exclusive. Short- and long-term goals should be defined for each athlete and reviewed at appropriate time intervals, depending on the injury. Appropriate clinical markers should be used to define the progression of rehabilitation.

Athletes should not be allowed to progress until they have, ideally, completed each stage without difficulty. Rehabilitation ladders or recipes should be used only as guidelines and each athlete should have a customized sport-specific and individually-negotiated rehabilitation plan.

Aerobic fitness and sport-specific motor control and co-ordination must be maintained where possible throughout rehabilitation.

The plan should be designed around what the athlete can do, rather than what they cannot.

Early phase (protection of the injured part)
- Strapping or bracing the injured part to prevent unwanted motion.
- Non- or partial-weight bearing with crutches may be necessary with lower limb injury, and a resultant antalgic gait. It is important to normalize gait.
- Relative rest.
- Protect, rest, ice, compress, elevate (PRICE).

Middle phase
- *Range of movement and flexibility:* aim to restore full range of joint motion (physiological and accessory) and muscle length.
- *Strength and conditioning*: motor control and re-education, strength, power, and endurance.
- *Proprioception:* aim to restore normal kinaesthetic awareness to the injured part.
- *Progression of proprioceptive exercises:*
  - Static → dynamic.
  - Conscious → automatic.
  - Decrease the base of support.
  - Decrease visual input.
  - Functional.

Late phase
- *Agility drills:* shuttle and sprint drills, cone, and ladder drills. Start with straight line work, progress to change of direction, cutting, and pivoting.
- Functional activities.
- Sport-specific skills.
- Power work.
- Plyometric training (where appropriate).
- Identification of a safe return to full training.

Determinants of outcome
- Age.
- Pre-injury activity level.
- Post-injury expectation.
- Motivation.
- Associated injury.

Further reading
About.com:Sports Medicine. Available at: http://sportsmedicine.about.com/od/sampleworkouts/a/Plyometrics.htm. Information on plyometric exercises and anterior cruciate ligament (ACL) injury prevention programme.

Elite athlete training services. Available at: ww.eliteathletetraining.com/Tips/Agility.aspx.

MyCoach Online. Available at: www.mycoachonline.com/. Covers predominantly American sports and is a coaching site, but many of the training drills shown here can be used for sport specific rehabilitation.

Sports Fitness Advisor. Available at: http://www.eliteathletetraining.com/agility-drills. Speed and agility drills, this site also has information on plyometric exercises.

You Tube Available at: www.youtube.com lots of online clips for training/rehabilitation in all sports.

Speed.Agility.Quickness. Available at: www.saqinternational.com/. Sports-specific training/rehabilitation for rugby, football, tennis, hockey, and cricket.

Sports-specific fitness tests

Cardiorespiratory fitness tests
Graded maximal exercise tests for aerobic capacity e.g. shuttle run or bleep test for oxygen uptake (VO_2 max).

Functional performance tests (FPTs)
Sporting activities require manoeuvres that demand a combination of vertical and horizontal force production. FPTs assess a variety of musculoskeletal parameters simultaneously:
- Joint laxity/mobility.
- Muscle extensibility (flexibility).
- Muscle strength and power.
- Proprioception.
- Neuromuscular control.
- Dynamic balance.
- Agility.
- Pain.
- Athlete confidence.

Functional tests can be done unilaterally or bilaterally, and progress may be measured (repetitions, time, distance). They may be used as baseline tests (pre-season), to monitor progress, or as an integral part of training. In rehabilitation they may be used to monitor progress or set targets for return to sport. Some common FPTs:
- One leg hop.
- Vertical jump.
- Triple hop.
- Side jump.
- Stair/slope running.
- Shuttle runs.
- Figure of 8.
- 6m hop.
- Cross-over hop.
- Vertical squat jump.
- Drop jump.

Types of skeletal muscle fibre

Type I or slow oxidative (SO) fibres
- These have a higher proportion of oxidative enzymes and mitochondria, and a greater capillary density and greater aerobic capacity.
- These fibres have a slow contraction time, are difficult to fatigue and good for prolonged, low-intensity work.

Type II
- Larger diameter, higher proportion of glycolytic enzymes, rather than oxidative enzymes, and fewer mitochondria.
- Greater anaerobic capacity.

Type IIa or fast twitch oxidative-glycolytic fibres (FOG)
These fibres have a fast contraction time and have the capacity for both aerobic and anaerobic activity. They have the ability to maintain contractile activity for relatively long periods of time.

Type IIb or fast twitch glycolytic fibres (FG)
These fibres are able to generate a lot of tension, but fatigue rapidly.

Features of skeletal muscle

Most muscles contain a mixture of fibre types. The nerve innervating the muscle determines the fibre type. Postural muscles tend to have more Type I fibres.

Functional unit is the motor unit—a single motor neuron and all muscle fibres innervated from it. The motor unit is the smallest part of a muscle that can contract independently. The number of muscle fibres forming a motor unit closely relate to the degree of control. Motor units show an all-or-nothing response.

The calling in of additional motor units in response to a greater stimulation of the motor nerve is known as recruitment.

The force a muscle can produce is dependent on the following:
- The length–tension relationship.
- The load–velocity relationship.
- The force–time relationship.
- Temperature.
- Pre-stretching.

Muscle training (isokinetic, isometric, isotonic)

During contraction, the force developed by muscle is known as muscle tension, and the external force acting on it is known as the load or resistance.

There are 3 types of muscle contraction:
- *Isometric*: tension is generated within the muscle without a change in muscle length.
- *Isotonic*: tension is generated within the muscle with a change in muscle length. During a concentric contraction the muscle shortens. During an eccentric contraction the muscle lengthens.
- *Isokinetic*: tension is generated within the muscle where the velocity of contraction remains constant.

Only isometric and isotonic contractions occur naturally. Greater tension can be generated by an eccentric contraction than a corresponding concentric contraction. Any isotonic contraction that results in a change in muscle length must initially have an isometric phase whereby enough tension is generated to overcome the load imposed.

Isokinetics can be used for training and assessment purposes.

The ability of a muscle to contract depends on the availability of adenosine triphosphate (ATP). Fatigue occurs when the ability to synthesize ATP is insufficient to keep up with ATP breakdown during contraction.

Muscle adaptation to exercise

Physiological adaptations
- *Neurogenic:* start slow—activate more motor units.
- *Myogenic:* onset after 6–8 weeks—hypertrophy.
- Increase in muscle size, strength, and power.
- Alter the mechanical properties of other connective tissues and bone.

Age-related changes

As we become older we lose strength. There is debate about the effect of ageing alone or disuse. Muscle mass decreases by 1%/yr after the age of 60. A decrease in the number of muscle fibres (preferentially type II), results in slower contractile properties. There is also a decrease in the number of motor units. Remaining units increase in size but the reduction in number compromises precision activities.

Principles of strength training

The fundamental principles of exercise training to optimize the response are overload, specificity, and reversibility. When a muscle adapts to a given stimulus, additional loads must be applied for further adaptation to occur, known as Specific Adaptation to Imposed Demand (SAID).

The parameters of a training programme include speed, resistance, repetitions, frequency, and duration; the recovery time between bouts; the form of the exercise; and the range through which the muscle works.

Overload

Intensity
- The greater the load, the higher the intensity.
- Normally expressed as a percentage of the 1 repetition maximum (1RM).
- A resistance of 80–95% 1RM is the optimal to maximize strength gains for most sports.
- This equates to 3–8 RM set.

Volume
- Volume = sets × reps × load.
- In general as intensity increases, volume decreases.

Rest intervals and recovery
- The total rest time between reps, sets, and exercises for the specific muscle being trained.
- Relates to the intensity of the training 2–3-min rest intervals between sets is common.

Frequency
- Strength can be maintained by 1 session per week.
- During rehabilitation when the emphasis is on regaining/maximizing muscle strength, this can be optimized by 2 or 3 sessions per week.

Mode
- Free weights.
- Resistance machines.
- Body weight.
- Variable resistance: sport cord, theraband.
- Isokinetic machines.

Specificity
The exercise chosen should target the specific muscle(s) with regard to its function during the specific activity/sport.

Reversibility
Any training adaptations will be reversed/reduced if training is stopped for 2–8 weeks.

Biomechanical assessment

Static

Observation while standing
- *Posture type:* kyphosis-lordosis, sway back, flat back, round back. Signs of scoliosis.
- *From the front:* anterior superior iliac crest (ASIS) levels, patella heights and orientation, femoral anteversion and tibial torsion, genu varum or valgum with feet together, forefoot to rear foot relationship, position of first ray.
- *From the side:* pelvic position, signs of genu recurvatum.
- *From the back:* equal levels of posterior superior iliac crest (PSIS) and gluteal and knee folds. Heel position—everted or inverted. Too many toes sign—increased lateral hip rotation.

Leg length discrepancy
- *Quick visual check:* supine, flex knees, subject lifts and lowers pelvis, knees straightened, check levels of medial malleolus.
- *Tape measure method:* measure ASIS to medial malleolus. Discrepancy should be less than 1.5cm.

Range of passive movement
- *Hip*: internal and external rotation with the hip at 90° and 0°.
- *Knee*: hyperextension or fixed flexion.
- *Ankle*: dorsiflexion with the knee at 90° and 0°—a difference may indicate gastrocnemius tightness, anterior drawer test.
- *Subtalar*: assess ROM. In subtalar neutral assess fore foot/rear foot positions and the eversion/inversion relationship.
- *First ray*: ROM and position in subtalar neutral and mid-tarsal pronation.

Dynamic
- *Bilateral knee bend in standing:* any compensatory movement in foot.
- *Single leg knee bend:* maintaining correct knee alignment and avoiding femoral internal rotation.
- *Gait analysis:* visual or video analysis.
- *Performance specific:* video analysis of training, competition, and specific sport techniques.

Orthotics

Indications for use
- Designed to correct abnormal foot/lower limb biomechanics.
- Have been shown to relieve symptoms where abnormal lower limb biomechanics are thought to be a causative factor, especially in overuse conditions, e.g. ilio-tibial band (ITB) friction syndrome, patellofemoral pain, patella tendinopathy, plantar fasciitis.

How do they work?
- Shock absorption.
- Mechanical control of subtalar and mid-tarsal movement.
- *Neural control:* afferent feedback from cutaneous receptors.
- *Muscle control:* reduce muscle activation required to control the foot.

Different types
- *Preformed:* heel cups or insoles normally bought off-the-shelf. Generally made of less durable material and provide less control. Do not last as long.
- *Custom made:* following biomechanical assessment and plaster cast taken of the foot. Generally made of more rigid material, provide more control, and last longer.

Choice of orthotics may depend on:
- Foot type.
- The sport played and the type of footwear used.
- The type of biomechanical problem.
- Weight of the patient.

Physiotherapy

Referral to a physiotherapist – what a patient might expect

A full and thorough history will be taken on a first visit. Patients may be frustrated as they feel they have already told a referring doctor, but these details may not have been relayed. It is necessary to establish what the problem is, if physiotherapy is likely to help, and what type of therapy to use.

The physiotherapist will test range of movement and how one moves, muscle strength, and timing of activation during specific tasks. With suspected referred pain they may examine the spine or more proximal joints.

Patients should take along relevant sports equipment including training shoes/rackets, etc., and any results of investigations such as X-rays, magnetic resonance imaging (MRI), blood tests.

Following assessment, the physiotherapist will define the problem and list therapy options. Physiotherapy may include:

- Manual techniques such as soft tissue therapy, mobilization and manipulation.
- *Exercise therapy:* a home exercise programme is useful in the management of most musculoskeletal conditions and the success of the treatment is dependent on the compliance with exercises and advice on posture and alignment.
- *Electrophysical agents:* heat/cold therapy, ultrasound, interferential, laser, etc.

Patients may feel sore after assessment or treatment, but it is important to inform the therapist, as they may modify management according to the response.

The aim of treatment is to restore normal function and prevent recurrence.

Each subsequent visit should include a reassessment for change in the condition; subjective and/or objective changes. Treatment will be modified according to the response. If the therapist is unhappy with progress or feels that the patient has reached a plateau, they may refer you on for further opinion to the relevant specialist or investigation.

Aims to restore normal function and return the athlete to their pre-injury activity level in the shortest possible time, using manual and exercise therapy and advice.

Manual therapy

- Joints can be mobilized passively or with active movement in their accessory or physiological range. Accessory mobilization is aimed at pain relief or restoring range of movement.
- Soft tissue techniques, including massage and muscle energy techniques, can be applied to muscles, tendons, ligaments, and fascia. They are used for pain relief by decreasing excessive tissue tension, stimulating large diameter fibres, and removal of substance P.
- Techniques that target myofascial trigger points are also be used for pain management. Other potential benefits include releasing adhesions or reducing excessive scar tissue, releasing tension and spasm and

promoting normal tissue length (e.g. myofascial release and PNF techniques).
- Neural mobilization techniques can be used as part of the pain management programme in isolation or associated with other pathology such as sciatic involvement with hamstring lesions. Their involvement can be assessed using neural tension tests (e.g. Slump test, upper limb tension test (ULTT)) as appropriate.

Manipulation

A small amplitude high velocity thrust normally performed on intervertebral joints at the end of the range. Normally performed where range of movement is limited by stiffness or in the acute locked neck. Care must be taken with cervical manipulation and vertebral artery screening should be conducted beforehand. Other contraindications include fracture, local malignancy or bony infection, *cauda equina*, rheumatoid arthritis of the cervical spine, pregnancy during the last trimester, recent whiplash, haemophilia, spondylolisthesis, and children with open ephiyseal plates. Can be applied to peripheral joints.

Exercise therapy

- *Motor control and re-education peripherally and centrally:* centrally, the 'core' muscles are transversus abdominis, multifidus, diaphragm, and the perineal muscles. Exercise programmes that enhance the timing and recruitment of these muscles under low and high load are widely employed as part of an athlete's regular training programme, as well as during rehabilitation. Central stabilization is essential for efficient control of the upper or lower limb. Peripheral exercises are aimed at those muscles primarily affected by the injury.
- *Good biomechanical alignment:* appropriate joint loading and muscle recruitment relies on good biomechanical alignment. Intrinsic and extrinsic factors need to be considered.
- *Good technique during specific sporting activity:* technique needs to be evaluated, often done in conjunction with a biomechanist and/or coach.

Electrophysical agents

A variety of these modalities are frequently used as an adjunct to treating soft tissue injury. The aim is to deliver physical energy to the tissue to help the natural healing process. Each modality appears to be dose dependant.

Low level laser therapy
Output less than 60mW, therefore, has no thermal effects. Two types—the gallium arsenide (GaAs) and helium neon (HeNe). Thought to alter cellular mechanisms that increase collagen synthesis. Used for pain management and the promotion of healing.

Ultrasound
The application of high frequency sound waves (1–3MHz), which produce thermal (continuous application) and non-thermal (pulsed) effects. Thermal effects increase local blood flow, non-thermal doses are thought to create mechanical and chemical effects that influence cellular permeability via cavitation and acoustic streaming. Frequency choice relates to the depth of the target tissue, 1MHz 2–5cm, 3MHz 1–2cm. The intensity and pulse ratio vary depending on whether the injury is acute, subacute, or chronic. For example, typical dose for an acute lateral ligament sprain 3MHz 1:4 (pulse ratio) 0.2W/cm^2 (intensity) for 10min.

Interferential
The application of 2 alternating medium frequency currents that creates a low frequency current where they 'interfere'. Thought to have 4 main effects:
- Pain relief.
- Increase in blood flow.
- Reduction of oedema.
- Muscle stimulation.

Frequency selected depending on the desired outcome (Table 3.1).

Table 3.1 Frequency range for stimulation of selected structures

Sympathetic nerve	1–5Hz
Smooth muscle	0–10Hz
Motor nerve	10–50Hz
Parasympathetic nerve	10–150Hz
Sensory nerve	90–100Hz
Nociceptive nerves	90–150Hz

Combination therapy
The simultaneous application of US and electrical stimulation, such as interferential. Little evidence to support any additional benefits compared with their application independently.

Gait analysis

Analysis of gait and other functional activities, such as running, golf swing, serving action; hurdle technique, for example, is an important part of assessment and athlete profiling. Observation is useful, but is subjective. Video analysis using software such as Silconcoach or Dartfish is a more objective measure of functional tasks in the field. Finally, some sophisticated systems measure multidimensional kinematic and kinetic parameters during the same activity.

Gait analysis is used to evaluate movement, highlight biomechanical anomalies and assess efficiency of movement. Some biomechanical abnormalities are associated with musculoskeletal injury. Over pronation, for example, is associated with patellofemoral pain syndrome (PFPS), tibial stress fracture, medial tibial stress syndrome and Achilles and tibialis posterior tendinopathy. Poor hip control, with resultant increased femoral internal rotation, has been associated with PFPS; poor lumbo-pelvic control with hamstring injury etc.

Biomechanical abnormalities may be identified, but it is more difficult to establish if abnormalities detected are relevant to the production of symptoms. Humans are not perfectly symmetrical and we do not all move the same way. In screening athletes one may find biomechanical anomalies in the absence of any symptoms. Should one intervene, do you try to fix something that is not broken?

In the presence of symptoms and biomechanical abnormalities, one may correct the abnormality and see if it changes the symptoms. If symptoms alter by changing the biomechanics, clinicians may advise biomechanical correction.

Injury prevention, screening, and prehab

The relationship between injury prevention, musculoskeletal screening and 'prehab' (in contrast to rehabilitation), is complex.

Injury prevention

We may identify risk factors, but eliminating these risk factors can only reduce the likelihood of injury and not completely eliminate injury. It may also be impossible to predict when an injury will occur.

Risk factors are commonly categorized into extrinsic and intrinsic risk factors:

Extrinsic risk factors include:
- Direct contact.
- Sport-specific skills.
- Level of competition.
- Shoes and equipment.
- Surfaces.
- Training errors.
- Overtraining.
- Environmental factors.
- Workplace design.

Intrinsic risk factors include:
- Movement dysfunction and muscle imbalance.
- Malalignment.
- Muscle weakness.
- Loss of flexibility.
- Poor proprioception.
- Intrinsic overload.
- Physical fitness.
- Age.
- Gender.
- Hydration and nutritional status.
- Inadequate warm-up.
- Previous injury.

Previous injury is the greatest predictor for a range of sports injuries. Thus, effective rehabilitation is essential in reducing recurrence.

Preventative strategies that address extrinsic risk factors include:
- Law change.
- Protective equipment.
- Better planning of training/competitive programmes.
- Athlete education.
  - Technique.
  - Preparation.
- Improve facilities.

Preventative strategies addressing intrinsic risk factors can be more difficult to implement and must be appropriate to the athlete and sport involved.

Screening/profiling

Musculoskeletal screening or 'profiling' is a detailed assessment of the athlete in an attempt to achieve the following aims:
- Identify predisposing factors to injury.
- Detect musculoskeletal impairments that may affect performance.
- Identify ongoing injuries, which may or may not be receiving treatment.
- Provide information to coaches on the management of ongoing injuries.
- Identify problems not responding to treatment.
- Follow-up to previous screening.
- Put in place appropriate measures to prevent injury and enhance performance.

Timing
Where possible, profiling should be carried out:
- Outside of the competitive season.
- As part of induction on entry to the elite athlete programme.
- At the end of the competitive season.
- On exit from the programme/club.

Personnel
Where possible, musculoskeletal profiling should be carried out by a chartered physiotherapist with:
- Sport specific knowledge.
- Experience in the management of musculoskeletal problems in sport.

Content
The profiling process should include the following elements:
- Personal details.
- GP contact details.
- Previous injury/illness history.
  - Nature.
  - Management/rehabilitation.
  - Recurrence.
- Anthropometric measures.
- Sports specific information.
  - Training.
  - Competitive cycle.
- Clinical tests to assess:
  - Posture (incl. alignment, etc.).
  - Flexibility.
  - Range of motion.
  - Joint systems.
  - Muscle tightness/inhibition.
  - Neural systems.
  - Neurological assessment (where appropriate).
  - Specific pathology (where appropriate).

It is also important that profiling includes a number of functional tests to assess:
- Muscle strength.
- Neuromuscular control.
- Motor control stability.
- Physical fitness.

Examples of functional tests (depending on the sport) that may be used are:
- Single leg squat.
- Overhead squat.
- Lunge.
- Gait analysis.
- Small knee bend.
- Prone hip extension.

It is important that any tests included in the profiling protocol are:
- Relevant.
- Quick and simple to perform.
- Reliable (intra- and inter-tester reliability).
- Valid.
- Provide quantitative and qualitative information.
- Ensure standardization of testing protocols and reporting mechanisms.

Example: selecting appropriate test to measure hamstring range
- Straight leg raise:
  - Indication of contracture of hamstring & other posterior hip tissues.
  - Does not give true indication of restrictions due to movement occurring at the pelvis and lumbar spine.
- Possible alternative:
  - Active knee extension test.[1,2]

Significance and consequence of findings
- Consider variations that exist within the normal population.
- Consider findings that may be advantageous to the relevant sport.
- Clinically relevant.
- Technically relevant.

Communication of findings
It is essential that the following people/groups are informed of profiling findings:
- Medical team.
- Coach.
- Sports science team.
- Governing body (where appropriate).

Following profiling it is necessary to formulate and implement an action plan to address issues identified. This should be carried out in conjunction with the multidisciplinary team and the following issues considered:
- How will the action plan be implemented? Consider:
  - The time of season.
  - Next competitive event.
  - Resources.
- Establish who is responsible for follow-up?
  - Doctor.
  - Physiotherapist.
  - Coach.

---

1 Fredriksen H, Dagfinrud H, Jacobsen V, Maehkum S. (1997). Passive knee extension test to measure hamstring muscle tightness. *Scand J Med Sci Sports*, **7**(5): 279–82.

2 Gajdosik R, Lusin G. (1983). Hamstring muscle tightness. Reliability of an active-knee-extension test. *Phys Ther* **63**(7): 1085–90.

- Performance manager.
- Athlete.
- How will implementation be monitored?
  - Identify person responsible.
  - Multi-disciplinary meetings.
- How will the results of intervention be assessed?

In order to ensure that the profiling process is beneficial the following potential problems should also be considered and avoided:
- Time intensive.
- Relevance of tests.
- Lack of follow-up.
- Lack of agreement between therapists regarding findings and interventions.
- Lack of communication with coaching staff.

'Prehab'

Exercise programmes that specifically address intrinsic risk factors in an effort to reduce the incidence of injury are commonly referred to as 'prehab'.

Prehab programmes should be based upon the findings of musculoskeletal profiling and should be tailored to the individual athlete and sport in which they are involved, and reflect the incidence of injury, the common injury mechanism, and probable causes of injury.

In sports, for example, where there is a high incidence of knee injuries, it is advisable to implement prehab programmes that focus on improving knee control and reducing the incidence of such injuries.

A number of prehab programmes have been shown to effectively reduce the incidence of knee, ankle and hamstring injuries.

Principles of prehab programmes

Technical components
- Correct technique is usually the biomechanically safest.
- Developing correct technique requires input from coaching staff, e.g.
  - Correct lifting technique for weight training.
  - Correct toss of the ball for tennis serve.
  - Correct body position during rugby scrum.
  - Correct movement mechanics for volleyball player.

Strength training
- Ensure adequate strength to achieve and maintain correct technique for specific sport, e.g. strengthening of hip abductors and external rotators can reduce the incidence of lower limb injury in athletes who are deficient in this area.
- Eccentric strength training is particularly effective in reducing muscle and tendon injuries, e.g. Nordic (Norwegian) hamstring curls significantly reduce incidence of hamstring injuries (*Note:* these are a high load eccentric exercise).

The athlete is in a kneeling position, with a therapist/training partner holding his/her feet. Maintaining a neutral lumbar spine and pelvis, the athlete drops forward, hinging at the knee joint, using eccentric hamstring control to slowly lower them down into a fully prone position.

Initially, most athletes will need to use their upper body to cushion them onto the ground.

The athlete stops at various points through the range. Extra resistance is used by the therapist, acting to push the athlete into a prone position.

Eccentric patellar tendon loading may help to prevent patellar tendinopathy in jumping sports:
- Eccentric unilateral squats are performed on a decline slope of 25°.
- Load is lifted concentrically using the contralateral limb and slowly lowered.
- 3 × 15 reps daily using a 10RM weight.
- Similar eccentric loading programmes can be used for shoulder external rotators and the Achilles tendon.

Balance and neuromuscular control training
Can significantly reduce the incidence of ankle and knee ligamentous injuries. Exercises used may include the following:
- Single leg standing—throw/catch ball:
  - Vary type of throw, e.g. underarm, overhead, side pass, chest pass.
  - Vary the direction of the pass receive, e.g. in front, from side, overhead.
  - Vary type of ball, e.g. tennis ball, medicine ball.
- Single leg standing on dynamic surface:
  - Folded towel.
  - Mini trampoline (rebounder).
  - Wobble board.
  - Balance pad.
  - Balance cushion.
  - Progress as for basic single leg stands.
- Manual perturbation from therapist/training partner.
- Pro-fitter exercises.
- Dynamic sport-specific drills with balance/control challenge included.

In order to reduce stresses on ligamentous structures, significant emphasis should be placed on dynamic movement control and the maintenance of correct limb alignment. Ensure that hip, knee, and foot are in correct alignment during movements such as:
- Hopping.
- Jumping and landing (bilateral and unilateral support).
- Lunging.
- Stepping.
- Planting and cutting drills.
- Sports-specific movements.

Flexibility
It is important to ensure that the athlete has adequate flexibility to enable them to complete the demands of their sport without placing excessive strain on the muscular system. Lack of flexibility will have been identified during the musculoskeletal profiling process.

Core stability
Appropriate core stability training is an important element of most prehab programmes. Core stability provides optimal control of the trunk,

supporting the effort and forces from the extremities, which in turn can contribute to safe, efficient, and effective limb function.

Core stability training should incorporate the following elements:
- Appropriate recruitment patterns of stabilizing muscles to facilitate and stabilize the rest of the kinetic chain.
- Focus on improved postural awareness and control.
- Emphasize perfect form.
- Appropriate load for the ability of the athlete.
- Performed in biomechanically correct position for muscle function of the extremities.
- Functional progression.
- Increase complexity as ability permits.
- Sports-specific skills.

In addition to specific prehab exercises to prevent injury, it is important to ensure that athletes are appropriately aerobically conditioned to participate in the sport. Other intrinsic elements that may contribute to the prevention of injury include:
- Nutrition.
- Hydration.
- Psychological preparation.

Cold therapy (cryotherapy)

Background
Cold therapy (cryotherapy) has traditionally been reserved for treating acute soft tissue injuries (e.g. sprains, strains and muscle contusions) to reduce pain, swelling, metabolism, and inflammation associated with secondary injury. Cold water immersion (CWI) is now used as to prevent muscle soreness and promote recovery after exercise.

Rationale
Potential effects include:
- *Anti-inflammatory effect:* reducing the potential for delayed onset muscle soreness (DOMS).
- *Vascular:* vasoconstriction (decreased blood vessel diameter) in the immersed musculature, stimulating blood flow and nutrient and waste transportation through the body after exercise.
- *Neural:* decreased nerve transmission speed and altered receptor threshold, cumulating in decreased pain perception.
- *Core body cooling:*
  - Employed in athletes with mild hyperthermia after exercising in extreme (hot/humid) environments.
  - Decreased subjective fatigue.
- *Psychological:* the body feels more 'awake' after exercise.

Practical application
CWI can be used in a range of environments, e.g. pitchside, changing room, rehabilitative facility. Choice of equipment should be guided by budget, rationale and the athletes' needs.
- Custom built temperature controlled spas:
  - Expensive.
  - Offer a range of water temperatures.
  - Usually more comfortable.
  - Many may have inbuilt jets to ensure water turbulence.
- Large containers filled with water and ice:
  - Low cost.
  - Inconvenience in terms of filling, emptying, and cleaning.
  - More difficult to control temperature.
  - Re-warm with repeated use, e.g. in team sports.

The duration of immersion, water temperature, and the depth/volume of body parts immersed are important factors to consider. These should be manipulated based on the environmental temperature, nature of the sport, athlete experience and physiological rationale. Popular treatment options include:
- Repeated short duration immersions at very low temperatures: 1 min immersion/1 min rest × 3 sets, 5°C water temperature. These are most likely to be associated with:
  - Moderate decrease in skin temperature.
  - Reflex vasoconstriction.
  - Increase in sympathetic nervous activity.
  - Psychological response.

- Continuous long duration immersions: up to 15-min immersions in higher water temperatures of up to 15°C. This approach may be of benefit after exercise in hot environment, and/or in collision sports involving high levels of body contact:
  - Large decreases in skin temperature.
  - Mild to moderate reductions in intramuscular/joint temperatures (dependant on levels of body fat).
  - Normalizing core body temperature (from mild hyperthermic levels).
  - Decreased levels of perceived exertion/fatigue.

Precautions

- *Open wounds/infection:* particularly important in team environments when individuals 'share an ice bath'.
- *Cold shock response:*
  - This occurs in the initial stages of immersion and is characterized by an inspiratory gasp, hyperventilation, hypnocapnia, tachycardia, and hypertension.
  - More pronounced with sudden, full body immersion or in athletes unaccustomed to CWI.
  - In extreme circumstances can cause syncope.
- *Cardiac:*
  - Arrhythmias.
  - Increased QT dispersion.
- *Oxidative stress and possible increase in free radical species:* may be more likely when using very low water temperatures and/or prolonged durations of immersion, e.g. when athletes are shivering.
- *Contraindication to cold:* e.g. Raynauds. Athlete does not tolerate cold temperature:
  - May relate to athletes with very low levels of body fat or with a psychological aversion to cold temperatures.
  - CWI should NOT be compulsory in team sports.
- *Athlete has no experience of CWI:*
  - Athletes will generally adapt to CWI over time.
  - Magnitude of the physiological response (e.g. cold shock response) will sometimes dampen.
  - Athletes may need a period of adaptation based on short duration immersion in more tepid water temperatures.
  - Long duration immersions and very cold water temperatures should be avoided in the inexperienced athlete.

Other recovery strategies

There are a number of other post-exercise recovery strategies. CWI can often be combined with other intervention strategies to achieve a cumulative effect.

- Rest/activity modification: DOMS usually resolves clinically after approximately 4–5 days. DOMS is more likely to occur with unaccustomed exercise or intense exercise involving eccentric muscle contractions (i.e. when the muscle is forcibly stretched when active).
- Active recovery (cool down): light jogging incorporating stretching and mobility exercises.

- Other water-based recoveries:
  - Contrast immersion—alternate cold and warm water immersions.
  - Hydrotherapy.
- Compression garments.
- Massage.

Chapter 4

Benefits of exercise

Introduction *96*
Physical activity or exercise? *97*
Health and physical activity *98*
Is physical inactivity a problem? *100*
Determinants of physical activity *102*
Understanding behaviour change *106*
Increasing population-wide participation in physical activity *109*
Clinical and community interventions to promote and support physical activity *110*
The way forward *115*
Overweight and obesity in children *116*
Epidemiology *120*

Chapter 4: Benefits of exercise

Introduction

The benefits of physical activity are widely recognized. The World Health organization identifies physical inactivity as the fourth leading risk factor for mortality—responsible for 6% of deaths globally after hypertension, (13%), tobacco use (9%) and high blood glucose (6%). Physical inactivity has been associated with 30% of the ischaemic heart disease, 27% of diabetes and, 21–25% of breast and colon cancer burden. Exercise has been described as the "best buy for public health"

Physical activity or exercise?

- Physical activity is an umbrella term and it refers to any musculoskeletal movement that result in energy expenditure. This energy expenditure is more than that normally expended at rest.
- There are five main types of physical activity that are currently measured in self-report physical activity recall questionnaires. These include:
  - Occupational activity.
  - House and gardening activity.
  - Sport and free time (leisure or recreational) activity.
  - Family activity (looking after a sick relative, actively playing with children).
  - Transport related activity (walking or cycling to get to and from places, e.g. school or work).
- Exercise is planned, structured, and repetitive bodily movement done to improve or maintain one or more components of health related physical fitness.
- The components of health-related fitness are muscular endurance, flexibility, aerobic capacity, muscular strength, and body composition.
- So, what's in a word? Most people perceive the term 'exercise' negatively, the word 'workout' with work and drudgery, while the phase 'physical activity' is perceived positively.
- A sedentary individual, for example, is someone who participates in little or no physical activity.
- We all need encouragement to get active and to remain active. To help us in this we need to view physical activity as pleasurable. We need to value the 'entire' process of participation in physical activity, as well as the final 'product' or benefits we may accrue.
- Whatever your age, ability or condition, you can benefit from being more physically active.

Advice in starting exercise
- Start low and build up exercise gradually.
- As a general rule, do not increase the intensity or volume of exercise by more than 10% per week.

The FITT principle
- Frequency (number of sessions per week).
- Intensity (effort, e.g. speed, resistance, hills).
- Timing (duration of exercise session).
- Type (less of an increase if cross-training added vs. more of the same exercise).

These same principles can be used for rehabilitation following any injury. Begin at a level that does not cause pain and slowly increase.

Health and physical activity

Health includes physical, social, and psychological components, each one of equal value. If an individual exercises purely for physical health reasons, for example, to lose weight and they pursue this to the detriment of their psychological or social health, then exercise is detrimental to their health.

The shift from an 'exercise training-physical fitness' paradigm to include the 'physical activity health' paradigm developed recently. This shift was due to scientific studies that showed that there was a reduced morbidity and mortality with an increase in moderate amounts and intensities of physical activity.

This evidence became known as the *dose–response curve*, and from this the concept of lifestyle physical activity interventions began to develop.

There is now little debate over the minimum amounts, intensities, and frequencies of physical activity required to confer health benefits. Most recommendations state that the intensity of the activity should be of at least moderate or vigorous effort.

- Moderate intensity activity is performed at 3.0–5.9 times the intensity of rest, roughly 50–60% of maximal effort.
- Vigorous intensity activity is equivalent to 6.0 times the intensity of rest for adults, and 7.0 times the intensity for children and youth. This equates to 70–80% of your individual capacity.

The World Health Organization's global recommendations on physical activity for health state that children and young people should be active, at a moderate or vigorous intensity, for a minimum of 60min daily. For adults, and older adults, this recommendation changes to 30min of moderate or vigorous intensity physical activity five days per week (or equivalent to 150min per week).

Additional minutes of health enhancing physical activity will confer extra health benefits. All individuals should also build muscle strengthening exercises, flexibility, bone strengthening, or balance activities into their daily routine.

The recommendations change if, for example, an individual wants to maintain or lose body weight, or if an individual has a disability. To maintain a healthy body weight, and avoid gaining weight, an adult would need to spend the equivalent to 60min of moderate intensity activity. To lose weight, the amount of activity is dependent on how much weight an individual wants to lose, how well they can adhere to a physical activity regime and what their physical condition is like. A guideline is to try to accumulate at least 60–75min of moderate intensity physical activity daily. However, it is important to remember that any activity is better than none. Every minute counts.

For individuals with a disability, taking into account what their disability allows, they should aim to follow the adult guidelines of a minimum of 30 min moderate intensity physical activity daily.

Although recommendations may be appropriate for prevention of disease and health promotion, as viewed from a biomedical model of health, participation in regular physical activity can provide much more than this.

A more humanistic or biopsychosocial understanding of physical activity is one that sees physical activity as a mixture of physical, psychological, and social factors. Regular physical activity can:
- provide a way to relax after work,
- be a way of having fun,
- help you to meet people,
- be an opportunity to play.

The positive elements of physical activity such as enjoyment, learning new skills, gaining in confidence, getting to know your body better, developing your mind and body, or just having fun should not be forgotten.

An understanding of personal preferences in relation to participation in physical activity is vital if we are to encourage *more people to be more active more minutes, more often.*

Is physical inactivity a problem?

Physical inactivity is now identified as the fourth leading risk factor for chronic disease mortality such as heart disease, stroke, diabetes, cancers. It contributes to 6% of deaths globally, and follows high blood pressure (13%), tobacco use (9%), and high blood glucose (6%). Overweight and obesity are responsible for 5% of global mortality.[1]

In general, people appear to know that regular physical activity is good for them, but they choose to remain sedentary. Two-thirds of the European population has insufficient activity to meet current recommendations. However, over 90% of the population of every European country believes that physical activity has numerous health benefits. There is little variation in these beliefs by age or socio-economic status. The gap between beliefs, or intentions, and behaviour represents a challenge.

In conclusion, inactivity is a problem. A difficulty is how to intervene to increase the percentage of the population who are physically active. Unless this is achieved, all the potential health benefits from regular physical activity available to individuals, communities, and populations may remain unrealized.

The *Toronto Charter for Physical Activity: A Global Call for Action* (May 2010) provides the beginning of a solution to this problem. It was written by the Global Advocacy Council for Physical Activity, International Society for Physical Activity and Health and can be downloaded from www.globalpa.org.uk. It is a call for action and it provides organizations and individuals, interested in promoting physical activity, with an advocacy tool to help influence decision makers, at national, regional, and local levels. It explains why physical activity is a powerful investment in people, health, the economy and sustainability. It provides guiding principles and a framework for action for population based approaches to increasing participation in physical activity.

---

[1] World Health Organization. (2009). *Global Health Risks: Mortality and Burden of Disease Attributable to Selected Major Risks*. Geneva: World Health Organization. Available at: http://www.who.int/healthinfo/global_burden_disease/en/.

Determinants of physical activity

It is important to know a person's reasons for being active, as well as any potential barriers that might prevent them from leading an active lifestyle.

Examples of reasons include:
- Good health.
- Reduction in stress.
- To meet people.
- Weight management.
- Fun and enjoyment.

Examples of barriers include:
- Perceived lack of time.
- Not motivated.
- No perceived need.
- Fear of injury.
- Not the fit or sporty type.

Equally, it is important to understand the determinants that increase or decrease one's likelihood of adhering to, or avoiding physical activity.

Factors, influences, or determinants, all interchangeable words, refer to variables for which there are established, reproducible *associations* or *predictive* relationships, rather than cause-and-effect connections.

It is important to know the determinants of physical activity so that we can:
- Revise and improve our theoretical basis for understanding physical activity involvement or avoidance.
- Identify inactive individuals easily and allocate scarce resources accordingly, e.g. rural women on low incomes.
- Design interventions that work better because they target key determinants, e.g. social support, enjoyment.
- Tailor-make interventions for specific populations—what works for city boys aged 15–17 might not work for country boys aged 15–17 (population subgroups).

The determinants can be divided into three key categories. These are:
- Environmental determinants.
- Personal determinants.
- Behavioural determinants.

The *environmental determinants* are made up of social (cultural, peers, family), physical (man-made/natural) and policy factors.

The *social environment* includes social support provided as formal and informal encouragement, assistance and/or information from individuals or groups. It can vary in frequency, durability, and intensity. It is provided by peers, family, friends or relatives, essentially significant others in your life.

The *physical environment* can actively and passively influence physical activity patterns. It represents an effective vehicle for increasing physical activity, as it has the potential to influence large groups, even entire populations.

Supportive physical environments possess features such as parks, cycling trails, and footpaths and are conducive to physical activity. Restrictive physical environments lack such relevant features and actively discourage physical activity

The *policy environment* examines how the presence or absence of, e.g. a national physical activity policy can impact on physical activity opportunities within a specific environment. A physical activity policy can provide direction, support, and coordination of the many different sectors involved in promoting physical activity. Without such a policy political commitment, at national, regional, and local level can be unclear.

One clear, single issue physical activity policy, accompanied by several related strands of physical activity policy embedded within other related agendas (e.g. in fields of education, transportation, parks and recreation, media, business and urban planning) will facilitate synergistic policy impacts. This will avoid duplication of effort, confusion about whose role or responsibility it is to promote physical activity and build partnerships for advocacy and action. If a population shift towards physical activity is to be achieved, this prioritization of physical activity is recommended.

The *personal determinants* are made up of cognitive/personality, demographics, and biological factors.

Cognitive/personality
- People who don't enjoy exercise don't do it 'I hate the gym, and therefore don't go'. Enjoyment is a positive determinant of physical activity.
- People who don't identify with exercise don't do it 'I'm not the sporty type'.
- Behavioural intention, attitudes, beliefs, knowledge, values, perceived competence, and self-efficacy—highly associated with physical activity.
- High levels of self-motivation are also highly correlated with adherence to physical activity. For example, when self-motivation was combined with % body fat, over 80% of subjects were correctly predicted as either an adherer or a drop-out.
- Individuals who are highly self-motivated are thought to be very effective at goal setting, monitoring, and rewarding progress and adjusting their exercise programme to their needs and abilities. These skills are learned through experience, but can also be taught to an individual.

Demographic
- Higher income, more education implies you are more likely to be physically active.
- Individuals earning less than 15K annually, 65% are inactive as compared with 48% of those earning 50K or more.
- 72% of individuals who have not completed secondary school education are inactive, as compared with 50% of university educated.

Biological
- *Gender:* boys are more active than girls.
- *Age:* activity levels decline with age.
- *BMI:* adolescent girls with higher BMI are much less likely to exercise than normal weight girls.

The *behavioural determinants* refer to our experience (past and present) with physical activity (in all its types) and how this may influence our current participation.

- Previous sport participation (recent participation is more predictive than childhood involvement).
- Past involvement in structured exercise programme is the best predictor of current participation 'once I was in the programme I knew what it took to stay active.'
- High intensity exercise is more stressful on the system than moderate or low intensity exercise. It is predictive of drop out for sedentary or unfit individuals and is linked to negative mood states.
- An exercise leader who is knowledgeable, likeable, and provides positive feedback regularly is more likely to encourage exercise adherence.
- Group exercise sessions can lead to increased social support, enjoyment, they provide an opportunity to compare progress and to tend to enhance commitment to the exercise programme as the individual becomes affiliated to the group. They are more likely to increase adherence than individual sessions.

Caution
- The relationship between the determinant and physical activity is not always clear.
- Higher exercise self-efficacy is more likely to lead to exercise involvement.

But
- Increased fitness due to exercise involvement can increase exercise self-efficacy.
- Determinants of physical activity are not isolated variables. They influence and are influenced by each other in terms of exercise.

Understanding behaviour change

Change is a dynamic process that occurs over time. As an individual changes their behaviour they progress through a series of five stages of change. Each stage of change has two components, one is behaviour and the second is intention or readiness to change.

Very few individuals are physically unable to take part in moderate or light physical activity. However, high proportions are not psychologically ready to take on board the challenges of changing their lifestyle to accommodate physical activity.

There are five stages of exercise behaviour change. These are pre-contemplation (sedentary individuals who have no intention of changing), contemplation (sedentary individuals and 6-month intention to change), preparation (irregularly active and 30-day intention to become more regularly active), action (regular physical activity for the last 6 months), and maintenance (regularly physically active for longer than 6 months).

In order to 'stage' an individual you must know their exercise behaviour and their behavioural intention.

Ensure you define regular health enhancing physical activity using guidelines of the minimum requirements for disease prevention and health promotion mentioned earlier. This incorporates both the moderate accumulative message and the continuous fitness message, and is worded to include frequency, intensity, time, and type of activity.

An active lifestyle does not require a regimented vigorous exercise programme.
- *Frequency:* most, preferably all days of the week.
- *Intensity:* moderate or above (e.g. brisk walking).
- *Time:* accumulating 30min or more per day.
- *Type:* any aerobic activity.

For an individual who wishes to develop and maintain aerobic fitness the continuous message recommends continuous aerobic activity 3–5 days per week, for a minimum of 20min per session, of at least a moderate intensity (60–90% of maximum heart rate).

Keeping these definitions in mind, an individual can be staged into one of the following five categories:

I currently …
- Do not exercise, and do not intend to start exercising in the next 6 months.
- Do not exercise, but am thinking about starting to exercise in the next 6 months.
- Exercise some, but not regularly (regular exercise = enough to meet the current recommendations). I intend to exercise regularly in the next 30 days.
- Exercise regularly, but have only begun doing so within the last 6 months.
- Exercise regularly, and have done so for longer than 6 months.

The time to progress through the stages of change is variable, the 'set of tasks' that have to be accomplished at each stage of change (SOC) are less variable.

Precontemplation

There is no intention to become active in the foreseeable future. Many individuals in this stage are unaware of their problem (physical inactivity). Resistance to recognize the problem is the hallmark of pre-contemplators.

Pre-contemplators need to acknowledge or take ownership of the problem, increase awareness of the negative aspects of the problem, and accurately evaluate self-regulation capacities.

Contemplation

Serious consideration of problem resolution is central to this stage. Individuals need to convince themselves to begin to take action to avoid a contemplative habit being established.

Contemplators need to take a firm decision to initiate physical activity, and engage in preliminary action to move to the next stage.

Preparation

Individuals' are intending to take action immediately and have initiated small changes in their behaviour.

Preparers need to set goals and priorities toward taking action. They are often already engaged in the processes which would increase self-regulation and initiate behaviour change.

Action

Individuals' modify their behaviour, experiences and/or environment in order to meet the minimum levels of physical activity required for leading an active lifestyle.

Actioners have to develop effective strategies to prevent lapses or slips from becoming complete returns to sedentary behaviours.

Maintenance

Individuals' work to prevent relapse and consolidate the gains attained during action. This is not a static stage, rather a continuation of change. Being able to remain free of the chronic problem and/or to consistently engage in a new incompatible behaviour (i.e. sustained or regular participation in physical activity) for more than 6 months is the criterion for Maintenance.

Maintainers require sustained behavioural change for periods of time from 6 months up to 3 or more years after the initial action.

Originally progression through the stages was conceived as linear, as individuals were thought to progress from one stage to another in a simple discrete fashion. A linear progression—although possible—has been identified as extremely rare, especially in some chronic disorders. This led to the model evolving to a spiral pattern.

In this pattern of change, each stage can be both stable and dynamic in nature depending on the individual concerned. For example, individuals are thought to progress through the stages of change at different rates with some individuals getting stuck at certain stages and others relapsing and sliding back to earlier stages.

The individuals that relapse (relapsers) may recycle into the model, or alternatively due to a variety of reasons, e.g. guilt, embarrassment, may return to pre-contemplation. Research suggests that a high number of relapsers recycle back to the contemplation or preparation stage. The spiral model suggests that most relapsers do not revolve endlessly in circles and that they do not regress all the way back to where they began. Instead, each time relapsers recycle through the stages, the potentially learn from their mistakes and can try something different the next time around.

Increasing population-wide participation in physical activity

Within the work of the Global Advocacy for Physical Activity (GAPA), a complimentary document, entitled 'Investments that work for physical activity' was published to support the Toronto Charter.[1] This document emphasizes the need for countries (not just individuals or organizations) to commit to a combination of strategies aimed at individual, social-cultural, environmental, and policy determinants of inactivity if they are serious at reversing the downward trend in physical activity.

Seven 'best investments' for which there is an evidence-base of effectiveness are explained. These investments are thought to have worldwide applicability and are as follows:

'Whole of School' programs
- Transport policies and systems that prioritize walking, cycling, and public transport.
- Urban design regulations and infrastructure that provide for equitable and safe access for recreational physical activity, and transport-related walking and cycling across the life course.
- Physical activity and non-communicable disease prevention integrated into primary health care systems.
- Public education, including mass media to raise awareness and change social norms on physical activity.
- Community-wide programs involving multiple settings and sectors and that mobilize and integrate community engagement and resources.
- Sports systems and programs that promote 'sport for all' and encourage participation across the lifespan.

---

[1] GAPA (2011). Global Advocacy for Physical Activity (GAPA) the Advocacy Council of the International Society for Physical Activity and Health (ISPAH). (2011). *NCD Prevention: Investments That Work for Physical Activity*. Available at: M www.globalpa.org.uk/investmentsthatwork

Clinical and community interventions to promote and support physical activity

Emphasis on individualism and lack of attention to the social and environmental factors that impinge on health could, in fact, increase rather than reduce the health gap in society. The seven investments identified by GAPA take into account the individual and their environment, ensuring that the full population can be targeted through the determinants of physical activity.

Effective physical activity interventions should adhere to a systematic approach to intervention design and evaluation.

Set an overall goal. Examples of outcomes generally include:

- Improvements in physical activity behaviour (e.g. increased time spent walking); and/or
- Increases in selected fitness measures (e.g. increased aerobic capacity or other components of health related fitness, e.g. muscular strength and endurance).
- Decrease in sedentary behaviour (e.g. number of hours spent watching TV).

Set specific objectives, linked to your goal, based on the SMARTER principles (Specific, Measurable, Accepted, Realistic, Time bound, Enjoyable, Recorded).

Frameworks

King (1994)[1] provided a framework for thinking about different interventions which aim to increase physical activity in the general population. There are four levels presented within this framework.

- Personal.
- Interpersonal.
- Organizational.
- Environmental.

Level one: personal approaches

The focus of level one is on individual change. Information delivered through a variety of sources. For this type of intervention to work it should be embedded into either: a primary health care system (GAPA investment 4), a community-wide program (GAPA investment 6) or a sport for all programme (GAPA investment 7).

Face-to-face, one-on-one consultations offer intensive, individualized attention by a trained professional and the opportunity for clients' behavioural prescriptions to be tailored to fit their needs. Office-based exercise consultations are an example of this type of intervention. A physician, exercise scientist, or health promotion professional generally conducts them. They have been shown to be very effective for clinical populations.

---

[1] King, A.C. (1994). Clinical and community interventions to promote and support physical activity participation. In: R. K. Dishman (ed.), *Advances in Exercise Adherence* (pp. 183–212). Champaign: Human Kinetics.

Mediated approaches include electronic (TV, radio, video) and/or print media (booklets, self-help kits, newspaper articles, newsletters). They provide advice and support to individuals on how to initiate, adhere to and maintain an active lifestyle. They, similar to a consultation, target key strategies to support and assist individual behaviour change. They are very useful for individuals who cannot make a face-to-face consultation.

Telephone plus mediated approaches are a combination of both of the above. They include supervised home-based programmes. They allow greater flexibility and convenience in choosing time, location, and setting for the consultation, they are more cost effective, yet still provide support from a trained professional for encouragement, advice and motivation to enhance physical activity levels.

The key ingredients for level one intervention are:
- Target the known determinants of physical (e.g. benefits vs. barriers, self-efficacy, exercise enjoyment, and choice).
- Explore behavioural change strategies to effect change in these determinants (e.g. goal setting, personal monitoring).
- Teach problem-solving for maintenance of physical activity and to avoid relapse into sedentary behaviours.

Advantages
- Individualized advice.
- Face-to-face feedback.
- Professional support.
- Learn specific problem solving skills.
- Learn relapse prevention.

Disadvantages
- Select few.
- Staff intensive.
- Expensive.
- Limited impact.
- Volunteer sample.
- Long-term effects are unknown.

Level two: interpersonal approaches

Interpersonal approaches use social forces to produce change. They are the most popular format for delivering exercise programmes in clinical settings, e.g. cardiac rehabilitation exercise programmes. Similar to the level one approaches, these intervention approaches should be integrated into the GAPA investments that work.

They are concerned with how leaders, teachers, and programme providers can create the most appropriate intra- and interpersonal climates, including various exercise choices, to encourage groups of people to increase or maintain activity.

They are primarily focused on the individual within the group setting. However, in order to be successful the emphasis should be on the how to build, strengthen, and maintain social networks that support, and promote initiation, and maintenance of physical activity.

The key Ingredients include:
- Enhanced feelings of group affiliation.
- Public support systems.
- Group problem-solving.

Support from peers, family, friends, teachers, coaches, instructors or co-workers are the hallmark of interpersonal interventions.

Advantages
- Large expert-to-client ratio.
- More cost effective.
- Visual modeling.
- On-site supervision.
- Set location/time/structure.
- Face-to-face encouragement by instructor.
- Group affiliation and support.
- Group problem-solving.

Disadvantages
- Inconvenient.
- Limited variety of activities.
- Expensive.
- Normative rather than individual advice.
- Social costs such as embarrassment at exercising in front of others.
- Need to recruit participants continually.
- Challenge of being a new exerciser in an established group.
- Group leader effect.

Examples
- Structured exercise groups/classes.
- Physical education classes.
- Classroom-based education focusing on information and development of skills, and reducing sedentary behaviours.
- Family-based social support.
  - Family record keeping of amount of physical activity undertaken by family members.
  - Family-orientated special events.
- Community-based social support.
  - Buddy systems.
  - Peer-led systems.

Level three: organizational or environmental approaches

The organizational or environmental level of the framework is focused on how communities and organizations, such as workplaces and schools, can change aspects of their setting or environment in order to promote physical activity. It includes personal and interpersonal levels, but adds approaches focused on organizational and environmental change. These approaches are aligned to the GAPA investments, such as 'the whole school approach' and the 'community-wide programmes'.

The key ingredients include:
- Physical and organizational structures rather than the individual.
- Influence organizational rules/policies.

- Increase availability of facilities for physical activity.
- Remove or minimize organizational or environmental barriers to undertaking physical activity.

Advantages
- Accessible and diverse population base.
- Convenience.
- Potential of group support.
- Systematic and organised format for promoting physical activity.

Disadvantages
- Limited to small group instruction.
- Short-term effects.
- Lack of a public health focus.

Examples
- Enhanced access to places for physical activity, combined with informational activities.
- Enhanced access to physical activity where we work, play, learn, and live. Workplaces, schools, day-care, and residential care centres for older adults, hospitals, places of worship are all community-based settings for exercise programmes.
- Re-evaluation of physical environment for physical activity.
- Point-of-decision prompts to encourage people to use the stairs, rather than the lifts.
- Traffic planning to reduce the amount of traffic congestion.
- Provision of cycle paths, foot paths, speed control measures, and adequate lighting.
- Safe routes to schools initiatives.
- Specific community initiatives such as family activity days, fun-runs, charity walks.
- Mass-media approaches combined with community based initiatives.

Level four: legislation or policy approaches
This level focuses on societal change. Its idea is to develop passive prevention strategies, ones that do not require action on the part of the individual in order to be effective. Physical activity is a participation behaviour and not a product (like alcohol, cigarettes), this makes it more difficult to develop passive prevention strategies. The key ingredients include:
- Policies to enhance physical activity participation.
- Legislative interventions that mandate changes to encourage and facilitate participation in physical activity, and/or remove barriers that restrict individual and community involvement.
- Institutionalization of programmes and strategies to affect change.

Examples
- Active transportation policies and systems that ensure people have a choice of, and access to, safe, clean, and adequately maintained cycling and pedestrian pathways, or public transport (GAPA, investment 2).
- Urban design regulations and planning approaches: zoning and land use, street, and living design to promote recreational physical activity, and transport-related walking and cycling across the life course (GAPA, investment 3).

- Policies for flexi-time to promote activity at work.
- Standard minimum qualifications/facilities and curriculum for physical education in schools.
- Standard qualifications for exercise specialists, for example the National Quality Assurance Framework for GP referral schemes.
- Countryside access which provides legal entitlement to the general public to use the countryside for recreation.
- Making the provision of recreation facilities a legal requirement for local councils, and providing monetary incentives for adequate public facilities for physical activity.

Summary
- Levels 1 and 2 suggest that short term increases in physical activity are relatively easy to achieve if people are ready to change; long-term adherence remains the challenge.
- Levels 3 and 4 offer best public health strategy (reach the most). There is now a strong body of evidence to support these approaches.
- Each level has major influence for increasing the effectiveness of an intervention.

The strongest intervention strategy is likely to include a multilevel approach. Using a combination of powerful personal strategies such as social support or self-efficacy in a community-wide initiative has the potential for substantial impact and change in physical activity behaviour.

The way forward

- Establish a comprehensive baseline of patterns of physical activity.
- Set realistic physical activity goals, objectives, and outcomes.
- Within key settings identify your partnerships for intervention: Local government, private and public sectors, agencies: those focused on health, exercise, recreation, transport, schools, worksites, political/legislative aspects of community.
- Guided by relevant exercise theories that explain the determinants of PA, e.g. transtheoretical model of behaviour change.
- Be aware of the different levels of intervention required to get a population more physically active. Aim for a multi-level approach where appropriate.
- Monitor change through robust surveillance systems.

Further reading

Bellew B, Schoeppe S, Bull FC, & Baumann A. (2008). The rise and fall of Australian physical activity policy 1996–2006: A national review framed in an international context. *Aust NZ Hlth Policy* **5**: 18.

Global Advocacy for Physical Activity (GAPA) the Advocacy Council of the International Society for Physical Activity and Health (ISPAH). (2010). *The Toronto Charter for Physical Activity: A Global Call for Action*. Available at: www.globalpa.org.uk

Overweight and obesity in children

The incidence of childhood overweight and obesity has increased dramatically over the past 20yr in the Western world. The current western culture nurtures obesity.

Epidemiology
- There has been a marked worldwide ↑ in prevalence of overweight and obesity in children.
- Childhood overweight and obesity rates are highest in the UK, Western Europe, North America, and Australia where they are between 20 and 30%.
- Childhood obesity (>3yr of age) is highly correlated with adult obesity.[1]
- Parental obesity more than doubles the risk of adult obesity among both obese and non-obese children <10yr of age.[1]
- Marked increase in incidence of Type 2 diabetes in adolescents.
- Progressive ↓ in physical activity after age 11.[2]
- ↓ Activity in girls before boys.
- Boys are more active than girls in every age-group.[2]

Possible causes
- Unstructured play time has been replaced with inactive pursuits such as watching television, playing video games and the Internet.
- Dominance of the car has meant that walking and cycling are less often used as a mode of transport.
- Safety concerns regarding places where children can exercise, i.e. local parks and streets.
- Desire for instant meals and the subsequent prevalence of fast food outlets (providing calorie dense food options).
- Advertising of unhealthy food choices directed at children.

Diagnosis
- International standards now exist for the definition of overweight and obesity in childhood (Table 4.1).
- BMIs at various ages for boys and girls which will pass through a BMI of 25kg/m^3 (overweight) or 30kg/m^3 (obese) have been determined.

Complications
- Dyslipidaemia and insulin resistance.
- Two-fold increase in risk of death from ischaemic heart disease (IHD). Over 57yrs if overweight in childhood.[3]
- Non-insulin dependent diabetes mellitus (NIDDM).
- Fatty liver disease.
- Sleep apnoea.

---

[1] Whitaker RC, Wright JA, Pepe MS, Seidel KD, Dietz WH. (1997). Predicting obesity in young adulthood form childhood to parental obesity. *N Engl J Med.* **337(13)**: 869–73.

[2] Australian Bureau of Statistics. (2011). *Sports and Physical Recreation: A Statistical Overview, Australia.* Availavble at: M (http://www.abs.gov.au/ausstats/abs/@.nsf/mf/4156.0)

[3] Gunnell DJ, Frankel SJ, Nanchahal K, Peters TJ, Davey Smith G. (1998). Childhood obesity and adult cardiovascular mortality: a 57 yr follow up study based on the Boyd Orr cohort. *Am J Clin Nutr* **67(6)**: 1111–18

Table 4.1 International cut off points for overweight and obesity

Age (yrs)	BMI 25 kg/m²		BMI 35 kg/m²	
	Males	Females	Males	Females
2	18.41	18.02	20.09	19.81
2.5	18.13	17.76	19.80	19.55
3	17.89	17.56	19.57	19.36
3.5	17.69	17.40	19.39	19.23
4	17.55	17.28	19.29	19.15
4.5	17.47	17.19	19.26	19.12
5	17.42	17.15	19.30	19.17
5.5	17.45	17.20	19.47	19.34
6	17.55	17.34	19.78	19.65
6.5	17.71	17.53	20.23	20.08
7	17.92	17.75	20.63	20.51
7.5	18.16	18.03	21.09	21.01
8	18.44	18.35	21.60	21.57
8.5	18.76	18.69	22.17	22.18
9	19.10	19.07	22.77	22.81
9.5	19.46	19.45	23.39	23.46
10	19.84	19.86	24.00	24.11
10.5	20.20	20.29	24.57	24.77
11	20.55	20.74	25.10	25.42
11.5	20.89	21.20	25.58	26.05
12	21.22	21.68	26.02	26.67
12.5	21.56	22.14	26.43	27.24
13	21.91	22.58	26.84	27.76
13.5	22.27	22.98	27.25	28.20
14	22.62	23.34	27.63	28.57
14.5	22.96	23.66	27.98	28.87
15	23.29	23.94	28.30	29.11

(*Continued*)

Table 4.1 (Continued)

Age (yrs)	BMI 25 kg/m²		BMI 35 kg/m²	
	Males	Females	Males	Females
15.5	23.60	24.17	28.60	29.29
16	23.90	24.37	28.88	29.43
16.5	24.19	24.54	29.14	29.56
17	24.46	24.70	29.41	29.69
17.5	24.73	24.85	29.70	29.84
18	25	25	30	30

Reproduced from: Establishing a standard definition for child overweight and obesity worldwide: International survey; Cole, TJ, Bellizzi, MC, Flegal, KM, Dietz, WH; Vol 320; pp 1240–43; 2000 with permission from BMJ Publishing Group Ltd

- Musculoskeletal concerns, e.g. slipped upper capital femoral epiphysis.
- Psychological disturbances including low self-esteem.

Strategies to ↑ exercise
- Involve the family in exercise interventions. Having both parents' support for physical activity increased participation rates of girls from 30 to 70%.[4]
- Carry exercise equipment in car for impromptu stops.
- Encourage habitual, daily exercise where possible. Walking to and from school or the bus-stop/train station is desirable.
- Introduce reward system for achieving short- and long-term activity goals.
- Link TV viewing (or other favoured sedentary activities) to exercise in reluctant exercisers.
- Encourage year round competitive sports participation as ↑ enjoyment, and ↑ intensity compared with unstructured exercise programmes.

Prevention and treatment
- Long-term results of current weight loss strategies have been disappointing.
- Treatments used have included: family therapy, cognitive behavioural therapy to promote dietary change and aerobic exercise, school-based interventions, pharmacological and surgical interventions.
- Prognosis is poor if one or both parents are obese.

Further reading
Wang Y, Lobstein T. (2006). Worldwide trends in childhood overweight and obesity. *Int J Pediat Obes* **1**(1): 11–252.

---

[4] Davison KK, Cutting TM, Birch LL. (2003). Parents' activity-related parenting practices predict girls' physical activity *Med. Sci. Sports Exerc*: **35(9):** 1589–95

Epidemiology

Epidemiology is the study of research methodology in humans. Clinical epidemiology is the application of these methods in research studies. Understanding epidemiology will help those interested in physical activity and injury prevention programmes adopt effective interventions, and avoid adopting ineffective or even harmful ones.

Experimental studies
- Researcher allocates treatment of interest (exposure) to one group, and a comparison treatment (control) to another group.
- Studies can also test several interventions at once.
- The allocation of individuals to a treatment or control group can be randomized or non-randomized.

Randomization
- Randomization should ensure that neither the researcher nor the subject influences the group assignment for the subject. Therefore, the person deciding should not know who the subject is that is being given the intervention (called allocation concealment).
- Often uses 2 different size blocks. If only blocks of 4 are used, researcher would know which group the 4th person would be assigned to.

Blinding
- Knowing that one is in the exposure group vs. control group may affect their response.
- The outcome evaluator should be blinded because most outcomes include a subjective component (e.g. ST depression on the EKG).
- In rehabilitation therapy, patient blinding is often not possible. One can sometimes (ethically) blind the patient to the study purpose.

Observational studies
- Exposure is not controlled by researcher (e.g. evaluating a new surgery) or subject (e.g. smoking).
- Several types of studies:
  - *Prospective cohort:* start with exposed and control groups and follow over time. Pro: good quality data. Con: requires time.
  - *Historical cohort:* use databases or chart reviews to determine exposed and control groups in past. Determine outcome today. Pro: immediate answer. Con: important data may be missing.
  - *Case-control:* categorize individuals as having the outcome or not. Then examine if they were exposed to the intervention or not. Pro: cost-efficient for rare disease. Con: difficult to choose appropriate controls, important data may be missing.
  - *Cross-sectional:* evaluate outcome and exposure of individuals at any one point in time. Pro: easy to obtain data. Con: unknown if exposure occurred before or after the outcome.
- The term prospective means that exposure and outcome data are obtained as they occur.
- The term retrospective can mean different things at different times and should be avoided. Sometimes, it means that the data was recorded in

the past and the researcher is retrieving the data (e.g. historical cohort study, case-control study). Sometimes it means the data is obtained by asking subjects about things in the past; this type of retrospective study is very prone to "recall" bias where affected subjects are likely to remember the past differently from unaffected subjects.
- Using the meaning referring to when the data is retrieved (as opposed to how it was retrieved), cohort and cross-sectional studies can be prospective or retrospective, but case-control studies are always retrospective.

Chapter 5

Exercise physiology

What happens when we exercise? *124*
Components of fitness *125*
Energy for exercise *126*
Muscle physiology *129*
Cardiovascular system and exercise *132*
Respiratory responses to exercise *136*
Oxygen uptake and lactate threshold *140*
Measuring exercise capacity *142*
Basic principles of training *152*
Aerobic endurance training *154*
Resistance training *158*
Anaerobic/sprint training *162*
Gender and performance *164*
Resistance training in children *166*
Exercise testing in children *168*

What happens when we exercise?

The individual response to exercise depends on a number of factors:
- Type of exercise stress encountered; level of training, conditioning, and nutritional and hydration status.
- Age, gender, body type, muscle fibre type ratios.
- Genetic factors and environmental conditions, psychological factors.

Physiological response to exercise stress varies according to the factors mentioned above. The complex interactions of the body's homeostatic mechanisms and responses can be briefly summarized in a time line:

Short-term—seconds to minutes (stress reaction)

- *Autonomic nervous system responses:* sympathetic nervous system (SNS) increase with parasympathetic nervous system (PNS) decrease resulting in predominance of fight and flight responses, and reduced vegetative functions.
- *Cardiovascular responses:* increased cardiac output to exercising muscles and reduced blood flow to other organ systems. Elevated core temperature increases blood flow to the skin to facilitate thermoregulation.
- *Respiratory responses:* increased rate and depth of respiration to meet demands for gas exchange.
- *Metabolic and respiratory responses:* buffering of lactic acid produced by the active muscles.

Medium-term—minutes to hours (resistance reaction)

Hormonal responses Accentuate and prolong the autonomic neural responses (above); release of catecholamines from adrenal medulla, adrenocorticotrophic hormone (ACTH) and growth hormone (GH) from pituitary, cortisol from adrenal gland increase substrate availability for energy metabolism to provide fuel for longer duration exercise. Activation of the renin angiotensin and antidiuretic hormone (ADH) mechanisms help preserve fluid and electrolyte balance and maintain BP.

Long-term—days to weeks (adaptation)

Repeated acute bouts of exercise (training) usually result in adaptation to exercise stimulus. Adaptation results from gene activation in the various tissues under stress. Cellular structural changes in muscle and other tissues result in strength and endurance changes; neural regulation changes optimize muscle activation patterns; renal mechanisms are responsible for changes in plasma volume and venous return leading to compensatory changes in cardiac dimensions.

Clinical note

Overtraining syndrome in athletes is defined by under-performance and is characterized by fatigue and physiological and psychological changes. It has been suggested that this is a maladaptive alternative 3rd stage of adaptation. Long term, may be useful as a protective physiological mechanism preventing damage from over-exercise when individual athletes train beyond the limits of physiological compensation.

Components of fitness

Stamina (aerobic conditioning, aerobic power)
All types of exercise require a base level of aerobic conditioning. High levels of aerobic conditioning enable more efficient use of fuel, greater tolerance of environmental extremes, quicker recovery during intermittent exercise and between training sessions, and are essential for long-term cardiovascular health. Important factors are: mechanical efficiency of the heart pumping blood (cardiac output, Q); the ability of muscle to extract and utilize oxygen (arteriovenous difference in oxygen concentration, a-vO_2 diff) and fuels.

Speed and strength (anaerobic power)
Sprint velocity, mass of weight lifted, or the distance of a throw depends on the maximum force that a muscle can exert through its leverage systems. Muscle forces depend on body size and type, biomechanics, muscle cross-sectional area, predominant fibre type, and rate of ATP resynthesis. Generally, the greater the muscle mass the more speed, force, or power that can be generated.

Skill (neuromuscular coordination)
Skills are co-ordinated neuromuscular patterns of activation, which increase efficiency, speed, and ease of movement. In neurological terms, highly developed skills are implemented subconsciously, which involve quicker neural pathways. Skills can be innate or learned, optimum acquisition is age dependent (9–12yr), but can be achieved with good training practices and high quality coaching at any age.

Suppleness (flexibility)
Flexibility or suppleness is the ability to move a joint through a full range of normal movement. Depends on joint type, joint surface congruity, tension in capsules, ligaments, and muscles. When a joint is forced outside its normal working range by external forces, greater flexibility may be protective against injury, and there is evidence that this and flexibility training may improve performance.

Psychology (mental fitness)
When the physiological and biomechanical components of fitness have been optimized, psychological factors become more important. At elite level, psychological factors may be the only difference between success and failure. Mental strength may be innate in some individuals, but aspects of psychological preparation can be learned and should be practiced as part of normal training. Preparation and training includes:
- Motivation to compete and train, and goal setting.
- Mental rehearsal of performance.
- Pre-competition routines to manage anxiety.
- Coping strategies for success or failure.
- Injury.

These are all important areas for professional athletes.

Energy for exercise

Exercise is powered by the high energy phosphate molecule ATP. Resting cellular energy processes provide a small amount of ATP for normal cellular homeostatic systems and in muscle cells ATP powers contractile elements. Cellular energy metabolic processes generate ATP rapidly for short bouts of high-intensity exercise and more steadily for longer-term exercise. Relative contribution of different metabolic energy systems depend on exercise duration, intensity, ratio of fast to slow twitch muscle fibre types and individual fitness levels of fitness.

Impulse energy (high energy phosphates/anaerobic)

This is the small quantity of energy (ATP) present in the cell at rest; it can provide the initial impetus for a throw, a jump, a punch, a serve in tennis, or the initial reaction off the blocks in a sprint. If high-intensity exercise is to continue the small amount of ATP present in the cell at rest must be rapidly regenerated.

Immediate energy (high energy phosphates/anaerobic)

$$CP \rightarrow creatine + Pi + energy \rightarrow ADP + Pi \mid ATP$$

The phospho-creatine system (ATP-PCR) is an ATP buffering system preventing short-term ATP depletion. Phosphate molecules are shuttled from creatine phosphate to adenosine diphosphate (ADP) regenerating ATP molecules rapidly. The high energy phosphate buffer can replenish cellular ATP levels for all out maximum efforts lasting ~6–7s or longer durations at lower intensity. A high percentage of fast twitch fibres replete with creatine stores (eat more red meat and oily fish or creatine supplementation) in addition to sprint and resistance training are factors, which optimize function of this system.

Short-term energy (anaerobic glycolysis)

A sustained high rate of ATP generation to power longer duration exercise require metabolism of fuels. Short-term (seconds to minutes) breakdown of glycogen or glucose anaerobically (substrate phosphorylation) provides a small amount of ATP rapidly.

$$\text{Glycogen or glucose} \rightarrow \text{pyruvic acid} \Leftrightarrow \text{lactic acid} \Leftrightarrow \text{lactate} + H^+$$

Advantage
Capable of high rates of ATP production to power high-intensity exercise for short periods.

Disadvantages
Inefficient as only small amounts of ATP are generated from fuel stores, relatively fast to fatigue, and the end product, pyruvate, is converted to lactic acid. Lactic acid dissociates, the hydrogen ion has to be buffered or cellular pH will fall inhibiting cellular enzyme activity, however lactate can be taken up by less active tissues and metabolized aerobically (extracellular lactate shuttle).

In healthy untrained subjects significant blood lactate (BLa) accumulation occurs at ~55% of VO_2 max and in highly trained endurance athletes this does not occur until ~85% of VO_2 max. A shift to anaerobic glycolysis and increased BLa is caused by increased exercise intensity, relative tissue hypoxia, and neural selection of fast twitch muscle fibres.

ATP-PCR and anaerobic glycolytic systems are the predominant energy systems for intense exercise lasting anywhere from 10–20s up to 90s, e.g. running 100–400m, 50–200m swim, or the short repeated sprints required during field sports. A favourable ratio of fast to slow twitch muscle fibres, correct training methods, and nutritional factors (high creatine level and adequate cellular carbohydrate (CHO) stores) will optimize function of these energy systems.

Long-term energy (oxidative phosphorylation/aerobic)

Prolonged or sustained activity (minutes to hours) utilizes more efficient metabolism of fuels with oxygen and greater energy yield. Aerobic breakdown of CHO and free fatty acids (FFA) to produce ATP requires mitochondrial enzymes and cofactors of the tricarboxylic acid cycle (TCA), and the electron transport chain (ETC). Glucose fully metabolized aerobically yields ~38 ATP and glycogen ~39 ATP, and although the rate of energy production is higher than for fat; intramuscular and liver stores of carbohydrate are limited.

NB During high intensity aerobic activity, such as marathon running at >19km/h pace, CHO is utilized for rapid aerobic ATP generation. If initial stores or intake of CHO in the race are inadequate after ~120min significant CHO depletion occurs, energy metabolism slows as fuel utilization switches to fat, pace rapidly falls, and the runner 'hits the wall'!

Energy yields from FFA metabolism are greater than CHO, due to greater numbers of CH_2 units in FFA chains. Aerobic metabolism of palmitic acid [$CH_3(CH_2)_{14}COOH$], for example, can generate 129 moles ATP. However, despite abundant availability of fat, rates of ATP synthesis from fat breakdown are much slower, greater O_2 is required, and a glycolysis is required to keep the TCA cycle turning … 'fat' is thus said to 'burn on a carbohydrate flame'. In the TCA cycle a series of enzymatically controlled steps strip the hydrogens from CH_2, the carbon combines with oxygen to form CO_2 and hydrogens combine with cofactors (nicotinamide adenine dinucleotide (NAD)/ flavin adenine dinucleotide (FAD)) and are transferred to the electron transport chain (ETC) where they are oxidized in a series of steps coupled to phosphorylation of AMP and ADP to produce ATP. Hydrogens finally combine with O_2 to produce water.

Aerobic production of ATP proceeds rapidly if muscle cells have large numbers of mitochondria replete with; oxidative enzymes, NAD/FAD cofactors, iron-containing cytochromes, and myoglobin. Greater capillarization of muscle cell improves O_2 and FFA delivery, and the removal of waste products; and, myoglobin within mitochondria draws in oxygen.

Factors affecting aerobic metabolism/endurance capacity
- Environmental effects on oxygen dissolved in solution (partial pressure of oxygen (pO_2)) (altitude or depth).
- Respiratory function (air pollution, bronchoconstriction).
- Oxygen transport (haemaglobin), delivery (heart function).
- Predominant muscle fibre types (ratio of slow twitch fibres (ST) and FOG to fast twitch fibres (FT)).
- Extraction of O_2 and fuel (capillary density and myoglobin level).
- Rate of utilization of fuel and oxygen (number/size of mitochondria, oxidative enzyme activity, stores/availability of co-factors, and fuel).

Muscle physiology

Structure
- Individual muscle fibres are multinucleated cells with a calcium rich transverse 'T' tubular system connecting outer sarcoplasmic membrane to sarcoplasmic reticulum enveloping the sarcomeres.
- Sarcomeres show the classic striated pattern of overlapping contractile elements of actin (thin) and myosin (thick) filaments plus associated anchoring proteins.
- Muscle fibres are further organized into progressively larger diameter fascicles and bundles, by envelopes of endomysium, perimysium, and finally a layer of epimysium encloses the whole muscle.
- Macroscopic structure—length, breadth, shape, and pennation (muscle fibre orientation to tendon) further determine function.

Excitation-contraction coupling
- α Motor neuron action potential→ neuromuscular end plate→ acetyl choline release→ depolarization sarcolemma/T tubule→ Ca^{2+} release.
- Ca^{2+} binds to troponin → conformational change in tropomyosin.
- Binding sites exposed on actin for myosin heads → cross-bridging.
- Myosin heads pivot on binding→ sarcomeres shorten.
- ATP then binds→ releasing myosin head from actin-binding site.
- Further cross-bridge cycling occurs as long as Ca^{2+} bound to troponin.

Fibre types are classified physiologically into slow twitch (aerobic) and fast twitch (anaerobic) fibres. FT to ST fibre ratio is genetically determined, and varies in different muscle groups according to function.

Slow twitch fibres
- Aerobic endurance fibres (red) have glycolytic and mitochondrial aerobic energy systems (TCA/ETC), stores of glycogen and a high muscle fibre to motor neuron ratio.
- If provided with constant fuel (FFA or glucose) and oxygen supply (capillarization/myoglobin) they fatigue slowly, but have low contraction speed and low unit strength.

Fast twitch fibres (FT_b)
- Speed and strength fibres (white) have highly developed cytoplasmic anaerobic energy systems: intercellular energy stores (creatine phosphate) and glycogen fuel stores, available for rapid turnover.
- FT_b fibres have high contraction speeds and greater unit strength but fatigue quickly due to rapid accumulation of lactic acid which is buffered or shuttled out of the cell during activity. Regeneration of creatine phosphate occurs in a small number of mitochondria.

Fast oxidative/glycolytic fibres (FOG/FT_a)
An intermediate fibre type also exists, which has both anaerobic and aerobic energy systems. Depending on training stimulus these fibres adapt, and behave more like ST or anaerobic FT_b fibres.

Muscle function (macro-level)

Muscles arise from a proximal bony attachment, and pass across one or sometimes two joints to a distal bony attachment. Muscles generate;
- Primary forces for movement (concentric shortening actions).
- Secondary forces to slow movement (eccentric elongating actions).
- Joint stabilizing forces (isotonic/isometric static co-contractions).
- Combination of all of the above to absorb externally applied forces.

Magnitude and direction of resultant force across a joint depend on:
- Muscle morphology (length/pennation).
- Type of muscle contraction (concentric/eccentric/isometric).
- Joint morphology (articular surfaces) and static restraints (ligaments).
- Dynamic actions of other muscles (synergists/antagonists).

Muscle actions can be evaluated in terms strength, power and endurance:
- Strength is the force a muscle or group of muscles can generate, measured as the greatest mass that can be lifted (1RM). Isokinetic dynamometry can profile isokinetic, concentric, and eccentric forces produced across a range of joints at varying speeds.
- Power [(force × distance)/time] is the functional aspect of the majority of muscle actions. In most sports, a combination of strength and speed of movement is the key determinant of performance. Peak power and power decline can be assessed using field- or laboratory-based sprinting tests.
- Muscular endurance is the ability to maintain a single contraction or repeated contractions at a given force over a longer duration assessed by number of repetitions possible at different percentage of the 1RM. It is also assessed in competitive races/time trials, and also in field and laboratory-based testing (12 min Cooper run, 2km rowing ergometer test, progressive incremental test to volitional exhaustion).

Cardiovascular system and exercise

Structure
- Fluid transport medium (blood) and central pump (heart).
- Distribution vessels (pulmonary and systemic arteries/arterioles).
- Exchange vessels (capillaries).
- Collection/return vessels (pulmonary and systemic venules/veins).
- Interstitial fluids return system (lymphatics).

Function
- *Delivery/removal*: oxygen and nutrients/CO_2 and waste products.
- *Transport/immunity*: hormones/antibodies and complement.
- *Homeostasis*: temperature, acid/base, fluid/electrolyte balance.

The heart produces a pressure head and volume flow of blood through the vascular system to enable capillary tissue exchange; during exercise: cardiac output increases, distribution of cardiac output is adjusted by arteriolar dilatation (working muscle/skin for cooling) and constriction (non-essential tissues), while baroreceptor and hormonally mediated homeostatic mechanisms maintain BP and circulating volume. Cardiovascular system (CVS) capacity partly determines aerobic exercise capacity, and training induces structural and functional adaptations in the heart, blood, arteriolar distribution of blood-flow, and autonomic and hormonal control mechanisms.

Summary CVS responses to exercise
- Muscular work→ ↑[metabolite]/↓pO_2/↑pCO_2/heat→ dilatation of muscle pre-capillary sphincters and arterioles→ capillary blood flow↑
- capillary blood flow↑ → transient ↓TPR→↓BP
- Baroreceptors→ autonomic nervous system (ANS) (brain) → ↑SNS/↓PNS activity…
- ↑SNS + ↑venous return (muscle pump)→ ↑HR and ↑SV →↑ cardiac output (CO).
- ↑SNS→↑arteriolar tone in non-essential organs →↑TPR.
- ↑CO and ↑TPR →↑BP →↑capillary hydrostatic pressure→ ↑delivery fuel and oxygen and ↑removal of waste products.
- Heat→ skin capillaries dilate/sweat rate ↑ → extracellular fluid (ECF) Na^+ and H_2O loss
- Fluid/electrolyte homeostasis (resistance reaction); ↑ADH/↑ACTH rennin/angiotensin systems maintain blood volume and BP by renal conservation of water and electrolytes, and by vasoconstriction.

Summary CVS responses to endurance training (~3/12)
- ↑Muscle capillary density →↑extraction O_2 and fuel.
- ↑Arteriolar control →↑blood flow muscle/skin→ ↑thermoregulation.
- ↑Stroke volume (SV) and ↓HR →↑cardiac efficiency, CO same, but ↓energy cost.
- ↑Plasma volume (renal mechanisms) and ↑red cell mass (RCC) but ↑PV > ↑RCC → haematocrit (Hct)↓ <0.42 and Hb fall[*]
- ↑Plasma volume (PV) →↓oxygen carrying capacity of blood, *but* ↓↓viscosity → ↓cardiac work (thinner blood is easier to pump!).

- *Cardiac adaptation:* upper limb/strength/speed sports →↑after-load (pressure work)→ concentric remodeling; whole body or lower limb aerobic endurance sports →↑pre-load (volume work) eccentric remodeling. In some sports both types of adaptation occur.

Heart rate

- HR is determined by sino-atrial node automaticity (80–100/min), atrial wall reflexes and balance of autonomic tone; at rest ANS tone mainly vagal, thus HR <80beats/min with exercise SNS/adrenergic tone predominates and HR ↑ with ↑work up to HR_{max} (180–220beats/min).
- *Resting HR:* usually measured on waking, is a useful marker of athletic fatigue, an ↑ 5–10beats/min over normal should alert the athlete to the possibility of training fatigue or inter-current illness.
- *Sub-maximal HR:* HR response to gradually increasing intensity exercise is curvilinear, i.e. a plateau phase at the beginning and end, but in the mid-range linear. At any fixed work intensity HR plateaus after at 2–3min, if work continues at this intensity for >4min HR will slowly rise (cardiovascular drift).
- HR_{max}: often given as 220 − age (yr), but this is a crude estimate given that variation in HRmax predicted by this method ~ ±12 beats.min^{-1}. HRmax determined by refractory period of conducting system in the AV node, HRmax falls by 1-2 beats/year starting in the 3rd decade, due to ageing effects in conducting system.
- HR zones for aerobic endurance training are often arbitrarily given as anywhere from 40–80% of HR_{max}, for elite athletes training zones are better interpolated from HR/BLa data directly recorded during exercise testing to exhaustion (see later sections) (see Box 5.1, i).
- *HR training response:* endurance training should ↓ resting HR and HR at sub-maximal work intensities by 5–10beats/min after 8–12 weeks; HR_{max} falls very little if at all from age predicted value ±12beats/min.

Stroke volume

- SV = end diastolic (EDV) − end systolic volume (ESV).
- EDV is determined by passive filling (70%) due to venous return/elastic recoil; and active filling (30%) due to atrial systole (see Box 5.1, ii).
- Emptying ESV is determined by pre-stretch of the ventricle causing a more forceful contraction (Frank Starling effect) and by effects on cardiac contractility of SNS and circulating catecholamines.
- In untrained athletes there is little increase in SV with increasing intensity exercise (70 → 80mL), during trained athletes SV at rest of 100–110mL can increase to 170–180mL during maximal exercise.
- SV is affected by exercise mode; greater SV in swimmers and lower in upper limb resistance work; and increases in SV with training are greater for whole body endurance sports, in strength/speed sports SV remains unchanged.
- *NB* in very high intensity exercise at HR_{max}, shorter filling time →↓SV.

Cardiac output

- CO (HR × SV) ~5L/min at rest →↑25L/min at end exercise.
- In elite cross-country skiers and tri-athletes CO data of greater than 40L/min have been recorded.
- CO increases linearly with increasing exercise intensity; in trained athletes up to 60% VO_{2max}, ↑CO mostly met by ↑SV, thereafter further ↑CO is met by ↑HR until a plateau phase is reached.
- Distribution of cardiac output depends on effects of smooth muscle tone in peripheral arterioles. Arteriolar radius (r) has profound effects on stroke volume resistance (SVR) to blood flow as SVR is proportional to r^4.
- In heavy exercise blood flow; rises ×20–25 in skeletal muscle, ×5 in cardiac muscle and skin; and, in non-essential tissues blood flow falls by ~×4 in abdominal viscera and kidneys.

Blood pressure

- Depends on site of measurement BP values lower limb < upper limb.
- Systolic blood pressure (SBP) ↑ with ↑ intensity exercise ~180–200mmHg.
- Very high SBP (>240mmHg) have been recorded in elite at athletes at very high work intensities with no ill effects.
- Diastolic blood pressure (DBP) little change during exercise 80 → 90mmHg, DBP represent changes in arterial wall compliance, changes from baseline of greater than 15mmHg may indicate disease.
- Mean BP (MAP) = CO × SVR ≈ DBP + *1/3 (SBP – DBP) ~ 94mmHg at rest rising to ~110–120mmHg with ↑intensity exercise.
- *Training effects:* at end exercise slight increase in SBP and MAP, but little or no increase in DBP; at rest and sub-maximal work intensities SBP may fall by ~10mmHg probably due to ↓ body mass and ↓SNS effects of training.

Cardiovascular drift

- In steady state sub-maximal exercise of >4min duration a slow upward drift is seen in HR to compensate for the effects of fluid shifts and PV loss due to sweating which reduce venous return and ↓ SV.
- If SV ↓ then to maintain or ↑ CO further, HR must ↑ and in longer duration exercise >30–45min, without fluid replacement, eventually CO and BP may gradually fall.

Blood viscosity

- Blood viscosity (η) also affects blood flow, in non-disease states viscosity is mainly related to haematocrit, ratio of red cells to plasma, increased viscosity increases the cardiac work and reduces flow.
- In response to aerobic endurance training, proportional increase in plasma volume is greater than the increase in red cell mass (athletic pseudo-anaemia), haematocrit falls, blood becomes less viscous and is subsequently easier to pump but has less oxygen carrying capacity (see Box 5.1, iii).

Box 5.1 Clinical notes

- (i) HR monitors are an essential for aerobic endurance training. Working in appropriate HR zones focuses work at intensities most likely to result in adaptation, lessens the likelihood of under or over-training, and by staying in the 'zones'; workload or running velocity automatically decreases when the athlete becomes dehydrated, overheated or fuel depleted.
- (ii) Athletes who develop atrial fibrillation lose 'atrial kick', the co-ordinated atrial systolic component of ventricular filling and pre-stretch before ventricular contraction. This leads to a marked decrease in cardiac output and although activities of daily living (ADL's) may not be affected, athletes are unable to raise CO for exercise and fatigue quickly.
- (iii) Athletes with very high haematocrit values >0.55 have a greater oxygen carrying capacity, an advantage in aerobic endurance sports but with dehydration this carries a higher risk of thrombosis. Consistently high haematocrit (>0.55) and haemaglobin levels (>16.5g/dL) in elite endurance athletes are unusual and although they may represent 'high normal' values, they should alert the sports physician to a possible blood disorder (haemachromatosis) or doping (erythropoetin (EPO)/autologous blood transfusions).

Cardiac work

- In the cardiac cycle, work is required—to raise pressure of volume of blood to that of the systemic circuit (pressure development), to eject/accelerate volume of blood into the aorta (volume flow) and to maintain tension in cardiac walls.
- Increasing SV and decreased HR with training reduces myocardial oxygen consumption and improves coronary blood flow at rest, and during sub-maximal and maximal exercise.
- Elastic recoil, wall tension, contractile properties, and cardiac dimensional indices are all important for normal function.
- Limitations of cardiac work (maximum cardiac output): electrophysiological factors (refractory period), reduced filling time at high HR, ability to fill elastic recoil/ventricular stiffness compliance, coronary blood-flow at very high HR shorter diastole reduced blood-flow.

Respiratory responses to exercise

Structure
- Airway: nose/larynx/trachea/bronchi/bronchioles/alveolar ducts.
- Gas exchange: alveoli/pulmonary capillaries.
- Ventilatory mechanism:
  - Chest wall: ribs and intercostal muscles.
  - Pleural cavity: parietal and visceral layers.
  - Respiratory muscles: diaphragm/intercostals.

Function
- 1. *Air movement*: pulmonary (V_E) and alveolar (V_A) ventilation.
- 2. *Gas exchange*: lung ↔ blood ↔ lung.
- Transport of O_2 and CO_2 (CVS).
- 3. *Gas exchange*: blood ↔ tissues ↔ blood.
- (1 and 2 = external respiration; 3 = internal respiration).

Mechanics of ventilation
- Elastic recoil of chest wall (ribs and intercostals) acting outward is counteracted by inward elastic recoil of lung tissue; produce a slight negative intrapleural pressure keeping lung surfaces apposed against inner chest wall.
- Chest wall movements cause small intrapleural/intrapulmonary pressure change (±2–3mmHg), which draw in or expel air from the lungs.
- Inspiration: scalene/external intercostals/diaphragm.
- *Expiration at rest:* passive elastic recoil of lung tissue
- *Forced expiration:* intercostals/abdominals for expulsive efforts (see Box 5.2, i).

Static and dynamic lung volume measures
Lung function test measure volume and velocity of air movement, volume of air moved per unit time, and peak rates of airflow. The ability to move air in and out of the lungs depends on 2 factors:
- Resistance to airflow in bronchi (proportional to fourth power of the radius) (Box 5.2, ii).
- Resistance of lung tissue to a change in volume (compliance).

Effects of training
There are no differences between the lungs of athletes and the normal population of similar gender, size, and stature. Athletes may wrongly think that static and dynamic lung volumes should be greater than the healthy untrained, and often equate a high forced vital capacity (FVC) with aerobic endurance capacity. Static lung volumes are genetically determined and in general do not change with training, with the exception of upper body sports like swimming, where muscular development in the chest wall is thought to increase thoracic wall dimensions. However, training does improve ventilatory endurance and endurance-trained athletes have a greater ability to sustain ventilation at sub-maximal workloads, reduced lactate production in respiratory musculature, and report less subjective feelings of breathlessness on exercise. Training makes the work of breathing more efficient.

Box 5.2 Clinical notes

- (i) *Valsalva manoeuvre:* forced expiration against a closed glottis, increases intrathoracic and intra-abdominal pressure, assisting abdominal and back muscles in stabilizing the trunk for heavy lifting. However, increase in intrapulmonary pressure can cause rapid increase in BP, accentuated baroreceptor responses, reflex fall in HR and CO, which is manifest clinically by dizziness, presyncope, and occasionally collapse.
- (ii) Objective evidence of a fall in FEV_1 (>10%) is *still* a requirement for athletes on *some* long-acting asthma medications (see updated World Anti-Doping Agency (WADA) list). Standard provocation procedures are; exercise of 8–10 min at 85% of HR max or 6 min eucapnic hyperventilation at V_E of 30 × resting FEV_1. FEV_1 is measured pre-, and at 5, 10, 15, and 30 min post-exercise or eucapnoeic voluntary hyperpnoea (EVH) challenge and responses recorded graphically.
- (iii) Endurance athletes should ensure adequate dietary sources of iron. Check iron stores annually (serum ferritin) and should not donate blood during important phases of aerobic endurance training or within 6 weeks of competitions.

Pulmonary ventilation (V_E) in exercise

Minute ventilation (V_E) is the product of RR and tidal volume (TV). With a RR of 12/min × TV of 0.5L/breath, the V_m at rest is about 6L/min. With exercise the RR increases to 60–70/min and TV can increase to 2.0–3.0 L, so that at the end of exercise V_E may reach 100L/min in untrained, 160L/min in trained, and >200L/min in highly trained athletes.

Effect of training on ventilation

Training shifts the respiratory responses to exercise by favouring depth of respiration, rather than rate, which is much more efficient in energy costs of breathing. Adjustment by alteration of the rate and depth of breathing to meet physiological demands of exercise is exquisitely well controlled. Attempts at readjustment of the rate and depth by entrained breathing are usually futile. At rest and during exercise athletes should be encouraged to breathe naturally.

Gas exchange

Gas exchange is dependent on solubility of gases (CO_2) and their partial pressure gradients. The alveoli provide a large surface area for gas exchange, lungs of volume ~4-6L, contain ~300 million thin/elastic-walled alveoli, and have a surface area ~ ½ a tennis court!

Approximately 250–300mL of blood is available for gas exchange in the pulmonary capillaries, at rest. 250mL O_2 passes from the alveoli to the capillary and 200mL CO_2 passes from the capillary to the alveoli. During exercise, gas exchange increases by ×20.

Gas exchange in the lung during exercise

Efficient gas exchange also requires effective matching of blood flow and aeration of the alveoli. In healthy lungs at rest perfusion/aeration mismatch has a negligible effect, and during exercise, opening of upper lobe capillaries and better ventilation of lower lobe alveoli ensure that effects of physiological dead space on gas exchange are minimal or non-existent in most circumstances. The normal lung therefore has more than enough capacity for gas exchange to meet the demands of exercise.

At the alveolar/capillary interface partial pressure of oxygen in the arterial blood (PaO_2) falls little below 100mmHg at maximal exercise and there is little change in partial pressure of carbon dioxide in the arterial blood ($PaCO_2$) (40mmHg). Although at maximum exercise pulmonary blood flow increases by 50%, opening of many more pulmonary capillaries ensures adequate gas exchange down diffusion gradients. Ventilation is adjusted to maintain alveolar partial pressures of O_2 and CO_2 according to metabolic requirements.

Oxygen transport

Oxygen is predominantly transported bound to the oxygen-carrying pigment haemaglobin, and a small amount is dissolved in plasma. Although O_2 solubility in plasma is very low at 0.3mL O_2 per 100mL plasma, physiologically it is very important as it determines:
- pO_2 of blood and tissue fluids.
- Partly determines regulation of breathing.
- Greatly influences O_2 binding to haemaglobin in the lungs.
- Offloading from haemaglobin in the active muscles.

Haemaglobin (Hb)

Fe-containing protein inside red blood cells (RBC; see Box 5.2, iii), increases O_2 carrying capacity of blood by ×60–70. Hb: male ~14–16g/dL; female ~13–15g/dL.

100mL blood carries ~20mL O_2 (19.7mL O_2 → Hb + 0.3mL O_2 → plasma).

Hb–O_2 binding is dependent on pO_2, alveolar pO_2 of 103mmHg Hb in blood leaving the lungs is fully saturated. When RBC/Hb reaches the tissues and lower PO_2 < 60mmHg → Hb-O_2 affinity↓ and O_2 is offloaded. In active muscle PO_2 is even lower (<40mmHg) and there is even greater O_2 offloading from Hb, see Fig. 5.1.

Myoglobin

Fe-containing protein found in mitochondria of cardiac and skeletal muscle, facilitates O_2 transfer to mitochondria, especially in early and intense exercise. Myoglobin has a greater affinity for O_2 at lower partial pressures than Hb (myoglobin 95% saturated at PO_2 40mmHg). When tissue pO_2 is less than 5mmHg, myoglobin offloads greatly. Training increases myoglobin levels in slow twitch fibres.

Arteriovenous difference (a-vO_2 diff)

At rest a-vO_2 diff ≈ 5mL, i.e. 15mL O_2 remains attached to Hb on venous side of capillary, during exercise with increased demand for O_2, tissue pO_2 falls lower, there is greater O_2 offloading from Hb, greater extraction and utilization by the active muscle such that in moderate exercise a-vO_2 diff → ↑ 10mL and at max → ↑ 20mL. Experimentally, after exhaustive exercise, blood taken from the venous side of large muscles contains no O_2 at all.

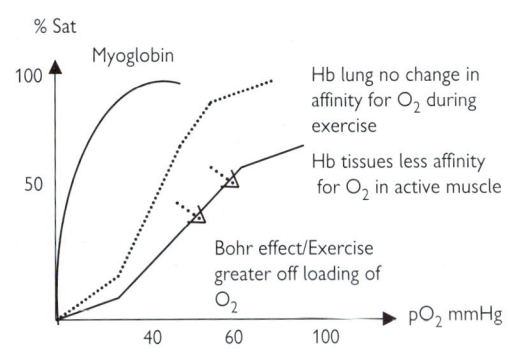

Fig. 5.1 Oxygen transport by myoglobin and haemoglobin showing oxygen diffusion at tissue level due to lower pO_2 (<40mmHg).

Hyberbaric oxygen therapy

Hyperbaric oxygen therapy (HBOT) is the breathing of O_2 at increased atmospheric pressure in order to increase plasma and tissue pO_2 (oxygen dissolved in tissue fluid or plasma). Typical HBOT interventions are; single or repeated exposures over a number of days in a hyperbaric chamber to 95 or 100% O_2 at 1.5–3 atmosphere absolute (ATA) for 30 to 120 min.

HBOT is clinically indicated in life and limb threatening conditions where benefits or increased tissue pO_2 are fairly obvious; decompression illness, carbon monoxide poisoning, severe crush injuries, nectrotizing fasciitis, burns, and to improve wound healing of devitalized or infected tissue.

However, use of HBOT in sports and exercise medicine is less clear and despite widespread use in professional and collegiate sports in the USA, HBOT as a treatment modality for acute and over-use closed soft tissue injury of muscle, ligament, and tendon; or use as an ergogenic aid pre-exercise, or as a post-exercise recovery strategy in training, remain controversial, and are not without risk of hyperbaric side effects.

Some reviews have recommended the use of HBOT within 24h to improve soft tissue injury recovery, but currently the balance of evidence from good to high quality studies, suggest that HBOT cannot be recommended for use in treatment of closed soft tissue injuries or in pre- or post-exercise training strategies.

Oxygen uptake and lactate threshold

Oxygen consumption (VO_2)
This is the product of CO and a-vO_2 diff. VO_2 and associated metabolic variables are typically assessed using on-line cardiopulmonary metabolic carts, with in-built analysers (O_2 and CO_2), which measure expired air gas concentrations on a breath-by-breath basis.

Maximal oxygen uptake (VO_2 max)
This is a quantitative measure of the ability of; the lungs to extract O_2 from inspired air, the circulatory system to transport O_2 to the tissues bound to haemoglobin (Hb), and the capacity of exercising tissues to extract and utilize O_2 in ATP regenerating processes. It is largely a genetic trait.

VO_2 max is measured during graded incremental tests to volitional exhaustion (GXT), and expressed in mL/kg/min or L/min at standard temperature and pressure for a dry gas (STPD). Maximum velocity or load attained during GXT is strongly related to an athlete's lactate profile and, along with HR and metabolic profiles, is used to design individualized training programmes and monitor performance across training cycles.

- Population VO_2 max ranges from 20–90mL/kg/min, with highest data recorded in endurance trained athletic populations.
- VO_2 max decreases with age and physical inactivity, and is generally higher in male vs. female volunteers.
- Training can improve VO_2 max by between 5–25%, capacity for improvement is dependent on initial fitness level, training frequency, intensity and duration, and genetic factors.
- VO_2 max does not necessarily confer competition success, in elite athletes with similar performance times, VO_2 max can vary significantly.
- Performance differences are due to; better pacing strategies, better economy of effort or efficiency of O_2 utilization expressed relative to velocity (mL/kg/m) for runners or load (mL/kg/W) for cyclists, rowers, and kayakers, both sub-maximally and at maximum exercise.

Aerobic-anaerobic threshold (TLac)
BLa accumulation during GXT is frequently used to define training intensities, evaluate effectiveness of training programmes and predict performance outcomes by identification of deflection points or TLac on BLa vs. load/velocity profiles.

BLa mirrors muscle lactate and indicates equilibrium between rate of production and utilization. Numerous definitions and models are used to assess lactate accumulation, including fixed lactate concentrations (2 and 4mmol/L), fixed increases above resting data, maximal lactate steady state models, exponential and logarithmic models, graphical, tangential, and maximum displacement (D_{max}) models.

TLac is highly related to endurance performance, and is a better marker of endurance capacity than VO_2 max. TLac data provide useful guidelines for exercise prescription and with appropriate training; velocity/load at TLac can increase significantly despite little or no change in VO_2 max.

Most of these models identify the same transition points: the workload or velocity where there is a sustained increase in BLa above resting data (generally at BLa > 2mmol/L). This part of the BLa response curve to exercise and reflects a shift from primarily oxidative to combined oxidative and glycolytic metabolism (BLa 2.5–5.5mmol/L).

BLa concentrations are affected by training, recovery, and nutritional status and therefore individualized thresholds are deemed more appropriate. Fig. 5.2 shows a graphical approach to interpolation of TLac during endurance performance in a standard laboratory-based GXT.

Respiratory-derived anaerobic threshold

Minute ventilation (V_E) increases disproportionately during exercise due to buffering of H^+ ions (produced by dissociation of lactic acid) by bicarbonate, leading to excess VCO_2. This produces a non-linear increase in V_E relative to VO_2.

Ventilatory thresholds are easier to detect using short rapid incremental protocols (40W/.min), when V_E is plotted as a function of VO_2, the initial non-linear increase (at ~50%VO_2 max) in V_E represents the aerobic threshold, and a second non-linear increase (at ~85% VO_2 max) in V_E represents the anaerobic threshold.

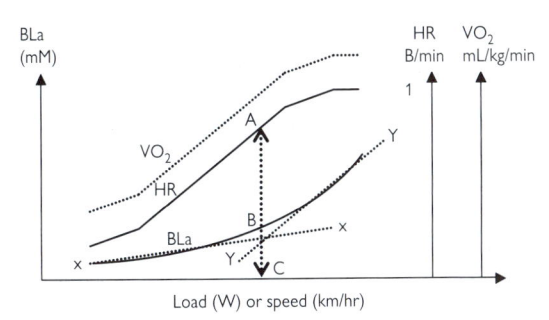

Fig. 5.2 Extrapolation of HR and load or speed at TLac from an incremental test data plot for an endurance athlete. Intersecting lines XX and YY are drawn through 2 points on the lactate curve below and above lactate threshold, respectively. The point of intersection are then used to derive HR at TLac (A), usually 80–90% of HR max; BLa at TLac (B), usually 2–2.5mmol./L; and load or velocity at TLac (C).

Measuring exercise capacity

Laboratory-based assessment

The purposes of laboratory-based physiological testing include:
- Opportunities for pre-season health check.
- Identification of strengths and weaknesses.
- Design of individualized training programmes.
- Evaluation of effectiveness of the training programme.
- Athlete education (nutrition, hydration, self-monitoring, and assessment).

Sport-specific testing
- The type of ergometer used and variables tested must be relevant to athlete's sport.
- Test protocols used must be highly sport-specific and relevant to the phase of the athlete's season.
- The variables tested must be sufficiently sensitive (precision) to infer training-induced adaptations, and data collection methods must be valid, reproducible and reliable.
- Assessments should be repeated at regular intervals (3–4 months) under identical test conditions, and where possible sub-maximal and maximal field-based self-assessments should be performed at monthly intervals.

Pre-test nutrition, hydration, rest, and exercise performed in previous 24h should be strictly controlled and the test administration itself should only be carried out by experienced and qualified personnel.

Test equipment must be regularly calibrated with daily quality control logs maintained to account for equipment variation over time.

Athlete's rights should be respected; all test data must be treated confidentially, with hard copies and electronic test data storage in line with standard medico-legal recommendations. All test results should be presented and interpreted to the athlete and their coach (if possible) immediately on completion of testing.

Laboratory testing may include the following assessments
- Anthropometric measurement of height, body mass, body composition, % body fat (skin-fold (SF) thickness technique), and estimation of lean body mass (kg) and body mass index (BMI, kg/m^2).
- Pulmonary function tests to rule-out pre-exercise respiratory limitation and post-exercise induced broncho-constriction.
- Haematology screen to rule-out sub-clinical infection, anaemia, and dehydration prior to exercise.

Measured variables assessed depend on the athlete's sport and phase of training and competition and may include
- Aerobic assessment to test endurance capacity using either a graded incremental test or a time to exhaustion test at fixed % of VO$_2$ max or maximum exercise capacity.
- Anaerobic tests to assess anaerobic power and capacity.
- Strength tests to assess gains induced by resistance training regimens and/or to assess for correction of muscle imbalance.

Anthropometric measurement

Stature
(Height in m) There are three general techniques—freestanding, stretch (removes minor effects of daily gravitational compression), and recumbent (used in infants and adults unable to stand). *NB* stature in any individual can vary by up to 10mm over the course of the day as fluid is extruded from the intervertebral discs. A wall-mounted stadiometer (measurement range 600–2100mm) used for freestanding and stretch methods—the individual stands feet together with heels, buttocks, and upper back touching the scale, head in the Frankfort plane (orbitale in a horizontal plane with the tragion). In the stretch technique the individual inhales maximally while maintaining their head in the Frankfort plane.

Body mass
Measured with a calibrated beam balance (accuracy <0.1kg), assess mass in minimal clothing. Body mass typically exhibits diurnal variation, normally assessed after fasting overnight and after voiding.

Body mass index
(Units kg/m^2), normal range 20–25kg/m^2, assessed from height and body mass by formula: BMI (kg/m^2) = mass (kg)/height^2 (m^2). Surface area, assessed from height and body mass using a nomogram or by formula: surface area (m^2) = 0.0072 × (mass (kg) × 0.425) × (height (cm) × 0.725). Lean body mass calculated from body mass and estimated fat mass.

$$\text{Lean body mass (kg)} = [\text{mass} - ((\text{mass} \times \%\text{fat})/100)]$$

Waist to hip ratio
Waist measurement recorded at the level of the umbilicus, hip measurement at the level of the greater trochanter. Ratio is an important predictor of future cardiovascular disease (female 0.7, male 0.8).

Body fat
Skin-fold thickness assessed using caliper or ultrasound are commonly used by most exercise physiologists to estimate percentage body fat, bioelectrical impedance testing is prone to measurement error, underwater weighing remains and whole body dual energy X-ray absorptiometry (DEXA) scanning are the gold standard.

Flexibility
The ability to move a joint through the complete range of motion, maintaining a joint's flexibility facilitates movement. Flexibility assessments routinely undertaken in an exercise laboratory include the active knee extension test at 90° of hip flexion to assess hamstring length and range of active knee extension, and the sit and reach (SAR) test of low back and hamstring flexibility, a non-specific test of overall flexibility. Active knee extension in the supple athlete should be at least 80°, and SAR should be beyond the toe line (>15cm).

Pulmonary function tests
Asthma is one of the commonest medical conditions producing exercise and performance limitation in athletes. Pre- and post-exercise lung function tests should be a routine part of physiological assessment, to detect

undiagnosed respiratory limitation prior to exercise testing and/or monitor control in athletes already on inhaler medications for asthma. All subjects with clinical evidence of asthma or exercise-induced bronchoconstriction (EIB), with FEV_1 values of 85–90% of predicted or less pre-exercise, or those who show a 10% fall in FEV_1 from baseline post-exercise, should be further evaluated and assessed.

An exercise challenge of 6–8min running outdoors in early morning cold air at 85% of HR max; or EVH, 6min hyperventilation through a mask system inspiring a gas mixture containing 5% CO_2 enriched air to prevent hypocapnia, at V_E of 30 times FEV_1, as provocation. Lung function tests are assessed pre-exercise and at 3, 5, 10, 15, and 30min post-exercise. Print outs of data from these tests are now required as objective evidence of EIB supporting applications (a therapeutic use exemption (TUE)) for permission to use inhaler medications as part of anti-doping regulations.

Routine blood tests

Mild infections, reduced oxygen carrying capacity (↓Hb), and reduced plasma volume due to dehydration will raise resting and sub-maximal HR, and influence exercise test results. Iron deficiency, usually due to vegetarianism and menstrual loss, is fairly common in female endurance athletes. A reduction of as little as 0.5–1.0g in Hb, even if still within the normal range, can produce significant performance decrements in elite athletes.

Measurement of aerobic capacity

The standard laboratory-based aerobic assessment is a graded incremental test to volitional exhaustion. The following variables are routinely assessed; heart rate, O_2 consumption, CO_2 production, BLa concentration, and associated respiratory variables. The normal protocol outline for graded maximal incremental test to volitional exhaustion is as follows:
- All tests preceded by 10min low intensity warm-up and self-stretching and concluded by 5–10min low intensity warm-down.
- Following a short period of data recording at rest, the test is started at a low sub-maximal velocity/load.
- Increment duration from 1–3min, usually 3min if steady state responses are desired, with average data collected over the final 60–90s of each increment. Fixed increments (W or km/h) for different genders, grades, and sporting disciplines vary accordingly.
- Increased loading or velocity (W or km/h) should result in VO_2 increases of ~2–3 MET or ~5–10 mL/kg/min with each increment.
- Total test time should be between 15–25min to control for cardiovascular drift, elevation in core temperature and self-motivation.

Measurement of anaerobic power and capacity

Peak power is the highest power output averaged over short periods of 1–3s, whereas anaerobic capacity is defined as the work performed during a short high-intensity sprint test. The main objectives are to accurately measure the rate and quantity of work under circumstances of minimal aerobic contribution.

MEASURING EXERCISE CAPACITY

Vertical jump test
- A measure of 'explosiveness' in physical fitness tests often used as an index of anaerobic capacity.
- Vertical jump height is the difference between standing height and jump height assessed using a vertical jump meter.
- Three jumps are used either from a crouched and held start or with a rapid counter-movement action from a knee angle of ~90° to assess the contribution of the stretch-shortening cycle.
- Power (W) = 21.67 × body mass (kg) × $v^{0.5}$, where v is jump height (m).
- Following suitable rest periods the test can be repeated with additional loading equivalent to 10, 15 and 20% body mass.

Wingate test
- A supra-maximal 30s cycle ergometer test performed with braking load proportionate to body mass (female 7.5%, male 8.5%).
- Assessment is made of maximum power, mean power, and power decline (fatigue index).
- Mean power data is calculated from pedal cadence and applied resistance over successive 1s intervals, because of the transient nature of the peak data (longer intervals reduce magnitude of measured data).
- Data for peak and mean power are corrected for body mass (W/kg) to account for gender, training status and muscle mass.
- Typical values for peak power range from 9–16W/kg.
- Power decline is calculated by expressing the difference between peak and minimum power relative to peak power, in percentage format.
- Power decline ranges between 35 and 50%.
- A major limitation is that there is a considerable aerobic contribution (25–30%) to the total work performed.

Margaria stair climbing test
This test purports to assess anaerobic capacity and the protocol involves:
- Sprint up a staircase (~1.8m) as quickly as possible, 2 steps at a time. Contact mats fitted at fixed steps on the stair to measure time taken.
- Power (W) = [9.81 × body mass (kg) × vertical displacement (m)]/time(s).
- Anaerobic capacity ranges from 700W (12W/kg) in poorly-trained females to >1500W (>18W/kg) in male sprint athletes.

Dal Monte sprint test
- This test is designed to assess speed endurance.
- Maximal repeated sprints are performed every 60s over a distance of 50m for male players, and 40m for goalkeepers and female players.
- Sprint distance must be completed in <7s.
- Decline in sprint time computed to assess speed endurance, minimal decline infers excellent speed endurance.

Continuous jump test
Similar in design to the Wingate test, this can be used to assess ballistic power and power decline, it involves:
- 10s of maximal counter-movement jumping (knee angle nominally 90°) on a specialized contact jump mat capable of assessing flight time.
- Body mass and flight time are subsequently used to compute maximum power and power decline in a similar manner to the Wingate test.

10 × 5m speed/agility test
- A sprinting and turning test performed at maximum velocity on a non-slip surface.
- Participant completes 10 shuttles of a 5m distance with both feet crossing end lines at each turn.
- Test stopped when participant crosses end line in the final shuttle.
- Performance time is recorded to 0.01s using either a stopwatch or, if possible, an infra-red beam timing apparatus.

Maximum accumulated oxygen deficit
- An assessment of anaerobic capacity based on extrapolation of the linear relationship between sub-maximal power and O_2 consumption.
- Once sub-maximal relationship has been quantified using loads equivalent to 40–85% VO_2 max, estimated O_2 consumption equivalents at intensities above VO_2 max are calculated.
- *Typical data:* endurance athletes 2.5–5.0L and sprinters 4.5–7.5L.

Other tests frequently used include sprints through infra-red timing gates over varying distances 10, 30, 50, 100 and 200m, rugby sprint shuttle test, and number of repetitions of exercises completed in fixed time (squat thrusts and push-ups).

Measurement of strength
Strength and power are sport-specific measures. Strength is the maximum force (N) or moment (Nm), whereas power is defined as the rate of work (force by velocity). Strength and power are applied in sport specific movements and postures, and at particular movement velocities.

The following should be considered when assessing strength:
- Reliability of the measurement protocol.
- Degree of correlation between test score and performance indices.
- Sensitivity of the measurement protocol to detect training adaptation.
- Prior effect of acute bouts of exercise.

Strength can be assessed either dynamically (isokinetic or isotonic/iso-inertial protocols) or statically (isometric) using open-or closed-chain models; each assessment type has particular advantages and limitations.

Isometric strength measurement
Static assessment of maximum voluntary capacity (MVC) uses strain gauges, load-cells or tensiometers at fixed joint angles. Isometric tests can also be used to assess endurance capacity, the time a fixed % of MVC can be maintained for, and the rate of force development (dF/dt) usually over range of 10–70% of MVC.

Advantages
- Isometric tests are easily standardized and inexpensive.
- Preferred when joint range of motion limited by bracing or pathology.

Disadvantage
Poor relationship to dynamic performance indices.

Isotonic (iso-inertial) strength measurement (gym-based testing)
Isotonic/iso-inertial and isokinetic assessment is across the full range of joint motion. Force-generating capacity is measured during both concentric and eccentric actions. Iso-inertial assessment reflects effort during a

weight-lifting task, and implies constant resistance to motion, rather than a constant resistance or load throughout the action. Normally assessed using free-weights or an elliptical cam-loaded variable resistance apparatus, the load applied to a muscle is only maximal at extremes of range, with forces decreasing to 40–50% of maximal capacity in mid-range. The maximum eccentric load applied is also limited by maximum concentric load.

Advantages
- Positive reinforcement from progressive increases in strength.
- Varying exercises can be included to test multiple joints simultaneously.
- Exercises are easily performed in weight bearing closed-kinetic chains.

Disadvantages
- Unable to quantify moment/torque, work or power.
- Strong muscles may compensate for weak muscle groups during closed-kinetic chain actions.

Isokinetic strength measurement

Using an isokinetic dynamometer, the velocity of joint movement can be controlled by an external motor enabling an accommodating resistance (Newton's 3rd law). This ensures that a maximum force can be applied at all angles both concentrically and eccentrically within the assessed range of movement. Assessment is made of force vs. angle profiles at different joint velocities in concentric and eccentric modes, and can also be made of bilateral instability (limb to limb differences) and functional reciprocal muscle group ratios (ratio of eccentric antagonist to concentric agonist).

Advantages
- Isolation of weak muscle groups.
- Quantification of movement/torque, work, and power.
- Accommodating resistance concept in addition to providing maximal resistance also ensures a functionally safe loading mechanism.

Disadvantages
- Assessment limited to isolated muscle groups acting through cardinal planes in non-weight bearing open-kinetic chains.
- Equipment costs are prohibitive and these assessments are mainly in a hospital-based rehabilitation setting and in academic institutions for research purposes.
- Minor reliability issues associated with subject re-positioning and stabilization in longitudinal rehabilitation and training studies.

Simple field-based tests of exercise capacity

Indirect protocols employing both maximal and sub-maximal effort can be used to predict VO_2 max. These basic predictive tests use steady state heart rate at sub-maximal workloads (exercise HR <85% HR_{max}) to estimate VO_2 max using multiple regression equations. HR_{max} may vary depending on body composition and in obese subjects HR_{max} is better predicted by the formula:

$$HR_{max} = 200 - (0.5 \times age).$$

Indirect sub-maximal tests to estimate aerobic capacity

Single stage walk test
- Walk for 4min at comfortable velocity on a motorized treadmill (nominal velocity 4.8–6.4km/h). Target HR of 100–120beats/min.
- Increase treadmill slope to 5% and continue walking for another 4min, but ensure that HR remains below 85% of age predicted HR_{max}.
- Record steady state HR at 30s intervals in final 2min (steady state HR implies a change of <5beats/min/min).
- Use the following multiple regression equation to predict VO_2 max:
  VO_2 max (mL/kg/min) = 15.1 + [13.6 × velocity (km/h)] − [0.327 × HR] − [0.164 × velocity × age] + [0.00504 × HR × age] + [5.98 × gender] (gender factor 0 = F, 1 = M).

Single stage jog test
- Walk for 4min at a comfortable velocity on a motorized treadmill (nominally 4.8–6.4km/h). Target walking HR of 100–120beats/min.
- Increase velocity to comfortable jogging pace (range 7–12km/h) depending on fitness.
- Ensure HR remains below 85% of age-predicted HR_{max}.
- Continue jogging for 4min, record HR at 30s intervals over final 2min while jogging.
- Use the following multiple regression equation to predict VO_2 max:

  VO_2 max (mL/kg/min) = 54.07 − [0.1938 × mass (kg)] + [2.79 × velocity (km/h)] − [0.1453 × HR] + [7.062 × gender] (gender factor 0 = F, 1 = M).

Sub-maximal two-stage jog test
This predictive test uses the relationship between sub-maximal VO_2 and HR to predict VO_2 max.
- Subject completes 2 stages each of 3min duration at fixed velocities depending on fitness (8.0, 9.6, 11.2, 12.0, 12.8, 14.4 or 16.0 km/h).
- Record HR over final 2min of each stage and convert treadmill velocity to equivalent oxygen cost (see Table 5.1).
- Use equation and age predicted HR_{max} to predict VO_2 max thus:

  VO_2 max (mL/kg/min) = SM_2 + [b × (HR_{max} − HR_2)].

  where b= $(SM_2 − SM_1)/(HR_2 − HR_1)$.
- SM_1 and SM2 = equivalent O_2 cost of 1st and 2nd stages, respectively.
- HRmax = age-predicted max HR, and HR1 and HR2 = heart rate during 1st and 2nd stages, respectively.
- NB Test is suitable for semi-sedentary and active populations only.

Sub-maximal cycle ergometer test (PWC170)
This predictive test uses the linear increase in HR with load during sub-maximal exercise.
- Exercise load at HR = 170beats/min is the estimated variable [original population were age ~20yr (85% of 220 − 20 = 170)].
- Adjust seat height and handlebar position on a stationary cycle ergometer to suit volunteer.
- Pedal at a constant cadence (60rev/min) at 3 sub-maximal loads (*NB* load (W) = cadence × braking mass).

Table 5.1 Table for calculation of equivalent O_2 cost of 1st (SM_1) and 2nd (SM_2) stages

Treadmill velocity (km/h)	Equivalent O_2 cost (mL/kg/min)
8.0	30.1
9.6	35.7
11.2	40.9
12.0	43.7
12.8	46.5
14.4	51.8
16.0	57.1

- Steady state HR is measured over last minute of each exercise element.
- Initial load (W/kg) is dependent on gender and fitness (see Table 5.2). Multiply body mass by relevant factor according to age and fitness level.

  PWC170 (W/kg) = $[\{((W_3 - W_2)/(HR_3 - HR_2))*((170 - HR_3))\} + W_3]/BM$,

  where HR_2 and HR_3 are the steady state heart rate data at loads 2 and 3; W_2 and W_3 are workloads in Watt at loads 2 and 3, respectively; and BM is body mass in kg.
- PWC 170 example: if HR at load 2 (96W) was 142beats/min and load 3 (136W) was 163beats/min and BM = 65 kg ⇒ PWC170 = $[\{((136 - 96)/(163 - 142))*(170 - 163)\} + 136]/65 = 2.29$W/kg.
- NB Test is suitable for sedentary and semi-sedentary populations.

Indirect maximal tests for estimation of aerobic capacity

The following are all maximal tests for indirect estimation of aerobic capacity. *NB* All maximal tests should only be undertaken after medical clearance.

Table 5.2 Table of gender and fitness factors for the PWC 170

	Obese/unfit	Normal	Fit
Male <18	0.75	1.00	1.25
Male >18	1.00	1.25	1.50
Female <18	0.50	0.75	1.00
Female >18	0.75	1.00	1.25

Maximal cycle ergometer test

This is an incremental cycling test to exhaustion. In non-cyclists, results for VO_2 max on the cycle ergometer are generally lower than for treadmill tests, due to the involvement of a smaller muscle mass.
- Load (W) = cadence (rev/min) × braking mass (kg); at 60rev/min with a frictional braking mass of 2kg the applied load is 120W.
- Adjust seat height and handlebar position to suit volunteer.
- Cycle at pedal cadence at 60rev/min throughout test.
- Start at a low workload 60W for 2min, with load increases of 30W every 2min until pedal cadence can no longer be maintained or volitional exhaustion.
- Load is then reduced to 60–90W for 5–10 min as cool down.
- ACSM cycle ergometer equation is then used to predict VO_2 max.
- VO_2 max = {12 × load (W) + 3.5 × body mass (kg)}/body mass (kg).
- If max load achieved was 300W and body mass was 80 kg ⇒:
- VO_2 max = {(300 × 12) + (3.5 × 80)}/80 = 48.5mL/kg/min.
- *NB* Test only suitable for active volunteers who are efficient cycling.

Leger and Lambert 20m shuttle test (20 metre shuttle test (MST)

This is an incremental running test to volitional exhaustion. The test tends to underestimate VO_2 max in individuals inefficient at rapid turning actions, more applicable to games players rather than distance runners.
- Athlete completes run between 2 lines placed exactly 20m apart in time to an audible signal.
- Running velocity initially slow (8.5km/h) and becomes progressively faster by 0.5km/h/min.
- As the velocity increases each minute, the test enters a new level.
- The test stops when the athlete can no longer maintain synchronization of their turning action at the ends of the runway with the audible signal.
- Number of completed levels and shuttles in the final level achieved is recorded as test score.
- Recorded score can be used as a basic measure of fitness or alternatively predictive tables can estimate VO_2 max in mL/kg/min.

Cooper 12 minute run test

This is a maximal 12 min running test performed on an all-weather track with marker cones placed at 10- or 20-m intervals:
- Distance completed in km (d) is recorded; number of completed laps plus number of completed 10m or 20m intervals in final lap.
- VO_2 max and velocity at lactate threshold are then estimated from the following equations.
- VO_2 max (mL/kg/min) = 22.4 * d − 11.4.
- Velocity at TLac (km/h) = 10.1 − 2.09* d + 1.03 *d^2.

All predictive tests, both sub-maximal and maximal, for assessing VO_2 max have some degree of predictive error associated with them, usually about ±5–10%. These predictive errors are due to differences between population under investigation and original study population used to derive the empirical formula using simple and multiple correlation analysis.

Soccer specific tests

Predictive tests reflective of the actions and intensity changes commonly associated with soccer have also been developed and validated; these tests include the Yo-Yo and Loughborough intermittent shuttle tests and soccer-specific Hoff test (performed with a football around a designated obstacle course).

Basic principles of training

Training is the use of progressive overload to stress the major energy systems used in an activity. Training usually results in adaptation of the energy system and improvement in performance (Table 5.3).

Overload
Greater than normal load with appropriate rest leads to adaptation. Exercise intensity should be near maximal and increased as fitness increases.

Progression
Frequency, intensity, time (duration), and type of training are manipulated to create a progression in load. Build up duration or volume of training, and with a basic foundation, reduce volume, but increase intensity and velocity.

Specificity
The metabolic and neuromuscular demands of exercise are usually specific to the sport or activity training must reflect sport specificity; train rowers in boats not on exercise bikes.

Individuality
Training load should be prescribed according to age, gender, level of skills, experience, and conditioning, and then adjusted according to individual response. Elite level training programmes should not be imposed on juniors, beginners, or intermediate level athletes.

Rest
Regeneration and adaptation occurs when resting. Rest should be an actively programmed part of training.

Periodization
Plan the season and build the necessary skills, strength, and endurance (distance) or speed systematically in a series of well-planned phases.

Table 5.3 Running distance, time and percentage contributions of energy systems

Event	Time	ATP/CP	Anaerobic	Aerobic
42km	135–180min	–	5	95
10km	28–50min	5	15	80
5km	14–25min	10	20	70
3km	8.5–16min	20	40	40
1.5km	3.6–6min	2	50	30
800m	2–3min	0	55–60	10–15
400m	45–90s	80	15	5
200m	20–35s	>90	<10	–
100m	10–15s	>95	<5	–

CP, creatine phosphate.

Aerobic endurance training

Training aims to maximize base aerobic capacity and develop the ability to maintain high aerobic power outputs without fatigue. Velocity or load at threshold and endurance capacity (how long threshold pace can be maintained) can still be improved even after VO_2 max has reached a plateau, and is the most important factor determining success in elite endurance sport. Aerobic capacity is built by long duration low intensity activity, interspersed with training at an intensity just below lactate threshold (TLac), for progressively longer and longer durations.

Aerobic training intensity, duration and frequency

Training intensity is usually prescribed in 2 or 3 aerobic HR zones, based on BLa vs. HR profiles from GXT (see Fig. 5.3) or empirically at fixed percentages of maximum heart rate or heart rate reserve [heart rate reserve (HRR) = HR_{max} − HR rest]. In endurance athletes heart rate at TLac ranges from 80 to 90% of HR_{max}, but prediction of individual zones based on heart rate formulae are prone to error (±10–15beats/min).

TLac for most endurance athletes occurs at BLa of 2–3mmol/L, but measuring BLa during training is impractical (see Box 5.3, i), and so HR training ranges equivalent to set BLa concentrations are interpolated from GXT data.

Aerobic base training (A1/A2)
- A1 pace usually HR of 120–140beats/min and BLa ≤ 1mmol/L. Train at this intensity for warm up/cool down routines, active recovery and fat burning, or when practicing technical skills.
- A2 pace usually HR of 145-155beats/min, BLa still below TLac (1–1.5mmol/L) and still predominantly aerobic and fat burning. Training for base aerobic training combines A1/A2 intensities: 10min warm up A1, 30min steady A2, 10min A1 cool down.

Lactate threshold training (A3)
- A3 pace is set just below TLac; HR ~160–180beats/min and BLa between 2–3mmol/L. Training at this pace burns a mixture of fat and carbohydrate fuels, the aerobic system is near its maximum limit.
- A small amount of lactate will accumulate at this pace, and therefore lactate transport mechanisms are also stimulated.

Recommended frequency
- Base aerobic/active recovery (A1/A2) 2–3 sessions per week.
- Aerobic endurance (A3) 2–3 sessions per week/non-successive days.
- Aim for one high quality training session per day, if just starting off; rising to 2 sessions on alternate days for the typical elite athlete.
- *NB* More than 1 session per day does not necessarily lead to greater performance gains if of poor quality, if already fatigued, inadequate fuel or fluid replenishment from previous session.
- Incorporate additional early morning easy A1/A2 (45–60min) to increase weekly mileage if needed.

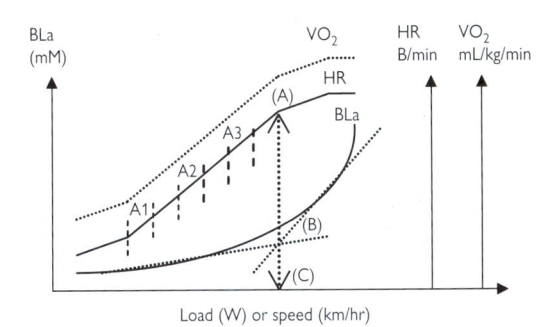

Fig. 5.3 Interpolation of aerobic training heart rate zones A1 to A3. (A) Heart rate at TLac, (B) BLa at TLac, (C) load or velocity at TLac. Aerobic training zones A1, A2, and A3.

Box 5.3 Clinical notes

- (i) It is now possible to profile lactate response during training using new hand-held BLa measurement devices. These offer a further useful tool alongside HR monitors for coaches/trainers to monitor exercise intensity in athletes during training. Although an advance when taken out of the controlled environment of the exercise laboratory there are obvious hazards such as infection and bruising at sample sites, blood contamination from incorrect disposal of lancets/sharps and test strips, incorrect sampling methods leading to erroneous data collection. Training to ensure safe use is essential.
- (ii) Endurance athletes training more than 12–14 sessions/14–16h/week represent a super elite group of usually international/Olympic standard performance and are part of highly regulated closely monitored programmes of work and recovery. Without these support structures this level of training should not be undertaken.

Training duration
- Aerobic base (A1/A2) is built gradually over 3–5 months initially 20–30min per session up to 60–90+min for elite endurance athletes.
- Lactate threshold (A3) initially 2 sets of 10min progressing to 2 × 12½, 2 × 15, 2 × 20, and 3 × 15 over a timeline of 3–5 months.
- Elite endurance athletes would be aiming for 3 × 20 min or 2 by 25min A3 pace by the end of main aerobic winter preparation phase.
- Overall weekly duration for all aerobic training elements should not usually exceed 12–14h/week for most athletes (see Box 5.3, ii).
- *NB* excessive endurance training above an optimum 8–12 sessions per week is usually non-productive and will result in over-use injury, athletic staleness, and burnout.

Long-term adaptive responses to aerobic training include;
- Improved O_2 efficiency (↓ O_2 consumption at fixed velocities/loads).
- Improved HR efficiency (↓ HR at fixed velocities/loads).
- Increased load/velocity at TLac.
- Decreased BLa data at sub-maximal exercise intensities.
- Increase in maximum load/velocity attained at VO_2 max.

Periodization for aerobic endurance athletes

Rest phase (normally 3–4 week)

Training is generally non-specific to keep generally active and maintain body mass near competition mass. Athletes may participate in alternative sporting activities for relaxation.

Preparation phase

Training programme with emphasis on increasing strength and muscular endurance in those muscles most directly involved in sporting activity. Low intensity long distance sessions, 2–3 times per week will help improve the aerobic base, and shorter sessions should target TLac—initially 2 per week. This phase usually takes place over winter months and can be broken up into 2 phase's Winter 1: Oct/Nov/Dec might emphasize base aerobic conditioning and slowly build duration at TLac, Winter 2: Jan/Feb/Mar would emphasize work and increase ability to work for longer durations at TLac.

Transition phase (4–6 week prior to competition)

Usually late April/May, athlete now prepares for specifics of competition, coaches may introduce speed-work, interval sessions and pacing work at actual race velocity, and overall a slightly higher intensity programme specific to the athlete's sport and predominant energy system.

This is a difficult phase to control as longer duration efforts must be reduced as intensity increases. It also involves early season racing, time trials, and selection races, and therefore the athlete needs to be monitored carefully to avoid fatigue.

In-season training

For the majority of athletes who compete regularly competition itself should maintain the increases in energy systems attained in pre- and off-season, provided they do not over-compete.

However, the training programme should still contain long slow distance (LSD) sessions, 1–2 per week plus sports–specific training sets directed towards upcoming-targeted races. The optimum in competition training cycles would comprise of a week of normal training week 1, including simulated competition at less than race pace followed by a tapering week (↓ duration/↑ intensity) and then a real competition and rest days at the end of week 2. Repeated 2 week cycles through the competitive season will avoid the athlete over competing and early season burn out.

Resistance training

Resistance training improves athletic performance by increasing muscular strength, power, and velocity. Training may induce hypertrophy, increase local muscular endurance, improve motor performance, and also improve balance and co-ordination.

Resistance training and competition
- *Power lifting*: muscle strength in squat, bench press, and dead lift.
- *Weightlifting*: muscle strength and power in clean and jerk, and snatch type lifts.
- *Bodybuilding*: building optimal muscle hypertrophy for definition and symmetry, while reducing percentage body fat to improve appearance.
- *Strongman*: improve muscle strength, power and endurance.
- *Athletics*: strength training to improve athletic performance.

Components of a resistance training programme

Programmes usually include dynamic concentric (CON) and eccentric (ECC) actions, isometric actions play a secondary role. Dynamic strength improvements are greatest when ECC actions are included.

When compared to CON actions, ECC actions produce:
- Greater force per unit of muscle size.
- Involve less motor unit activation for a fixed force.
- Require less energy for a fixed force.
- Are critical for optimal hypertrophy.
- Result in greater delayed onset muscle soreness (DOMS).
- Greater potential for injury if exercises are performed incorrectly.

Types of exercise in resistance training

Free-weights and machine exercises are used in single or multiple joint exercises. Single joint exercises stress one joint or muscle group (leg extension/leg curl) and are thought to pose a lower injury risk as less skill is involved. Multiple-joint exercises stress more than one joint and muscle group (bench press, squat, power cleans) involving complex neural activation and coordination due to the involvement of a larger muscle mass, and are the most effective resistance exercise type for increasing strength and power. Snatch and power clean exercises are the most effective for increasing muscle power because they require fast force production to successfully complete each repetition.

Metabolic and hormonal responses

Exercise stress of multiple large muscle groups will show the greatest acute metabolic responses. Dead lifts, squat jumps and Olympic lifts produce greater testosterone and HGH responses compared with simple bench press and seated shoulder press. Metabolic demand and anabolic hormonal response have direct implications for improvements in local muscle endurance, lean body mass, and reducing percentage body fat. Sequencing of exercises and number of muscle groups trained effects acute expression of muscle strength.

Basic resistance training workouts

Total body workout (>3 sessions.wk^{-1})
- Stress all major muscle groups.
- Normally 1–2 exercises per group.
- Commonly used for general fitness by athletes and Olympic weightlifters.

Upper/lower body routines (2–3sessions/week)
- Exercises are split into upper body during one session and lower body during the next session.
- Used by athletes for general fitness, in power lifting, and body building.
- Large muscle groups before small, multiple joint before single joint, rotate opposing agonist/antagonist exercises.

Muscle group split routines (1–2sessions/week)
- Exercises are targeted at specific muscle groups during the same workout; for example, chest/triceps workout—all exercises for chest performed and subsequently all exercises for triceps are performed.
- Workouts common among body builders or individuals striving to maximize muscle hypertrophy.
- 3–4 exercises performed compared with 1 or 2 during a total body regimen.
- Multiple joint before single joint, perform higher intensity (higher percentage of 1RM) before lower intensity exercises.

Exercise sequence
Train large muscle groups before small, multiple joint before single joint, for power training exercise order (most to least complex) before basic exercises, such as squat or bench press, rotate upper and lower body exercises, or opposing agonist/antagonist exercises.

Loading
Loading describes the amount of weight lifted and is highly dependent on: exercise order, volume, frequency, muscle action, repetition speed, and rest interval. Optimal strength, hypertrophy, and local muscle endurance training requires the systematic usage of various loading strategies.

Load prescription depends on training status and goals:
- Power training at >85% of 1RM stresses the ATP-PC system.
- Hypertrophy training at 70–80% of 1RM stresses the adenosine triphosphate-phosphocreatine (ATP-PC) and glycolytic systems, with minor contribution from aerobic metabolism.
- Local endurance training <70% of 1RM involves a high aerobic component. Loads <70% of 1RM rarely increase maximal strength, but are effective for increasing local muscle endurance.
- Training continuously at one intensity, high risk of training plateaus, or over-training.
- 80% of IRM corresponded to 10RM for bench press, leg extension, and lat pull-down (latissimus dorsi); 6RM for leg curl; 7–8RM for arm curl; and 15RM for leg press.

Rest interval
- Rest interval length is dependent on training intensity, goals, fitness, and targeted energy system utilization.
- The amount of rest between sets significantly affects: metabolic, hormonal, and cardiovascular responses to an acute bout of exercise, as well as performance of subsequent sets and training adaptations.
- Rest interval influences relative contribution from the energy systems.
- When training for absolute strength and power rest periods of 3–5min are recommended.
- Rest interval appears to be a potent stimulator for anabolic hormones and local blood flow, and results in significant lactate production.
- Training to increase local muscle endurance requires the athlete to perform high reps, have a long duration workout and minimize recovery between sets. Minimizing recovery between sets is an important stimulus for improving local muscle endurance (increased mitochondrial and capillary number, increased buffer capacity and fibre type transitions).
- Rest intervals vary for each exercise within a training session; consider fatigue associated with previous exercises when performing exercises later in a workout.

Velocity
The velocity that dynamic repetitions are performed at affects responses to resistance training. Moderate velocity training produces the greatest strength increases across all test velocities. Training for local muscle endurance, and in some aspects hypertrophy, may require a spectrum of velocities with various loading strategies.

Frequency/recovery
The number of training sets and number of times certain exercises or muscle groups are trained per week affects subsequent resistance training adaptations. Frequency is dependent on several factors: volume and intensity, exercise selection, level of conditioning/training status, recovery ability, nutritional intake, and training goals.

Heavy ECC training may require 72h recovery, whereas large/moderate loads require less recovery time. Advanced weightlifters and bodybuilders use high frequency training (4–6day/week). Double-split routines, 2 sessions per day with emphasis on different muscle groups, are common and this can result in the completion of up to 8–14sessions/week.

Olympic weightlifters typically perform 18sessions/week. Short sessions followed by recovery, supplementation, and food intake allows for high intensity training via maximal energy utilization, and reduced fatigue during exercise performance.

Anaerobic/sprint training

Anaerobic/sprint training involves a series of repeated bouts of high intensity exercise alternated with periods of relief (rest or low intensity exercise).

Energy system
ATP-PCR supplies more ATP than anaerobic glycolysis, during intermittent short duration efforts when compared to short duration continuous efforts.

Training
- Overload is applied by manipulating intensity, distance, number of repetitions, rest interval between repetitions, activity during rest interval, and training frequency (sets per week).
- Typical anaerobic/sprint training includes:
  - Longer duration intervals at moderate intensity.
  - Medium duration intervals at moderate-high intensity.
  - Very short intervals at close to maximum intensity.
- Longer duration (4–5min) anaerobic/sprint training sessions are used to induce improved lactate tolerance with HR during exercise > HR at TLac from mid-interval onwards.
- Medium and short (1–2min) duration intervals; exercise intensity based on recent time-trial (TT) performance time, nominally 92–95% effort during week 1 and 2, and 95–97% effort during week 3, repeat TT at end of recovery week to assess improvement.
- Relief time nominally 150% of exercise interval, if necessary adjust relief time to ensure that exercise time remains constant across successive repetitions.
- Number of repetitions decreases as exercise duration increases (12 × 400m, 6–8 × 800m or 5–6 × 1000m).

Metabolic adaptations
Anaerobic training increases resting levels of anaerobic substrates and key glycolytic enzymes.
- Free creatine ↑ 32–40%, PCR ↑ 5–20%, ATP ↑ 16–18% and glycogen ↑ 30–60%.
- No change or increase in glycolytic enzyme activity (phosphofructokinase (PFK), lactate dehydrogenase (LDH), hexokinase (HK)).
- No change in ATP turnover enzymes (myokinase (MK), CPK).
- Decrease in mitochondrial volume (density) due to an increase in size of myofibrils and sarcoplasmic volume.
- Selective hypertrophy of FT + FOG and an increase in FT + FOG to ST fibre ratio.
- Increased BLa during all-out exercise probably due to enhanced glycogen storage and increased glycolytic enzymes following anaerobic training, in addition to improved motivation and pain tolerance.
- In addition to the metabolic and biochemical changes noted above, imprecisely identified nervous system changes also occur (better motor unit recruitment patterns and synchronization).

Types of anaerobic training

Strength/resistance training for improved running velocity include short interval sprints, hill training, and weight training. Heavy weights (small number of lifts) or light weights 50–60% 1RM (large number of lifts with short rests).

- *Fartlek:* alternating fast and slow running over natural terrain, informal interval training lacking precise control of exercise or relief elements.
- *Sprints to develop ATP-PCR system*: repeat sprints at maximum velocity (duration 5–6s, distance 40–50m to experience running at V_{max}), longer relief intervals (30+ s) required to ensure almost complete phosphagen recovery.
- Interval sprints alternate 50m sprints and 50–70m jog for 3–4 km, because of onset of fatigue after several sprints subsequent sprints are not run at V_{max}.
- Acceleration sprints, gradual increase in running velocity (from jog-stride-sprint) over a distance of 50–100m followed by 50–100m walk phase, recovery almost complete before subsequent sprint phase.
- Plyometrics bounding type exercises and drop jumps to improve neuromuscular synchronization and explosiveness.
- Sprint training for games players sprint distance 40–50m, including backward and lateral movement patterns typical of athlete's sport, stop-and-go sprints over 5–10m with sports-specific elements completed during each stop phase.

Short interval sprints (30–50m) facilitate maximum and synchronous recruitment of fibres. Increased recruitment may lead to muscle damage because of force generated, normally prevented via central inhibition initiated by stretch receptors and Golgi tendon bodies. Central nervous system (CNS) overrides and prevents maximum recruitment, over time sprint training desensitizes central inhibition.

ATP and PCR storage and glycolytic flux increased by inducing biochemical changes in key enzymes in cytosol (phosphorylase, PFK and LDH).

Long interval sprints (100–200m) improved usage of PCR, ↑ ATP/PCR and total Cr storage, ↑ lactate tolerance and buffering capacity, initial improvements primarily neural—strength gains without muscle hypertrophy.

Gender and performance

Gender issues in sport and exercise embrace genetic, hormonal, anatomical, physiological, psychological, and sociological aspects, as well as those of sports performance and body image. World record performances in women's sports have improved rapidly for a variety of reasons, including greater numbers participating and better training practices. Female world record performances are still however only 90–95% of that of male athletes, and in all but a minority of sports female performance will probably never equal or surpass male performance. Anatomical and physiological reasons for this are discussed here.

Stature and body mass
- Female athletes are on average of shorter stature, 1.6m as opposed to male athletes where average height is 1.7m.
- Girls are briefly larger and stronger between the ages of 10–12yr, due to an earlier growth spurt.

Skeletal differences
- Women have narrower shoulders, shorter arms with a wider carrying angle, broader hips, and shorter legs.
- Shoulder arm difference and smaller muscle mass in women accounts for weaker upper body compared with lower body strength in women than men.
- Broader hips cause greater angle of the femur to the knee (genu valgum), causing many women to throw their heels out when running.

Centre of gravity
- Shorter stature and body shape differences lead to a lower centre of gravity.
- In adults; centre of gravity is 55% of standing height in women (S1 level) and 56–57% in men.
- Consequently in gymnastics women have better balance and are better suited to floor and balance beam exercises.

Flexibility
- Women have better flexibility than men.
- Advantageous in gymnastics and dance.
- *NB* Hypermobility of the joints can bring problems.

Body fat percentage
- Females have higher % body fat (23–28%) than males (12–18%).
- This is advantageous in cold climates, during starvation, and may improve performance in long distance swimming events.
- However greater percentage body fat is a major disadvantage in weight bearing sports involving running and jumping.

Muscle
- There is little difference in muscle quality between genders.
- Strength differences between genders due to greater cross-sectional area, greater overall muscle mass (androgen effects), and longer levers.

- Low grade muscle endurance is better in female athletes when performing repetitions at 20–30% of 1RM.
- This may benefit female athletes in ultra-distance events, swimming, and cycling.

Cardiovascular system
- Women have proportionately less blood than men (65 vs. 75mL/kg) and lower Hb (13.9 vs. 15.8g/dL).
- Women tend to have smaller hearts, smaller left ventricular mass, and smaller stroke volume.
- Despite hearts being 8% smaller in female volunteer's maximum heart rates are similar across gender.
- At maximum levels of aerobic work female athletes need to pump 7L of blood for every litre of oxygen consumed, whereas male athletes require only 6L.
- This affects maximum oxygen intake, highest recorded data are between 85–90mL/kg/min for male endurance athletes and 75–80mL/kg/min for female endurance athletes.

Motor control, vision, and hearing
- Women have better fine manipulative skills, but worse visual acuity than men.
- Women have better colour discrimination, especially in the blue-grey range, and are able to perceive quieter sounds.

Thermoregulation
Thermoregulation in male and female volunteers is slightly different.
- Total body water to body mass ratio is 50–55% in women and 55–60% in men.
- Body temperature is higher in the luteal phase of the menstrual cycle, but this is thought not to have any effect on performance.
- Men sweat more per m^2 of skin (800 vs, 600mL/h/m^2).
- Women tend to lose more heat through radiation.
- Change in sweat patterns and sweat electrolytes in response to training are similar in both genders.
- Unfit female volunteers lose heat more by radiation and onset of sweating is earlier in trained female athletes.
- Well-trained male and female athletes respond in a similar manner in warm temperatures with low humidity.
- Women therefore are benefited in warm humid conditions and men in warm dry conditions.
- Women may be able to work and survive better in the cold than men because they are better insulated.
- However, surface area to body mass ratio (SA/M) also determines heat loss and women have a larger SA/M ratio than men.
- Women lose heat more rapidly in the cold, especially if immersed in cold water.

Resistance training in children

Resistance training in children has always been a controversial topic. The detractors say that it is injurious and does not produce strength improvements in the pre-adolescent child, but studies now show that it can produce strength gains even in pre-adolescent children and, when well-supervised, the injury risk is low.

Part of the controversy surrounding weight training in children stems from confusion as to the difference between weight training and weight lifting.

Weight-lifting refers to a competitive sport where maximal lifts are performed. Most authorities agree that this sport is unsuitable for children before skeletal maturity or Tanner Stage 5.

Weight training (also called strength training or resistance training) involves repetitive sub-maximal muscle contractions with the aim of improving strength.

Effects
- Resistance training (RT) has been shown to improve muscle strength in pre-adolescents and adolescent volunteers although the mechanism by which it works appears to differ.
- In the pre-adolescent, strength gains are thought to be the result of improved motor co-ordination and neural adaptations, which increase motor unit activation and recruitment.
- In the adolescent, muscle hypertrophy is largely responsible for the strength gains which occur.
- There is some evidence that RT improves aspects of motor performance, but no good evidence that it improves overall sports performance or reduces incidence of injuries.
- Improves body composition in overweight and obese children and adolescents
- Can result in improvements in bone mineral content

Risks
When compared with other sports played in the same age group, there is no evidence that a well-supervised RT program has any greater injury rate than sports participation.

Guidelines for RT in children
- Must be well supervised by an adult familiar with RT in children.
- Focus on good technique
- Gradual progression of loads (5–10%).
- Start with low loads and high repetitions (2–3 sets of 12–15 reps).
- If using weight machines, ensure that the lever length is appropriate for children.
- Train agonist and antagonist muscle groups equally.
- Include core strengthening as a component of the programme
- Train 2–3 times/week for strength gains on non-consecutive days
- Have 'circuit' set up to encourage cardio-respiratory training at the same time.
- Stress that RT should be just one part of overall exercise regimen.
- Avoid lifting maximal loads before Tanner stage 5.

Further reading

American Academy of Pediatrics Council on Sports Fitness, McCambridge TM, Stricker PR. (2008). Strength training by children and adolescents. *Pediatrics* **121**(4): 835–40.

Faigenbaum AD, Kraemer WJ, Blimkie CJ, *et al.* (2009). Youth resistance training: updated position statement paper from the national strength and conditioning association. *J Strength Condit Res* **23**(5 Suppl.).

Young WK, Metzl JD. (2010). Strength training for the young athlete. *Pediat Annl* **39**(5): 293–9.

Exercise testing in children

Physical activity (PA) of children and adolescents is a major health issue. PA plays a critical role in determining cardiovascular, respiratory, skeletal and psychological health of children. In adults; PA strongly related to VO_2 max, fit have lower morbidity and mortality rates, in children; PA only weakly related (r = 0.16) to aerobic capacity.

Important to note that *children are not small adults.*

NHANES reported that >20% of children in USA were overweight, but over past 30yr the number of obese children had doubled. Overweight children were 2.4 times more likely to have high cholesterol, LDL cholesterol, triglycerides, and elevated BP, low high density lipoprotein (HDL), cholesterol, and fasting insulin, and adults that were overweight as children had increased mortality and morbidity rates irrespective of their adult weight. While causes of childhood obesity are complex, low PA and unhealthy diet are important contributing factors.

A recent review of PA and skeletal health in children concluded that a lifelong commitment to PA was needed: weight-bearing activities are ideal, short intense daily activity better than prolonged infrequent activity; activities that increase muscle strength also enhance bone mineral density (BMD). Activities should work all large muscle groups, immobilization and periods of immobility should be avoided (even brief daily weight bearing movements can minimize bone loss).

In adults a high relative VO_2 max infers good endurance performance, not true in children. VO_2 max (mL/kg/min) in boys remains relatively constant from age 6–16, in girls declines continuously, especially at puberty. Although VO_2 max (mL/kg/min) remains relatively constant, endurance performance steadily improves.

Before puberty, VO_2 max (L/min) slightly higher in boys vs. girls and improves with age and growth in both genders. Following puberty, relationship changes, boys increase VO_2 max (L/min) with age and growth of their pulmonary, cardiovascular and skeletal systems, in girls of similar age VO_2 max (L/min^{-1}) remains relatively constant. Differences in VO_2 max are possibly attributable to increase in non-metabolic mass (fat mass) and decreasing daily PA.

Contraindications for maximal testing in children are similar to adults. Terminate the test if systolic >240mmHg or diastolic >120mmHg, progressive decrease in systolic BP, pallor or clamminess of the skin, pain, headache, dyspnea, or nausea.

Criteria of plateau in VO_2 max is extremely difficult in children, as they stop because they fatigue. Peak VO_2, rather than VO_2 max is better terminology. Typical criteria for determining peak VO_2 include; 95% age-predicted HR_{max}, respiratory exchange ratio (RER) >1.05, rate of perceived exertion (RPE) > 18 on Borg 6 to 20 scale.

Additional criteria include subjective signs of exhaustion; stopping because of fatigue. BLa of 6–7mmol/L for 7–8-yr-olds or 4–5mmol/L for 5–6-yr-old.

Children must understand that a maximal effort is required, reassure with constant verbal encouragement. In children peak HR and VO_2

higher during treadmill running, RER at maximal effort higher using cycle ergometry.

Most treadmill protocols (maximal or sub-maximal) are modifications of adult protocols. Comfortable running velocity (5–8km/h) and increase gradient by 2% every 2min to volitional fatigue or maximum criteria attained. Cycle ergometer protocols also similar to adult, normally cadence lower at 50–60rev/min. Adams sub-maximal cycle protocol similar to PWC170 and consists of 3 × 6-min stages, HR is monitored and mechanical load at HR of 170beats/min, computed as index of aerobic fitness. Modifications have included 3-min stages and a maximum HR of 190beats/min.

Field-based tests commonly used to predict VO_2 max in children include 1.6 km run/walk test or the shuttle running test (20MST). For the 20MST the start velocity 8.5km/h and the increment is 0.5km/h/min.

VO_2 max (mL/kg/min) = $[3.24*(V_{max})] - [3.25*(age) + 0.15*(V_{max}*age)] + 31.025$,
where V_{max} (km/h) = 8.5 + 0.5 (number of stages completed).

To assess anaerobic capacity using the Wingate test for legs or arms, use 50m run time. However, note that results of run tests can be influenced by running experience, genetics and motor performance, use standing vertical jump and reach test, measured data are recorded in cm used to compute peak power.

Peak power (W) = $[78.5 \times VJH (cm)] + [60.6 \times mass (kg)] - [15.3 \times height (cm)] + 431$

Body composition

Hydrostatic weighing not recommended, as it is known that children undergo changes in their chemical composition of fat free mass especially during puberty. Protein increases by 5% and water content decreases by 9% from birth to adulthood, consequently, adult equations overestimate by between 7 and 13%.

Skin-fold thickness

Slaughter et al.[1] derived equations using 2 sites (calf and triceps or calf and subscapularis), percentage fat using triceps and calf skin-fold in male (1 + (0.735 × SF), in female (5 + (0.610 × SF). Bioimpedance not recommended for use in children because of rapid growth rates and body chemistry changes. BMI is the easiest and least invasive technique, weakness is the inability to distinguish between muscle and fat mass. DEXA is safe, reliable, and valid for estimating percentage body fat in both children and adults.

Flexibility

Flexibility declines with age, boys decrease their flexibility after age 10, girls after age 12, and generally girls are more flexible than boys. Trunk extension test; prone position (toes pointed and hands under thighs) lift upper body off the floor in a slow controlled manner to a maximum height of 30cm. SAR test, standard test assess hamstring and low back flexibility. Back-saver SAR test, similar to traditional SAR except that each leg is tested separately. This modified test causes less pressure on the anterior portion of the lumbar vertebrae.

Exercise prescription

Integration of exercise science/physiology with training resulting in the long-term development and attainment of training goals, challenging in adults and very difficult in children. In general, children should be physically active as part of play, games, sport, transportation, recreation, physical education, or planned exercise.
- Older children should engage in moderate to vigorous activity using large muscle groups, running, cycling and swimming—3day/week for 30–60min at intensity equivalent to 75%HRR.
- Young children—30–120+min/day using age and developmental appropriate activity, include periods of moderate to vigorous activity interspersed with short rest periods.

Chapter 6

Metabolic

Cellular recovery after exercise *172*
Bodyweight *173*
Energy requirements *174*
Food and exercise *176*
Recovery after exercise *180*
Exercise and the environment *182*
Overtraining syndrome *194*

Cellular recovery after exercise

Exercise increases the generation of oxygen free radicals and lipid peroxidation which have harmful cellular effects. The rate of oxygen consumption and the presence of cellular antioxidant systems influence the magnitude of cellular damage occurring as a result of exercise.

Free radicals generated during exercise may arise from three potential sources:
- The mitochondria from which oxygen radicals have escaped.
- The capillary endothelium through hypoxia.
- Inflammatory cells mobilized from tissue damage.

Skeletal muscle has adapted to protect against further cell injury following exercise. Normal cellular adaptation occurs in response to an appropriate stimulus, and ceases once the need for adaptation has ceased. These adaptations include:
- Biochemical changes such as an increase in antioxidant enzymes and production of heat shock proteins.
- Response to increased work demands by changing their size (atrophy or hypertrophy), number (hyperplasia), and form (metaplasia).

Exercise, repair, and recovery

Exercise training reduces the susceptibility of muscles to further damage by increasing the activity of antioxidant enzymes, such as superoxide dismutase, catalase, and glutathione peroxidase. The ability of cells to respond to stress by increasing the content of cytoprotective proteins is blunted over time by the ageing process.

Physical damage to muscle cells from repeated muscular contractions (particularly eccentric contractions) is repaired in the following sequence:
- During days 2–4, there is invasion by phagocytic cells and prominent degeneration of cellular structures.
- During days 4–6, regeneration of muscle begins by the activation and migration of satellite cells. These satellite cells migrate into the damaged area, differentiate to form myoblasts, and fuse to form multinucleated myotubes, which develop into mature skeletal muscle.
- Rapid repair of plasma membrane disruption is essential to cell survival and involves a complex and active cell response that includes membrane fusion and cytoskeletal activation. Tissues, such as cardiac and skeletal muscle, adapt to a disruption injury by hypertrophy. Cells adapt by increasing the efficiency of their re-healing response.

Bodyweight

Total energy intake must be raised to meet the increased energy expended during training. Maintenance of energy balance can be assessed by monitoring bodyweight, body composition, and food intake.

Weight gain

For those athletes who wish to gain bodyweight, caloric intake should exceed energy expenditure. Increased muscle mass, from physical training, can lead to increased bodyweight even with a reduction in body fat percentage.

Weight loss

For those athletes who wish to lose weight, caloric intake should not exceed energy expenditure. The caloric deficit will dictate the amount of weight that can be lost. To maximize the loss of fat and minimize the loss of lean tissue, weight loss should be limited to 500–1000g per week. This would require an energy restriction of 2–4MJ per day. The body, however, acts as a homeostatically regulated system so that attempts to lose weight by calorie restriction or increased energy expenditure will usually generate hunger and the desire to eat more rather than weight loss. The most effective weight loss is achieved by reducing the carbohydrate content of the diet by increasing fat and protein intake. This reduces circulating insulin concentrations which regulate the body fat mass by stimulating fat and glucose uptake and storage by insulin sensitive fat cells.

The use of diuretics and laxatives should be discouraged.

Fluid status will affect bodyweight. Volume depletion will present as 'weight loss', while hyper-hydration can present with bodyweight gain. These fluid gains and losses are transient and can be detrimental to health if performed for the wrong reasons (i.e. 'making weight' in sports which require weight classes for competition).

Body mass index

BMI is generally used as a descriptive tool for assessing health risks. BMI can be calculated with imperial or metric units:

Weight in pounds/[(height in inches)^2] × 703;

or

Weight in kg/[(height in m)^2].

Energy requirements

The main component of daily energy turnover in an average person is the basal metabolic rate (BMR).

Basal metabolic rate (BMR) represents the *minimum* amount of energy expenditure needed for ongoing processes in the body in the resting state, when no food is digested and no energy is needed for temperature regulation. The most variable component of daily energy turnover is the energy expenditure for activity (EEA) which can range between 15–25% of the BMR in moderately active persons.

For sports such as gymnastics, dancing, diving, and running in which a lean physique is desired, athletes will routinely restrict their caloric intake or chose a diet with a higher protein/fat content with fewer calories to achieve a leaner body composition. Caloric restriction reduces the metabolic rate and may lead to conditions such as menstrual dysfunction (amenorrhoea), iron deficiency (anaemia), and a decrease in bone density (osteoporosis/osteopenia); complications not present when a higher fat/protein diet is ingested.

A chronic negative energy balance will result in a loss of fat free (muscle) mass as well as a loss of body fat. Lethargy from the excessive loss of lean body mass and depletion of glycogen stores generally limits performance and the ability to train properly, making an athlete more susceptible to illness and injury. These complications are not seen when fat loss is achieved by modifying the macro-content balance by reducing the carbohydrate intake.

An increase in lean body mass will increase energy requirements for basal activities and vice versa. Athletes who sustain hard and vigorous activity for prolonged periods of time must supplement their caloric needs by ingesting more energy dense foodstuffs to sustain exercise and match energy demands during exercise. While increased energy consumption can be achieved by ingesting primarily more carbohydrate-rich solid food or liquid carbohydrate formulas, increases in fat and protein ingestion are also part of a healthy mixed diet.

The higher the intensity of the exercise and the more muscle groups that are activated, the more energy requirements of that activity are increased.

Food and exercise

Physically active individuals must meet their energy requirements by ingesting a variety of foodstuffs both: before, during, and after exercise.

For most individuals the consumption of a normal mixed diet consisting of 50% carbohydrate and 10–30% fat, with the difference made up with protein, is adequate. Athletes who are unable to maintain the desired fat mass on this diet should reduce their carbohydrate intake by eating proportionately more fat and protein.

The only reason to consume protein or fat several hours before exercise or exercise performance is to provide satiety, which can influence performance by promoting a sense of well-being. If carbohydrate stores are adequate, the choice of food before exercise should be based on the past experience of the athlete in so much as that the food choice should minimize hunger yet not interfere with the exercise mode and duration.

Habituation to a high-fat diet decreases the amount of muscle glycogen used during exercise by increasing the body's ability to use and mobilize fat. The increased ability to oxidize fat for fuel may enable an athlete to continue exercising for longer periods at intensities of 70% of VO_2 max or less which may be beneficial in events lasting days or weeks. However, habituation to a high-fat diet is associated with a reduced performance ability during high intensity exercise performance, such as when attempting to elevate power output during hill climbing in endurance cycling or running events.

Carbohydrate needs

The CHO needs of individuals vary depending on their mass and the level of physical activity. Larger and more active individuals will require generally more energy and, therefore, more CHO. However, in the normal exercising population the CHO needs will be met by consuming a normal mixed diet as described above. Athletes with insulin sensitive fat cells will have greater difficulty maintaining an ideal weight if their diets contain excessive amounts of carbohydrate.

Protein needs

The protein needs of individuals also vary with mass and activity level, but are also generally met when one is consuming a normal mixed diet. Although the recommended daily allowance (RDA) for protein is 0.8g/kg of body mass, highly active endurance athletes may require up to 1g per kg of body mass, while those striving to build large amounts of muscle mass or to lose body fat may require in excess of 1.5g/kg of body mass. Usually, these requirements are adequately covered by the increased energy intake stimulated by physical activity, and it is often unnecessary to increase actively the protein content of the diet by eating selectively protein-rich foodstuffs. Protein is the macronutrient that most affects satiety so that a higher protein intake promotes fat loss, in part by reducing calorie intake, but also by reducing elevated circulating insulin concentrations produced by a higher carbohydrate intake.

Pre-event diet

Carbohydrate loading has been shown to increase muscle glycogen content before exercise and delay the time at which low muscle glycogen concentrations are reached. The main effect of this practice is to decrease the amount of fat oxidized during exercise. Carbohydrate loading is achieved by eating a high carbohydrate diet (75–90%) for 3 days prior to the competitive event. To achieve this, athletes should consume approximately 8g CHO or more per kg of body mass.

Pre-event meal

The pre-event diet aims to optimize muscle glycogen and liver glycogen stores that maintain blood glucose levels during exercise. The ingestion of carbohydrate before an event will stimulate carbohydrate oxidation and inhibit fat oxidation. Evidence suggests that performance is improved when 200–300g CHO is consumed 3–4h before prolonged exercise, compared to when no food is ingested.

Immediately prior to the event

Foods that are consumed immediately prior to an event should be low in fat, protein, and fibre, and should not cause GI distress.

Foods ingested 4–6h before an event should be of a low to moderate glycaemic index to minimize the insulin response. If the muscles are not fully stocked with glycogen (because of recent exercise or a low CHO diet), however, then foods with a moderate to high glycaemic index are preferred prior to an athletic event.

Food supplements

Numerous well-controlled studies have concluded that individuals eating a well-balanced diet do not need to supplement their diet with vitamins, minerals, or trace elements when undertaking an exercise programme. The ingestion of these supplements on physical performance has not been clearly shown to have benefits.

Vitamins

Vitamins are divided into water- and fat-soluble categories. Water-soluble vitamins such as thiamin, riboflavin, B-6, niacin, pantothenic acid, biotin, and vitamin C are involved in mitochondrial metabolism. Folate and vitamin B-12 are primarily involved in DNA synthesis and RBC development. Fat-soluble vitamins include vitamins A, K, E, and D with vitamin E being the most widely studied as an ergogenic aid. Vitamin E has antioxidant properties, as do vitamins C, A, and beta carotene. There is a linear relationship between energy intake and vitamin intake, thus vitamin intake should exceed the RDA provided that a varied diet is consumed. Mega doses of both fat and water-soluble vitamins have been shown to have toxic effects.

Minerals

Minerals are divided into macrominerals and microminerals (trace minerals). Macrominerals include calcium, magnesium, phosphorous, sulphur, potassium, sodium, and chloride with calcium, phosphorus, and calcium each constituting 0.01% of total bodyweight. Trace minerals include iron, zinc, copper, selenium, chromium, iodine, fluorine, manganese, molybdenum, nickel, silicon, vanadium, arsenic, and cobalt with each constituting less than 0.001% of total bodyweight. Iron, zinc, copper, selenium, and chromium have been proposed to enhance physical performance and may improve physical performance if an athlete is deficient in that certain mineral, or if an increased level of this mineral would boost the body's natural response to enhance performance.

Amino acids, electrolytes, and herbal supplements have not been shown to improve physical performance in well-controlled scientific studies.

Iron

Iron is a necessary component of haemoglobin and myoglobin, and facilitates the transport of oxygen through the bloodstream as well as the transfer of electrons in the electron transport chain system. 60–70% of iron is found in haemoglobin with the remainder found in bone marrow, muscle, liver, and spleen.

Organ meats, black strap molasses, clams, oysters, dried legumes, nuts and seeds, red meats, and dark leafy vegetables are good exogenous sources of iron. Symptoms of an iron deficiency include generalized fatigue and anaemia. Liver damage can occur from iron excess.

Iron deficiency anaemia in athletes may result from a poor diet, excess blood loss (through menstruation in females), footstrike haemolysis, and through sweat loss. Although numerous studies have documented that athletes, particularly endurance athletes, are iron depleted, the degree and percentage of iron depletion is similar between athletes and non-athletes.

Pseudoanaemia occurs in athletes secondary to an increase in plasma volume, which occurs as an adaptation to training. This increase in plasma volume 'dilutes' an otherwise normal red blood cell count into falsely low levels. Hence, this is an artificial lowering of haemoglobin rather than a true anaemic response, which is a common laboratory finding in endurance athletes.

The recommended daily allowance for iron intake for males is 10–12mg/day and 15mg/day for females.

Calcium

Calcium is required for the formation and maintenance of hard bones and for the conduction of nerve impulses. Calcium activates enzymes responsible for the transmission of membrane potentials as well as for muscle contraction. 99% of calcium is found in the skeleton with the remainder found in extracellular fluid, intracellular structures, and cell membranes.

Dairy products, sardines, clams, oysters, turnips, broccoli, and legumes are good exogenous sources of calcium. Osteoporosis and fractures can occur from a deficiency in calcium intake over decades. Constipation, kidney stones, and chelation with antibiotics and other nutrients (such as iron and zinc) can occur with calcium excess.

Weight-bearing exercise has been shown to increase bone density, especially when undertaken at critical growth periods (8–14yr). Oestrogen has been shown to reduce urinary calcium excretion, increase intestinal absorption of calcium and increase the secretion of calcitonin which reduces bone resorption. Calcium also can be lost through sweat, which may increase an athlete's total daily requirement if exercise is regularly performed in hot and humid environments.

The recommended daily allowance for calcium is 800–1200mg/day for both men and women.

Creatine

Creatine is a naturally occurring compound in the body, specifically in the muscles.

Creatine supplementation is widely practised by professional and recreational athletes. The benefits and side effects are varied and debatable. Purported benefits include increased mass, improved rate of recovery after exercise, and increased power or speed. Side effects include cramping and water retention.

Although much research has been devoted to creatine and its effects, the real value of creatine supplementation remains uncertain. Untrained persons undertaking a weight training programme for the first time appear to benefit the most. Elite athletes who eat diets with adequate protein intake may benefit less.

Recovery after exercise

Recovery after exercise is most important if another bout of physical activity will shortly follow. Full recovery after exercise is also important in reducing the risk of overtraining, although the training volumes required to produce overtraining are usually achievable only by highly trained individuals.

Recovery is also an important part of adapting to exercise training, because the physical adaptations that are stimulated by exercise training occur during the rest and recovery phase.

Recovery appears to be aided by the ingestion of carbohydrate- and protein-rich foodstuffs within 30–60min after the termination of exercise.

Exercise and the environment

Different environmental conditions will affect exercise tolerance and capacity in different ways. There are three overriding environmental factors to which athletes may be exposed in either training or racing, or both—heat, cold, and reduced oxygen content in the inspired air as occurs at increasing altitude.

In order to survive, humans require to regulate their body temperatures at between 35 and 41°C, and to maintain the partial pressure of oxygen in their blood in excess of about 40mmHg.

Environmental conditions, in particular the environmental temperature, the wind speed, and the water content of the air (humidity) determine the rate at which heat is lost from the body. The normal average human skin temperature is 33°C. At any lower environmental temperature, heat will be lost from the skin to the environment in the process of heat conduction. The rate at which this heat will be lost by conduction from the body will, in turn, be determined by the magnitude of the temperature gradient—the steeper the gradient, the greater the heat loss—and the rapidity with which the cooler air in contact with the skin is replaced by colder air. Continual replacement of warmed air by cooler air causes loss of heat from the body, by means of convection. Convective heat loss rises as an exponential function of the speed at which air courses across the body, in effect the prevailing wind speed. With high humidity, sweat loss by evaporation is reduced.

Body temperature

At rest, humans regulate their body temperatures within a narrow range of between 36.5 and 37.5°C. During exercise, this safe thermoregulatory range is increased to up to 41.5°C. Heat–acclimatized human athletes have a superior capacity to exercise without apparent distress even up to body temperatures of 41.5°C.

The human body temperature represents a balance between the rate of heat production by, and heat loss from the body. Hence, changes in the rates of either heat production or heat loss, or more commonly both, determine whether an abnormal rise in body temperature (hyperthermia leading to heat stroke) or an excessive fall (hypothermia) is likely to develop and under what conditions. The principal physiological challenge that athletes face during exercise is how to lose the excess body heat produced by muscle contraction. The control of body temperature during exercise is, however, homeostatically-regulated so that the exercise behaviour is modified to ensure a safe body temperature. Thus athletes slow down when exercising in the heat; this reduces their rates of heat production when environmental conditions become too severe.

Hypothermia

When environmental conditions are particularly cold, for example (i) during winter conditions at latitudes above about 50° in either hemisphere, (ii) when cold is associated with windy and especially wet conditions, or (iii) when the athlete exercises in cold water for prolonged periods, the risk arises that the athlete will lose heat faster than he or she can produce it. Under these conditions, the body may be unable to maintain its core body temperature which may fall progressively, leading to hypothermia (core temperature <35°C) and the risk of death from the exposure/exhaustion syndrome or drowning (if swimming).

Low body temperatures of 35°C occur frequently in swimmers exposed to cold water temperatures for many hours, for example, in long distance Channel swims. This occurs because water is an excellent conductor of heat, approximately 30 times more effective than air. As a result, the naked body exposed to a body of water that is colder than the normal body temperature of 37°C is unable to produce heat as rapidly as it is lost by conduction to the surrounding water. If exposed for sufficiently long, the human body will be cooled to the temperature of the surrounding water which is seldom more than 20°C except at the tropics. Wearing more appropriate clothing, in particular, dry or wet suits that maintain a layer of insulating water or air heated to body temperature, is the only way to prevent the ultimate development of a fatal hypothermia when exposed to cold water for any protracted period (hours).

Prevention of hypothermia

When exercising in cold conditions, hypothermia can be prevented by continued activity, adequate clothing that is dry and waterproof, and the presence of insulating layers. There is a high rate of heat production during exercise. Thus, as a general rule, continuing to move reduces the risk that hypothermia will develop. However, once the subject becomes too exhausted to continue, his or her rate of heat production falls sharply and the risk of hypothermia rises dramatically.

The important practical point is that continuing to exercise will protect against hypothermia if it maintains the rate of heat production that equals or exceeds the heat loss. In contrast, once the hiker, runner, or mountain climber starts to walk or stops walking altogether, the rate of heat production falls dramatically, providing the necessary conditions for hypothermia. The change from running to walking, for example, has a marked effect on the clothing needed to maintain body temperature, even at relatively mild temperatures. Thus, clothing with at least 4 times as much insulation is required to maintain body temperature at rest at an effective air temperature of 0°C than when running at 16km per hour. Thus, extra clothing should always be available if there is any possibility that fatigue will develop when exercising in cold conditions.

Air is a poor conductor of heat and, hence, a good insulator, but water is a very poor insulator. Thus, the thin layer of air trapped next to the skin by clothing is rapidly heated to the skin temperature, thereby producing a layer of insulation. However, the saturation of clothing with water removes this insulating layer and essentially exposes the skin to whatever the external temperature is. Under these conditions, the exposed human must either find dry, warm clothing, and a warm shelter, or he/she will cool to the prevailing environmental temperature. This loss of insulation caused by water explains why saturated, wet clothing experienced by runners, climbers, or hikers in windy, wet conditions or alternatively swimmers in cold water, predisposes to the development of hypothermia.

Experience with the English Channel swimmers has shown that body build, especially the body muscle (but also the body fat) content, is a critical factor determining the rate at which a swimmer will cool down during a long-distance swim in water temperatures below about 24°C. It is probable that the same applies in out-of-water activities; subjects who are more muscular and fatter are likely to cool down more slowly when exposed to very cold conditions.

Thus, appropriate fitness, proper clothing including water repellent outer garments, adequate nutrition to prevent premature fatigue, early recognition of danger, and an avoidance of extreme environmental conditions, are crucial to ensure that exercise can be safely undertaken in cold, wet, and windy conditions.

Diagnosis of hypothermia
- Rectal temperature <37°C (usually much lower).
- Exposure to cold conditions for prolonged periods.
- Fatigue.
- Muscle weakness and loss of co-ordination.
- Desire to stop exercising.
- Disorientation, leading to coma.

Treatment of hypothermia
- Removal from the cold environment, application of dry clothing and/or blankets.
- External heating in the form of hot water bottles, warm water bath, radiant heat, convective heat, or even the body heat of other humans.
- In severe hypothermia, consider using heated intravenous fluids or extra-corporeal blood warming techniques.
- Warming efforts should continue until the body temperature exceeds 35°C. since a person with hypothermia is not 'cold and dead' until they are shown to be 'warm and dead'.

Special note
⚠Be aware that ventricular fibrillation is a common complication of treatment for hypothermia, especially during rapid re-warming, and should be treated appropriately.

Hyperthermia

Hyperthermia describes an increase in body temperature above the normal resting upper limit of 37.5°C. Elevated body temperatures of up to 41.5°C are frequently measured in healthy winners of short distance (5–15km) running events contested in hot, humid, windless environmental conditions. Such high body temperatures occur because the rate at which elite athletes produce heat when running at their maximum pace can exceed the capacity of the hot environment to absorb that heat for short periods until homoestasis is regained. Fortunately, the brain also has protective mechanisms that reduce the allowable rate of energy production (exercise intensity/speed) during exercise in the heat. As a result, incidences of severe heat injury (heatstroke) are remarkably uncommon in sport despite the frequency with which sport is played in severe environmental conditions.

During exercise, the chemical energy stored in the muscles in the form of ATP, is converted into the mechanical energy of motion. However, this process is inefficient so that only 25% of the chemical energy used by the muscles produces motion; the remaining 75% is released as heat that must be lost from the body if the body temperature is to be safely regulated. Thus, when elite ultra-marathon runners run at an average pace of about 16km per hour during races of 90–100km, they use approximately 56kJ of energy every minute or about 18,480kJ in the 5.5h that they require to complete these races. However, of the total amount of KJ used, only about 4000kJ actually transport them from the start to the finish of their races. The remaining 14,480kJ serve only to overheat the runners' bodies. To prevent their temperatures from rising to over 43°C causing heatstroke, these athletes have to lose more than 90% of the heat they produce.

The humidity of the air determines the extent to which heat can be lost to the environment in the form of sweat, which evaporates from the skin surface and, to a lesser extent, from the respiratory membranes. This process of evaporation is the predominant source of heat loss in exercising humans, especially in the heat since each gram (mL) of water so evaporated removes 1.8kJ from the body. As the humidity of the air rises, the efficiency of heat loss by evaporation falls so that the ease of maintaining heat balance becomes increasingly difficult as the humidity rises above 60–70%.

Sweating is an extremely efficient mechanism for heat loss. Thus, provided the humidity is low, well trained, and heat-acclimatized humans can regulate their body temperatures and prevent dangerous hyperthermia even when they exercise at high intensities in hot environmental conditions (up to 34°C) or at lower even up to 43°C, provided the humidity is low. It is high humidity that poses the greatest threat since heat loss by sweating is markedly impaired in humid conditions.

The brain provides the final mechanism that protects humans from unsafe hyperthermia when exercising in hot, warm, and humid conditions. Feedback from sensors throughout the body to a central regulator in the brain monitor both the extent of the environmental stress to which the body is exposed, as well as the rate at which the body stores heat during exercise in those environmental conditions. Since it is safe to exercise only to a body temperature of less than 42°C, immediately on exposure to the prevailing environmental conditions at the onset of exercise, and on the basis of the rate at which heat will be stored and the expected duration of the exercise, the brain calculates the rate at which work can be safely performed under those specific environmental conditions. This central governor therefore pre-sets the number of motor units in the active muscles that can be recruited in order to ensure that a safe rate of heat production is allowed for the expected duration of the exercise. At the same time, the brain pre-sets the rate at which the perception of effort increases during the exercise bout so that the perceived effort of continuing to exercise becomes intolerable before the body temperature is elevated to dangerous levels.

In this way, the brain ensures that dangerous hyperthermia including heatstroke occurs uncommonly during exercise. When heatstroke does occur during exercise, the presence of pathological precursors must be considered. These include the presence of a pre-existing medical condition including a muscle disorder that predisposes to excessive heat production during exercise (exercise-induced malignant hyperthermia), any condition that elevates the body temperature before the onset of exercise, or the use of drugs, especially amphetamines or cocaine, that prevent the normal function of the central governor mechanism by reducing the sensations of discomfort during exercise.

Exercise in the heat

Hot (>30°C) and humid (>50% relative humidity) environmental conditions will reduce exercise capacity and performance, although represent no immediate danger to an individual.

Acclimatization and the heat

In addition to the general adaptations that occur with exercise training, individuals can also adapt to exercise in hot and humid environments. This is referred to as heat acclimatization and can be achieved with a specific programme of exercise and conditions.

General terminology

Wet bulb (WB)

Temperature value derived from specialized thermometer that is used to measure the amount of water vapour pressure in the air. Commonly referred to as the wet bulb or relative humidity (RH). WB is less than the dry bulb (DB) in proportion to the environmental humidity. When the RH is 100%, the WB and DB are the same.

Dry bulb

Temperature value derived from a normal thermometer, and from which the ambient temperature is obtained. Commonly referred to as the dry bulb.

Black globe

Specialized thermometer to measure the radiant heat load. It consists of a dry bulb thermometer enclosed inside a black, metal sphere. Commonly referred to as the globe temperature (GT).

Wet bulb globe temperature (WBGT)

An index system used to rate the combined environmental variables of temperature, radiation, and humidity, as measured with the above terms. Calculated with the equation

$$WBGT = 0.7\ WB + 0.2\ GT + 0.1\ DB$$

Heat acclimatization

Complete heat acclimatization requires 7–10 consecutive days of low to moderate intensity exercise of 60–120min in ambient temperatures above 30°C and 50% RH. A large proportion of the adaptations occur within the first 5 days, but 7–10 days are required for full acclimatization. A number of general adaptations occur with heat acclimatization.

Earlier onset of sweating

Sweating begins at an earlier core temperature, representing an increased ability to dissipate heat.

Decreased sweat sodium concentration

To conserve Na^+, the body produces more dilute sweat. Unacclimatized sweat Na^+ concentration is approximately 75mmol/L Na^+.

After acclimatization this can decrease to 20–30mmol/L Na^+ of sweat or even lower (>10mmol/L Na^+) in those eating a low Na^+ diet

Cardiovascular adaptations
After acclimatization, the heart rate and core temperature at the same given exercise intensity will be lower compared with pre-acclimatization levels.

Fluid retention
The amount of fluid in blood (plasma volume) increases.

Heat-related illness in children

In the past, children were thought to be significantly disadvantaged compared with adults when exercising in the heat.

The reasons for children's possible ↑ susceptibility are:
- Higher SA to body mass ratio means that children absorb more heat from the environment in hot conditions.
- They are less efficient exercisers, i.e. produce more heat for a given workload.
- Lower cardiac output therefore less able to divert blood to the skin for cooling.
- Lower sweat rate.
- Higher sweating threshold.
- Slower to acclimatize.
- Children tend to voluntarily dehydrate and need to be reminded to drink while exercising. Despite the above factors however, there is no epidemiological data to suggest that children have higher heat-injury rates than adults and a number of recent studies examining thermoregulatory responses to a given workload in children vs. adults have revealed no differences in core temperature.

Children have a different process of thermoregulation

- Larger SA results in increased reliance on dry heat dissipation (radiation, convection, conduction) and increased skin blood flow, rather than evaporative heat loss. Children may be more advantaged with high humidity which favours non-evaporative heat dissipation.
- Sweat rate, when corrected for body mass, does not change with age or maturity suggesting that thermoregulatory differences between children and adults are quantitative not qualitative.

Children may be more vulnerable under extreme conditions, but are probably not under most ambient conditions.

Signs and symptoms of heat-related illness

The signs of heat-related illness represent a continuum from heat exhaustion (at the early stage) to heat stroke (a medical emergency).

Early signs of heat exhaustion include:
- Headache.
- Dizziness.
- Nausea.
- Muscle fatigue.

The signs of heat stroke include:
- Tachycardia.
- May or may not be sweating.
- Altered mental state (confusion → seizures → coma).
- Rectal temp >40°C.

Children at particular risk include:
- Obese children.
- Children with previous history of heat-related illness.
- Children with diabetes, cystic fibrosis, and cardiac conditions.
- Children taking certain medications including antihistamines, phenothiazines, and anticholinergics.

Treatment of heat-related illness in children
- Remove child to shady area and remove unnecessary clothing.
- Measure rectal temperature.
- Give cool fluids if conscious.
- If altered consciousness or rectal temp. >40°C, this is a medical emergency and child should be immediately transferred to hospital facility.
- Cooling and rehydration, however, should commence immediately.
- Early treatment is important for a favourable outcome.

Prevention of heat-related illness in children
- Avoid scheduling children's events for the heat of the day.
- Ensure adequate hydration by providing cool drinks with flavouring as these appear to be associated with increased consumption.
- Ensure appropriate clothing, i.e. light-coloured, permeable materials.
- Early identification of symptoms.

Further reading
Falk B, Dotan R. (2008). Children's thermoregulation during exercise in the heat: a revisit. *Appl Physiol Nutr Metab* **33**(2): 420–7.

Exercise at altitude
Altitudes exceeding 1500m above sea level will have an effect on exercise tolerance and capacity by reducing the maximal oxygen consumption in a curvilinear fashion. High altitude poses two distinct physiological challenges for the human body.

Increasingly lower amount of O_2 in the air as one ascends to higher altitudes
As the altitude above sea level increases, the barometric pressure falls. As a result, the number of oxygen molecules in each litre of air falls. In order partially to compensate for this, humans breathe more often and more deeply at altitude. However, as the altitude increases, the partial pressure of oxygen in the blood falls, reaching values that are not compatible with sustained human life at altitudes much above about 7000m. That some humans are able to reach the summit of Mount Everest (8840m) attests to the phenomenal biology of some humans; to the value of oxygen inhalation for others; and the quite remarkable ability of most humans to adapt to the stresses to which they are exposed for weeks to months.

Originally, it was argued that exercise performance at altitude was 'limited' by the production of excessive amounts of lactic acid by the oxygen-starved muscles. However, early studies showed that this could not be the case, since blood lactic acid during maximal exercise are as low at the summit of high mountains as they are at rest at sea level. This finding is paradoxical since, according to the traditional understanding, exercise in the increasing levels of hypoxia that occur at altitude should cause an increased skeletal muscle anaerobiosis with an increased production of lactic acid. Elevated lactic acid concentrations would then explain why the capacity to exercise is substantially reduced at increasing altitude. In addition, the maximal cardiac output is also much reduced during exercise at altitude. This too is paradoxical since a higher cardiac output should be advantageous, as it would increase blood and oxygen delivery to the exercising muscles to offset the effects of the progressive reduction in the amount of oxygen stored in each unit of arterial blood.

Increasingly harsh ambient conditions due to the cold and wind

Fortunately, at the temperatures at high altitude, water exists in the form of ice and snow so that the environment is usually dry. As a result it is easier to keep clothes dry than it is in the cold and wet conditions that predominate at lower altitudes. On the other hand, the presence of high winds at altitude markedly increases the coldness of the environment by increasing the wind chill factor and promoting heat loss by convection to the environment. Many deaths at altitude occur not as a result of fatal falls, but are caused by hypothermia.

Studies show that the ability of the brain to recruit the muscles is regulated by a number of variables including, at increasing altitude, the partial pressure of arterial oxygen which is a direct function of the barometric pressure. Thus, as the barometric pressure falls the brain reduces the mass of muscle that it will allow to be activated during exercise. The end result of this control is to reduce the maximal exercise capacity at altitude specifically to prevent a reduction in the arterial oxygen partial pressure to levels that cannot sustain normal brain function.

Hypoxia

As humans ascend to increasing altitude, they are exposed to a progressively lower partial pressure of oxygen in the inspired air. As a result the partial pressure of oxygen in the blood supplying their brains also falls. Whilst there are a number of physiological adaptations that increase this pressure, ultimately each human will reach an altitude at which they are no longer able to survive, since their blood oxygen pressure falls below that required for those crucial brain functions necessary for sustaining life. Exercise at altitude is also 'limited' by the brain to ensure that no exercise intensity is undertaken that will produce a blood oxygen partial pressure at which unconsciousness develops.

Altitude acclimatization

Acclimatization to altitude can be achieved with a gradual ascent to higher altitudes over a number of days or weeks. The regulator of exercise at altitude appears to be the PaO_2. When the PaO_2 falls below some critical value (different between individuals, perhaps on the basis of genetic factors or the extent of the adaptation to altitude), the brain prevents the continuing recruitment of motor units in the exercising limbs so that exercise must terminate. Effective adaptations to altitude must increase the PaO_2 at any altitude (barometric pressure), maintain higher PaO_2 during exercise, and adapt the brain so that it is able to maintain the recruitment of an appropriate muscle mass at the same or lower PaO_2, without risking brain damage from hypoxia.

Specific adaptations to altitude
- Increase ventilation rate.
- Rise in arterial pH as arterial CO_2 is reduced (due to hyperventilation which drives the reaction ($H^+ + HCO_3^- \rightarrow H_2O + CO_2$) to the right).
- Kidney retention of H^+ compensates for this respiratory alkalosis.
- Increased PaO_2 (due to hyperventilation).
- Increase in blood haemoglobin concentration due to an initial fall in blood volume.
- Increased excretion of erythropoietin by the kidneys in response to the reduction in PaO_2.
- Progressive increases in the red cell mass (for up to 3–12 months) with more prolonged exposures above about 3250m. This is due to increased erythropoietin (EPO) production at altitude.
- Oxygen dissociation curve of haemoglobin shifts to the left, favouring increased haemoglobin oxygen saturation at any PaO_2.
- No change in pulmonary diffusing capacity at moderate altitude, but becomes impaired at very high altitudes.
- Increased pressure in the pulmonary circulation due to pulmonary arteriolar vasoconstriction; develops in proportion to the reduction in PaO_2.
- Potential right ventricular hypertrophy when pulmonary hypertension is sustained.
- Increased cerebral blood flow in response to the reduction in PaO_2. (The extent to which cerebral blood flow increases is limited by the cerebral arteriolar vasoconstriction which occurs in response to the fall in $PaCO_2$ induced by hyperventilation).
- Increased secretion of adrenal cortical hormones and activation of the sympathetic nervous system.
- Increase in the blood concentrations of sodium and water conserving hormones (renin, aldosterone and ADH) especially in response to exercise. These hormones favour increased fluid retention.
- Increased respiratory water losses in response to hyperventilation and the low humidity of the air at altitude.

As a result of these adaptations, exercise performance capacity at altitude improves, but is always less at altitude compared to sea-level.

Altitude sickness
Occurs in about 25% of people acclimatized to moderate altitude on acute exposure to altitudes in excess of about 2500m. In about 5%, symptoms will be sufficiently severe to require bed rest. The incidence of symptoms, including incapacitation requiring bed rest, increases with increasing altitude and may be 100% in those who ascend rapidly to above 3000m. Although acute altitude sickness is usually no more than an illness

of inconvenience, progression to high altitude pulmonary oedema or cerebral oedema can occur. Thus, all persons with the condition must be observed until symptoms disappear.

Symptoms
Symptoms are most intense for the first 48h after arrival at altitude, lessening thereafter and disappearing within 5–8days. Symptoms are worse in the morning, perhaps as a result of increased hypoxaemia during sleep. Headache, insomnia, lassitude, and anorexia are often associated with nausea and vomiting.

Aetiology
Unknown, but may be related to cerebral hypoxia and an increased cerebral blood flow. May also be related to excessive water retention since the condition shows common features with the encephalopathy associated with exercise associated hyponatraemia (EAH), also caused by water intoxication.

Prevention
- Avoid rapid ascension to altitudes above 2000–2500m.
- Ascend slowly with stops at intermediate altitudes.
- Avoid vigorous exercise on the first few days of arrival at altitude. Rather emphasize rest during that period.
- The use of acetazolamide (125–250mg bd) beginning 48h before ascent to altitude and continued for the first 5 days after arrival at altitude is the only proven efficacious medication.
- Low flow oxygen at night may be helpful if available.

Treatment
- Treat mild symptoms with appropriate medications.
- If symptoms progress, oxygen at high flow should be administered.
- If available, a hyperbaric bag can be used.
- If symptoms progress further despite these interventions, urgent evacuation to a lower altitude is essential.
- Descent to a sufficiently low altitude cures the symptoms.

Cerebral/pulmonary oedema

A potentially fatal, but preventable condition that develops rapidly and with little warning in persons unacclimatized to altitude, but who ascend rapidly to altitudes in excess of about 2500m and who, on arrival at altitude, often partake of vigorous exercise. Easier access to high altitudes for unacclimatized mountain climbers, skiers, and trekkers has increased the incidence of the condition with about 20 deaths/yr reported annually around the world.

Aetiology (pulmonary oedema)
Uncertain, but probably involves hypoxic pulmonary arteriolar vasoconstriction with thrombotic obstruction of some parts of the pulmonary vascular bed.
- Over perfusion of non-obstructed capillaries increases capillary shear forces.
- Increased shear forces injure capillaries causing leakage of red cells and protein into the alveoli.
- Individual susceptibility (as repeat attacks occur in some individuals).

Aetiology (cerebral oedema)
Increased cerebral blood flow with capillary damage induces leakage of oedema fluid into the brain.

Symptoms (pulmonary oedema)
- Dyspnoea, cough, weakness, chest tightness, and occasionally haemoptysis, usually within the first 3 days of arrival at altitude.
- In more severe cases, alterations in consciousness may occur.

Symptoms (cerebral oedema)
Symptoms of central nervous system dysfunction including ataxia, headache, lethargy, and irrational behaviour indicate the impending development of high altitude cerebral oedema. Coma indicates the presence of advanced cerebral oedema.

Signs (pulmonary and cerebral oedema)
- Cyanosis, tachycardia, tachypnoea, and pulmonary rates.
- Papilloedema.
- Abnormal reflexes.
- Altered level of consciousness.

Treatment
- Oxygen at high flow rates.
- Use of a hyperbaric bag if available.
- Immediate evacuation to lower altitudes.
- Bed rest, oxygen, and nifedipine should be given at lower altitudes if rapid clinical improvement does not occur.
- Descent to lower altitude cures the condition.
- Deaths usually occur only when the initial diagnosis is delayed; the emergency nature of the condition is not appreciated and descent to lower altitude either does not occur, or occurs too late in the course of the illness.

Overtraining syndrome

History and examination

A condition of fatigue and underperformance that occurs following a period of hard training and competition. It affects mainly endurance athletes. The symptoms do not resolve after 2 weeks adequate rest, and may be associated with frequent infections and depression. No causative medical condition can be identified.

Normal training is usually cyclical (periodization) allowing adequate time for recovery, and with progressive overload to improve performance. During these cycles there may be transient symptoms and signs of overtraining known as over-reaching.

With overtraining syndrome, there may have been a sudden increase in training, prolonged heavy training, and other physical and psychological stresses. Most athletes recover fully after 2 weeks of adequate rest, but the diagnosis of overtraining syndrome is made when the symptoms and signs persist after 2 weeks of relative rest. The main complaint is of underperformance, but there are other associated features:

- Sleep disturbance is common.
- There may be loss of competitive drive, loss of appetite, and increased emotional lability, anxiety, and irritability.
- Athletes may complain of frequent upper respiratory tract infections or other minor infections, sore throats, and lymphadenopathy, myalgia, arthralgia, and heavy legs. The athlete may also report a raised resting heart rate.
- There may be symptoms of depression and reduced concentration. There may be loss of libido.

Clinical examination is frequently normal.
- Cervical lymphadenopathy is common, but non-specific.
- Increased resting heart rate.
- Increased postural fall in BP and postural rise in HR.
- Slow recovery of pulse rate to normal after exercise.
- Reduced sub-maximum oxygen consumption.
- Reduced maximum power output.

Investigations

There is no specific diagnostic test. Clinical investigations exclude other causes of fatigue and reassure the athlete. The basis of this condition is likely to reside in the CNS for which no test has yet been derived.

- *Routine haematological screen:* many athletes have a relatively low Hb and packed cell volume. This athletic anaemia is physiological due to haemodilution and does not affect performance.
- Creatine kinase levels are often high reflecting the intensity, volume, and type of exercise.
- Post-viral illness is confirmed by appropriate viral titres.
- *Stress hormones:* e.g. adrenaline and cortisol are generally higher in over trained athletes compared with controls. A low testosterone: cortisol ratio has also been noted in underperforming athletes.
- Low levels of glutamine have been found in over trained athletes compared to controls.

Treatment

Reassure the athlete that there is no serious pathology and that the prognosis is excellent. The symptoms normally resolve within 6–12 weeks, but can persist if athletes return to intensive training too quickly.

- Relative rest for a minimum period of 6 weeks.
- Exercise aerobically at a pulse rate of 120–140 for a short period each day, depending on the clinical picture and rate of improvement with the emphasis on volume not intensity of exercise.
- Avoid own sport and use cross training to prevent too rapid an increase in exercise intensity.
- Vitamins and supplements are recommended, but there is no evidence that they are effective.

Prevention and monitoring

Athletes tolerate different levels of training, competition, and stress throughout the season. There is no single test to detect overtraining, but athletes can monitor fatigue, muscle soreness, sleep, and perceived exertion during training, and performance. Because it is difficult to predict those athletes who will progress from overreaching to becoming over trained, adequate rest is essential. Training intensity and periodization are the most important factors in minimizing the risk of overtraining. Awareness of the condition and monitoring the response to training may help to prevent overtraining syndrome.

- The profile of mood states (POMS) may be helpful, but is not a reliable diagnostic tool.
- Laboratory investigations are not reliable enough for routine monitoring of athletes.
- Athletes can monitor their heart rate, but this is non-specific.

Chapter 7

Aids to performance

Ergogenic aids *198*
Performance-enhancing drugs *198*
Stimulants *200*
Dietary ergogenic aids *202*
Doping and prohibited drugs *206*
Drug testing *210*

Ergogenic aids

Sports people have long used performance-enhancing substances (or *ergogenic aids*) in an attempt to gain advantage, and many believe that most of their competitors are taking such substances. Media influences, financial rewards, and pressure from coaches, peers, and families can encourage a competitor to attempt to cheat by using drugs or other ergogenic aids. Those using such methods tend to have genuine concerns regarding their own health, but believe that taking the substances increase their chances of being successful.

Apart from supplements and drugs, other examples of ergogenic aids might include:
- Psychology imagery.
- Custom-fitted shoe orthoses.
- Blood or gene doping.
- Some of the pharmaceutical and physiological aids are outlined below.

Performance-enhancing drugs

Anabolic steroids

These are natural or synthetically-made derivatives of the hormone testosterone. Their ergogenic effects are:
- Reduced recovery time after training.
- Increased lean body mass.
- Increased aggression (seen as a benefit in some contact sports).

Anabolic steroids are used orally, as a cream, or injected.

Needle sharing carries risks of HIV, hepatitis B or C, and needle abscesses are seen from contaminated injection sites.

Despite this catalogue of adverse effects, anabolic steroid abuse is still widespread as sports people and bodybuilders risk their health in the pursuit of success. Polypharmacy and massive doses of multiple drugs is common.

Commonly abused steroids include stanozolol, nandrolone, clembuterol, and dihydrotestosterone. Tetrahydrogestrinone, a new synthetic 'designer' steroid, specifically produced to be difficult to detect in urine samples, was discovered in 2003. See Table 7.1 for side effects of anabolic steroid use.

Table 7.1 Side effects of anabolic steroids

Male	Female	Both sexes
Breast enlargement	Male pattern baldness	Acne
Testicular atrophy	Deepening of voice	↑ BP
Sperm count	Enlarged clitoris	↑ LDL/total cholesterol
	↑ Facial hair	↑ Risk of premature ischaemic heart disease/death
	Irregular menses	Liver abnormalities

Erythropoetin

This is a glycoprotein, produced naturally in the body by the kidneys in response to hypoxia. EPO can be prescribed in a recombinant form and is licensed to treat or be used in renal failure, some cancers, and in acquired immune deficiency syndrome (AIDS). It is administered by subcutaneous injection.

Effects of EPO
- EPO exerts a direct effect on bone marrow to increase RBC production, particularly in the presence of iron.
- Hb levels increase so improving aerobic performance by enhanced oxygen-carrying capacity of blood.

Adverse effects
Side effects of EPO include:
- Potential life-threatening thrombosis or embolism.
- Cerebrovascular accidents.
- Seizures and encephalopathy.
- Myocardial infarction.
- Iron overload causing liver or cardiac disease.

Effects similar to using EPO can be obtained by high altitude training, blood doping, and by the use of hypoxic, hypobaric chambers at ground level.

Until 2000, EPO was undetectable. Individual sporting federations, such as cycling and triathlon have instigated blood testing with upper limits of haematocrit levels being deemed as acceptable, leading to an indirect test 'failure'. At present, blood and urine tests are based upon transferrin receptor and ferritin concentrations.

Several sports are now also using 'biological passports' for some athletes that monitor for fluctuations in serial full blood counts over a period of time.

Growth hormone

GH is produced from the anterior pituitary and acts to:
- Increase protein synthesis and fat breakdown.
- Increase hepatic glucose production.
- Stimulate the liver to produce insulin-like growth factor-1 (IGF-1), which helps muscle and bone growth.

GH is now available commercially as a recombinant product, but previously was made from pituitary glands extracted post mortem. This latter process carried a risk of the recipient developing human variant Creutzfeldt Jakob Disease (CJD). GH works synergistically with testosterone. Many of its effects rely on insulin, and the two drugs are often abused in combination. Recently, a seemingly reliable blood test for recombinant GH has allowed its direct measurement. Over-production or over-dosage of GH causes acromegaly, glucose intolerance, and hypertension.

Stimulants

Amphetamines
Sports people have abused amphetamines for over 70yrs and several high profile deaths have been linked to their use. The main ergogenic benefits of amphetamines are:
- Increased awareness and delayed fatigue.
- Enhancement of speed, power, endurance, and concentration.

Adverse effects of amphetamines
- Amphetamines are highly addictive.
- Delirium.
- Paranoia.
- Aggression.
- Risk of cerebral haemorrhage.

Possession and supply of amphetamines in the UK is a criminal offence.

Modafinil
Recently, Modafinil, a stimulant, licensed to treat the familial condition of narcolepsy has become a drug of abuse in sport. The drug is not thought to be performance-enhancing, but there is speculation that its main use is as a masking agent for new 'designer' steroids.

Sympathomimetics
Sympathomimetics are readily available 'over-the-counter' remedies, used as treatments for the common cold. Many of these drugs are not performance-enhancing, but have been abused for years to increase energy.

Adverse effects of sympathomimetics
- Anxiety.
- Agitation.
- Headaches.
- Hypertension.
- Tremor.
- Cardiac arrhythmias and myocardial infarction.

Most of the drugs in this group were removed from the WADA banned list in 2004, although ephedrine remains included. Athletes who require a 'cold cure' should be advised always to check with a doctor before taking any such drug, even if purchased through a pharmacy. Different countries may have the same preparation on sale, but there can be a variance in the constituents which can lead to an inadvertent doping offence particularly when travelling.

Caffeine
- No longer on the WADA banned list of drugs.
- Has been shown to be ergogenic—appears to improve endurance.
- Spares glycogen and, therefore, delays the onset of fatigue.
- Exerts its effect by stimulating adipose tissue to release fatty acids, and also stimulates adrenaline production from the adrenal medulla, so in turn further facilitating fatty acid release.
- Caffeine has also been shown to enhance motor unit recruitment.

Beta-2 adrenoceptor agonists
- Include the drug salbutamol and related compounds.
- Potent treatments used in everyday practice to treat asthma.
- Orally, beta-2 agonists are not permitted in sport.
- No evidence that these drugs, in inhaled form, are ergogenic in the non-asthmatic athlete.
- Salbutamol (up to 1600mcg/day) and Salmeterol are allowable in inhaled form. Other beta-2 agonists require that the sports person has submitted a therapeutic use exemption (TUE), and that the TUE has been approved by their national anti-doping organization or their international governing body.
- TUE must be completed by a doctor, and include a full medical history and findings of a clinical examination, as well as document laboratory evidence proving the diagnosis. The TUE should be sent to the sport's governing body with laboratory evidence confirming the diagnosis of exercise-induced asthma (EIA). In the UK the appropriate body is UK Anti Doping (UKAD)

Tests for exercise-induced asthma
There are two approved bronchoprovocation methods by which sports people with EIA can meet the diagnostic criteria to obtain a TUE:
- Spirometry pre- and post-exercise challenge, showing an increase in airway obstruction, reversed by inhaled beta-2 agonist.
- Eucapnic voluntary hyperpnoea—EVH test: this is used by WADA as the optimal laboratory challenge to confirm EIA. The subject has to hyperventilate dry air containing 5% carbon dioxide for 6 min. An increase in airway obstruction of greater than 10% measured by FEV_1 confirms the diagnosis.

Further reading
Further information is available at: http://www.ukad.org.uk/support-personnel/about-TUE

Dietary ergogenic aids

Problems with ergogenic aids
- Many supplements contain substances that are not contained on the label.
- Many supplements do not contain ingredients in sufficient amounts.
- In the 1990's significant number of athletes tested positive for nandrolone.
- IOC studied risk of contamination and found that in supplements that were tested, out of the 634 products analysed, 15% were found to be contaminated with steroids

IOC Consensus statement, 2003
Athletes are cautioned against the indiscriminate use of dietary supplements. Supplements that provide essential nutrients may be of help where food intake or food choices are restricted, but this approach to achieving adequate nutrient intake is normally only a short-term option. The use of supplements does not compensate for poor food choices and an inadequate diet. Athletes contemplating the use of supplements and sports foods should consider their efficacy, their cost, the risk to health and performance, and the potential for a positive doping test.

Informed sport
- Quality assurance programme run by HFL to provide athletes with an informed choice regarding supplements
- *Never* possible to provide a 100% *guarantee* that any product is absolutely free of contamination.
- Programme certifies products and/or ingredients have been tested for banned substances by an ISO 17025 lab (HFL).
- Only products that are registered with informed sport can bear the logo.[1]

Carbohydrates
- The primary energy source for anaerobic activity.
- Athletic diet should include 55–70% of total calories as carbohydrate, (approximately 5–10g/kg body weight).

Proteins
- Recommended daily intake varies depending on the demands of the sport in which a person participates, with the range between 1.2 and 2g/kg body weight.
- Strength and power athletes tend to require a larger intake than those who undertake endurance exercise.
- Protein supplements are useful to gain strength during conditioning and are used post-exercise to aid recovery.

Dietary supplements
- Widespread use of supplements in sport is controversial.
- Little evidence to support the use of supplements as ergogenic aids.

---

[1] Further information is available at: www.informed-sport.com.

- Risk of contamination of supplements by banned substances is a concern.
- A recent study, found that as many as 19% of supplements produced in a selection of countries contained banned substances that were not mentioned on the product label.

Many high-profile sports stars have blamed their failed drug tests on a contamination of their supplements, taken in good faith. Athletes should be strongly advised to be extremely cautious about the use of these—any supplements taken by an athlete are at their own personal risk of liability.

Creatine monohydrate
- Physiologically active substance needed for muscle contraction.
- Present in the normal diet, particularly in meat.
- Also synthesized in the body (liver, kidneys, and pancreas).
- Increases phosphocreatine production, theoretically increasing the available energy during maximal exercise.
- Studies have found that creatine ingestion can significantly increase exercise performance through the maintenance of force or work output during exercise (especially interval and sprint training programmes).
- Causes weight gain, although this may be due to water retention, rather than muscle mass gain.
- Individuals vary in response to creatine with some not responding at all.

Adverse effects
Include muscle cramps, GI disturbances. Avoid if renal or prostate disease. Long-term health effects are unknown.

Antioxidants
- Vitamins and other compounds that occur naturally in the diet.
- Act to destroy free radicals in the body.
- Free radicals are produced as a by-product of high intensity exercise and increased oxygen consumption, or as part of the normal process of inflammation and tissue healing.
- Free radicals are known to damage DNA and RNA and to destroy important enzymes, and are linked to arteriosclerosis, some cancers, and ageing as well as exercise-associated muscle damage.
- Antioxidants such as beta-carotene (vitamin A pre-cursor), vitamins C and E, selenium, and glutathione all are present in a normal healthy diet, which should contain at least five portions of fruit and vegetables daily. Such a diet is likely to give the athlete their recommended daily allowance (RDA) of vitamins.
- Most commercial multivitamins will also contain ample to satisfy the RDA. The potential benefits of taking a simple multivitamin probably outweigh any risks, but there is not enough evidence to recommend taking supplements to reduce post-exercise muscle damage.

Chromium
- Potentiates insulin action, and therefore cellular glucose and amino acid uptake.
- In theory might produce muscle mass gain, but lack of evidence.
- Also has the potential to induce iron and zinc deficiency, by competition for binding sites and reduced absorption.

Magnesium
- An essential mineral and a co-factor in many enzymatic reactions.
- A typical Western diet may be deficient in magnesium, but as yet supplementation has not been proven to be performance-enhancing.
- Only use if subject has been shown to be magnesium deficient.

L-carnitine
- Detoxifies ammonia, a by-product of metabolism associated with fatigue.
- In theory, muscle glycogen will be spared and fatty acid oxidation increased, but studies are inconclusive.

Beta-hydroxy-beta-methylbutyrate (HMB)
- A bioactive metabolite produced from breakdown of the amino acid leucine.
- May increase fatty acid oxidation and reduce protein loss during stress by inhibiting protein catabolism.
- Used by resistance-trained athletes.

Glutamine
- A non-essential amino acid, which is synthesized in the liver, lungs, adipose tissue, and skeletal muscle.
- Stored in muscle, and is used for immunity, as a fuel for cells, protein synthesis, and to maintain acid-base balance.
- It has been hypothesized that intense exercise can increase demand for glutamine, leading to its depletion and so an increased susceptibility to infection.

Iron
- Athletes may have higher requirements than the general population (training loads, losses in sweat or blood) and vegetarian diet.
- Lack of published evidence to support its use, but it is claimed that glutamine enhances immune cell function in those at risk by undertaking high intensity exercise.

Fish and seed oils
- Athletic diets have tended to be low in these oils, which contain omega-3 oils and essential fatty acids.
- Omega-3 oils are known to have a cardioprotective effect, and it may simply be good advice for general health reasons for an athlete to include oily fish in their diet.

Lactic acid
- A by-product of anaerobic glycloysis, which builds up in muscle and blood during exercise.
- Recently, has been found to also act as a fuel during sub-maximal exercise, particularly by the heart, liver, and kidneys, to generate ATP.
- The liver uses any remaining lactic acid for gluconeogenesis in an attempt to restore glycogen levels and maintain glucose levels.

Sodium bicarbonate
- Neutralizes metabolic acids, including lactic acid.
- Supplementation is said to produce an alkaline reserve, to neutralize the hydrogen ions produced in anaerobic glycloysis and so reduce the onset of fatigue.
- *Adverse effects:* GI upset; urine pH may take hours to return to normal meaning long waits in doping control!

Beta alanine
- May offer an alternative or an addition to bicarbonate loading as an intracellular buffer by increasing carnosine levels.
- 4 weeks supplementation needed for performance effect.
- Main adverse reaction is paraesthesiae which last 5–10min caused by activation of neurons in the skin.

Caffeine
- Shown to produce performance benefits in a wide variety of high intensity and endurance sports.
- Improves reaction time, concentration, and alertness.
- *Adverse effects:* increased HR, poor sleep patterns, over-arousal, headache, tremor, and dieresis

Vitamin D
- Diet contains little vitamin D.
- Sunlight activates endogenous production of vitamin D via skin exposure to UVB. The amount of exposure needed is: arms, hands, face for 20–30min 2–3× per week. Production is reduced with increased melanin in skin, regular SPF >15 screen use, indoor lifestyle.
- Supplementation should contain vitamin D3 (cholecalciferol).

Doping and prohibited drugs

Doping has been defined on many occasions, but the current definition on the WADA website (http://www.wada-ama.org) is:
- The presence of a prohibited substance in an athlete's sample.
- The use or attempted use of a prohibited substance or method.
- Refusal to submit a sample for collection after being notified.
- Failure to submit athletes' whereabouts information and missed tests.
- The tampering with any part of the doping control process.
- The possession of a prohibited substance or method.
- The trafficking of a prohibited substance or method.
- Administering or attempting to administer to an athlete prohibited substance or method.

Brief history
- *1968:* drug testing first started at Grenoble Winter Olympics.
- *1974:* semi-reliable tests for anabolic steroids became available.
- *1976:* 8 athletes tested positive for anabolic steroids. Rumours were rife of widespread use by athletes and swimmers despite the small number of positive tests.
- *1983:* urine test developed to determine the ratio between testosterone and epitestosterone. These isomers usually exist in the body in a 1:1 ratio, so any exogenous testosterone taken would alter this. A ratio of 6:1 implies suspicion that an athlete has taken an anabolic steroid, although 10:1 is more likely to produce a 'guilty' verdict in a court of law. Exogenous epitestosterone has also been abused in an attempt to mask any changes in the ratio caused by taking anabolic steroids.

World Anti-Doping Agency

The banned list is no longer operated by the International Olympic Committee, and responsibility has passed to WADA, established in 1999 after the World Conference on Doping in Sport in Lausanne recognized the need for an independent agency. The aims of WADA are to set unified standards for anti-doping work and to co-ordinate efforts against doping, seeking to foster a drug-free culture in sport.

Out-of-competition testing is conducted by independent parties and in 2003, the World Anti-Doping Code was accepted and most sports have now agreed to implement the code. This code was revised in 2009. In the UK, UK Ant-Doping (UKAD) was set up in December 2009 and is responsible for drug testing and education. UKAD fully supports WADA and the code.

Anti-Doping Administration and Management System (ADAMS)

ADAMS has four Web-based primary functions
- *Athlete whereabouts:* allows athletes to enter information from anywhere in the world. Shares whereabouts information; athletes can also modify their whereabouts by sending SMS messages.
- *Information clearing house:* all data is stored, including laboratory results, TUE authorizations and anti-doping rule violations. Permits sharing of

information among relevant organizations. Allows anti-doping activities to be performed with highest level of transparency.
- *Doping control planning:* the ADAMS doping control database provided to Anti-Doping Organizations (ADOs) is an essential tool for managing both an in- and out-of-competition doping control program. Stakeholders can use ADAMS to plan, co-ordinate and order tests, as well as manage test results. Coordination of doping control programmes in the ADAMS system helps to avoid duplication of testing efforts.
- TUE management

Where can the banned list be seen?
The Prohibited List is available online at the WADA website, along with educational pages: ℘ http://list.wada-ama.org.

Important note
It must be stressed that it is the athletes' responsibility to adhere to WADA regulations and that ignorance is not considered a defence.

Outline of the banned classes of drugs
Substances and methods banned at all times
Non-approved substances
Any pharmacological substance that is not addressed by any of the subsequent sections of the List and with no current approval by any governmental regulatory health authority for human therapeutic use (i.e. drugs under preclinical, or clinical development, or discontinued) is prohibited at all times.

Anabolic steroids
Testosterone derivatives and related compounds.

Peptide hormones and analogues
- Erythropoetin.
- Growth hormone.
- Insulin.
- HCG.

Beta-2 agonists
- Oral use *not* permitted.
- All are prohibited except inhaled salbutamol and Salmeterol.

Anti-oestrogens (banned in males only)
- Tamoxifen.
- Clomiphene.

Masking agents
- Probenecid.
- Diuretics.
- Epitestosterone.

Prohibited methods
- Blood doping.
- Chemical manipulation.

- Self-catheterization.
- Gene doping

Substances and methods banned in competition only
Stimulants
- Amphetamines and related drugs.
- Epinephrine and related drugs.
- Ephedrine.
- Cocaine.
- Methylexaneamine: a legitimate medicine until 1970's, in 2010 started appearing in supplements and has been subject to inadvertent use by athletes

Narcotics
Morphine and related drugs—note that codeine is not banned.

Cannabinoids
Hashish and marijuana banned in competition.

Glucocorticosteroids
These drugs are banned orally, rectally, IV, or IM, although exemptions for genuine medical illness on production of evidence may be granted.

Prohibited in certain sports
- Alcohol.
- Beta-blockers (shooting, archery).

Advice to doctors prescribing for athletes

Doctors who prescribe for sports people who may be liable for drug testing must be aware of the banned list of substances. Most doctors will be able to access Internet resources and a valuable site is the UK Sport Drug Information Database, available at: www.globaldro.com.

This site will allow almost any drug, bought anywhere in the world, to be identified and classified as either permitted, restricted, or banned. The advice is also sport-specific and can be printed out for safekeeping. Although the athlete is ultimately responsible for whatever substance is found on drug testing, incorrect prescribing by a sports doctor is a potential medico-legal issue.

If in doubt do not prescribe!

Blood doping

Blood doping occurred more commonly in the 1970s and 1980s than now, and the need for this practice has been largely superseded by the abuse of erythropoetin. Blood doping was banned by the International Olympic Committee (IOC) in 1986 and involved the IV transfusion of blood into an individual in order to increase red cell mass and therefore improved oxygen carrying capacity. In many cases, autologous transfusions were used, which involved taking two units of blood from an athlete, 6 weeks prior to competition (often whilst training at altitude), then re-infusing the blood on the day before competition. It is reported that this process could increase an individual's haematocrit by 5–10%.

Gene doping

The future of doping seems certain to involve genetic manipulation. WADA defines gene doping as 'the non-therapeutic use of genes, genetic elements, or of the modulation of gene expressions, having the capacity to improve athletic performance'. Gene therapy is already used to treat muscular dystrophies, and experiments in mice show that genetic manipulation can increase muscle mass by 25%. The modified gene works via insulin-like growth factor 1 (IGF-1) to increase muscle cell division. The gene is attached to an inert virus, causing 'infection' in muscle cells, but no disease process in the host. Scientists are currently working on tests to detect gene doping.

Drug testing

Random out-of-competition testing started in the UK in 1981. Its aims were to deter athletes from gaining an unfair advantage, to catch athletes who had taken performance-enhancing substances, and to remind them of the regulations and the inadvertent use of banned substances.

Testing procedure (from UKAD guide to drug testing procedures)

- At an event, during training, or at an out-of-competition location, athlete is notified of selection for a drug test, using an official sample collection form. Once informed, the athlete must stay in full view of the Doping Control Officer (DCO). World-class athletes in the UK's registered testing pool are required to be available for testing anytime, anywhere and must be prepared to provide a sample when notified.
- Athlete is required to report to doping control station as soon as possible and no later than one hour after notification. Sealed non-alcoholic drinks are available. Privacy and integrity should be maintained.
- Athlete will be asked to select a sealed sample collection vessel. This collection vessel must be kept in sight at all times.
- Athlete provides a sample of urine observed directly by the DCO, in order to avoid any manipulation of the sample.
- Athlete selects a sealed urine sampling kit from a choice of such kits stored in tamper-evident packaging. The security seal should be intact.
- Athlete divides the sample between two bottles, labelled A and B, which are then tightly sealed (by the athlete). A small residual amount of urine is left in the collection vessel to enable testing of pH and specific gravity. The athlete should then invert the sealed sampling bottles to ensure that there are no leaks.
- If pH or specific gravity is outside the required limits, this is recorded on the sample collection form.
- DCO records the A and B sample numbers on the sample collection form, and the athlete is asked to declare any medications, substances, or supplements taken in the past 7 days. Athlete then checks that all information on the sample collection form is correct and, together with the DCO, signs the form. The athlete is given a copy of the signed form.

Drug test result reporting

Negative result
In the UK, following analysis of the A sample, the result is reported to UKAD, and after processing this is passed to the relevant authority, who will notify the athlete.

Positive result
If a prohibited substance is found in the A sample, UKAD is notified of the finding. After confirmation of the accuracy of supporting documentation and supporting evidence has been confirmed, the relevant authority will notify the athlete of the result. The athlete may be suspended from competition at this point and will be invited to explain the finding. The athlete may challenge the A sample finding, and is entitled to be present at the

analysis of the B sample. If this second test confirms the A sample result, the athlete must attend a disciplinary panel, which may decide on a suspension, or, in some cases, a lifetime ban from competition. The athlete may appeal against any decision reached.

Blood testing

Blood testing is used in some sports to check for unusual blood profiles, such as an elevated haematocrit, using much of the same procedure as outlined for urine testing, apart from the DCO taking blood by venepuncture, rather than observing the passage of a urine sample.

Chapter 8

Disability

What is a disability? *214*
Physical activity recommendations *214*
Organization of sport for people with disabilities *216*
Technology *218*
Classification *219*
Disability groups *220*
Elite sport talent identification and profiling *224*
Thermoregulation *224*
Travel issues *225*
'Boosting' *225*
Doping issues *226*
Useful resources and further reading *226*

What is a disability?

The Disability Discrimination Act of 1995 defines it as 'physical or mental impairment which has a substantial and long-term adverse effect on his ability to carry out normal day-to-day activities.'

Sport and disability evolution

Sport for people with disabilities evolved rapidly over the last century, from an archery tournament at Stoke Mandeville hospital on the opening day of the Olympic Games in London in 1948, to 4000 athletes from over 146 countries competing at the Beijing 2008 Paralympic Games in 20 different sports.

Reasons for increased participation

- Increased acceptance of rights of people with disabilities within society, e.g. Disability Discrimination Act 1995.
- Increased recognition of sporting capability of people with disabilities:
  - High jump >2m by a single leg amputee.
  - Wheelchair marathon time below 1h 30min.
- Increasing recognition of importance of physical activity for health for all the population, including those with a disability, e.g. reduced healthcare costs for active paraplegics vs. sedentary paraplegics.

Physical activity recommendations

How much activity?

- The accumulation of at least 30min of moderate intensity activity on most days of the week and at least five days of the week is equally applicable to someone with a disability.[1]
- The same principles of training apply, i.e. the graded increase induration, intensity, and frequency of activity.
- More thought may be required as to the mode of exercise according to the disability.
- The social and psychological benefits of exercise and sport participation.
- Major improvements in self-esteem and social integration may occur through an active lifestyle.

Advice on choosing a sport/exercise

It is important to try and marry the potential benefits of exercise participation and enjoyment for maximizing long-term increases in physical activity behaviour, with various aspects of the individual's disability.

- *Personal preference of the individual:* important for adherence
- *Characteristics of the sport:*
  - *Physiological demands,* e.g. aerobic, anaerobic.
  - *Collision potential*—increased risk of injury, e.g. osteopenic limbs in paraplegia.

---

[1] Department of Health (2004). *At Least Five a Week—Evidence of the Impact of Physical Activity and Its Relationship to Health*, A report from the Chief Medical Officer. London: DoH.

- *Team or individual*—preference of individual, social interaction.
- *Co-ordination requirements*—e.g. tremor or ataxia would limit performance in some sports.
- *Potential effects of the medical condition:*
  - *Beneficial aspects*—e.g. cardiovascular disease (CVD) risk reduction, improved bone density.
  - *Detrimental*—e.g. excess cardiac risk in high intensity sport where a cardiac defect is present, fracture risk.
- Conditions associated with the condition, e.g. syndromic conditions may have physical limitations to sport participation, but may have other associated medical issues that need consideration, e.g. Down's syndrome, and cardiac anomalies or atlanto-axial instability.
- *Cognitive ability*: impaired cognition may limit participation in certain activities or reduce safety.
- *Social skills of the person:* ability to follow rules and interact with others.
- Availability of facilities in the locality.
- Availability of appropriate coaching and support staff (e.g. lifting and handling).
- Equipment availability and cost.

Barriers to physical activity
- Cultural.
- Medical or parental over-protection.
- Social factors.
- Lack of opportunity during education.
- Facilities.
- Accessibility.

Organization of sport for people with disabilities

Disabilities may be physical, sensory, or intellectual or a combination of each of these. There are consequently a large number of organizations that promote and support sport for people with disabilities.

These organizations may be:
- Local.
- Regional.
- National.
- International.
- Disability specific.
- Multi-disability.
- Encouraging participation.
- Elite sport.

The International Paralympic Committee (IPC)

The IPC unites these disability-specific organizations globally with the exception of the hearing impaired. The hearing-impaired hold a games termed the 'deaflympics' every 4yr and this is held in a non-Olympic Games year. The Paralympic Games involves sport at the elite level and is held just after, and in the same city as, the Olympic Games for the following disability groups:
- Spinal cord-related disability.
- Amputee.
- Visually impaired (VI).
- Cerebral palsy (CeP).
- Les Autres: other physical disabilities not falling into the other categories, e.g. muscular dystrophy, multiple sclerosis.
- Intellectual disability (or learning disability).

Sports

People with disabilities can take part in most sports and activities but the number of sports in summer Paralympic Games is limited to the following:
- Archery.
- Athletics.
- Boccia.
- Cycling.
- Equestrian.
- Football 5-a-side.
- Football 7-a-side.
- Goalball.
- Judo.
- Powerlifting.
- Rowing.
- Sailing.
- Shooting.
- Swimming.
- Table Tennis.
- Volleyball (sitting).

- Wheelchair basketball.
- Wheelchair fencing.
- Wheelchair rugby.
- Wheelchair tennis.

There are also Winter Paralympic Games with Alpine and Nordic events as well as wheelchair curling and sledge hockey—a form of ice hockey using a seated sledge.

The Special Olympics is a separate event that involves people with intellectual disability with less emphasis on elite performance and more on participation.

Technology

Wheelchair design
Initially, people with disabilities took part in sports or activities using a standard wheelchair, but became increasingly frustrated at the lack of performance capability and needs for the specific sport. As a result sport-specific chairs developed. Racing chairs owe much of their design to cycle technology, and are ergonomically designed and individually customized for the user. Wheelchair tennis and basketball chairs have a much larger wheel camber to facilitate rapid turning, and may have a rear wheel to prevent tipping over. Rugby chairs have fenders and guards for attacking and defensive manoeuvres. New technological developments will occur to meet the needs of wheelchair users over time to enhance performance.

Prostheses
People are unable to run using the traditional single-axis prosthetic foot as they cannot push off from the foot flat position. To improve function and reduce fatigue an energy-storing, spring action prosthetic foot can be used to simulate normal gait. As the athlete lands on the prosthetic limb energy is stored and released back on push-off much in the same way as the normal Achilles tendon would. Computer-controlled knees for above knee amputees can produce automatic swing-phase adjustments relevant to their activity level.

Classification

To enable athletes to compete on an equal basis relative to their impairment, athletes are classified into groups for competition. In some sports this is disability-specific groups, e.g. cerebral palsy or spinal injury. In other sports, such as swimming, a functional classification system is used so swimmers with different disabilities compete against each other based upon physical disability and functional performance of the sport. The process is not always straightforward and many medical tests are open to subjective interpretation. Classification for intellectual disability has been particularly problematic, but competition in limited events will be re-introduced in London 2012. There are 'minimum disability' criteria within a sport for a person to become eligible to participate in competitive sport.

Disability groups

Spinal cord-related disability
This may be congenital, e.g. spina bifida, or acquired, e.g. trauma or disease. Of the spinally injured 60% are in the 16–30 age group with a male to female ratio of 4:1. The majority of these are from road traffic accidents with about 15% occurring in sport. Common activities include diving, rugby, horse riding, and skiing. The injuries can be divided by the level of neurological loss and whether the lesion is complete or partial (incomplete paralysis).

The spinal injury results in a number of problems:
- *Motor loss:* loss of muscle function relating to the level of injury.
- *Sensory loss:* increasing the risk of pressure sore.
- *Loss of autonomic control:* e.g. sweating affecting thermoregulation (see later).
- *Effects on cardiac function in exercise:* sympathectomized myocardium in higher spinal lesions gives reduced HR max of 110–130beats/min. There is limited:
  - Cardio-acceleration.
  - Myocardial contractility.
  - Stroke volume.
  - Cardiac output.
- *Respiratory function:* loss of intercostal muscle function.
- Recurrent urinary tract infection (UTI) from a neuropathic bladder.

Amputee or limb deficiency
This may be congenital, e.g. developmental or acquired. Acquired lesions are usually due to:
- *Disease:* e.g. tumour, vascular disease.
- *Trauma:* road traffic accident (RTA), workplace injury.

An athlete with a limb deficiency may compete:
- With a prosthesis, e.g. running.
- Without a prosthesis, e.g. swimming, high jump.
- In a wheelchair, e.g. tennis, basketball.

The fitting and alignment of the prosthesis is important for both function and reducing the risk of musculoskeletal injury. Impact injury or skin chafing of the residual limb are common problems. The leg length discrepancy necessary to allow the toe of the prosthetic limb to clear the ground on swing through may cause problems further up the kinetic chain producing hip, pelvic, or back pain.

Cerebral palsy
CeP is a group of disorders affecting body movement and muscle co-ordination, and is due to an insult or anomaly of the developing brain. Any damage to the developing brain, whether caused by genetic or developmental disorders, injury, or disease may result in CeP. It may be classified according to the number of limbs affected (see Fig. 8.1) and/or by the type of movement disorder.
- *Spastic CeP:* is the most common type and is caused by damage to the motor cortex. Spastic muscles are tight and stiff, which limit movement.

- *Choreo-athetoid CeP*: results from damage to the basal ganglia or cerebellum, and leads to difficulty in controlling and co-ordinating movement.
- *Mixed-type CeP*: when areas of the brain affecting both muscle tone and voluntary movement are affected.

The classifications of movement disorder and number of limbs involved are usually combined (e.g. spastic diplegia). Athletes with CeP may also commonly have associated problems:
- Epilepsy.
- Visual defects.
- Deafness.
- Intellectual impairment.

Approximately half of athletes with CeP compete in wheelchairs. The spasticity associated with the condition may be important for function, and without that tone the athlete may not be able to stabilize their trunk. Hence, the normal practice of stretching pre-exercise may not be appropriate for all athletes with CeP. Maintaining range of movement with flexibility exercises is important, but may not be appropriate immediately prior to competition.

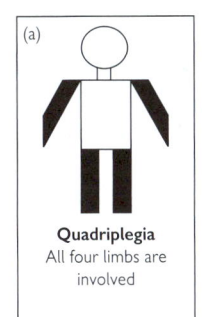

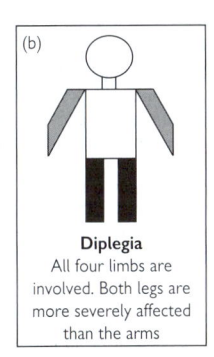

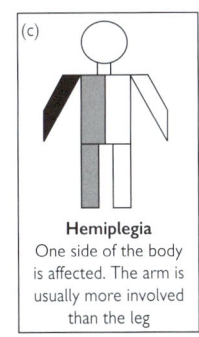

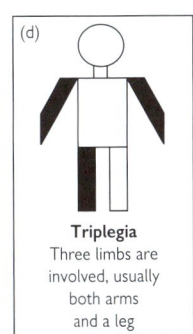

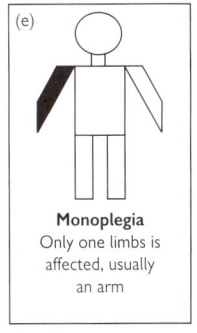

(a) **Quadriplegia** — All four limbs are involved

(b) **Diplegia** — All four limbs are involved. Both legs are more severely affected than the arms

(c) **Hemiplegia** — One side of the body is affected. The arm is usually more involved than the leg

(d) **Triplegia** — Three limbs are involved, usually both arms and a leg

(e) **Monoplegia** — Only one limbs is affected, usually an arm

Fig. 8.1 Classification of cerebral palsy.

Visually-impaired

Visually-impaired athletes are classified by ophthalmology examination and the classification reflects both visual acuity and field of vision.

- *B1:* from no light perception in either eye, but inability to recognize the orientation of a 100M Single Tumbling E target (height: 145mm) at a distance of 250mm (STE LogMAR: 2.6).
- *B2:* from being able to recognize the orientation of a 100M Single Tumbling E target (height: 145mm) at a distance of 25cm (STE LogMAR: 1.6) to being unable to recognize the orientation of a 40M Single Tumbling E target (height: 58mm) at a distance of 1m, and/or a visual field constricted to a diameter of less than 10°.
- *B3:* from being able to recognize the orientation of a 40M Single Tumbling E target (height: 58mm) at a distance of 1m (STE LogMAR: 1.6) to having a visual acuity of less than LogMAR: 1.00 (6/60) when with an ETDRS chart or other LogMAR chart presented at a distance of 1m or Class.
- All classifications must be made by measuring the best eye and to the highest possible correction. This means that all athletes who use contact lenses or correcting glasses normally must wear them during classification, whether or not they intend to use them during competition.

Sports for the visually-impaired include athletics, judo, and swimming. In cycling, a sighted pilot rider is used on a tandem. Guide runners may be used in athletics where a tie or band is used to link a sighted runner to the athlete. The guide runner cannot run in advance of the athlete and 'pull' them along; doing so brings disqualification for the athlete. In bi-athlon the skier will follow a guide skier and use a rifle that produces a high tone when aimed at the centre of the target for the shooting component of the event. Injuries in visually-impaired athletes often occur following falls, collisions, or misplaced footing.

Les autres

This group encompasses a variety of physical disabilities that does not fit easily within a specific category and encompasses a number of conditions such as:

- Congenital disorders: e.g. spondyloepiphyseal dysplasia, Stickler syndrome.
- Limb deficiencies.
- Muscular dystrophies.
- Multiple sclerosis.
- Arthritis of major joints.

The variety of conditions and in particular the variety of rare syndromes encountered in disability sport makes care of these athletes a challenge for the physician.

Intellectual disability

These athletes are largely able-bodied unless the disability results from, e.g. a head injury where there may be physical changes also. As such, they are susceptible to the same sport-related injuries as able-bodied athletes. However, the challenge for the treating doctor is in taking the history and then explaining the diagnosis and management of the condition and supervising the rehabilitation. Training errors are more common and correcting technical problems may be more difficult. Athletes with an intellectual disability may be over keen to please their coach in training and may be susceptible to abusive practices. The duties of care issues are important with these athletes.

Elite sport talent identification and profiling

In able-bodied sport there is a large body of scientific evidence, and profiles of the physical characteristics of the elite athlete help identify the future champions by talent identification. Although elite disability sport is gaining more credibility worldwide, there is still a shortage of research and documentation of these athletes' performance capabilities that makes talent identification and profiling more difficult. This is compounded by:
- Multiple disability groups that may take part within a single sport.
- Wide range of abilities within the same disability, e.g. different levels of spinal injury.
- Different physiological responses to exercise, e.g. paraplegics vs. quadriplegics.
- More research exists for rehabilitation and/or exercise therapy rather than performance-related sport.
- Limited exposure to good quality coaching.

Injury issues

The literature is limited in data on the epidemiology of injuries in disability sport, but it is clear there are different aspects:
- Sport-specific injuries similar to able-bodied athletes, e.g. shoulder injuries in swimmers or throwers.
- Disability sport-related injuries to technical or training factors—wrist injuries from repetitive pushing of the chair, e.g. causing nerve compression injuries.
- Disability related injuries, e.g. existing spinal injury aggravated by repetitive strain of training, skin abrasions from rubbing of the chair on skin without pain sensation, osteoporotic fractures from minimal trauma.

Thermoregulation

The spinally-injured athlete has impaired thermoregulation, which may impair performance or increase the risk of heat illness. There are several factors contributing to this:
- Loss of peripheral receptor mechanism function.
- Loss of autonomic control on the sweating effector mechanism.
- Loss of control of the ability to appropriately vasoconstrict or vasodilate the peripheral vasculature.

Cold conditions may also adversely affect the spinally-injured athlete—as there is impaired perception of temperature the athlete can become hypothermic without feeling symptoms before an adverse reaction occurs. Precautions regarding wearing appropriate clothing should be taken and a vigilance to consider the possibility of hypothermia developing.

Travel issues

The international nature of disability sport now means that many athletes will face long-haul travel on a regular basis. In addition to the problems of travel fatigue, deep vein thrombosis (DVT), and jet lag there can be additional problems that can occur of which the accompanying physician should be aware:

- *Skin breakdown of skin pressure areas:* prolonged sitting in airline seats.
- *Dehydration:* increasing the risk of exacerbations of urinary tract infections.
- *Dependent oedema:* occurs frequently in long haul travel but is worse when there is no active muscle pump.
- *DVT:* there is no evidence that the incidence of DVT is increased for someone with a disability than an able-bodied person.
- *Autonomic dysreflexia:* is an exaggerated autonomic response caused by a painful stimulus below the level of the spinal lesion, resulting in high blood pressure that occurs in people with high spinal cord injuries (thoracic level 6 and above). It can cause seizures, cerebral haemorrhage, and death. The stimulus may come from prolonged seating in an uncomfortable position and may occur during travel.
- *Medications:* the timing of taking medications, e.g. anticonvulsants needs to be assessed for athletes crossing multiple time zones.

'Boosting'

Some athletes have intentionally-induced the state of autonomic dysreflexia as they found that they had reduced perception of effort during exercise, allowing them to push harder and faster than otherwise. Methods to induce this state may include applying tight straps to the legs or clamping the urinary catheter to distend the bladder. Because of the medical dangers of inducing this response it was originally banned as a 'doping method' by the IPC, but is deemed to be a medical safety issue, rather than doping. Athletes can have their BP taken during the pre-race period and may be withdrawn from competition if the pressure is above 180mmHg systolic on the grounds of medical safety.

Doping issues

The IPC is a signatory of the world anti-doping code and, as such, the list of substances prohibited by the code is the same as for able-bodied athletes. Athletes with disabilities are more likely to be taking medications for medical conditions as a result of their disability, but the same rules apply for therapeutic use exemption (TUE) where an athlete can apply to take medication on the prohibited list for a specific reason. TUE requires that:
- The athlete would experience a significant impairment in health if the substance were withdrawn.
- The substance would produce no additional enhancement of performance.
- There is no reasonable therapeutic alternative.

Other differences in doping regulations or procedures include:
- Sample collection procedures differ where catheter or condom/leg bag urine collection is used.
- Visually impaired and intellectually impaired athletes need to be accompanied by a representative during the procedure.

Useful resources and further reading

Cerebral Palsy International Sport and Recreation Association (CP-ISRA). Available at: www.cpisra.org

Comité International Sports des Sourds (CISS). Available at: www.ciss.org

Fallon KE. (1995). The disabled athlete. In: Bloomfield J, Fricker PA, Fitch KD *Science and medicine in sport* (pp. 550–51). Oxford: Blackwell Science, Carlton.

International Blind Sport Federation (IBSA). Available at: www.ibsa.es

International Paralympic Committee. Available at: www.paralympics.org

International Sports Federation for Persons with Intellectual Disability (INAS-FID). Available at: www.inas-fid.org

Webborn N. (2009). In: Caine D, Harmer P, Schiff M. (eds) *Paralympic Sport in Epidemiology of Injury in Olympic Sports*, Volume XVI of *The Encyclopedia of Sports Medicine*, An IOC Medical Commission Publication. Oxford: Blackwell Publishing.

Webborn N. (2010). The travelling athlete. In: Goosey-Tolfrey V. (ed.), *Wheelchair Sports* (pp. 87–98). London: Human Kinetics.

Webborn N. (2011). In: Speed C, Hutson M. (eds) *Disability Sports in Sports Injury*. Oxford: Oxford University Press.

Webborn N, Willick S. (2010). Sports medicine. In: Vanlandewijck Y. (ed.) *The Handbook of Paralympic Sports. The Encyclopedia of Sports Medicine*. An IOC Medical Commission Publication. Oxford: Blackwell Publishing.

Chapter 9

Arthritis

Osteoarthritis 228
Osteoarthritis: management 236
Inflammatory arthritis 240
Investigations 242
The acute hot joint 246
Inflammatory arthritis: management 248
Rheumatoid arthritis 252
Crystal arthropathy 254
Seronegative arthritides 256
Miscellaneous conditions 257

Osteoarthritis

The term osteoarthritis (OA) refers to a heterogenous group of conditions with similar pathological and clinical features. OA is the most common cause of disability amongst adult populations and exists radiographically in more than 80% of those aged over 75. The association between exercise and OA starts with the well-documented association between OA and joint injury, and ends with the evidence that patients with OA benefit from exercise therapy.

Definition

Historically arthritic disorders were divided into atrophic and hypertrophic disorders. The hypertrophic group are synonymous with what we think of as OA, the atrophic disorders referring to inflammatory arthropathies.

The American College of Rheumatology defines OA as a 'heterogenous group of conditions that lead to joint symptoms and signs which are associated with defective integrity of articular cartilage, in addition to related changes in the underlying bone at the joint margins'. In simple terms, OA can be thought of as representing age-related joint changes that reflect joint insult or injury. In essence the clinical and pathological consequences of OA are caused by attempted (possibly failed) repair following joint failure (injury).

Prevalence

Hand OA occurs most frequently (75% of women aged 60–70 years). Knee OA occurs in 30% of those over 75, and is more common in females with female:male ratios between 1.5 and 4. Not as common as hand OA, but the most significant cause of disability in elderly populations. Hip OA, least common of the 'big three', probably occurs equally in men and women, although some studies suggest a male excess.

Pathogenesis

The aetiology of OA remains obscure, but it is likely that a combination of local and systemic risk factors are responsible for the structural features and that these, certainly as far as symptom reporting is concerned, are variably influenced by central neurological factors. The importance of individual risk factors on the risk of developing OA will vary from individual to individual and joint to joint, and will partly reflect the interaction between risk factors, e.g. menisectomy is a well-known local risk factor for knee OA, but is more likely in those with generalized OA.

Local risk factors

The most important individual local risk factor is joint injury, which may occur in a number of ways including:
- Joint fracture.
- Chondral fracture.
- Ligament tear, e.g. cruciate.
- Meniscal injury.
- Developmental injury, e.g. slipped femoral epiphysis.

The most prevalent example of trauma causing OA is the relationship between knee OA, cruciate ligament rupture, and meniscal tear. The risk increases with advanced age, time since injury, and any background hereditary predisposition.

In global terms, however, altered joint biomechanics play an important role and repetitive 'micro-injury' may be a result of a number of factors that may or may not be a consequence of traumatic injury:
- Joint laxity.
- Joint malalignment.
- Muscle weakness.
- Joint shape, e.g. dysplastic developmental abnormalities.

Joint shape
The shape of the hip and knee joint predispose to OA. The most obvious example in is someone with developmental abnormalities, e.g. Perthes' disease, slipped femoral epiphysis or joint dysplasia (e.g. acetabular) predisposing to hip OA. It is probable that some normal variants of joint development contribute to the risk of OA. Premature hip OA in runners may be associated with the so called 'bullet' shaped appearance of the femoral head.

Systemic risk factors
A number of constitutional or generalized risk factors may predispose to OA. The most important of these in impact terms is probably heritability, however, in terms of reversibility, the lifestyle, and environmental factors listed below achieve greater importance.

Heritability
Strong heritability has been demonstrated for OA of the hand, knee, hip, and spine. This susceptibility probably results from multiple unidentified genes, but individual genetic abnormalities may cause OA, e.g. abnormalities of the *Col2A1* gene predispose to premature widespread OA.

Age
Stating the obvious, but age is clearly an important risk factor for OA—the older you are the more likely you are to have OA joints.

Obesity
Obesity is associated with knee OA, there is still debate about its association with hip and hand OA. There appears to be a linear relationship between BMI and the risk of knee OA. Furthermore, the prognosis of knee OA, once developed, is worse in patients with a higher BMI.

Gender
OA affecting the hand and knee is more prevalent in females, although the exact explanation for this has yet to be confirmed. It has been suggested that female sex hormones modify chondrocyte function.

Occupation
Repetitive activity in work has been shown to increase the risk of OA. Examples of this are:
- Increased OA in the dominant or non-paretic hand.
- Knee OA in manual workers, especially those whose work requires prolonged kneeling or squatting. Knee OA has been approved for industrial compensation in coal miners.
- Hip OA in agricultural workers, possibly related to heavy lifting and walking on uneven ground. Again, industrial compensation has been approved.

Exercise and sport
Joint movement is essential for normal joint health. There is no evidence that exercise is damaging to a healthy joint. However, significant injury to a joint, e.g. meniscal tear, which may have been sustained through exercise, does predispose that joint to premature OA. Exercise, in particular excessive loading of a damaged joint, almost certainly further increases the risk of OA, although what constitutes excessive loading is unknown. Debate also exists as to whether subtle alterations to biomechanics when exposed to excessive loading, as might be seen in endurance runners, predisposes to OA. Even if a certain form of exercise does predispose a susceptible individual to OA, the well documented benefits of exercise would have to be considered against any perceived risk.

Hypermobility
Hypermobility is found in normal healthy populations, as well as being a feature of certain inherited conditions, e.g. Ehlers-Danlos. It is uncertain to what effect joint mobility has on the risk of OA.

Bone density
High bone density, while helpful in reducing fracture risk, is associated with OA at the hip and knee.

Smoking
Smoking seems to have a protective effect, not that anyone would advocate this as a preventative strategy.

Systemic illness
In addition to the above factors, a number of systemic conditions are associated with OA, e.g.:
- *Haemochromatosis:* iron overload. Worth checking ferritin levels in younger individuals with OA, especially if associated with calcium pyrophosphate deposition (chondrocalcinosis).
- Acromegaly.
- Ochronosis.

History
The typical features of any joint pathology—pain, stiffness, swelling, and loss of function—hold true for OA. In addition, patients frequently complain of instability and crepitus.

Pain
Pain is the most important symptom of OA. Typically, pain is activity-related, but with variations on a weekly if not daily basis. The nature and severity of pain is poorly-correlated with radiographic features of OA, but is associated with female gender, evidence of psychological distress, and affected joint. Patients are most likely to complain of hip pain and least likely to complain of hand pain for any given severity of X-ray change. Rest and night pain is usually indicative of more severe OA.

OA joint pain is multifactorial and may be influenced by the following physical factors in addition to the psychological factors:
- Altered biomechanics due to structural change, e.g. osteophytes.
- Bone pain possibly related to raised IO pressure.

- Synovitis: mild synovitis is common. Occasionally patients will present with severe flares of pain related to significant inflammation—sometimes related to the presence of calcium pyrophosphate crystals (pseudogout).
- Secondary pain from other structures, e.g. bursitis, tendinopathy.
- Referred muscular pain, usually involving muscles directly responsible for joint movement.

Examination

The osteoarthritic joint will vary in its appearance depending on the severity. You should assess the joint for the following generic signs:
- Functional movement patterns, e.g. gait.
- Appearance (standing and at rest):
  - Deformity.
  - Wasting.
  - Swelling (bony and soft tissue/joint effusion).
  - Scars.
- Active and passive ROM:
  - Pain.
  - Tenderness.
  - Crepitus.
- *Palpation:* palpation may be least useful, however, it does help identify those patients with generalized tenderness, rather than specific joint tenderness. The former usually have a functional element to their symptoms with evidence of psychological distress.
- *Related joints:* you will have been taught to examine the joints above and below the painful joint because of the tendency for joint pain to refer, e.g. it is not uncommon for hip OA to present with knee pain. Referred pain is not always as simple as joint above and below, and further you should look for evidence of a more generalized arthropathy.
- Assess *joint function:* e.g. gait for lower limb joints, manual function for hand joints.

Hand osteoarthritis

- More common in women.
- Peak incidence in middle age.
- Predominantly affects distal interphalangeal (DIP) joint and 1st carpometacarpal (CMC) joint (base of thumb).
- DIP joint involvement thought to be attributable to stress through these joints. CMC involvement due to ligament (and thereby joint) instability.
- Metacarpophalangeal (MCP) joint involvement unusual. If present consider traumatic cause, e.g. previous fracture.
- Involvement of 2nd and 3rd MCP (usually symmetrically) a feature of chondrocalcinosis, consider haemachromatosis.

Knee osteoarthritis

Knee OA commonly affects athletes (or ex-athletes) because of its association with joint injury:
- Three major joint compartments, which can alone or in combination, be affected by OA (medial and lateral tibiofemoral and patellofemoral).
- Strongly associated with previous injury to cruciates or menisci.
- Medial compartment takes greatest load during activity. In flexion patellofemoral joint may take over twice the load of tibiofemoral joint. Medial tibial plateau and lateral patella facet therefore most frequently involved.
- Medial OA causes varus (bow) deformity, while lateral causes valgus (knock) knee deformity. Deformity increases asymmetrical load thereby accelerating OA process.
- Complex relationship between knee pain and radiological evidence of OA with psychosocial factors playing an important role.
- Acute effusions may develop and are associated with severe pain. Sometimes these acute flares are triggered by chondrocalcinosis.
- When pain increases acutely consider osteonecrosis.

Hip osteoarthritis

A frequent new presentation of OA to a sports medicine clinic. In particular, younger patients complaining of groin pain with markedly restricted hip movement whose X-rays have confirmed premature OA.
- Three different patterns described; superior pole (commonest), medial pole, and concentric (affects whole joint uniformly and more frequently associated with generalized OA).
- Not usually associated with OA in other joints.
- Usually presents as groin pain, but referral to the thigh and knee not uncommon.
- Usually develops slowly and may even show spontaneous improvement.
- Rapid clinical deterioration either from onset of first symptoms or after years of clinical stability not uncommon.
- May be complicated by osteonecrosis (bone collapse), which presents as sudden deterioration.

Nodal osteoarthritis

- Hereditary variant strongly associated with women.
- Presents in middle age.
- Characterized by extensive involvement of DIP joint and proximal interphalangeal (PIP) joint with Heberden's (DIP) and Bouchard's (PIP) nodes.
- Associated with knee OA.
- Joint erosions may be seen in affected joints. Bone characteristically shows hypertrophic change on X-ray (osteophytes), which help differentiate from inflammatory arthritis.

Spine

Spinal degenerative change is common on X-ray and usually bears no relationship to patients reporting to back pain. OA affects the spinal apophyseal (facet) joints and is associated with disc degeneration. C5 and L3–5 most frequently affected. In some patients, OA changes are sufficient to cause pressure on the spinal cord (spinal stenosis) or exiting nerve roots.

Other joints
It is possible for any joint to be affected by OA. Involvement of other joints, e.g. shoulder, elbow, temporomandibular joint is usually a reflection of local factors altering biomechanical stress on the index joint, e.g. previous joint injury, abnormal development, avascular necrosis.

Non-osteoarthritic joint pain
Not all joint pain is due to 'wear and tear', yet there is an increasing tendency for doctors to apportion this non-diagnosis to musculoskeletal symptoms that elude an immediate diagnosis. A term like undifferentiated joint pain may be more appropriate. Most people accept that the majority of headaches do not have a pathological or diagnostic explanation, so why not joint pain.
- OA does not cause red flag symptoms and, if these develop in a patient with OA, consider an alternative explanation for a patient's symptoms and investigate appropriately.
- It is increasingly common to see patients with generalized non-inflammatory musculoskeletal pain. While OA may be a contributing factor, such symptoms reflect a tendency to chronic pain and psychological distress. Patients should be advised and managed accordingly.

Radiological features
The radiological assessment of OA is usually confined to X-ray examination. Rarely is there a requirement to proceed to US, MRI, CT, or isotope imaging unless an alternative diagnosis is being considered. OA is characterized by the following features seen on plain X-ray.
- Normal mineralization.
- Non-uniform joint space narrowing.
- Osteophyte formation.
- Subchondral new bone formation (sclerosis).
- Cyst formation.
- Abnormal bone contour.
- Absence of erosions (although OA of the DIP and PIP joints can be associated with joint erosion).
- Joint subluxation.

Practical points
- Ask yourself whether an X-ray will alter your management. X-rays expose a patient to a small amount of radiation and are associated with a cost in terms of time (patient and health care professional) and resources.
- It is important to appreciate that a radiology report is only as good as the clinical information provided.
- Always try to review X-rays that you have requested, although I appreciate this is not straightforward for those working outside of a hospital setting.

CHAPTER 9 **Arthritis**

- Treat your patients and not their X-rays. Severe knee pain, normal knee movement, and a normal X-ray may be a hip problem.
- Request the correct X-ray and consider function:
  - In the patient described above perhaps if the patient had been properly examined an unnecessary knee X-ray would have been avoided, a hip X-ray requested, and the diagnosis confirmed.
  - There is little point in carrying out non-weight bearing knee X-rays in the context of OA. We don't walk lying down, non-weight bearing films give false reassurance of joint space.

Osteoarthritis: management

The standard response to, 'How do you manage OA?' is: painkillers, and if they don't work, refer to an orthopaedic surgeon. Fortunately for the health care professional with the time and the patient with the motivation, there is considerably more that can be advised to assist the OA sufferer.

The management of the individual patient with OA will clearly depend on a number of variables, including joints affected, functional impact of OA, and patient co-morbidity. Generic treatment principles may be tailored to an individual. Treatment strategies are non-pharmacological, local pharmacological, systemic pharmacological, and surgical.

Non-pharmacological

Education
Patient education is essential. Confirm diagnosis:
- Emphasize self-management approach.
- Reassure patient that being active is a good thing.
- Reassure patient that pain is not an indicator of doing harm.
- Do not avoid the thorny issue of weight management. It is vital that your patient is fully aware that being overweight will have a negative impact on their OA.
- Discuss breadth of treatment options.

Weight management
Irrespective of how 'badly' you think your patient will respond to a discussion on weight management, you are doing them a disservice by not drawing their attention to the need to lose weight. You must be supportive and empathetic, it is difficult to break out of the overweight—joints hurt, don't exercise, comfort eat, gain weight vicious circle. Exercise physicians have a considerable role to play in advising on the role of exercise to help manage a weight problem, and there is no better place to start than with your overweight OA sufferer.

Joint rehabilitation
The OA joint should be viewed as a dysfunctional unit in which one or more of the components has failed. In simple terms, you have a two-pronged approach, reduce the stress on the joint, e.g. weight management, footwear modification, or increase the capacity of the joint to withstand that stress. Joint rehabilitation to try and restore more normal joint function, or to ensure that other structures, e.g. muscles are more able to compensate for OA changes, is central to OA management. Basic rehabilitation principles should be followed with, if possible, an achievable functional outcome that is patient-centered.

Exercise
You should differentiate between exercise aimed at joint rehabilitation and general aerobic exercise. Aerobic exercise aims to improve overall fitness and may well have a positive effect on self-esteem, psychological wellbeing, and thereby symptoms. In addition, exercise will help with weight management. Exercise prescription for OA follows generic principles, most important of which is that it must be tailored to the individual.

OSTEOARTHRITIS: MANAGEMENT

Footwear

The ground reaction forces going through the lower limb during walking are considerable, as much as 4 times body weight on walking alone. Patients should be encouraged to wear shoes with good shock absorbing properties. Ideally, shoes should also have a flat sole (particularly for knee and hip OA). You will not win the battle over fashion shoes, but most patients accept the logic of 'sensible' shoes for long-term use and fashion footwear for restricted use at appropriate times.

Orthotics

Orthotics may offer a number of benefits for the patient with OA:
- Shock absorbing insoles may be helpful in improving the comfort of shoes without a specialized insole.
- Heel wedges can be useful in counteracting the effects of either a varus or valgus deformity in knee OA.
- Patients with OA have impaired proprioception and feelings of instability, which might be improved by the use of orthotics.

Aids to daily living

A walking aid (usually a more acceptable term to patients than a walking stick) will reduce lower limb joint loading, improve balance and stability, and perhaps most importantly restore confidence. For patients with severe OA, a walking aid can enable modest levels of daily living activity, which would otherwise be impossible. For patients with mild OA who wish to remain active, walking poles are a convenient way of increasing walking exercise capacity particularly where slopes are concerned. An essential part of the rambler's kit.

Some patients find knee braces helpful, particularly if stability is a concern.

Diet

Diet is frequently mentioned by patients. A well-balanced diet should provide all the essential nutrients and is sufficient to ensure an ideal weight is maintained. Some patients swear by supplements, e.g. cod liver oil, or green lip mussel extract, although there is no scientific evidence of their effectiveness.

Acupuncture

Acupuncture undoubtedly helps some patients and may be useful if pain control is proving problematic.

Miscellaneous

Standard 'first aid' approaches with a RICES regimen will help in certain situations. Cooling will certainly help an inflamed joint. Heat will help with joint or muscular stiffness, e.g. wax treatment, wheat bag (great for troublesome neck pain).

Relaxation techniques and similar modalities can prove useful for some patients.

Local pharmacological

Topical NSAIDs

Topical NSAIDs are on the whole safe and well-tolerated, and do help some patients.

Capsaicin
Capsaicin is the active ingredient in chilli peppers. It is thought to work as a painkiller by depleting substance P. It has been shown to be effective in patients with knee OA. Patients must be advised that it will sting initially, but if used regularly this will resolve. It is very irritant to the eye and care must be taken to wash hands thoroughly after application.

Intra-articular steroid
Corticosteroid injections have their place. They appear to work best for:
- The inflamed OA knee where there is a definite effusion (depomedrone 80mg or triamcinolone 40mg). A joint effusion has a significant negative impact on muscle function and aspiration/injection prior to rehabilitation can prove very useful.
- The massive knee effusion; when a combination of joint aspiration and steroid injection can have a dramatic effect.
- The patient with severe OA of the thumb base (1st carpometacarpal joint). Surgery (trapeziectomy) also offers good results and should be considered in patients requiring repeated injections.

Intra-articular hyaluronic acid
Hyaluronate has been shown to improve symptomatic knee OA. Hyaluronate injections are increasingly used for OA in other joints, although anecdotal reports seem favourable, there is no published evidence of their use. A number of different hyaluronic acid preparations exist with varying molecular weights, and there is debate about the influence of patient selection and preparation. Most treatments require between repeated injections on a weekly basis. NICE does not currently support the use of hyaluronic acid injections in OA.

Systemic pharmacological

Pain is generally unpleasant and is associated with negative emotions. Occasional pain, e.g. a headache, can be perfectly well treated by occasional painkillers. Patients with regular pain, of which OA is a good example, should anticipate their pain, rather than playing catch up. Encourage patients to take regular analgesia to control their pain.

Glucosamine
Glucosamine and chondroitin sulphate have been used widely in managing OA pain, but the evidence is variable and NICE doesn't currently recommend their use in OA.

Paracetamol
An excellent analgesic, but under utilized because it is available over-the-counter (OTC). Patients with regular OA pain should be encouraged to take paracetamol regularly up to 1g qid daily. If necessary, regular paracetamol can be topped up as required by the use of the following:

Compound analgesia
This term encompasses the wide range of drugs that contain varied combinations of weak opiate-based drugs, e.g. codeine phosphate and paracetamol. These preparations add little in terms of analgesia to paracetamol alone and can be associated with problematic side-effects.

Opiate analgesia

There are a wide range of opiate-based analgesics some of which are used in the treatment of OA, e.g. the mid-range opiates. Opiate patch technology has advanced in recent years on the basis that they offer the analgesic properties of stronger opioids without the side effects. Low dose patches are now available and are being aimed at the OA market. Their role is probably best restricted to selective patients where other treatment options have been exhausted.

Non-steroidal anti-inflammatory drugs

If alternative analgesics have been tried then NSAIDs offer the next stage in analgesia. The clinician and patient need to weigh up the relative balance between the benefits and side effects of NSAIDs. Use the lowest dose required, ideally supplementing prn NSAIDs with regular simple oral analgesia to minimize NSAID requirements. Gastroprotection should be considered in at risk patients. The cardiovascular risks need to be balanced against the potential benefits. In patients requiring chronic NSAIDs an annual full blood count (FBC) and urea and electrolytes (U&E) is appropriate.

Disease modifying agents (DMARDs)

The role of disease-modifying drugs in the management of inflammatory arthritis is well established. These drugs have been used in managing patients with OA, where there appears to be a significant inflammatory component, e.g. nodal/erosive OA. Specific disease-modifying OA drugs are in development. They aim to inhibit cartilage breakdown. None has been shown to have a clear benefit in human OA.

Surgical

A variety of surgical approaches are utilized in managing the osteoarthritic joint including arthroscopic washout/debridement, soft tissue procedures, arthroplasty, and arthrodesis. While the success of well-established joint replacement operations, e.g. knee and hip is not in doubt, recent evidence suggests that arthroscopic washout/debridement of the knee was no more beneficial than sham procedures. The potential for chondrocyte transplantation remains under investigation in specialized centres.

The surgical approach will depend on the joint concerned and a number of patient specific factors.

NICE has produced evidence based guidance on managing OA.[1]

---

[1] NICE (2008). *Osteoarthritis: The Care and Management of Osteoarthritis in Adults.* NICE Clinical Guidelines 59. London: NICE. Available at: http://www.nice.org.uk/nicemedia/pdf/CG59NICEguideline.pdf

Inflammatory arthritis

Athletes frequently present with joint pain, usually attributed to musculoskeletal trauma, but joint inflammation should not be discounted, particularly as management will have to be modified accordingly. A careful history and examination will help the sports physician identify those patients who require referral to a rheumatologist for a second opinion.

Arthritis is simply joint inflammation but, to avoid any confusion with OA, the term inflammatory arthritis is used. Inflammatory arthritis may present acutely, acute on chronically, or chronically. Joint inflammation is characterized by:
- Pain
- Swelling
- Heat
- Redness/erythema
- Loss of function.

In addition joint inflammation is usually associated with:
- Prolonged early morning stiffness
- Inactivity stiffness.

History

Most clinicians focus on the musculoskeletal features of inflammatory arthritis, but conditions associated with inflammatory arthritis may have systemic features and, therefore, a full history is necessary. In particular, the following will help in establishing your differential diagnosis:
- Pattern of joint involvement.
- Spinal involvement.
- Red flag signs:
  - Constitutional symptoms (fever, weight loss, night sweats).
  - History of malignancy.
  - Neurological symptoms, especially bladder and bowel dysfunction.
  - Extremes of age (<16, >65).
- Pre-existing connective tissue disease (CTD).
- Evidence of any recent infection, in particular streptococcal infection, infectious gastroenteritis, and sexually-acquired infection.
- *Chlamydia* infection deserves special mention because of the implications of undiagnosed *Chlamydia* to female fertility as a result of pelvic inflammatory disease. *Chlamydia* infection is often asymptomatic and a careful and sensitive history is essential. Referral to a GU medicine department should be considered in all patients—a history of monogamy does not exclude polygamy in the partner!
- History of established inflammatory bowel disease (IBD) or symptoms suggestive of IBD. Diarrhoea, rectal bleeding, rectal mucus, abdominal pain, weight loss.
- Psoriasis or 1st degree family history of psoriasis.
- Ocular inflammation.
- Family history of inflammatory arthritis or CTD.

Examination

A good history will direct your examination.
- Pain may be referred.
- The importance of the kinetic chain—the presenting symptom may not be the problem.
- Exercising patients frequently justify musculoskeletal symptoms by recounting an injury.
- The inflammation of inflammatory arthritis is not confined to the intra-articular (IA) space, all components of the joint including capsule and bone are involved. Inflammation may be present at the enthesis or within the tendon sheath.
- Systemic features may not be appreciated by the patient, e.g. a patient may not be aware they have psoriasis or a sexually-acquired infection.
- Inflammatory symptoms fluctuate, asking a patient to provide photographic evidence of joint swelling is frequently helpful.
- Pain is not a good indicator of inflammatory symptoms. A number of chronic pain disorders present with joint pain, the key is usually the presence of definite joint swelling or a proven inflammatory response.

As with the history a thorough examination is usually required given the systemic nature of inflammatory arthritis and CTD.

Investigations

Investigations help in establishing the correct diagnosis, although may require specialist interpretation.

Blood tests

FBC
Joint inflammation may produce an anaemia of chronic disease and a thrombocytosis. This gives some measure of chronicity. Several CTDs are associated with leucopenia, neutropenia, lymphopenia, or thrombocytopenia.

Erythrocyte sedimentation rate (ESR)
The ESR is useful as a non-specific indicator of inflammation.

C-reactive protein (CRP)
CRP is an acute phase protein produced by the liver and is a non-specific indicator of inflammation. It is very sensitive to change and will reflect improvement or deterioration more responsively then the ESR.

ESR and CRP are particularly useful in patients with few clinical signs, but the following should be considered when interpreting acute phase markers:
- The ESR normally increases with age.
- An elevated ESR may be seen in patients without inflammatory disease.
- Most patients with inflammatory arthritis will have a raised ESR or CRP, although normal results do not exclude inflammation.
- A single inflamed large joint will affect the ESR and CRP to a far greater degree than 10 inflammed small (e.g. MCP) joints and therefore, the ESR and CRP are not always indicative of severity.
- A raised ESR and normal CRP may be suggestive of a connective tissue disorder, e.g. lupus.

Routine biochemistry
Renal, liver, and thyroid function are all worth checking to exclude conditions that may present with musculoskeletal pain and, prior to starting medication, might affect organ function.

Bone biochemistry
Calcium, alkaline phosphatase (usually included with liver function tests (LFTs)), and vitamin D levels are useful in more non-specific musculoskeletal pain. Hypovitaminosis D is increasingly being diagnosed even in populations not traditionally deemed to be at risk, e.g. young Caucasians.

Blood cultures
If septic arthritis is suspected, blood cultures are mandatory. They may be positive in 30% of cases.

Creatinine phosphokinase
A metabolic or inflammatory myopathy may present with symptoms of inflammatory arthritis. A raised CPK is associated with exercise and elevated levels must be considered in the light of a patients exercise history.

Immunoglobulins (urine for Bence–Jones protein)
Multiple myeloma may present with features of inflammatory arthritis. A polyclonal increase in immunoglobulins is invariably seen in inflammatory arthritis.

Bacterial and viral titres
Reactive arthritis is common. If there is a history of infection then objective evidence of recent infection is useful.

Uric acid
Uric acid levels have poor sensitivity and specificity for gout, and therefore neither confirm nor exclude the diagnosis. However, if gout is confirmed on analysis of synovial fluid, serum uric acid level may help with treatment and its monitoring.

Ferritin
Haemochromatosis may present with acute arthritis related to calcium pyrophosphate crystals (pseudogout). Untreated haemochromatosis is associated with systemic complications including diabetes, hepatic, and cardiac dysfunction, and has an autosomal recessive inheritance pattern. Detection is therefore important for the patient and their family.

Autoantibody profile
The diagnosis of inflammatory arthritis and connective tissue disease is a clinical one. Autoantibodies generally have poor specificity and/or sensitivity, and therefore patients may have false negative or positive results. Autoantibodies only become important in a patient with an appropriate history and examination.

The discovery of antibodies against citrullinated protein (CCP) has however proved particularly helpful in the diagnosis of rheumatoid arthritis, and a positive test is now included in the 2010 ACR-EULAR classification criteria for rheumatoid arthritis (RA).

Radiology

Imaging is an important extension to musculoskeletal examination but never replaces careful examination.

Plain X-rays
Plain musculoskeletal X-rays have traditionally been the first line investigation for a patient with suspected inflammatory arthritis, although with alternative imaging techniques, especially US and MRI, one could reasonably ask if that should still be the case.

The decision to image a potentially inflamed joint is made for the following reasons:
- To exclude serious pathology, which may mimic inflammatory arthritis, e.g. infection, tumour, or fracture.
- To assess the 'health' of the joint in question and the degree of joint inflammation or damage.
- To identify the differing radiological features of inflammatory arthritis which might help with confirming a diagnosis.
- To reassure the patient, or doctor.

MRI and US will answer most of these questions and will frequently provide far more information than is available on plain X-ray. However, until MRI and US is widely available, plain X-rays remain the first line investigation.

Ultrasound
US is increasingly used to establish a diagnosis, to direct treatment, and to monitor response to treatment. US is far more sensitive to articular cartilage and bone damage than X-ray, and will reveal joint erosions before changes are seen on plain films. This is increasingly useful in the assessment and monitoring of drug treatment. US is also useful in assessing inflammation in other synovial lined structures, e.g. bursae and tendon sheaths.

MRI
MRI is useful to establish the extent of synovitis and involvement of soft tissue structures, e.g. tendons, enthesis, bursa, capsule, and muscle. MRI is also very helpful if tumour or infection is considered, and the location of pathology is known. Like US, MRI is far more sensitive for articular cartilage and bone damage than X-ray.

Isotope bone scan
Bone scintigraphy is useful if you are unsure where a patients pathology (inflammation, tumour, or infection) is located and the potential area concerned is too large to allow straightforward MRI examination, e.g. in patients with pelvic pain, or if multifocal inflammation, tumour, or infection is suspected. In either case you may need to proceed to focused investigation with MRI once the site of pathology has been established.

Bone scintigraphy is also helpful if you wish to exclude significant musculoskeletal inflammation in patients without clear symptoms or signs.

CT
Musculoskeletal CTs are rarely helpful in the assessment of patients with inflammatory arthritis.

DEXA
Osteoporosis is a complication of arthritis and its treatment, especially systemic steroids. There are several ways in which bone density can be assessed, although the most validated method in terms of establishing fracture risk is DEXA.

Multi-system examination
Inflammatory arthritides and connective tissue diseases are systemic conditions that will therefore require systemic assessment. A number of radiological techniques may assist in this process.

Synovial fluid analysis
Normal synovial fluid has a very pale yellow hue, is transparent, and has a normal viscosity. Progressive levels of inflammation are associated with increasing levels of cellularity with increasing turbidity (increasingly yellow with loss of clarity), and loss of normal viscosity. Inflammatory arthritis is usually associated with a deeper yellow colour and some clarity, whereas pus, the hallmark of septic arthritis, is thick, a deep mucky yellow with

no transparency. Unfortunately the appearances of synovial fluid from non-infectious synovitis, particularly that associated with crystal arthritis, can be identical to septic arthritis and some forms of infectious arthritis (e.g. tuberculous), which are associated with a minimal cellular response.

The presence of blood is usually due to the leaking of erythrocytes as part of the inflammatory response within inflamed synovial fluid, or a traumatic aspiration, rather than reflecting a bleed into a joint (haemarthrosis). A haemarthrosis is usually a sign of trauma, although consider a bleeding diathesis, over-anticoagulation and minor trauma to intensely vascular synovial hypertrophy, e.g. pigmented villo-nodular synovitis.

Microbiological analysis is essential if septic arthritis is considered. A septic joint is not always obvious clinically, and given the consequences to the joint (irreversible joint destruction) of failing to make a diagnosis, send synovial fluid for analysis. This should be done prior to giving antibiotics and be followed by IV antibiotics (to cover likely pathogens) until culture results are available. Histological analysis of synovial fluid can be extremely helpful in specialist hands.

Monosodium urate and calcium pyrophosphate crystals in synovial fluid are diagnostic for gout and pseudogout respectively. Urate crystals are usually very obvious (rod-shaped strongly negatively birefringant), and their absence almost certainly means the diagnosis is not gout. Calcium pyrophosphate crystals are very difficult to see even in experienced hands.

The acute hot joint

An athlete may present with acute joint inflammation to a team or squad physician. The differential diagnosis includes almost every condition capable of causing synovitis, however, there are a number of simple rules, which will help with your immediate management.

Septic arthritis is a diagnosis of exclusion
Although septic arthritis is unusual in an otherwise healthy young athlete, the consequences of delaying a diagnosis are catastrophic to both the joint and the patient.

History
- Symptoms/signs of localized infection, e.g. skin injury or excoriating rash, foreign body injury, e.g. urchin spines, wood splinters.
- Symptoms/signs of systemic infection that might cause a bacteraemia or reactive arthritis, e.g. upper respiratory tract infection (URTI), chest, urogenital, GI.
- Constitutional symptoms, e.g. weight loss, fever, night sweats.
- Past medical history (PMH) of arthritis, psoriasis, systemic inflammation, e.g. eyes, bowels.
- Family history (FH) of arthritis, psoriasis.
- A history of trauma is clearly important, but beware the patient who tries to justify acute joint pain and swelling with a history of what sounds like minor trauma.

Examination
- Clinical examination of the joint will rarely add useful information over and above confirming that your patient has an inflamed joint. The degree of inflammation is not a good discriminator of infectious and non-infectious causes. In particular, it is impossible clinically to differentiate septic arthritis and gout.
- Systemic examination to look for more generalized signs of infection or systemic illness.

Investigations
- Septic arthritis must be excluded and, unless certain on clinical grounds that a patient does not have septic arthritis, the joint must be aspirated, and a synovial fluid sample sent urgently to a microbiology department for microscopy, culture, and sensitivity. Atypical myobacterial infections may present in this way and you should request mycobacterial cultures.
- An FBC, ESR, and CRP are useful, although they will not always discriminate between septic arthritis and inflammatory synovitis.
- Blood cultures will be positive in about 30% of cases of septic arthritis, even when synovial fluid cultures are negative.
- An acutely inflamed joint in a patient without a history of inflammatory arthritis should be X-rayed.

Immediate management
- If septic arthritis is a possibility then, after synovial fluid aspiration, give high dose IV antibiotics until culture results are known. In a non-hospitalized patient who is otherwise well *Staphyloccus* and *Streptococcus* are the most likely infecting organisms and your antibiotic regime should reflect this.
- Patients with suspected septic arthritis require hospitalization and specialist review.
- If septic arthritis is highly unlikely or has been excluded then aspirate to reduce IA pressure and at the same time inject the joint with steroid.
- NSAIDs are usually helpful.
- Oral steroids maybe helpful where rapid resolution is desirable, however, this decision should only be reached after discussion with a rheumatologist, and will require the completion of a TUE in a competitive athlete.
- Most cases of mono-arthritis should be discussed with a rheumatologist, and certainly in someone whose occupation depends on normal joint function a specialist opinion should be sought.
- Most cases of mono-arthritis are iatrogenic, and a good proportion (up to 30% of reactive arthritis) becomes chronic requiring long-term rheumatological care.

Inflammatory arthritis: management

Inflammatory arthritis is a descriptive term, rather than a diagnosis, although sometimes the expression undifferentiated inflammatory arthritis will be used in the absence of clear diagnostic criteria. Many diseases may cause or be associated with an inflammatory arthritis.

Inflammatory arthritis—generic principles

The underlying principle of managing synovitis is that joint inflammation causes irreversible joint damage, which causes disability and handicap.

- An athlete's sport must be considered as their occupation. Whatever the occupation/sport, an individual who aspires to high-level performance will become disabled much earlier than an individual whose physical requirements are less demanding. A professional tennis player with knee synovitis is potentially no different to a self-employed builder. On any given day, both individuals may be equally affected by their condition.
- The important difference between the tennis player and the builder rests with the relative importance of that day's employment:
  - For the tennis player, that day may be the final of a major tournament, whereas for the builder at worst it might mean a 24-h delay in completing a job.
  - An average professional tennis player's career may span 10–14yrs with perhaps only a fraction of that time when the player is truly competitive. An average builder might be expected to have a working life of 40–45yrs.
  - The tennis player will require 100% confidence in his knee to be competitive, whereas the builder, even if required to climb ladders, may be functional with a partial response to treatment.

It is appreciating these subtle differences between a professional athlete and a non-athlete that is central to the successful management of arthritis, and where the sports physician's skills as the athletes advocate will be required.

Controlling synovitis

The control of joint inflammation is imperative to preserve joint function. Drugs that have been shown to control synovitis and prevent or attenuate joint inflammation and subsequent damage fall into 3 categories—DMARDs, biological therapies, and steroids.

NSAIDs reduce pain, swelling, and stiffness but do not influence the underlying inflammatory process in terms of reducing joint damage, and should only be used for symptom control.

DMARDs

A number of DMARDs have been used to treat inflammatory arthritis, however, the most commonly used drugs in current practice are methotrexate, leflunomide, and sulphasalazine. They all broadly share the same characteristics:

- They are slow-acting, may take up to 3–6 months to have their full effect.
- They only work in about 70% of patients.
- Their side effect profile requires the regular monitoring of blood tests (FBC, U&E, LFT).
- They may be used alone or in combination.

- Treatment is escalated in terms of dose and combinations until control of synovitis is achieved.
- Full remission of arthritis is unlikely.

Biological therapies

Biological therapies are designer drugs aimed at blocking particular components of the inflammatory cascade. The biologics widely used in clinical practice are drugs that reduce or block tumour necrosis factor (TNF) activity, IL6 receptors or CD20 (to suppress B cell activity). They all broadly share the same characteristics:
- All work quickly (usually within 4 weeks, although the B-cell blockade can take longer).
- They are all given parenterally (infusion or subcutaneous (SC) injection).
- Research suggests that they are effective in 70% of patients, although clinical observations suggest a more positive response rate.
- They are more effective if co-prescribed with methotrexate.
- They require monitoring with regular blood tests.
- Their main side effect is an increased risk of serious and non-serious infection, in particular tuberculosis (TB) and soft tissue infection.
- In the UK their use is rationalized by NICE guidelines, when conventional DMARDs have failed.
- Current evidence increasingly suggests that for selective patients they should be considered as first line treatment with methotrexate.
- Complete remission is achievable in some patients.

Steroids

Steroids can be given as injections (IA, IV, IM) or in oral form. Their use may require the completion of a TUE depending on the route of administration.
- Injectable steroids have a rapid onset of action and are widely used, particularly IA steroids. In the context of mono or oligo (<4 joints) arthritis an IA steroid injection can be extremely effective. Some rheumatologists pulse patients with IM or IV steroids at times of a generalized arthritis flare.
- Oral steroids have been used in rheumatological practice for many years. They are very effective at reducing inflammation, but unfortunately their long-term use is limited by dose-dependent side effects. Consequently, most rheumatologists would not use long-term doses greater than 5–7.5mg daily. With the advent of biological treatments the use of long-term oral steroids has decreased significantly.

Medical aspects of managing inflammatory arthritis

Specific medical roles include:
- Prevention of disease or treatment-associated side effects, e.g. preserving bone health, pro-actively managing cardiovascular risk factors.
- Liaison with surgical colleagues to ensure surgical referrals are made expeditiously.
- Specialist medical referral, e.g. genito-urinary (GU) medicine referral if sexually transmitted infection causing reactive arthritis is possible, dermatology referral for problematic psoriasis, gastroenterology referral if occult inflammatory bowel disease causing arthritis is suspected.

Joint rehabilitation

An inflamed joint will undergo the same functional deterioration as an injured joint and therefore rehabilitation is vital to restoring normal joint function. With the exception of an acutely inflamed joint, when pain rather than any evidence that exercise induces damage is the limiting factor, patients with inflammatory arthritis should be encouraged to rehabilitate pro-actively. The greater challenge is often in trying to control the athlete's enthusiasm to prevent overly aggressive rehabilitation.

Multi-disciplinary care

The doctor is only one member of team which includes nurses, physio- and occupational therapists, podiatrists, orthotists, and psychologists.

Monoarthritis

Patients with acute inflammatory monoarthritis may go on to develop a chronic arthropathy. The management of chronic mono-arthritis follows the principles outlined above. There are a number of differences which can be summarized:
- Initial management will utilize joint-specific, rather than systemic treatment modalities, e.g. IA steroid and physiotherapy modalities.
- Patients who fail to respond to targeted treatment will probably have to consider systemic drug treatments. Depending on the joint concerned the impact of monoarthritis on physical function and athletic performance may be no less than that of polyarthritis. DMARDs are uniformly slow acting, which is very frustrating for any patient, but particularly a professional athlete.
- Current rationing guidelines for the NHS prescription of biological treatments only apply when traditional DMARDs have failed and when NICE severity criteria have been met, which precludes their use in monoarthritis.
- Consequently the use of anti-TNF treatments for monoarthritis would have to be made on the basis of a case of exceptional need or alternatively paid for privately. This is disappointing as in my experience biological treatment offers the individual the greatest chance of returning to full competitive sport.
- The importance of rehabilitation cannot be over emphasized.

Oligoarthritis

Oligoarthritis is a term used to describe arthritis that affects no more than 4 joints. It is characteristic of the seronegative arthropathies. The management of an oligoarthritis falls somewhere between that of a monoarthritis and a polyarthritis. Intra-articular steroids are widely used but the early introduction of DMARDs would be normal clinical practice.

Spondyloarthropathy

Spondyloarthropathies are inflammatory conditions of the axial skeleton and in particular the sacroiliac joints. Bilateral sacroileitis is therefore a diagnostic feature. The clinical assessment and management of these conditions differ from peripheral arthritis in a number of ways:
- Symptoms usually start as a young adult, but not always.
- Strong predilection for male gender.
- Diagnosis is frequently delayed because symptoms are misinterpreted.

- Inflammatory back pain is characterized by early morning stiffness and improvement with activity, contrary to mechanical pain, which is usually eased by rest.
- Bilateral sacroiliac joint involvement is diagnostic. X-rays taken during the early phase of the condition are frequently normal, MRI is the investigation of choice in early disease if radiological diagnostic confirmation is required.
- Unilateral sacroileitis is unusual and infection should be excluded.
- Peripheral joints may be affected but by definition not in isolation.
- Associated with characteristic extra-articular features (Table 9.1).
- NSAIDs help manage symptoms but do not prevent ankylosis (fusion) of the spine.
- Peripheral arthritis may respond to standard DMARDs, axial symptoms do not.
- Anti-TNF medications have been shown to dramatically improve axial symptoms and reduce spinal damage.

Table 9.1 Non-infectious inflammatory arthritis

Descriptive term		Associated conditions	Notes
Seropositive arthritis		Rheumatoid arthritis	RA is not always seropositive
Seronegative arthritis	Monoarthritis	Psoriasis	Seronegative arthritides are frequeny associated with characteristic extra-articular features e.g. uveitis, genitourinary symptoms, skin rashes.
	Oligoarthritis (less than 4 joints affected)	Inflammatory bowel disease	
		Reactive arthritis	
	Spondyloarthropathy	Ankylosing spondylitis	Inflammatory arthritis involving the sacroiliac joints and spine in addition to peripheral joints. All seronegative arthropathies are associated with HLAB27.
		Psoriasis	
		Inflammatory bowel disease	
		Reactive arthritis	
Crystal arthropathy		Gout Pseudogout	Confirmation of crystals in synovial fluid is the gold standard for diagnosis.
Connective tissue disease		Systemic lupus scleroderma	Arthritis is only one feature of these multi-system illness but this highlights the importance of taking a full history when presented with an acute arthritis.
Systemic vasculitis		Wegener's granulomatosis Polyarteritis nodosa	
Multi-system illness		Sarcoidosis	

Rheumatoid arthritis

RA is the most common type of inflammatory arthritis, affecting approximately 1% of the UK population. The following points are worth emphasizing:
- The diagnosis should be made on clinical grounds, but subtle inflammation can be overlooked and hand/foot US is increasingly being used to identify early inflammatory arthritis.
- A positive anti-CCP antibody is very specific for RA. Rheumatoid factor (RF) is unhelpful in proving the diagnosis, but is associated with a worse prognosis.
- Other investigations should only be seen as providing supported evidence, e.g. elevated inflammatory markers, anaemia suggesting chronicity.
- It usually presents as an acute symmetrical inflammatory polyarthritis affecting most of the large and small joints (classically affecting the MCPs and PIPs).
- It can initially present as a mono- or oligoarthritis, but will usually evolve into a polyarthritis.
- It is more common in females and classically presents in middle age, although it can present at any age.
- The cause of RA is unknown. Genetic factors only account for 30% of its aetiology. A family history is interesting but neither confirms nor excludes the diagnosis.
- Systemic features, e.g. weight loss, fatigue, and even a low grade fever are not uncommon.
- The management of RA is that of an inflammatory polyarthritis.
- Inflammation produces joint damage and therefore the emphasis is on early aggressive treatment to switch off joint inflammation as quickly as possible.
- RA is a multisystem disease and is associated with complications that can affect all of the major organs.
- RA is associated with increased mortality. This seems to be largely attributable to increased cardiovascular mortality, hence there is an increasing appreciation of the importance of managing cardiovascular risk factors.
- The use of biological medications has revolutionized the management of RA. These drugs will likely be used first line in the future to try and induce remission.

Crystal arthropathy

Gout and pseudogout are the most common forms of crystal arthritis. Gout, in particular, is associated with a number of medical conditions for which exercise should be prescribed or recommended. The most important associated feature of pseudogout is OA, which is both a consequence of joint injury and another condition for which exercise has an important therapeutic role. The following may help you assess and manage a patient with crystal arthritis.

- Gout is caused by monosodium urate crystals and pseudogout by calcium pyrophosphate.
- Gout is usually a result of the under excretion of urate.
- Both conditions cause acute and dramatic joint inflammation with severe pain, marked swelling, and erythema. The clinical features are indistinguishable from septic arthritis.
- The classical presentation of gout is podagra, acute inflammation of the first MTP joint. Pseudogout typically presents with knee involvement. Both conditions may present with acute inflammation of any synovial lined structure including tendon sheaths. It is therefore not uncommon for both conditions to be initially diagnosed as cellulitis and treated with antibiotics.
- Although monoarthritis is typical, polyarticular involvement may occur.
- There are no serological diagnostic tests for gout, or pseudogout. A normal uric acid level does not exclude, and a raised level is not diagnositic. Synovial fluid analysis is the gold standard for diagnosis.
- An acute attack is best treated with NSAIDs (with appropriate gastrointestinal protection). For patients who do not respond or can't take NSAIDs then colchicine is a useful alternative.
- Colchicine causes diarrhoea (use a maximum dose of 500mcg bd or tid to control symptoms.)
- IA steroids can work extremely well, and unlike NSAIDs and colchicine, are not associated with any systemic side effects. At the same time the joint can be drained to provide immediate comfort and synovial fluid sent for examination under a polarizing microscope. Septic arthritis must be excluded.
- In resistant or polyarticular disease the use of a 1–2-week course of low dose oral steroids (10mg) can be extremely effective.
- Both conditions may be triggered by environmental stress, e.g. dehydration and joint injury.
- There is no prophylaxis for pseudogout.
- Gout maybe caused by a high purine diet (and in particular alcohol) as well as drugs, e.g. diuretics. Patients should be encouraged to reduce alcohol consumption, modify their diet (low calorie and carbohydrate restricted), and where possible drug regimes altered.
- The decision when to introduce gout prophylaxis is best left to the patient given the need for daily treatment (assuming there are no features of articular or non-articular damage, uric acid is associated with a nephropathy and raised serum levels may be a cardiovascular risk factor). Drugs either reduce uric acid production (e.g. allopurinol)

or increase its renal excretion (uricosuric drugs). Allopurinol is the treatment of choice.
- In otherwise healthy individuals (normal renal function) it is usual to start allopurinol 100mg daily and increase the dose in 100mg increments until the serum uric acid < 300μmol/L . Allopurinol may cause hypersensitivity skin reactions and affect renal function. Patients should have their renal function checked after starting or changing dose.
- Paradoxically, allopurinol may cause an attack of gout. This must be explained to the patient and, unless contra-indicated, co-prescribe a NSAID or colchicine for the first month after starting or changing dose.
- Gout is associated with diabetes, hyperlipidaemia and hypertension and these should be screened for and managed.

Seronegative arthritides

The sports physician is most likely to encounter athletes with a seronegative arthritis. Dactylitis, the uniform sausage like swelling of a digit, is diagnostic of seronegative arthritides. Enthesitis is another typical feature and may be overlooked as a mechanical tendinopthy unless an inflammatory cause is considered.

Psoriatic arthritis
- Psoriatic arthritis can present as a monoarthritis, oligoarthritis, spondyloarthropathy, arthritis confined to the DIP joints, and a severely destructive polyarthritis.
- 10% of patients with psoriasis may develop an arthritis.
- There is no association between the severity or location of psoriasis and the nature or pattern of the arthritis. Psoriatic plaques may be well hidden on the scalp or around the umbilicus or confined to nail dystrophy, such that the patient may not even appreciate they have psoriasis.
- To complicate matters further, psoriatic arthritis may precede the development of the rash or only be present in a first degree relative.
- A number of drugs used to treat arthritis are also extremely effective for psoriasis, e.g. methotrexate, leflunomide and anti-TNF preparations.

Enteric arthritis
- Arthritis associated with IBD is more common than widely appreciated. It mainly presents as a monoarthritis, oligoarthritis, or spondyloarthropathy.
- Uncontrolled arthritis is frequently an indication of active bowel inflammation, which may not be clinically apparent. (Crohn's disease in particular.)
- Steroids are frequently used to treat IBD and the arthritic symptoms may only reveal themselves upon steroid reduction.
- NSAIDs may exacerbate IBD so should be used cautiously.
- A number of drugs are effective in the treatment of arthritis and IBD, e.g. azathioprine, anti-TNF preparations (Crohn's).

Reactive arthritis
- With an acute arthritis consider an infectious cause.
- Streptococcal infections and those causing infectious gastroenteritis and GU infection are most common, although the viral URTI is probably most often to blame, but is usually self-limiting, although potentially devastating to the competing athlete.
- Monoarthritis is the most common presentation.
- *Chlamydia* infection is often asymptomatic and a careful and sensitive history is essential. Referral to a GU medicine department should be considered in all patients, a history of monogamy does not exclude polygamy in the partner!
- Treatment of the infectious cause does not enhance resolution of the arthritis or improve long-term prognosis of the arthritis, with the possible exception of Lyme disease. In some series up to 30% of patients developing reactive arthritis may develop chronic synovitis.

Miscellaneous conditions

The aetiology of inflammatory arthritis is too diverse to discuss fully in this context, however, there are a number of other potential causes that deserve mention.

- *Red flag conditions:* the importance of local sepsis (e.g. osteomyelitis) or tumour (primary, secondary, and haematological) presenting as an arthritis is worthy of emphasis.
- *Erythema nodosum:* usually associated with troublesome lower and sometimes upper limb distal arthritis.
- *Pigmented villonodular synovitis:* usually presents with a blood-stained effusion, MRI is diagnostic.
- *Osteoid osteoma:* still overlooked in patients with chronic joint/bone pain. Triple phase bone can, CT, and MRI all have diagnostic utility.

Chapter 10

Cardiorespiratory

Coronary artery disease 260
Treatment of coronary heart disease 262
Exercise and coronary artery disease 263
Physical inactivity, exercise, and coronary artery disease 264
Cardiac rehabilitation 265
Phases of rehabilitation 266
Secondary prevention 268
Exercise referral 270
Exercise and adult congenital heart disease 272
Guidelines for exercise and sport in congenital heart disease 274
Factors in individual congenital conditions 276
Marfan syndrome 278
Hypertension and exercise 282
Natural history of hypertension and prognosis 283
Exercise and left ventricular hypertrophy 283
Exercise capacity and hypertension 284
Exercise and heart failure 286
Treatment of cardiac failure 288
Exercise in cardiac failure 289
Exercise testing 289
Effects of exercise in heart failure 290
Exercise and treatment of cardiac failure 291
Sudden death 292
Intensity and type of exercise performed in specific sports 298
Exercise-induced bronchoconstriction 300

Coronary artery disease

- Coronary artery disease (CAD) remains a major cause of morbidity and mortality in developed countries.
- One million people in the USA sustain myocardial infarction yearly. A major increase in incidence is occurring in developing countries.
- Death rate has declined in developed countries by 30% in last 10yr.
- 50% of deaths with acute myocardial infarction occur within 1h attributable to ventricular fibrillation.

Clinical presentation of coronary heart disease

- *Stable angina pectoris:* predictable onset of anginal symptoms on exercise or stress following imbalance of increased myocardial demand over supply.
- *Unstable angina and non-ST elevation myocardial infarction (non-STEMI):* new onset, changing pattern or episodes of angina at rest. May be associated with release of cardiac enzymes. Troponin T and I used to make diagnosis or to exclude myocardial damage.
- *STEMI:* presentation with rest pain, typical serial electrocardiogram (ECG) changes and enzyme release. Complicated by arrhythmias, associated with myocardial damage and left ventricle (LV) dysfunction or failure.
- Sudden death associated with acute infarction or as an arrhythmic event.
- Cardiac failure secondary to recurrent infarction or ischaemic cardiomyopathy.

Pathophysiology

Development of atheromatous plaques

- Long pre-clinical phase of development with rapid change at time of plaque rupture.
- Principally affect the proximal portions of coronary arteries, therefore, large muscle beds influenced by stenosis or occlusion.
- Human coronary arteries are end arteries with little collateral development unless stimulated by reversible myocardial ischaemia or previous occlusion and infarction.
- Distribution of arterial narrowing's confers prognosis. Increasing mortality through single, double, and triple vessel or left main disease.

Plaque dynamics

- Thrombogenic lipid rich core covered with fibrous cap of smooth muscle and inflammatory cells.
- Inflammation may occur stimulated by oxidized lipid accumulation in the intima. CRP is an inflammatory marker. If elevated confers increased risk of further events.
- Macrophages and T-lymphocytes are present in fatty streaks and mature plaques, cytokines, and growth factors are secreted.
- Adhesion molecules interact with inflammatory cells.
- Plaque rupture leads to platelet deposition and thrombus formation which may precipitate total obstruction and infarction.

CORONARY ARTERY DISEASE

- Unstable plaques may be angiographically insignificant but can rapidly progress in significance.
- Plaques may stabilize after rupture.
- CAD is episodic in clinical presentation.

Aetiology
Atheroma associated with risk factors; subject to primary and secondary prevention.

Class 1 interventions
- Hypertension.
- Hypercholesterolaemia.
- Cigarette smoking.
- Cardiac protection with aspirin, beta-blockers, and angiotensin converting enzyme (ACE) inhibitors.

Class 2 interventions
- Diabetes.
- HDL and triglycerides.
- Physical inactivity.
- Obesity.
- Moderate alcohol consumption.

Class 3 interventions
- Diet.
- Psychosocial factors.

Investigations

History of cardiac pain
- Resting ECG.
- Exercise stress testing for exercise capacity and evidence of myocardial ischaemia (ST depression).
- Increasing use of functional imaging testing with pharmacological challenge.
- Radionuclide scanning for distribution of perfusion defects and assessment of LV function.
- Echocardiography for assessment of LV function. Stress echo techniques may be applied.
- Multislice CT coronary angiography used as baseline noninvasive examination for anatomy.
- Coronary arteriography to determine anatomical distribution of obstructive lesions and for coronary interventions.

Treatment of coronary heart disease

Pharmacological agents
- *Nitrates*: act as venous dilators, reduce preload and systolic wall stress, used sublingually, orally, or by parenteral route in unstable patients. Tolerance may occur.
- *Beta blockers*: act on cardiac beta receptors, reduce HR, contractility, systolic wall stress, and BP at rest and on exercise. Used to alter supply-demand ratio in stable angina, and after myocardial infarction as secondary prevention for anti-arrhythmic action. Consider other agents to reduce heart rate.
- *Calcium channel blockers*: vasodilating action on coronary and peripheral arteries. Main therapy for increased vasoactivity such as Prinzmetal angina.
- *Nicorandil*: potassium channel blocker, vasodilating action, but no tolerance. Action may be related to preconditioning.
- *Anti-platelet therapies*: given as long-term therapy, (aspirin) as adjunct to coronary artery intervention acutely (abciximab) or as continuing treatment (clopidigrel, tigagretor).
- *Thrombolytic therapy*: administered to patients with ST elevation myocardial infarction presenting early in absence of facilities for primary reperfusion therapy with angioplasty.

Interventions
Coronary interventions may be applied to each of the clinical presentations. Choice of intervention is determined by coronary artery anatomy on angiography.
- Coronary artery bypass surgery generally applied to patients with left main or triple vessel involvement.
- Increasing application of percutaneous coronary intervention (PCI) with balloon angioplasty and stenting in patients with stable angina with severe symptoms, unstable presentations, or in ST elevation myocardial infarction (primary angioplasty).
- Primary angioplasty is treatment of choice if possible within 90min of attendance at a PCI equipped centre or within 120min of first presentation. Intervention associated with better short- and long-term outcomes with this system.

Exercise and coronary artery disease

Potential benefits of exercise
- Reduced body weight and component of fat.
- Reduced HR, systolic BP, lactic acid production, and muscular blood flow at equivalent work rate.
- Increased exercise capacity and endurance Increased VO_2 max by 10–15%.
- Increased A-VO_2 diff at maximal exercise.
- Reduced total cholesterol and low density lipoprotein (LDL).
- Reduction in triglycerides.
- HDL and HDL2 increased, reduction in fibrinogen and platelet aggregation at rest.
- Enhanced fibrinolysis.
- Improved endothelial dysfunction, decreased systemic inflammation.

Exercise prescription
- Used as major component of rehabilitation following acute myocardial infarction.
- May be applied to subjects with stable angina. Should have pre participation exercise test.
- Non-pharmacological management of angina leads to increased functional capacity and angina threshold.

Potential adverse effects
- Enhanced catecholamine release, increased HR contractility, and systolic wall tension; main determinants of myocardial oxygen consumption.
- Potassium release may predispose to arrhythmias.
- Rise in free fatty acids.
- Enhanced platelet activation during exercise.
- May induce onset of angina, myocardial infarction, or sudden death.

Physical inactivity, exercise, and coronary artery disease

Epidemiological observations
- Occupational physical activity protective. IHD less in bus conductors than drivers, but drivers obese, raised cholesterol, and BP.
- Sedentary workers who participate in vigorous exercise have 50% fewer coronary heart disease (CHD) events than inactive colleagues.
- Indirect relationship of level of exercise and CHD; 3 times mortality in light workers compared to heavy workers. Shows dose–response for positive effects of exercise.
- Lifelong exercise protective, late exercisers assume low risk.
- Leisure time vigorous exercise protective.
- General increased level of cardiovascular fitness protective against coronary events.

Cardiac rehabilitation

Definition
A long-term process by which patients with cardiac disease are encouraged and supported by multidisciplinary professionals to achieve optimal physical and psychosocial health. Used as vehicle for paint specific secondary prevention.

Evidence of benefit
- In patients with myocardial infarction. Individual studies of exercise-based or comprehensive cardiac rehabilitation programmes are equivocal, but meta-analyses confirm 20–25% reduction in mortality and 28% reduction in fatal re-infarction at 2–3yr. No effects on non-fatal re-infarction or revascularization.
- 30–50% increase in exercise capacity and peak oxygen uptake of 10–20%. May not be sustained in long term.
- Improved sub-maximal exercise capacity, reduced rate of perceived exertion, and delayed onset of lactate threshold.
- Delayed onset of angina by reduced rate pressure product.
- Improved psychological well-being and quality of life.
- Improved physical activity but long term effects determined by compliance.
- Programme of exercise and information sessions that help patient to get back to everyday life as quickly as possible.
- It aims to help by understanding the problem, aiding recovery from a heart attack or surgery, make changes to lifestyle to improve heart health and reduce the risk of further clinical events.

Phases of rehabilitation

Phase 1: in-patient
Key elements are evaluation, reassurance, education, risk factor assessment, mobilization, and discharge planning. Applied after myocardial infarction, unstable angina, cardiac surgery, or angioplasty, or cardiac failure. To engage the patient and partner and identify particular problems prior to hospital discharge, and tailor the rehabilitation programme according to individual needs. Can be used after a step change in clinical condition. Encourage a positive attitude and introduce educational material.

Exercise prescription
Engage in self-care activities, general range of motion exercise, and walk short distances.

Phase 2: early outpatient recovery after discharge
Programme commencing 2–4 weeks after discharge lasting 4–12 weeks. Support from hospital or community-based health professionals through home visits or telephone contact. Education for risk factor modification and behavioural change. Medical evaluation for future management.

Exercise prescription
Undertake daily living activities and gradually increase the duration, frequency, and intensity of walking to increase functional and endurance activity.

Phase 3: intermediate outpatient
Generally comprises an exercise training programme undertaken in hospital gym with self-monitoring. Can be accommodated in community or home-based setting. Generally up to 12 weeks.

Exercise prescription
20–30min of low to moderate intensity aerobic exercise, e.g. walking, cycling, circuit training on 3 days a week and moderate intense physical activity, e.g. walking, on days when not participating in formal exercise programme.

Phase 4: long-term maintenance
Continued education after exercise period. Long-term rehabilitation may involve self-help groups, exercise leaders, or buddy programme. Community-based programme out of the hospital setting with most care delivered in primary care. Patient's clinical status, medication, and risk factor modification undertaken by GP or other health care professional.

Exercise prescription
A minimum of 20min of moderate intensity exercise on 3 days per week, and/or accumulate 30min or more of moderate intensity physical activity on at least 5 days a week. Use of local facilities.

Components at all phases
- Education to improve adherence to preventive therapies.
- Smoking cessation.
- Counselling.
- Exercise training.
- Psychology.
- Secondary prevention.

Initially, patient group with myocardial infarction and revascularization with coronary artery bypass graft (CABG). Total cardiovascular events and hospitalizations reduced after CABG. Angioplasty patients who participate in cardiac rehabilitation have a 50% better long-term survival.

Secondary prevention

Rehabilitation now used as vehicle for delivery, and exercise is one component. Encourage life style changes including diet and smoking.

Target risk factors with pharmacological agents to treat:
- Hypercholesterolaemia.
- Hypertension.
- Diabetes.
- Use of anti-platelet compounds, beta-blockers, and ACE inhibitors.

The multidisciplinary team includes doctors, nursing staff, physiotherapists, dieticians, and exercise consultants. Co-ordinate the programme for the maximum benefit of the individual.

Adherence strategies

High level of dropouts (9–49% from short supervised programmes). Factors include social class, angina, reduced ejection fraction, inactive leisure habits, current smoking, transport problems, medical problems, work, or domestic commitments, lack of motivation, inconvenient timing of programmes, anxiety, and depression.

Factors to improve maintenance of exercise
- Compliance improved by addressing travel problems.
- Membership of cardiac support groups and buddy systems.
- Community programmes.
- Home based programmes using local facilities.
- Use of electric or paper resources. Information from National Audit of Cardiac Rehabilitation.

Exercise referral

Exercise referral has now been widened to a larger group of subjects. With recognition that most individuals do not take adequate exercise, exercise prescription is now more widely applied.

Physical activity guidelines: exercise prescription for healthy adults

- 1990 American College of Sports Medicine (ACSM) exercise recommendation to improve and maintain cardio-respiratory fitness a minimum of 3 times 20 min of continuous moderate to vigorous intensity aerobic exercise per week. (60–90% of maximum HR or 50–85% of maximum aerobic capacity.)
- 1995 ACSM and Center for Disease Control (CDC) physical recommendation to promote health and prevent disease. Accumulate at least 30min of moderate intensity physical activity on five or more days per week. This activity would include alterations of daily routine of walking short distances or climbing stairs, and includes activities such as gardening, housework, or washing the car.
- Physical Activity Guidelines for Americans 2008:
  - Children and adolescents (6–17 yrs) should do 1h or more of physical activity every day. Most activity should be moderate or vigorous intensity aerobic physical activity. Vigorous intensity and muscle strengthening and bone strengthening activity should occur on at least 3 days a week.
  - Adults (18–64 yrs) Should do 2h and 30min a week of moderate intensity or 1h and 15min a week of vigorous intensity aerobic physical activity in episodes of at least 10min. Additional health benefits may occur by doubling the duration of exercise activities. Muscle strengthening exercises should be performed on 2 or more days a week.

Benefits of exercise

Mechanism of increased exercise capacity
Peripheral effects of skeletal muscle and vascular adaptations; increase in a-vO_2 diff, increased extraction, increased blood flow, and aerobic metabolism in skeletal muscle, increased fibre area, capillary density, and oxidative activity. Cardiac effects increased ejection fraction, cardiac output, stroke volume.

Clinical benefits
Lower risk of early death, heart disease, stroke, type 2 diabetes, high BP, adverse blood lipid profile, metabolic syndrome, colon, and breast cancers.

Prevention of weight gain, weight loss when combined with diet, improved cardiovascular and muscular fitness, prevention of falls/reduced depression and better cognitive function

New patient groups

Sedentary low risk groups have risk factors but no clinical symptoms nor overt disease. After screening for symptoms these patients are seen for exercise consultation.

High-risk patient groups have evidence of previous disease with a previous history of angina, myocardial infarction, or revascularization, but no ongoing exercise programme. Appropriate programmes of exercise are prescribed after pre-participation health and symptom questionnaires and exercise testing.

Information regarding facilities and sources
Exercise networks and sites of delivery are collated and advertised in public places, primary care facilities, and websites to provide the widest possible public access.

Exercise and adult congenital heart disease

The live birth incidence of congenital heart disease is 7–8 cases/1000 and 96% survive into adult life. Survival patterns have changed and exercise plays a role in assessment. Common heart defects include atrial septal defect, ventricular septal defect, patent ductus arteriosis, coarctation of the aorta with or without additional disease, valvular aortic stenosis, pulmonary stenosis, Fallot's tetralogy, and transposition of the great arteries. Many have interventions, but some complicated disease states have palliation and supportive therapy, including those with pulmonary hypertension including Eisenmenger circulation.

Areas for advice include employment, insurance, and driving. In particular we are concerned with advice re-exercise, activity level, sports participation, and the risk of sudden death.

Patient groups include:
- No previous surgery, but may be needed in future, e.g. aortic stenosis.
- Previous surgery with possible risk of arrhythmia, e.g. Fallot's tetralogy.
- Patients with palliation, further intervention required, e.g. Mustard procedure for transposition of great arteries (TGA).
- Inoperable subjects, consideration of heart- or heart-lung transplant.

Uses of exercise testing
- To evaluate symptoms and perception of functional capacity and decide if exercise prescription is indicated.
- To identify underlying cardiac lesion severity. Abnormal ventilatory response to exercise relates to cyanosis and predicts survival. Low peak oxygen uptake predicts hospitalization or death over the following year.
- To assess effectiveness of treatment or interventions.
- To assess functional capacity prior to recreational or athletic activity.

Information available from exercise testing
- Functional capacity including workload, oxygen consumption and anaerobic threshold.
- Heart rhythm including atrial and ventricular arrhythmias induced by exercise or heart block.
- BP response on exercise. (May induce fall in obstructive lesions or abnormal rise in patients with coarctation, with or without previous intervention.)
- Induction of myocardial ischaemia in patients with valvular disease.

Causes of limitation of exercise capacity
- Limitation of rise in cardiac output; Fontan repair, obstructive lesions of valves or ventricular outflow tract, or regurgitant lesions.
- Associated with chronotropic incompetence, inadequate stroke volume, and ventricular filling.
- Inadequate peripheral compensation and conditioning.
- Associated pulmonary disease.
- Psychological barriers of perceived limitations.

Exercise prescription
- Individual programme for each patient.
- Use of prescreening exercise test and use of target HR.
- Advice regarding type and duration of exercise according to nature of structural lesion.
- Education regarding symptoms and heart rhythm.
- Maintenance of fluid balance and avoidance of hypotension.

Guidelines for exercise and sport in congenital heart disease

- Advice should be in keeping with the nature of the exercise challenge, including whether the exercise is recreational or competitive, and also including the personality of the participant.
- Factors will include type, intensity, and duration of training and competition related to individual sports.
- Special consideration of the influence of bodily contact in subjects with valve replacements.
- Special limitation in sports if risk of loss of consciousness.
- Classification of sports is required in terms of isotonic and isometric components.

High risk
- Compromised ventricular function.
- Significant cardiomyopathy.
- Critical obstructive lesions.
- Severe regurgitant lesions.
- Severe pulmonary hypertension.
- Exercise induced ventricular arrhythmias.

Light exercise permitted
- Moderate obstructive lesions.
- Moderate regurgitant lesions.
- Moderate pulmonary hypertension.
- Systemic hypertension.
- Uncorrected cyanotic heart disease.

Minimal restriction to exercise
- Mild obstructive lesions.
- Mild regurgitant lesions.
- Shunts in the absence of pulmonary vascular disease.
- Corrected cyanotic patients with minimal anatomical abnormality.

Factors in individual congenital conditions

Coarctation of the aorta
Rigid proximal aorta leads to inappropriate BP response to exercise. Even after repair, 10% of those normotensive at rest have abnormal exercise or 24h BP responses. Nature of repair determines the long-term risk of aneurysm development or risk of rupture.

Pulmonary stenosis
Determine if mild, moderate, or severe. If major obstruction, gradient >50mmHg then recommend mild intensity of exercise and short duration. May be unrestricted post operation.

Atrial septal defect
In those without surgery—a small shunt in absence of pulmonary hypertension, no limitation. If pulmonary hypertension, then low intensity. In those following surgery, if pulmonary vascular resistance remains low, then no restriction. If post-operative pulmonary pressure is elevated then restrict. Atrial arrhythmias may occur on exercise.

Ventricular septal defect
Advice depends on the size of defect and pulmonary vascular resistance. Post-operative advice depends on pulmonary artery pressure, exclusion of ventricular arrhythmias on exercise, and 24h monitoring.

Patients with associated pulmonary vascular disease
If severe, low level exercise may lead to marked dyspnoea. Exercise may increase the left to right shunt. Local tissue acidosis occurs. Exercise induced syncope may occur.

Tetralogy of Fallot
If uncorrected, advice depends on exercise capacity associated with the degree of obstruction to the right ventricular outflow tract and increase in right to left shunt. Particular risks may occur with isometric exercise.

After repair, exercise influenced if residual shunt, induced pulmonary regurgitation following outflow tract repair, stenosis of pulmonary artery at site of previous Blalock shunt, or induction of arrhythmias which may occur in any patient with previous ventriculotomy.

Transposition of great arteries (Mustard repair)
Venous pathway obstruction may reduce exercise capacity. Baffle leaks may induce desaturation on early phase of exercise.

Depression of systemic right ventricle limits increase in cardiac output.

Sinus node dysfunction. Atrial and ventricular tachyarrhthmias or abnormal atrioventricular (AV) conduction may occur. General guideline of no more than mild to moderate isotonic exercise.

Fontan circulation

Circulation devoid of a functional sub-pulmonary ventricle. Function depends on nature of sub-aortic ventricle, which may be morphological left or right. Exercise performance reduced with lowered aerobic capacity, HR reduction, and post-operative hypoxaemia. Exercise capacity may be improved by total caval pulmonary connection.

Marfan syndrome

- Mutations in a single gene affects components of the extracellular matrix, leading to a disorder of the connective tissue.
- Autosomal dominant disease of connective tissue with variable expressibility. Frequency 1 in 20,000; 25% represent new mutations.
- Mutation on chromosome 15 in *fibrillin-1* gene (*FBN-1*) affecting the extracellular matrix glycoprotein present in the aorta, suspensory ligament of the lens, and connective tissue of tendons and ligaments.
- Molecular analysis of complement deoxynbp nucleic acid and deoxynbo nucleic acid on fibrillin 1 gene from skin fibroblasts culture shows reduced, absent, or structurally abnormal fibrillin and excessive transforming growth factor beta TGF-β.

Challenges

- Diagnosis made on clinical grounds with abnormalities in two systems.
- Genetic counselling, particular problems with pregnancy.
- Life style advice, body habitus may allow sports participation, e.g. basketball or volleyball.
- Cardiovascular surveillance aimed predominantly at aortic size and mitral valve.

Diagnosis

Skeletal system

Major criteria

- Pectus carinatum, pectus excavatum requiring surgery.
- Reduced upper to lower segment ratio or arm span to height ratio >1.05.
- Wrist and thumb signs.
- Scoliosis of >20° or spondylolisthesis.
- Reduced extension at the elbows (<170°).
- Pes planus.
- Protrusion acetabulae (on X-ray).

Minor criteria

- Pectus excavatum of moderate severity.
- Joint hypermobility.
- High-arched palate with crowding of teeth.
- Typical facial appearance.

Ocular system

Major criteria
Ectopia lentis.

Minor criteria

- Flat cornea (keratometry).
- Increased axial length of globe (ultrasound).
- Decreased miosis.

Major criteria

- Dura.
- Lumbosacral dural ectasia by CT or MRI.

Family/genetic history
Major criteria
- Having a parent, child or sibling who meets the diagnostic criteria independently.
- Known mutation in *fibrillin 1* gene.
- Haplotype of *FBN-1* is inherited and known to be associated with unequivocal Marfan syndrome in the family.

Cardiovascular system
Major criteria
- Dilatation of ascending aorta including sinuses of Valsalva.
- Dissection of ascending aorta.

Minor criteria
- Mitral valve prolapse.
- Unexplained dilatation of main pulmonary artery <40yr.
- Calcification of mitral valve annulus <40yr.
- Dilatation or dissection of descending thoracic or abdominal aorta <50yr.

Pulmonary system
Minor criteria
- Spontaneous pneumothorax.
- Apical blebs (chest X-ray).

Skin and integument
Minor criteria
- Unexplained stretch marks.
- Recurrent or incisional herniae.

Diagnostic criteria for Marfan syndrome

Negative family/genetic history
Major criteria in at least two different organ systems and involvement of a third system, or known genetic mutations plus one major criterion and involvement of a second organ system.

Positive family/genetic history
One major criterion in an organ system and involvement of a second organ system.

Cardiac problems
- Early mortality in 4th and 5th decades.
- Children are more affected by mitral valve disease.
- Aortic problems progressively more likely in adolescents and older.
- Mitral complications more common in females than males.

Higher risk of deterioration (25%) in this group of mitral valve prolapse than in normal population.

Mitral valve disease
Mitral annulus dilatation stretching, may occasionally rupture chordae. 10% have associated calcification. Repair of the valve is often successful.

Factors influencing the results of surgery: Valve cusp extremely redundant, marked chordal damage, degree of calcification. There is an increased risk of dehiscence of prosthetic valve if replacement required.

Aortic root involvement
May be dilated at birth, rate of progression variable. Prediction of dissection is difficult. Screening with trans-thoracic echo sufficient if dilatation limited to proximal ascending aorta. Usual rate of change is slow. If dilatation of descending aorta, trans-oesophageal echo and serial MRI required. Aortic valve regurgitation usually accompanies dilatation of 50mm. Consideration of surgical intervention if aorta 45mm

Positive family history may influence the decision

Treatment
Beta-blockers should be introduced as early as possible at the highest tolerated dose. Possible benefit of angiotensin 11 receptor blockers to reduce TGF-β.

Valve surgery
Approach to repair dilated aortic root, and preserve the aortic valve to avoid risks of endocarditis and anticoagulation.

Aortic root replacement
Elective root repair low operative mortality. Emergency results much poorer.

Aortic dissection
Most arise above the coronary ostium (type A Stanford). Some may extend the entire length (type 1 deBakey scheme). 10% distal to left subclavian (type B or 111). Rarely may be limited to abdominal aorta.

Follow-up to exclude progression requires MRI, transoesophageal echocardiography (TOE), and CT scan if prosthetic valve. Angiography and stenting procedures may be required for further dissection.

Pregnancy
- High risk of affected child.
- Dilatation of aortic root with aortic regurgitation and cardiac failure.
- Heightened risk of dissection. In third trimester, at parturition, and first month post-delivery.
- Risk highest if previous dilatation or dissection.
- Risk much less if aorta <40mm.

Preconception counselling
- If dilated or previous dissection consider termination.
- Avoid physical activity.
- Beta-blockade.
- If problems elective section.

Indications for monitoring
- Aortic root size must be monitored by echocardiography or MRI if echo window inadequate.
- If aortic root diameter is 4cm then investigations should be undertaken 3-monthly and if diameter is 4.5cm then prophylactic surgery will be considered.
- If aortic root is normal and no family history of sudden death then dynamic exercise may be undertaken in low and moderate static/low dynamic competitive sports, but isometric exercise should be avoided.

Hypertension and exercise

Prevalence
20% of adults over 40yrs have a BP > 140/90. Prevalence rises with age to >60% over age 60. Risks rise progressively over whole range of BP.

Diagnosis
- To establish level of BP, 3 readings should be taken in a relaxed environment over 3 months. If borderline, 24h ambulatory monitoring should be performed or home BP recordings performed using automatic recorders by patients on 4 week days on four occasions These values correlate better with target organ damage.
- Transient or persistent increases in BP may occur associated with stress, but have normal values at other times (e.g. white coat hypertension). This may occur in some 20% of subjects and is not related to cardiovascular events.
- There is considerable variability over 24h with a normal nocturnal dip. Loss of dip associated with more serious target organ effects.
- Exercise-induced hypertension may occur. Systolic BP rise >60mmHg after 5min, >70mmHg after 10min, or diastolic rise >10mmHg at any time is associated with the development of hypertension and an increased risk of cardiovascular events.

Aetiology
- Primary, essential, or idiopathic (90–95%).
- Secondary, associated with (a) renal disease (b) endocrine abnormalities, including Cushing's syndrome.
- Coarctation of the aorta.
- Pregnancy.

Natural history of hypertension and prognosis

- Established increase in diastolic BP (5–10mmHg) associated with a 34–56% increase in cerebrovascular accidents and a 21–37% increase in CAD.
- Absolute risk small 3.5% over 8yrs.
- Cause of death in hypertension; 50% CAD, 33% cerebrovascular accident (CVA), 10–15% chronic renal failure.

Symptoms and signs

- Uncomplicated high BP asymptomatic.
- End organ complications include left ventricular hypertrophy, abnormalities in renal function and hypertensive retinopathy.
- Decision on treatment is based on the overall cardiovascular risk including total cholesterol, low HDL, cigarette smoking, glucose intolerance and left ventricular hypertrophy (LVH).
- LVH is a cardiovascular risk factor. LVH independent predictor of cardiovascular death, cardiovascular events, and all cause mortality. Earliest change in LV is diastolic dysfunction. Then asymmetrical septal change, followed by concentric hypertrophy. Regression can occur with therapy.

Exercise and left ventricular hypertrophy

- Endurance exercise causes eccentric LVH; isometric exercise leads to concentric LVH.
- Posterior left ventricular wall increases with age, LVH more prevalent in some ethnic groups. LVH more common in males than females.

Vascular accelerated or malignant phase:
- Haemorrhagic stroke.
- Congestive heart failure.
- Nephrosclerosis.
- Aortic dissection.
- May reflect accelerated atherosclerosis; CAD including sudden death.
- Arrhythmias.
- Thrombotic stroke.
- Peripheral vascular disease.

Exercise capacity and hypertension

- Gradient in exercise capacity; increased from control, to those with no LVH, to those with LVH.
- Reduced ejection fraction if LVH.
- Significant reduction in exercise capacity, even in moderate hypertension and reduced oxygen consumption.
- Higher levels of systolic BP at each level of exercise.
- Independent inverse and grade association between fitness level and mortality risk.

Exercise haemodynamics, exercise capacity

- Inverse correlation between O_2 consumption, mean arterial pressure, and age.
- Inverse correlation between stroke volume and cardiac output and mean arterial pressure at rest.
- Cardiac output and HR inversely correlated with age.
- LVH not associated with maximum oxygen consumption.
- In people with hypertension, post-exercise BP reduced for up to 12h due to enhanced vascular compliance. Post-exercise hypotension occurs even with low intensity short duration exercise.

Treatment of hypertension

For mild rise in BP, introduce life-style changes.
- Prevention of obesity.
- Moderate reduction in Na intake.
- Higher levels of physical activity.
- Avoid excess alcohol.

Exercise as treatment for hypertension

Effects of exercise for 20–60min at 60–80% maximum HR, 3 times weekly.
- Reduction in sub maximum HR.
- Increase in peak VO_2.
- Reduction in maximum BP (systolic and diastolic and sub maximum BP). Associated with reduction in LV mass and LV mass index.
- Meta-analysis of randomized controlled trials. 29 trials including 1533 subjects. Small consistent reduction in BP with aerobic exercise (systolic 4.7, diastolic 3.1).
- Little difference according to intensity of exercise.
- Little effect of number of training sessions.

Drug treatment of hypertension

Agents and specific indications for comorbidites

- *Diuretics*: heart failure, elderly and systolic hypertension.
- *Beta-blockers*: angina, post-myocardial infarction, and tachyarrhythmias.
- *ACE inhibitors*: heart failure, LV dysfunction, post-myocardial infarction, and diabetic nephropathy.
- *Calcium antagonists*: angina, elderly patients, and systolic hypertension.
- *Alpha blockers*: prostatic hypertrophy.
- *Angiotensin 11 antagonists*: ACE inhibitor cough.

Exercise and heart failure

Definition
The pathophysiological state in which an abnormality of cardiac function is responsible for failure of the heart to pump blood at a rate sufficient for the requirements of the metabolizing tissues.

Epidemiology
- Prevalence in European population 0.4–2%. The prevalence increases with age: 1% at 25–54yrs, 4–5% at 64–74yrs, 6.6–7.9% at 89–90yrs.
- Five-year mortality 50%. 10 million cardiac failure (CHF) patients in EU countries (ESC Taskforce on Heart Failure 2001). Frequent hospitalization, requirement for help with daily living, but with high economic cost.

Aetiology and clinical presentation
- High output failure secondary to anaemia, pregnancy, thyrotoxicosis, AV fistula, Paget's disease.
- *Low output failure:* acute or chronic.
- *Volume overload:* regurgitant valve or high output state.
- *Pressure overload:* systemic hypertension, outflow obstruction, e.g. aortic stenosis.
- *Loss of muscle:* acute following myocardial infarction.
- Chronic cardiomyopathy with longstanding IHD.
- *Infective:* endocarditis, viral myocarditis, infiltrative.
- *Metabolic:* nutritional.
- Drug-induced adriamycin, 5-fluorouracil and daunorubicin.
- *Restricted filling:* pericardial disease, restrictive cardiomyopathy.

Classified as per New York Heart Association with increased symptoms on exercise.
- *Grade 1:* no limitation, but objective evidence of cardiac dysfunction VO_2 15–20mL/kg/min.
- *Grade 2:* limited on moderate physical exertion, e.g. hills and stairs VO_2 10–15mL/kg/min.
- *Grade 3:* limited on normal daily activities, e.g. bathing, cooking VO_2 5–10mL/kg/min.
- *Grade 4:* limited at rest on minimal exertion, e.g. rising from chair VO_2 < 5mL/kg/min.

Left ventricular failure
Dyspnoea may extend to orthopnoea or paroxysmal nocturnal attacks with pulmonary oedema. Increased respiratory rate, tachycardia, S3, and basal crepitations.

Right ventricular failure
Peripheral oedema—site related to posture. Breathlessness, fatigue. Signs of right ventricular hypertrophy, elevated JVP.

Central haemodynamics
- Systolic dysfunction usually associated with LV dilatation.
- Reduced stroke volume and ejection fraction.

- Diastolic dysfunction may predominate.
- Reduced cardiac output.
- Elevated end diastolic pressures, with increased preload.
- *Compensatory neurohormonal activation:*
  - *Increased sympathetic activity*—increases HR and contractility, but leads to increased arteriolar constriction and afterload and increases oxygen consumption.
  - *Increased renin angiotensin aldosterone*—leads to salt and water retention with increased venous return, but associated with vasoconstriction and increased afterload.
  - *Increased vasopressin*—enhances venous return, but increases vasoconstriction.
  - *Increased endothelin*—vasoconstriction, but increased afterload.
  - Increased interleukins and TNF $\propto$.

Investigations
- Clinical examination.
- Electrocardiography including exercise testing.
- Echocardiography transthoracic echocardiography (TTE), or TOE.
- Chest X-ray.
- MRI.
- Invasive investigations including coronary arteriography.

Treatment of cardiac failure

Drug treatment
- Diuretics.
- ACE inhibitor.
- Beta-blocker.
- Spironolactone.
- Angiotensin receptor blocker.
- Digoxin if atrial fibrillation or severe heart failure.
- Consider aspirin and statin.

Devices: CRT, implantable cardioverter defibrillator (ICD), and LV assist devices.

Lifestyle modification
- Stop smoking.
- Fluid restriction.
- Reduce salt intake.
- Eat more fresh fruit and vegetables.
- Monitor body weight.
- Reduce alcohol intake.
- Lose weight.
- Regular moderate exercise.

Exercise in cardiac failure

LV performance, cardiac output, and myocardial oxygen consumption are determined by: (a) HR, (b) preload, (c) contractility, (d) afterload.
- *Preload:* in a normal heart, ventricular systolic performance is related to the degree of end diastolic fibre stretch or preload. This is influenced by end diastolic pressure and volume. In heart failure, further stretch is associated with decreased function.
- *Contractility:* force and velocity contraction can be assessed in isovolumic or ejection phases. May be expressed as the ejection fraction.
- *Afterload:* force resisting myocardial shortening, i.e. resistance—the LV must overcome to eject stroke volume.

Reduction in exercise capacity in CHF
- Cardiac insufficiency, poor left ventricular function and resulting reduced cardiac output, decreased exercise tolerance, and reduced peak VO_2.
- Pulmonary changes with increased respiratory rate reduced tidal volume, and ventilation perfusion mismatch.
- Skeletal muscle dysfunction secondary to hyper perfusion with reduced oxidative enzymes, and increased glycolytic enzymes. Impaired oxygen utilization during exercise.
- Further changes due to detraining and development of abnormal mitochondria.
- Metabolic receptor activation may lead to increased ventilation and increased sympathetic tone with vagal withdrawal and reduced baroreceptor sensitivity.

Exercise testing
- Exercise time determined using treadmill or bicycle ergometer protocol. Use of ramp protocol most appropriate with workload increasing continuously. Optimum duration 8–12min. Breath-by-breath analysis shows that Ve/VCO_2 peak exercise: rest correlates with exercise time and anaerobic threshold.
- Peak VO_2 is the best indicator of prognosis in heart failure, although correlates poorly with haemodynamic measurements at rest, which do not reflect functional reserve.
- Peak VO_2 < 10mL/kg/min, 77% 1yr mortality. Peak VO_2 10–18mL/kg/min, 10.1% 1yr mortality.

Six-minute walk test
Simple non-invasive test, which is a good predictor of morbidity and mortality in patients with mild-to-moderate CHF.

Distance walked in 6min is an independent predictor of mortality and hospitalization in advanced heart failure.

Effects of exercise in heart failure

- No significant change in left ventricular ejection fraction.
- Improvement in diastolic function.
- Increased cardiac output at peak exercise with increased peak leg blood flow.
- Increased exercise tolerance. Peak VO$_2$ increased by 12–31%.
- Reduced chronotropic response to exercise.
- Minute ventilation reduced, slope of minute ventilation to rate of CO$_2$ production reduced. Improved ventilatory threshold.
- Reduction in activity of ergo receptors with reduction in excessive ventilation.
- Reduced catecholamine levels and sympathetic tone. Increased vagal activity.

Altered skeletal muscle function

- Decreased lactate production at sub-maximal exercise.
- Decrease in early acidosis and phosphocreatinine depletion on exercise. Enhanced capacity for oxidative synthesis of adenosine triphosphate.
- Increased volume density of mitochondria.
- Restoration of flow dependent endothelium mediated vasodilatation in exercising limbs.

Exercise and treatment of cardiac failure

- *Moderate exercise training*: improved functional capacity, quality of life, and outcome in patients with stable CHF after 2 months No further improvement after 1yr. Addition of full cardiac rehabilitation with lifestyle education and behavioural modification associated with improved survival for patients with left ventricular dysfunction.
- *Three months of low level exercise training*: increased peak VO_2. Reduced perceived dyspnoea during exercise and improved quality of life score. Improved exercise tolerance of >2min, peak O_2 uptake of 2mL/kg/min.

Beneficial actions are additional to actions of angiotensin-converting enzyme inhibitors (ACEI) and beta-blockers.

- *Randomized trials*. Exercise training in heart failure is beneficial in improving functional capacity. Quality of life improves. Reduced need for hospital admission. Mortality reduction.
- *Cost effectiveness*. Exercise prolonged survival by additional 1.82yrs at a relatively low cost per year of life saved.
- *Selective respiratory muscle training*: improves ventilatory muscle endurance and reduces perceived dyspnoea.

American Heart Association (AHA) exercise recommendation in cardiac failure

- Include adequate warm up of 15min.
- Individualized approach.
- Aim 70–80% peak VO_2 for 20–30min.
- Severely debilitated—unaccustomed to exercise. Aim 60–65% peakVO_2.
- Builds progression into prescription.
- 3–5 exercise periods/week.
- Initial session supervised.
- Cool down session advised.

Alternative use of low intensity physical training, home exercise programme and localized arm training programmes.

Sudden death

Sudden death in sport is uncommon, but has major media interest. Two cases occur per 100,000 subject years. Five in 100,000 of the sporting populations have a predisposing cardiac condition. 10% of those at risk die suddenly. The causes reflect the age of participant, structural, and electrophysiological abnormalities in the young, CAD in older groups.

Pre-participation screening

This remains controversial. The main aim is to identify causes of sudden sporting death, with screening applied to the whole participating population. Alternative strategies have been suggested for those with:
- A family history of sudden death.
- Premature CAD.
- Counselling of patients with known abnormalities—education about warning symptoms including syncope, pre-syncope, palpitation, chest pain, and dyspnoea.

Guidelines may be required for disqualification from competition.

Methods of pre-participation screening
- Use of health questionnaires; includes symptomatic enquiry for warning symptoms and family history. May include aspects of respiratory and orthopaedic health as part of wider screening programme.
- ECGs may be taken as routine.
- Echocardiography and exercise testing may be used in those with suggestive symptoms or with abnormal ECG. May require tests in 30% of population.

Conditions with known cardiovascular risk <35yrs
- Hypertrophic cardiomyopathy.
- Idiopathic concentric LVH.
- Anomalies of coronary arteries.
- Aortic rupture.
- Right ventricular dysplasia.
- Myocarditis.
- Valvular disease.
- Arrhythmias and conduction defects.

Hypertrophic cardiomyopathy
- Leading cause of sudden unexpected death in young athletes.
- Autosomal dominant with high degree of penetrance.
- Some echocardiographic features present in 1 in 500 of the population.
- Symptoms may include chest pain, palpitation, syncope, and dyspnoea.
- Predisposition to supraventricular and ventricular arrhythmias.
- Clinical signs include a jerky character pulse, double apex beat, and a fourth heart sound often present.
- Ejection systolic murmur at left sternal border.
- Abnormal ECG in 90%.

Echocardiography Hypertrophied non-dilated left ventricle with no predisposing cause for LVH. Chamber size reduced. Impaired diastolic filling.

Left ventricular outflow tract obstruction with hypertrophy of sub-aortic septum and systolic anterior motion of the mitral valve.

Adverse prognostic factors include:
- Family history of sudden death.
- Documented ventricular tachycardia.
- Young age of onset of symptoms.

Concentric left ventricular hypertrophy
- Concentric hypertrophy of left ventricle in the absence of hypertension.
- Associated with cardiac death.
- Significant incidence in black athletes, which might reflect athletic training.
- If present, expect deconditioning for 6 months, may show regression.

Coronary artery anomalies
- Significant anomaly of left coronary artery arising from the right coronary cusp maintaining an acute angle with the aorta.
- Aortic dilatation on exercise causes obstruction to flow.
- Other anomalies may include the absence or under-development of major coronary branches.
- Symptoms of chest pain, syncope, or sudden death.

Investigations
- Resting ECG.
- Exercise testing or evidence of exercise-induced reversible ischaemia.
- Radionuclide assessment for regional perfusion.
- Coronary arteriography.
- Treatment and transplantation of coronary artery may be undertaken using cuff of peri-coronary artery tissue.

Marfan syndrome
- Connective tissue derangement if fibrillin reduced or defective.
- Autosomal dominant with variable penetrance, 15% sporadic.
- Gene on the long arm of chromosome 15.

Systems involved:
- Musculoskeletal.
- Ocular abnormalities.
- Cardiovascular system.

Cardiovascular abnormalities
- Mitral valve prolapse.
- May develop significant mitral regurgitation.
- Aortic root dilatation.
- Aortic regurgitation.
- Aortic dissection may occur in ascending, descending, or abdominal aorta.Investigation.
- Echocardiography for aortic valve and ascending aortic root sizing.
- MRI of individual aortic segments.
- *Medical therapy*: beta-blockade shows slowing of aortic dilatation. Possible additional action of A11 inhibitors.
- *Aortic root dilatation*: screening for change on 3-monthly intervals.
- If 4.5cm consider prophylactic valve sparing surgery.

Right ventricular dysplasia
- Right ventricular cardiomyopathy.
- Unusually high incidence in northern regions of Italy.
- Pathological change of fibro-fatty replacement, with irregular muscle disruption.
- Malignant re-entrant ventricular tachyarrhythmias.
- *Symptoms:* reflecting right ventricular dysfunction, palpitation, and syncope.

Investigation
- Clinical signs of right ventricular dysfunction.
- ECG shows inverted T waves in right ventricular leads.
- Echocardiography shows global right ventricular enlargement with increased residual volume and (RV) wall motion abnormalities.
- Investigations may include right ventricular angiography and endomyocardial biopsy.
- Treatment for right ventricular dysfunction and arrhythmias.

Myocarditis
- Variable illness associated with symptoms of viral infection.
- Myocardial lymphocytic infiltration with focal necrosis leading to cardiac dysfunction and conduction system problems.
- Symptoms non-specific, like cold or flu.
- *Clinical examination:* tachycardia, supraventricular or ventricular extrasystoles. May progress to cardiomegaly and frank signs of cardiac failure.
- *Diagnosis:* ECG—non-specific changes with ST-T wave changes, arrhythmias, heart block.
- Echocardiography shows signs of chamber dysfunction.
- *Management:* broad spectrum of severity. Treat cardiac failure and arrhythmias in severe cases. If objective signs present on investigation return to sport when ECG normal, left ventricular contraction normal, and absence of arrhythmias.

Valvular disease
- The aetiology may be congenital, acquired, or degenerative (atherosclerotic in older age group).
- Type of valve disease identified clinically.
- Severity assessed on clinical examination.
- Electrocardiography for evidence of atrial or ventricular chamber hypertrophy with ST–T wave changes of strain pattern.
- Chest X-ray for identification of chamber enlargement.
- Echocardiography and Doppler assessment for chamber size, assessment of stenosis, and regurgitation of individual valve, calculated gradients, and regurgitant volume.
- MRI shows detailed assessment which may be complementary to echocardiography.

Aortic stenosis
- Valve lesion associated with cardiac sudden death in sport.
- Management depends on presence of symptoms of chest pain, syncope, and breathlessness.
- Advice re exercise. If mild, all sports can be undertaken. If moderate, low intensity or moderate static and dynamic exercise.

Mitral valve prolapse
- Variable condition.
- May be a normal variant in 6% of the population.
- Often with non-specific symptoms.
- Clinical examination: may be evidence of click murmur.
- ECG non-specific.
- *Echocardiogram:* evidence of 'floppy mitral valve leaflets'.
- *Complications:* TIAs in small proportion.
- Progressive mitral regurgitation.
- Association with supraventricular and ventricular arrhythmias.
- Predisposition to endocarditis.
- *Management:* pragmatic. If asymptomatic and no family history of cardiac complications, no limitation in activity.

Arrhythmias and heart block
- The mechanism of sudden death is arrhythmic, almost always ventricular fibrillation.
- Predisposing factors of enhanced automaticity, conduction, or repolarization in the electrophysiological tissues of the heart.
- Autonomic changes may occur during exercise, baseline vagal activity leading to bradycardia and heart block.
- Sympathetic activity during exercise: may lead to catecholamine-induced serious arrhythmias.
- Arrhythmias may be associated with structural abnormalities such as hypertrophic cardiomyopathy, or right ventricular dysplasia. Structural abnormalities associated with valvular and other congenital heart disease including those with previous right ventriculotomy.
- Arrhythmic symptoms include palpitation, syncope or presyncope, breathlessness, sudden death.

Investigations
- ECG for evidence of pre-excitation, prolonged QRS or evidence of myocardial ischaemia or structural abnormality.
- Exercise electrocardiography used to induce symptoms.
- Continuous ECG monitoring (minimum duration 24h) period expanded according to symptoms. If rare occurrence, but significant symptoms, use of symptom or event triggering monitoring.
- Invasive investigation by programmed electrical stimulation, with intracardiac sensing electrodes.
- *Management:* anti-arrhythmic therapy, intracardiac ablation techniques for ectopic sites of electrical activity, or pulmonary vein ablation for atrial fibrillation. Device implantation may be required.

Pre-excitation in Wolff–Parkinson–White syndrome
- ECG confirms short PR interval, <0.12s.
- Wide QRS complex, initial slurring of the QRS complex (delta wave).
- Commonest tachycardia 150–250beats/min.
- Rarely atrial flutter or fibrillation, which may conduct through anomalous pathway to predispose to ventricular fibrillation in those with accessory pathways with short refractory periods.

- If symptomatic, assessment of accessory pathway undertaken. In high-intensity sports, electrophysiological studies should be undertaken, atrial fibrillation (AF) induced and shortest RR interval assessed.
- If rapid ventricular rates drug therapy or ablation.

Prolonged QT syndrome
- Repolarization abnormalities and prolonged QT syndrome. Symptoms associated with emotion or physical stress.
- QT prolongation to more than 0.44s corrected for HR in the absence of other causes of prolongation (drugs and electrolyte abnormalities) leads to ventricular tachycardia, including torsades de pointes.
- Bradyarrhthmias common on ECG monitoring. T wave alternans may be induced by emotion.
- Therapy beta-blockade, surgical sympathectomy if treatment failure. Occasional pacing therapy.
- Avoidance of competitive athletics and sympathetic stimuli.

Brugada syndrome
- Commonest cause of sudden death in young men without underlying cardiac disease.
- 20% associated with mutations in gene *SCN5A* on short arm of third chromosome, which encodes for sodium ion channel.
- Autosomal dominant with variable degrees of penetration and expression.

Diagnosis
Characteristic pattern on electrocardiograph which may be present at all times or elicited by administration of class 1c antiarrhythmic agents. (ajmaline or flecainide.) Diagnostic pattern of persistent ST elevation in leads V1-V3 with RBBB pattern. ECG influenced by autonomic balance and exercise.

Treatment
- ICD for ventricular arrhythmias, polymorphic ventricular tachycardia, or ventricular fibrillation.
- Possible prophylactic use of quinidine.

Coronary artery disease
- Major cause of death in those >35yrs.
- Most deaths occur in vigorous sports.
- Previous symptoms suggestive of coronary atherosclerosis may be recognized, including anginal symptoms on exertion.
- Established risk factors for CAD often present, including hypertension and hypercholesterolaemia.
- Victims often perceived as being very fit with type A personality.
- Pathological studies confirm the presence of obstructive CAD.
- Myocardium may show previous healed infarction.
- Sudden death is not prevented by extreme forms of conditioning.
- Investigations of resting ECG, exercise stress testing, assessment of left ventricular function, and coronary arteriography.
- Management by risk factor modification.

- Education concerning warning symptoms of chest pain, palpitation, or syncope.
- In subjects with structural abnormalities including valvular disease or congenital lesions, operated or not, then advice on exercise participation will be directed by the classification of the physical needs of each activity.

Intensity and type of exercise performed in specific sports

Type A
- Moderate or high dynamic and static demands: boxing, cross-country skiing, cycling, downhill skiing, fencing, ice hockey, rowing, rugby, running (sprinting), speed skating, US football, water polo, and wrestling.
- *Moderate to high dynamic and low static demands:* badminton, baseball, basketball, field hockey, lacrosse, orienteering, race walking, racket ball, running (distance), soccer, squash, swimming, table tennis, tennis, and volleyball.
- Moderate to high static and low dynamic demands: archery, auto racing, diving, equestrian, field events (jumping and throwing), gymnastics, karate or judo, motor cycling, sailing, ski jumping, water skiing, and weightlifting.

Type B
- *Low intensity (low dynamic and low static demands):* bowling, cricket, curling, golf, and shooting.
- *Danger of bodily collision:* boxing, ice hockey, karate or judo, lacrosse, rugby, soccer, US football, and wrestling.

Increased risk if syncope occurs
Auto racing, cycling, diving, downhill skiing, equestrian events, gymnastics, motor racing, polo, ski jumping, water polo, water skiing, and weightlifting.

Exercise-induced bronchoconstriction

Definition
- *EIB:* also sometimes called exercise-induced bronchospasm. A transient, reversible increase in airway obstruction that occurs in association with vigorous exercise.
- *Intrinsic asthma (IntA) or allergic asthma:* chronic airway restriction assumed to be due to some endogenous cause such as allergies.
- Contraction of airway smooth muscle, airway swelling (oedema).
- Excess mucous production coupled with inflammatory exudates.
- Thickening of the airways (remodelling)—not fully reversible.
- 'Triggers' of IntA include:
  - *Allergens:* indoor (house-dust mites, pets, fungi); and outdoor (pollens, grasses, moulds, etc.).
  - *Pollutants:* indoor (cigarette smoke—passive and active smokers, chloramines in swimming pools); and outdoor (air pollutants, dust).
  - Cold air, exercise.
  - Respiratory infections.
  - *Drugs:* beta-blockers and NSAIDS.
- The term EIA—should *not* be utilized interchangeably with EIB. If used at all, it should refer to exercise-induced bronchoconstriction in patients with intrinsic asthma.

Epidemiology
- Asthma is the most common medical condition affecting Olympic athletes—greater than 7% confirmed in 2006, 2008, 2010 Games.
- EIB occurs in 80–90% of asthmatic persons and 40–50% of those with allergic rhinitis.
- EIB can also occur in non-asthmatic persons (can be found in more than 10% of the general population).
- EIB has an incidence of 11–50% in elite athletes, 90% in those with IntA.
- Incidence of EIB is greater in athletes participating in:
- *Swimming*—exposure to chlorinates/chloramines in indoor pools.
  - *Summer endurance sports*—high minute ventilation, pollutants.
  - *Winter sports*—found in approximately 50% of Olympic Nordic or cross-country skiers (cold dry air and high minute ventilation).
  - Over time, endurance athletes training in cold climates may be at risk of sustaining injury to airways (remodelling). Partly irreversible?
  - *Speed skating, ice hockey, figure skating*—may be from exposure to pollutants from diesel powered ice-resurfacing machines (zamboni).
- Scuba diving is best avoided by those with chronic asthma (and maybe those with EIB): combination of physical exertion, inhalation of dry, cold compressed air, and the possibility of inhaling fresh or salt water. Can cause airways obstruction, air trapping, hyperinflation of lungs, increasing the chance of pulmonary barotrauma and pneumothorax during ascent to the surface, possibly even fatal air embolism.

Aetiology
Exact cause is not well understood. May be multiple aetiologies specific to the individual. The airways are much more sensitive in EIB than in normal individuals, although normal people can have exercise-induced bronchoconstriction under the right conditions (i.e. cold air, infections).

- *Hyperventilation as a cause of airway drying:*
  - EIB is worsened in some individuals when exercising in cold dry air.
  - Evaporative water loss results in drying and cooling of the airways.
  - The increased osmolarity of the mucous somehow causes a release of inflammatory mediators (prostaglandins, cysteinyl-leukotrienes), which cause bronchoconstriction and altered vascular permeability.
  - Hyperventilation alone can cause bronchoconstriction.
  - Hyperventilation with moist warm air inhibits bronchoconstriction (explains why indoor swimming is thought to be non-asthmagenic).
- *The osmolarity of airways does not recover immediately after exercise:*
  - Prostaglandin E2 may be protective.
  - Leukotriene B4 is increased following exercise.
  - Leukotriene inhibitors have been shown to decrease and prevent bronchoconstriction during exercise.
- *Post-exercise rewarming as a source of bronchoconstriction:*
  - Rapid rewarming may cause reactive hyperemia and edema in the airway mucosa and submucosa.
  - This may result in luminal narrowing and reactive asthma.
- *Air pollution:*
  - Primary pollutants and secondary pollutants have been identified: ozone, sulphur dioxide, nitrogen oxides, particulate matter (PM).
  - Hyperventilation also increases the amount of allergens and pollutants that may reach the pulmonary tree and lower airways.
- Exercise-induced mediator release from mast cells and basophils.
- Parasympathetic mediation through vagus nerve innervation.

Definition of pulmonary/lung function tests (PFTs):
- FEV_1 = forced expiratory volume (L) in 1s after full inspiration.
- FVC = total volume of air forcefully exhaled out of the airway when the breath continues (usually for period of 6 or more seconds)—effort dependent.
- PEFR = peak expiratory flow rate—maximal flow rate of air (L/s or L/min) out of the airways—also effort dependent.
- FEV_1/FVC ratio—decreases in obstructive lung disease (i.e. asthma, pulmonary fibrosis); remains normal in restrictive lung disease.
- FEF_{25-75} = flow between 25% and 75% of FVC.
- Levels should be at least 80% of predicted values to be considered 'normal', and FEV_1/FVC ratio should also be above 80%.

Clinical presentation
- In normal people and in those with EIB with no baseline PFT changes, exercise increases PEFR and FEV_1 by less than 5%.
- In those with baseline obstruction it may increase by more than 25%.
- 28–52% of those with EIB experience a decline in PFTs by the end of exercise; may intensify over 3–20min and may last 20–30min.
- After exercise there may be a decrease in pulmonary function by up to 10% in normal subjects (this decrease is higher in EIB).

Refractory period
- After exercise, approximately 50% of patients with EIB are resistant to further bronchoconstriction.
- This usually lasts less than 3h.
- Mechanism is not readily understood.
- Can be used by athletes as a non-pharmacological therapy in preparation for training and/or competition.

Late phase reaction
- A second increase in airway reactivity may be seen in up to 50% of children 4–12h after the acute episode.
- The release of inflammatory mediators (such as eosinophilic chemotactic factor of anaphylaxis, platelet activating factor, and leukotrienes) by bronchial smooth muscle has been theorized as a cause.

Diagnosis

History

The athlete may be unaware of any bronchoconstriction (Table 10.1):
- More significant symptoms include dyspnoea (shortness of breath,) cough, lack of endurance, or wheeze, during or immediately after sustained vigorous exercise (peaks about 5–10min afterwards).
- Athletes may feel vague chest tightness or feel 'out of shape'.
- Children may simply avoid strenuous play or exercise, have chest pain, or experience abdominal pain.
- History of symptoms is a poor predictor of occurrence of EIB.
- There is much evidence that EIB is underdiagnosed.
- Multiple stimulants have been identified (Table 10.2).

Pulmonary function tests
- Medications are withheld for 8–24h before testing.
- Baseline PFTs are done first and should be within 80% of predicted values (or intrinsic asthma may be present).
- Most athletes with EIB have normal baseline spirometry

Bronchodilator test

Can confirm airway hyper-responsiveness (AHR) with bronchodilator test, positive if a 12% or greater increase in FEV_1 occurs after inhalation of rapidly acting beta2 agonist.

Challenge tests: direct

Methacholine challenge test
- If suspicion is high for EIB and/or exercise challenge testing is negative, a methacholine challenge test may be performed.
- Increasing doubling concentrations of drug are used.
- Concentration or dose that creates a 20% fall in FEV_1 from baseline is expressed as the PC or PD20.
- Positive test: 20% drop (PC20 < 4mg/mL or PD20<2μmol)
- More sensitive test, but less specific.
- Done in a hospital setting, must have intubation equipment available.

Histamine challenge test
- Not as commonly performed, may not be as sensitive for EIB.
- Positive test is 20% or greater fall in FEV_1 at a histamine concentration of 8 mg/mL or less during a graded test of 2min.

Table 10.1 Clinical clues to exercise-induced bronchospasm (may be present during or after exercise)

Obvious clinical clues	Subtle clinical clues
• Wheezing • Cough • Dyspnoea on exertion • Chest tightness	• Abdominal pain • Athlete feels 'out of shape' • Cannot run 5min without stopping • Chest congestion • Chest discomfort or pain • Increased difficulty in cold air • Problems with running but not swimming • Lack of energy • Frequent 'colds'

Table 10.2 Stimulants that can contribute to exercise-induced bronchospasm

- Exercise
- Cold air
- Low humidity
- Respiratory infections
- Fatigue
- Emotional stress
- Athletic overtraining
- Primary pollutants
- Secondary pollutants
- Other pollutants
- Strong odors and other airborne irritants
- Allergens

Challenge tests: indirect

Laboratory-based exercise challenge
- Use treadmill, bicycle, or rowing ergometer for exercise stress (or whatever activity is most asthmagenic).
- Athlete exercises until 80–90% of maximum HR is achieved.
- HR is maintained for 6–8min.
- PFTs are measured before and immediately after exercise, and then every 5min for 20–30min.
- EIB is present if there is a 10% or more decrease in PEFR or forced expiratory volume after one second (FEV_1).
  - 10–20% decrease is mild EIB.
  - 20–40% decrease is moderate EIB.
  - >40% decrease is severe EIB.

Field-based exercise challenge
- An example is the Free Running Asthma Screening Test (FRAST).
- Spirometry before and after exercise in the challenging environment.
- Sensitive and specific for cold weather athletes.
- Inexpensive, easily performed (minimal equipment), not standardized.

Eucapnoeic voluntary hyperpnoea
- Also called isocapnic hyperventilation test.
- Athlete hyperventilates a mixture of cold dry air containing 5% CO_2, 21% O_2, and 74% N_2.
- Hyperventilation for 6min: EVH test relies on athlete being able to attain and maintain ventilatory flow equivalent to 85% of maximal voluntary ventilation (MMV)—approximately 30 times baseline FEV_1.
- Positive test is 10% drop in FEV_1.
- Not always available: relatively expensive, need to control inspired gases and humidity, and accurately monitor minute ventilation.

Osmotic challenge tests (mannitol or hyperosmolar saline)
- Inhaled substance develops an osmotic gradient across airways.
- Positive test is 15% fall in FEV_1 after hyperosmolar challenge.

Mannitol
- *Dry powder inhalation test:* comes in standardized test kit with prefilled capsules in escalating doses and hand-held powder inhaler device.
- Can be used safely in pre-hospital setting.
- Not available yet in all countries.

Hyperosmolar saline
- Administration of nebulized hypertonic saline.
- Spirometry before and after nebulization.

Differential diagnosis
Vocal cord dysfunction
- Paradoxical adduction of the vocal cords.
- Inspiratory stridor (wheeze) and throat tightness.
- Highest incidence is among young females.
- Flow-volume loops may show inspiratory blunting.
- Definitive diagnosis requires direct visualization of vocal cords during exercise (fibre optic videolaryngoscopy)—on cycle ergometer.
- Treat with breathing retraining exercises, speech pathology.

Other conditions
- Deconditioning, obesity.
- Hyperventilation syndrome, anxiety.
- Cardiac abnormalities (congestive heart failure, CAD, dysrhythmias, hypertrophic cardiomyopathy, valve disease).
- Pulmonary vascular diseases, such as pulmonary hypertension or pulmonary arteriovenous malformations.
- Pulmonary disease (asthma, chronic obstructive pulmonary disease (COPD), cystic fibrosis, interstitial lung disease, scoliosis, pectus excavatum, tracheobronchial malacia).
- Gastroesophageal reflux disease (GERD).
- Myopathies: muscular dystrophies, disorders of muscle energy metabolism.

Exercise-induced anaphylaxis
- Exercise-induced or cholinergic urticaria: can sometimes lead to hypotension and collapse.
- Often associated with pre-exercise exposure to food allergen.
- Spectrum of disease can be associated or confused with EIB.

Treatment of EIB
See Table 10.3.

Table 10.3 Treatment for exercise-induced bronchoconstriction (EIB)

Non-pharmacological corrections (see text)
EIB continues
⇓
SABA
EIB continues
⇓
Add cromolyn or nedocromil if paediatric, a late responder, or previous history of response to cromolyn (may double B2A and cromolyn if needed)
EIB continues
⇓
Add LABA and inhaled glucocorticosteroid
EIB continues
⇓
Add leukotriene inhibitor
EIA continues
⇓
Add inhaled glucocorticosteroid
EIB continues
⇓
Add ipratropium bromide. By now most asthmatics should be controlled. If not, consider oral steroid burst, alternative cause, or referral
⇓
Effective control of EIA
(check inhaler technique and lung function regularly)

Non-pharmacological
- *Regular exercise programmes:*
  - Regular exercise programmes produce a significant reduction in bronchoconstriction.
  - Increased tolerance and threshold levels for exercise.
  - Decreased medication needs.
  - Decreased absenteeism.
  - Improvement in aerobic capacity (increased VO_2 max).
  - Enhancement of self-image.
  - Greater recognition and acceptance by peers (removes negative image).
- *Considerations:*
  - Wearing a facemask for outdoor exercise may increase air temperature and humidity, and help to filter out allergens and pollutants. Not usually practical during competition.
  - A warm shower immediately after exercise may reduce the bronchoconstriction.
  - Avoid exercise in early morning or late evening if conditions are cold.
  - Encourage indoor sport in winter.
  - Avoid areas where pollutants and allergens are high.
  - Encourage water sports or sports that allow intermittent rest periods (most team sports, tennis, weightlifting, racquetball, etc.).
  - Short bursts of activity can produce refractory periods that last up to 3h.
  - Warm up before any exercise for 10–15min and cool down for 8–10min.
  - Nasal breathing may increase temperature and humidity of inspired air.
  - Encourage the athlete to try to 'run through' their asthma to take advantage of the refractory period.
- *Nutritional strategies:*
  - Low sodium diet for 1–2 weeks has been shown to reduce EIB.
  - High-dose omega-3 fatty acids (fish oil) supplementation.
  - Increasing vitamin C intake.

Pharmacological (consult up-to-date doping guidelines)
- Short-acting beta2 agonist (SABA), measured dose inhaler (MDI) (albuterol or salbutamol), terbutaline, metaproterenol, bitolterol.
  - Drug of choice for prophylactic and acute treatment.
  - Initial treatment is with a beta2 agonist MDI 15–60min before exercise prophylactically, also for 'rescue'.
  - Effective in about 95% of patients.
  - May provide protection for 3–6h.
  - May cause tachycardia or slight tremor, less commonly headache.
- *Glucocorticosteroids:* oral or intravenous, and inhaled (beclomethasone, budesonide, ciclesonide, flunisolide, fluticasone, triamcinolone).
  - Those athletes with a baseline obstruction on PFT (and maybe late phase reactors) should be on an inhaled bronchodilator and an inhaled glucocorticosteroid (GCS).

- Oral (an/or IV) glucocorticosteroids are used acutely and in emergencies for gaining control in inflammatory asthma (but will require notification to relevant authorities for Doping Control).
- Inhaled glucocorticosteroids are used for maintenance of control, and as first line therapy for IntA.
- Both will decrease the reactivity of the airways.
- *Long acting beta2 agonists (LABA), MDI (salmeterol, formoterol):*
  - Taken 45–60min before exercise.
  - May give protection for up to 6h.
  - Cannot be used for acute episodes.
  - Expensive.
  - May get tachyphylaxis (tolerance), including lessened response to SABA as 'rescue' medications.
  - Not recommended as monotherapy: should always be used in combination with inhaled corticosteroids (ICS).
- *Mast cell stabilizers, MDI (cromolyn sodium and nedocromyl sodium):*
  - MDIs have been discontinued—due to withdrawal of chlorofluorocarbon propellants; cromolyn still available as a nebulized solution.
  - If paediatric, a late responder, or has responded to cromolyn in the past, add cromolyn 15–30min before exercise.
  - 70–80% are protected.
  - May prevent late phase reaction and therefore may be more effective in children.
  - Decreased duration compared to beta2 agonists.
  - Not effective for acute attacks.
  - May be most effective in combination with beta2 agonists.
- *Leukotriene inhibitors, oral (montelukast, zafirlukast, zileuton):*
  - Leukotriene receptor antagonists.
  - Shown to improve airway edema, smooth muscle constriction and reduce inflammation.
  - Block leukotrienes D4 and E4 as well as slow-reacting substance of anaphylaxis.
  - Recently advocated as prevention/treatment for EIB.
  - Monteleukast is the most commonly used: daily single dosing at bedtime; rapidly absorbed—peak plasma levels in 2.6–4h, mean bioavailability 58–73%, higher in chewable tablets.
  - Others may have some drug interactions, liver toxicity (zileutron).
- *Theophylline, oral:*
  - May be of some benefit in some patients.
  - Serum levels must be monitored.
  - Toxic in high doses.
  - Not presently used often for EIB.
- *Anticholinergic agents, MDI (ipratropium bromide):*
  - Add ipratropium bromide 1–2h before exercise.
  - Not effective in all patients.
  - Especially effective for COPD, bronchitis, and emphysema.
  - May be used for acute attacks.
- *Antihistamines:* no significant role in EIB.
- *Nasal cortisosteroids:* in athletes with allergic rhinitis, may decrease EIB.

- *New agents under study:*
  - Alpha-1 agonists.
  - Inhaled calcium channel blockers.
  - Inhaled heparin.
  - Inhaled diuretics.
  - Gene therapy.

General management principles for IntA and EIB
- Written instructions: 'Asthma Action Plan' and 'EIB Action Plan'.
- All asthmatics should purchase an inexpensive peak flow meter or FEV_1 meter, and monitor their lung function on a regular basis:
  - *'Green Zone'*—peak expiratory flow (PEF) values 80–100% of personal best—no asthma management changes needed.
  - *'Yellow Zone'*—PEF values are between 50% and 80%, caution is warranted and use of medications is required.
  - *'Red Zone'*—PEF values are less than 50% of personal best—refrain from exercise, emergency action needed, may require hospital visit.
- Athletic trainers and other medical and/or para-medical personnel working with athletes 'on the sidelines' should also have a peak flow meter available, as well as extra doses of short-acting beta2 inhalers.
- Proper use of inhalers is essential to ensure medication is administered into lungs, not oropharynx—use of a 'spacer' with MDI is helpful.
- Regular washing of mouthpiece and spacer is important.
- Rinsing out mouth after using ICS may help prevent *Candida* infection.

Prevention of EIB
- Obtain good control of any underlying intrinsic asthma with ICS.
- Add LABAs and when necessary, leukotriene inhibitors, chromones, anticholinergics (rarely).
- Pre-exercise warm-up.
- Pre-exercise medication: SABAs, leukotrienes and/or chromones.
- Avoid unfavorable environmental conditions when possible.
- Use warming face mask to reduce effects of cold air while training.

Anti-doping rules and regulations
- Inhaled salbutamol (albuterol) and salmeterol, are both permitted, without any need for Declaration of Use (since January 2011).
- No convincing ergogenic effects have been documented with either inhaled SABAs or LABAs, or inhaled GCS.
- Systemic beta agonists are not permitted.
- If an athlete takes enough of an inhaler (greater than the maximum 1600micrograms over 24h), and tests over the urinary threshold level of 1000ng/mL—giving an adverse analytical finding (AAF)—may need to prove that the AAF was the consequence of the use of a therapeutic dose, through a controlled pharmacokinetic study.
- Inhaled ICS are permitted (without Declaration of Use). Should be used as first-line therapy for asthma, with short-acting beta agonists used for treatment/rescue. (See non-pharmacologic strategies to help prevent exercise-induced bronchoconstriction or EIB.).
- Oral or intravenous glucocorticosteroids require a full application for a TUE; but in the event that there is a need to use such medications in an emergency situation—an application can be made for a retroactive TUE.

- Terbutaline is still a prohibited medication, whether administered orally, by inhalation, injection or by nebulizer. Therefore it will still require application for a full TUE, with the criteria set out by the WADA (http://www.wada-ama.org).
- However, as of January 1, 2012, formoterol is no longer prohibited when taken by inhalation and at a dosage under 36 micrograms over 24 hours (i.e. a physician-prescribed dosage).
- The accepted bronchial provocation tests are those that are listed.
- Long-acting beta agonists should not be used for mono-therapy - because of the risk of developing tachyphylaxis, and also decreased response to short-acting beta agonists. This can be reversed by ceasing inhaled beta agonists for a few days.
- Combination inhalers containing a long-acting beta agonist and a glucocorticosteroid are approved for use without restriction. Since formoterol is now permitted at a therapeutic dosage - Symbicort (which contains formoterol and budesonide) is acceptable, as is Advair (fluticasone and salmeterol).
- Most TUEs should be applied for well in advance, at least 30 days prior to the national or international event.
- Most TUEs for asthma medications are valid for a period of 4y, with annual review of the treatment plan by a pulmonary specialist, or a physician knowledgeable in the treatment of asthma.

Chapter 11

Infectious disease

Effects of exercise on immunity *312*
Why are athletes prone to infection? *313*
Upper respiratory tract infections *314*
Common viral infections *315*
Viral hepatitis *316*
Other infections *317*
HIV *317*
Otitis externa *317*
Malaria *318*
Diarrhoea *320*

Effects of exercise on immunity

Benefits
Regular, moderate levels of exercise improve resistance to most infections, particularly those affecting the upper respiratory tract (URTI).
Possibly because of mild elevations in:
- T-cell lymphocytes.
- Interleukins.
- Endorphins.

Adverse effects
There is good evidence that athletes undertaking intensive training (e.g. endurance runners covering >90km/week) are more prone to minor infection, particularly URTI. This is thought to be due to reduction of:
- Salivary IgA, which plays an important role in resistance to some viruses.
- IgM.
- Natural killer cells, which show increased activity during exercise, only to fall in the first few hours of recovery.

Supplementation with carbohydrate, vitamin C, glutamine, and zinc may reduce the immunosuppressive effect of heavy exercise.

Why are athletes prone to infection?

Stress/overtraining/under recovery
Symptoms may include:
- Poor performance.
- Depressed mood.
- Insomnia.
- Frequent URTIs.
- Cervical lymphadenopathy may be present.
- High cortisol or low testosterone levels are sometimes seen.
- Lack of recovery time in training programmes can lead to lowered IgA levels, reducing resistance to viral infection, and lowered T and B lymphocytes (cortisol driven).

High level and endurance athletes are particularly at risk of training excessively, due to their competitive nature.

Treatment includes rest and education about the need for increased training recovery time, optimization of nutrition, psychological monitoring and support, and gradual re-introduction of training.

Close contact with other athletes
On tours and in training/competition camps, the inevitable close contact between athletes, coaches, and support staff can encourage the spread of respiratory and GI infections.

Sexual activity
Like the population as a whole, athletes are at risk of sexually-transmitted diseases if practicing unsafe sex.

Trauma
Traumatic injury can predispose to infection, especially if wounds are open.

Foreign travel
Hepatitis B is endemic in many third world countries, and travelling athletes should be considered for immunization (particularly in contact sports). Travel also carries risk of tropical diseases, such as malaria and diarrhoea.

Upper respiratory tract infections

Although a small proportion of URTIs will be caused by group A streptococcus, most are caused by a virus such as:
- Echovirus.
- Adenovirus.
- Coxsackie viruses A and B.
- Influenza.

Investigations may include a throat swab and a monospot or Paul-Bunnell test for infectious mononucleosis (glandular fever).

Treatment of URTIs
- *Analgesia*: paracetamol—effective and safe in correct dosage.
- *Decongestants*: nasal sprays can help. Doctors and sports people need to be aware that some decongestants are still on the WADA banned list and, if in doubt, the drug should be checked using the UK sport drug information database. Menthol or eucalyptus inhalants will relieve most symptoms of congestion and are not banned.

Prevention
Team groups especially are at risk of outbreaks of influenza, and vaccination can be offered every winter to the team members and attached staff. There is some evidence that zinc lozenges taken orally can reduce the duration of symptoms, and that certain probiotics drinks or colostrum can reduce risk of picking up URTI's.

Dangers of URTIs
Coxsackie virus can cause inflammation of heart muscle (myocarditis) in exercising athletes. If a sports person has a combination of the following symptoms, they should be advised not to train or play:
- Resting tachycardia (>10beats/min above normal).
- Myalgia.
- Lethargy.
- Oral temperature >38*C.
- Cervical lymphadenopathy.

Advise athlete that premature return to training/playing will delay recovery and there is a small risk of myocarditis and cardiac arrhythmias.

'Neck check' guidelines for athletes
- If all of the symptoms are above the neck (stuffy or runny nose, sneezing, watery eyes, and/or scratchy throat), it is okay to start your usual workout at about half speed.
- Do not work out if you have a fever or symptoms below the neck (aching muscles, a hacking cough that seems to resound deep within the chest, nausea, vomiting, and/or diarrhoea). Working out under those conditions is risky, and you'll recover much faster from your illness if you rest.[1]

---

[1] Eichner ER. (1995). Contagious infections in competitive sports, *Sports Sci Exch* **8**(3).

Common viral infections

These can be caused by several viruses, particularly:
- Epstein–Barr virus (infectious mononucleosis).
- Toxoplasma.
- Cytomegalovirus (CMV).
- Primary HIV disease.

They commonly occur in younger age groups, and are linked to the development of chronic fatigue syndrome. Splenomegaly occurs and participation in contact sports carries a risk of traumatic splenic rupture.

Infectious mononucleosis (InfM)
- Spread by intimate close contact.
- Symptoms of sore throat, cervical lymphadenopathy.
- Fatigue—can last 2–6 weeks acutely.
- Maculopapular rash sometimes seen.
- Splenomegaly may be present (confirmed on US).
- 5% can have significant complications.
- Up to 40% of traumatic splenic rupture linked to InfM.
- Paul-Bunnell blood test positive.
- 15%+ atypical lymphocytes on blood film.
- Epstein-Barr virus IgM positive for approximately 2 months.
- Most can return to sport at 4 weeks.
- Gradual re-introduction of exercise as symptoms settle.
- Chronic fatigue (>3 months) is a complication especially if recovery is rushed.

Toxoplasmosis
- Fever.
- Hepatosplenomegaly.
- Generalized lymphadenopathy.
- Picked up from cats' faeces.
- 60% with positive serology have no history of illness.
- Recent infection diagnosed on IgM serology.
- Self-limiting. Return to sport usually in 6 weeks.

CMV
Similar symptoms to toxoplasmosis, but less common.

Lyme disease
- Tick-borne, spirochaete infection (*Borrelia*).
- Common in spring and summer, especially in USA.
- Rash (red rings), malaise, myalgia, arthralgia, headaches.
- Diagnosed on serology.
- Treatment with doxycycline or amoxycillin orally.

Viral hepatitis

Hepatitis A
- Oro-faecal spread.
- Relatively common especially in travellers.
- Can be sub-clinical, often in childhood.
- Fever, nausea, abdominal pains.
- Jaundice after 3–7 days.
- Hepatosplenomegaly and lymphadenopathy may be present.
- Abnormal LFTs and Hep A IgM positive 20+ days after exposure. Hep A IgG positive lifelong.
- Effective vaccination recommended.
- Treated symptomatically and full recovery ensues.
- Self-limiting illness. No chronic liver disease after infection.
- Safe to return to sport when clinically better, although some derangement of LFTs may persist.

Hepatitis B
- Endemic in Africa and parts of Asia.
- Spread by blood or sexual contact, IV drug use.
- Highly infectious. Incubation period 30–180 days.
- Clinical features similar to Hep A, but may have associated arthralgia and urticarial.
- Most cases will recover spontaneously.
- 5–10% of sufferers will become carriers with high risk of transmission especially in contact sports, and if diagnosed are excluded from boxing, wrestling, and rugby.
- Abnormal LFTs and Hep Bs antigen positive 1–6 months post-infection. Hep Be antigen positive suggests high infectivity.
- Treated symptomatically and require careful follow-up
- Graded return to exercise only when LFTs are back to normal.
- Complications include chronic active hepatitis, cirrhosis and liver failure, and hepatocellular carcinoma.
- Vaccination available and strongly advised for all participants in contact sports.

Hepatitis C
- Often transmitted in blood transfusions or from IV drug abuse. Less infectious than hepatitis B.
- May be asymptomatic at time of infection.
- 85% develop chronic infection.
- High incidence of cirrhosis and also hepatocellular carcinoma.
- Same symptoms as other forms of viral hepatitis.
- No available vaccine.
- Treated with interferon-α.

Other infections

Panton-Valentine leukocidin (PVL)
- Has been reported in rugby union players.
- Produced by *Staph. aureus* and can cause severe skin disease with multiple deep furuncles and abscesses, as well as severe infection.
- 90% of primary skin abscesses can be positive for PVL.

HIV

- Spread by blood or sexual contact, IV drug abuse.
- No risk from sweat.
- Present in saliva, but no reports of spread by this route.
- 100 times less infectious than hepatitis B.
- Initial symptoms are 'flu-like'.
- May then be asymptomatic for months/years.
- Eventually develops into AIDS.
- HIV antibodies found in blood at approximately 12 weeks after exposure and infection.

Note
Risk of transmission of Hepatitis B, C, or HIV during sport is extremely low. The viruses cannot be transmitted via showers or shared drinks bottles. Vaccination against hepatitis B and the following infection control measures help reduce risks even further:
- Wear protective gloves when giving first aid to a bleeding player.
- Wipe any blood from the face or limbs of players.
- Blood-stained towels should not be re-used. Put blood-stained clothing in a plastic bag for disposal or laundering.
- Players should not be allowed to continue in the game until bleeding has stopped, and the wound is cleaned and covered.
- If there is concern about cross-infection, contact a doctor straight away.

Otitis externa

- Inflammation ± infection in ear canal.
- Common in swimmers and can be very painful.
- Moistness of ear canal predisposes to the condition.
- *Pseudomonas* often grown on swab.
- Treated with antibiotic ± corticosteroid eardrops, although can sometimes require aural toilet by suction to remove debris in canal.
- Prevention using 70% alcohol drops before and after swimming is best.

Malaria

- 2000 new cases/annum in UK after foreign travel (7 deaths).
- Most cases have failed to take adequate prophylaxis.
- Natural immunity wanes on leaving endemic area.
- Prevention is better than cure.
- Obtain up-to-date anti-malarial drug advice before departure to a high-risk area.
- All travellers to be supplied with and comply with prophylaxis advice.
- Anti-malarial drugs can have adverse reactions and any doctor travelling with a team to a high-risk area should be aware of these.
- Advise all competitors and staff to wear long sleeves and trousers in the evening and use DEET mosquito repellents.
- Symptoms can present up to 12 months after return from high-risk area, and should always be considered in cases of pyrexia of unknown origin.

Diarrhoea

Diarrhoea of infectious origin is a major cause of morbidity in sports people who travel the world to compete. These athletes are as much at risk of the development of travellers' diarrhoea as the general population.

Symptoms of travellers' diarrhoea
- Are defined as passing three or more unformed stools over 24h, during or shortly after, a period of travel.
- Can be accompanied by fever.
- Can be very disruptive to training and competition, on average lasting 4 days.

High-risk destinations for diarrhoeal illness include most of Asia, Africa, and South America.

In most cases, no pathogen is found and possible causes include:
- Change in diet/fluid intake.
- *E. coli* (commonest bacterial pathogen).
- Rotaviruses.
- Salmonella and *Campylobacter*.
- *Shigella*.
- *Giardia* and *Entamoeba*.

Advice for sufferers
- Usually no treatment is required.
- Maintain fluid and electrolyte balance with replacement drinks.
- Stick to simple starchy foods.
- Seek medical advice if diarrhoea is bloody, accompanied by fever, or lasts more than 14 days.

Advice to travellers to prevent diarrhoea
- Wash hands after going to toilet/before eating or handling food.
- Consider taking daily pre- and pro-biotics.
- Drink only sealed bottled water or boil your own.
- Avoid ice in drinks.
- Avoid salads and cold vegetables.
- Peel all fruits if uncooked.
- Avoid shellfish—seawater may be contaminated by sewage.
- Eat only hot, well-cooked food. Avoid any food that has been kept warm or food from street vendors.

Investigation of diarrhoea
Anyone who suffers from chronic diarrhoea will need investigation to rule out other medical causes, such as:
- Infection/food poisoning.
- IBD.
- Food intolerances (e.g. gluten or lactose).
- Cancer.
- Irritable bowel syndrome.

History and examination are particularly important. Initial simple investigations will include:
- Stool microscopy and culture (evidence of infection).
- FBC (check for anaemia and abnormal MCV).
- Vitamin B12/folate and ferritin levels to look for evidence of malabsorption.
- U&E (low K^+).
- CRP/ESR (inflammation/infection/cancer).
- Anti-endomysial antibodies (suggestive of gluten enteropathy).

Pharmacotherapy
- *Loperamide* can reduce stool frequency and ease stomach cramps in cases of diarrhoea.
- *Codeine* is a narcotic analgesic, but is no longer on the WADA list of banned substances. It is a very effective analgesic and anti-diarrhoeal agent, but may cause drowsiness.
- *Alverine citrate* is a useful additional treatment in the presence of bloating and cramping symptoms.
- The vast majority do not require antibiotic therapy, but *Ciprofloxacin* 500mg as a single dose has been shown to reduce duration of illness (*NB* This drug has been linked to the tendinopathies and should be used with caution in sports people). *Trimethoprim* is an alternative.
- *Probiotics*, which contain viable micro-organisms, are sometimes taken prophylactically and also to treat diarrhoeal illness. Their mechanism of action is unclear, but their use may reduce the length of acute diarrhoea. The widespread use of probiotics is not advocated at present, but travelling sports persons commonly use them, and they appear to have few side effects.

Tip for doctors travelling to high-risk areas
A useful preventative tip

In many high-risk countries, river water is used on playing fields and after playing/training, players or competitors should be instructed to wash hands thoroughly before eating. Alcohol-based gel is very useful as a readily available hand sterilizer in the absence of clean running water.

Chapter 12

Dermatology

Description of terms in dermatology 324
Problems caused by friction 326
Benign skin conditions 329
Sun and heat-related problems 330
Cold-related injuries 334
Fungal infections 336
Bacterial infections 340
Viral infections 346

Description of terms in dermatology

See Table 12.1 for a description of common terms used in dermatology.

Table 12.1 Description of terms in dermatology

Terminology	Description	Example
Macule	A discoloured spot or patch on the skin, neither elevated nor depressed, of various colours, sizes, and shapes.	Vitiligo Café au lait spots Petechiae
Papule	A solid lesion elevated above the plane of the surrounding skin. Often precede vesicles and pustules. Generally considered less than 1cm in diameter.	Measles Acne vulgaris
Ulcer	An open sore or lesion of the skin or mucous membranes where there has been destruction of the overlying epidermis and upper papillary layer of the dermis resulting in the formation of a crater.	Decubitus ulcers Venous stasis ulcers Aphthous ulcers
Nodule	A palpable solid round or ellipsoidal lesion deeper than a papule and present in the dermis, SC tissue, or epidermis. The depth, rather than the diameter differentiate it from a papule.	Bouchard's and Osler's nodes Warts Squamous cell carcinoma Basal cell carcinoma
Wheal	A rounded or flat-topped pale red elevation in the skin that is evanescent, disappearing within hours, and often intensely pruritic. A result of oedema in the upper layer of the dermis.	Urticaria Insect bites
Bulla	A large blister or skin vesicle filled with serum, lymph fluid, blood, or extracellular fluid. They are located within the epidermis, or the epidermal-dermal interface. Usually more than 0.5cm in diameter.	Blisters Pemphigus
Vesicle	A small blister filled with serum, lymph, afluid, blood, or extracellular fluid. They are located within the epidermis, or the epidermal-dermal interface. Usually less than 0.5cm in diameter.	Herpes zoster Herpes simplex Variola Varicella
Pustule	A circumscribed elevation of the skin that contains a purulent exudate that may be white, yellow, or greenish-yellow. May be associated with a hair follicle. Vesicles may become pustules.	Acne vulgaris Impetigo

(Continued)

Table 12.1 (Continued)

Terminology	Description	Example
Plaque	An elevation above the skin surface that occupies a relatively large surface area in comparison with its height above the skin. It may be formed by a confluence of papules.	Psoriasis Mycosis fungoides
Lichenification	Like a plaque, but the elevation above the skin surface is due to proliferation of the keratinocytes and stratum corneum due to continued irritation. The skin appears thickened, and skin lines are accentuated.	Eczematous dermatitis
Scales	Due to an increased rate of proliferation of epidermal cells the stratum corneum is not formed normally, causing the skin to peel in visible sheets or flakes.	Eczema Seborrhoea Psoriasis
Crusts	Result when serum, blood, or purulent exudate dries on the skin surface. They may be thin, delicate and friable, or thick and adherent.	Impetigo Ecthyma

Problems caused by friction

Blisters

Description
- Fluid filled bullae that form at the site of friction.
- Usually caused by a change in training pattern, or ill-fitting equipment.
- Location and history are main clues to the diagnosis.

Risk factors
- Early in the workout season.
- Hard playing surfaces.
- Repetitive activities.
- Role of sweating—friction combined with moisture.

Treatment
- Treat 'hot spots' with ice and protection.
- May use protective socks (or two pairs of socks), petroleum jelly, or mole skin ('doughnuts'), antiperspirants for treatment and prevention.
- Superglue may be painted on hot spots for protection from irritation, but may increase traction on the site.
- Commercial products like Second Skin™ are helpful—can leave top layer of plastic on, so dressing will last longer.
- Drain in a sterile manner only if tense or large, leave overlying skin on.
- Antibiotic ointment or hydrocolloid if open.

Differential diagnosis
- Pemphigus.
- Pemphigoid.

Calluses

Description
- Thickening of the outer layer of skin (hyperkeratosis) with no central core as seen in verruca vulgaris.
- Skin lines are maintained.
- Caused by repetitive friction.
- Possibly ill-fitting equipment.
- May be painful and lead to blisters or subdermal haematoma.

Risk factors
- Hard playing surfaces.
- Repetitive activities.

Treatment
- Properly fitting shoes and equipment.
- Pumice stone or paring down.
- Salicylic acid preparation.
- Use gloves or equipment to protect skin.
- May use protective socks, petroleum jelly, or mole skin.

Differential diagnosis
- Warts.
- Bunion.

Court abrasions and turf burns

Description
- Superficial epidermal abrasion or frank ulceration into dermis.
- Propensity to become infected.

Risk factors
Sports where collision with the court, turf, or ground are common—football, rugby, volleyball, cyclists ('road rash').

Treatment
- Irrigation with high pressure (50cm^3 syringe with 20G needle).
- Thorough washing with antibacterial cleanser (such as chorhexidine, hexachlorphene, or providone-iodine).
- Ice, topical lidocaine for anesthesia while cleaning.
- Sterile protective dressing (Op-site, Duoderm, Tegaderm).

Prevention
- Wearing long sleeves.
- Appropriate protective padding.

Subungual haematoma (black toe, runners toe, tennis toe)

Description
- Splinter haemorrhage underneath the nail bed, usually involving the first or second toe.
- Develop acutely after pressure from tight shoes or from sudden deceleration.

Risk factors
- Most often seen in racquet sports, football, and distance runners.
- Downhill running.
- Long or malformed toenails.
- Tight shoes, especially the toe box.

Treatment
- Close trimming of toenail proximal to the distal aspect of the toe.
- Properly fitting shoes with adequate room in the toe box.
- Use of orthotics to lift arch and pull toes away from end of shoe.
- Change of running style/route.

Differential diagnosis
- Subungual melanoma.

Plantar petechiae (black heel, black dot syndrome, talon noir)

Description
- Intra-epidermal bleeding and petechiae of the heel.
- Occurs on the heel at the edge of the foot pad.
- Caused by shearing forces and sudden stops.
- With paring, skin lines are maintained and no additional bleeding is seen.

Risk factors
- Seen in volleyball, racquet sports, running, lacrosse, and basketball.
- Poor fitting shoes.
- Repetitive trauma (cutting or stops).
- Black palm or tache noir seen in athletes who apply pressure to hands—such as gymnasts, racquet sports players, weightlifters, golfers.

Treatment
- Properly fitted shoes.
- Use of a 'soft' shoe.
- Thick socks.
- Heel pads.

Differential diagnosis
- Melanoma.

Benign skin conditions

Piezogenic pedal papules

Description
- Skin-colored or yellowish papules along lateral plantar surface.
- Become obvious upon prolonged standing or exercise.
- Herniation of subcutaneous fat through small tears in plantar fascia.
- Occasionally painful.

Risk factors
- Common in long-distance runners.
- Can be seen in non-athletes, particularly obese people.

Treatment
- Elevation of feet often provides relief.
- Heel cups in shoes can help during exercise.

Striae distensae or stretch marks

Description
- Continuous and progressive stretching of skin can lead to striae or stretch marks.
- Often around lower abdomen, also in axillae.
- Initially reddish colour, fade with time to a more silverish colour.

Risk factors
- Intense sports such as weightlifting, body building, and football.
- Can occur during pregnancy, weight gain, rapid growth spurts.
- Commonly seen with anabolic steroid use.

Treatment
- Topical tretinoin or laser therapy may be helpful.

Differential diagnosis
- Cushing's disease.

Sun and heat-related problems

Sunburn

Description
- Excessive exposure to UVA and UVB light.
- Acute sunburn caused by UVB (wavelengths 290–320nm), and peaks 24–48h after a single exposure.
- Photosensitized reactions caused by UVA (wavelengths 320–400nm), require 48h or more to develop fully.
- May cause up to second degree burns.
- Increases risk of skin cancers.

Risk factors
- Water sports, outdoor sports.
- Early during the warm season (even on cloudy days).
- Increased risk with reflection off water, snow, ice.
- High altitude (mountaineering, skiing), low latitudes.
- Duration of exposure (marathons).
- Lack of clothing (board sailing, beach volleyball).
- Medications (tetracycline, sulfa, phenothiazines, thiazide diuretics).
- Photosensitizing plant oils containing psoralens (lime, parsnip, celery and others)—cause phytophoto dermatitis.
- Fair complexion, blue eyes.

Treatment
- Cool compresses.
- Aloe vera lotions.
- Topical anaesthetics and/or antihistamines.
- Antibiotic ointments if second degree burns.
- Oral fluids.
- Maintain the integrity of the overlying skin.
- Oral and topical steroids may be required for moderate to severe burns, to control inflammation and discomfort.

Prevention
- Sun screen/sun block (sweat proof/waterproof).
- Sun protective factor (SPF) at least 15: PABA-esters protect mainly against UVB exposure; if athlete intolerant, or requires protection from UVA range—PABA-free products—benzophenones, cinnamates.
- Apply half an hour before exposure, again after sweating or swimming.
- Protective clothing and hats.
- Avoid midday sun.
- Gradual exposure to develop protective tan (tanning booths may be a more controlled environment).
- Provide shade near workout area.

Differential diagnosis
- Sun sensitizing medication.
- Flushing.
- If unusually severe or persistent sunburns, look for photosensitive disorder such as systemic lupus erythematosus (SLE).

Photodermatitis

Ranges from nodular (sun poisoning) to solar purpura, to solar urticaria.

Description
- Immune reaction directed against the skin caused by sun exposure.
- Often requires a co-factor to trigger the reaction (medications, etc.).
- May present as hive-like lesions, nodules, purpura, to generalized oedema.

Risk factors
- Outdoor sports.
- Medication use.

Treatment
- Difficult to treat.
- Avoidance of sun exposure is best.
- Psoralen with UVA (PUVA).
- Antihistamines.
- Severe cases may require IV steroids.

Differential diagnosis
- Sun-sensitizing medication, such as tetracycline, sulfonamides, griseofulvin, diuretics, phenothiazides, first generation sulfonylurea agents, diphenhydraminel, and some cosmetics.

Atopic dermatitis

Description
- Eczematous eruption that is itchy, recurrent, flexural, and symmetric.
- It generally begins early in life, follows periods of remission and exacerbation, and may resolve by the age of 30.
- Infants have facial and patchy or generalized body eczema.
- Adolescents and adults have eczema in flexural areas and on the hands.
- Polygenic inheritance.
- May be aggravated by heat, sweat, or exertion.

Risk factors
- Exposure to heat, sweat, allergens, and exertion.

Treatment
- May be improved by sun exposure.
- Emollients.
- Avoidance of radical temperature changes.

Differential diagnosis
- Seborrhoeic dermatitis, psoriasis, contact dermatitis, tinea corporis.
- Can be associated with true asthma.

Miliaria rubra (prickly heat)

Description
- Due to occlusion of eccrine sweat duct in the mid to lower epidermis.
- Presents as small scattered papules and vesicles with surrounding erythema and sparing of hair follicles.

- Pustular lesions may result from sterile accumulation of leukocytes or secondary staphylococcal infection.
- Associated prickling stinging sensation induced by onset of sweating.

Risk factors
- Profuse sweating and equipment causing local increase in skin humidity and temperature.

Treatment
- Air-conditioning.
- May be able to maintain intense activity if athlete can spend prolonged daily periods or rest in cool, dry, air-conditioned living quarters.
- Adjustments in equipment and practice time.
- In severe cases, athlete might require a week or so of rest from sweating to allow the epidermis to heal.

Hyperhidrosis

Description
- Excessive perspiration.
- May be congenital or stress-related.
- May cause problems with grip, vision, self-confidence.

Risk factors
- Exposure to heat, physical exertion, and stressful situations.

Treatment
- Aluminum chloride.
- After several weeks, may only need application 1–2 times per week.
- Iontophoresis units.

Differential diagnosis
- Anxiety.
- Excessive heat exposure.
- Hyperthyroidism.
- Very severe condition—hidradenitis suppurativa—chronic relapsing inflammatory disease of the skin with recurrent draining sinuses and abscesses, found in skin-folds carrying terminal hairs and apocrine glands (skin of axillae and inguinoperineal regions).
- Treat with topical (clindamycin) or systemic antibiotics (tetracyclines, clindamycin), topical antiseptics, and intralesional corticosteroids.
- May require surgical removal of involved tissues.

Xerosis (asteatotic dermatitis)

Description
- Dry stinging skin: 'winter eczema'.
- Xerosis and defatting of skin.
- Often on extensor surfaces of limbs.
- Skin is dry and finely fissured some erythema.

Risk factors
- Low absolute humidity of heated winter air.
- Athlete who showers frequently, swims or sweats heavily.

Treatment
- Showers short and not too hot.
- Use super-fatted cleansers (Dove bar, etc.)
- Avoid antibacterial and highly alkaline hard soaps.
- Pat skin dry after showering, apply moisturizer/lubricant.
- Wear cotton and soft synthetics, avoid wool next to skin.
- Humidification of room air.
- May need moderate strength topical corticosteroid.

'Cholinergic' urticaria

Description
- Heat-induced—caused by exercise, sweating, and hot showers or baths.
- Sweat glands are innervated by cholinergic nerve fibers.
- Urticarial lesions are small and intensely itchy.
- If severe, may cause hypotension and syncope.
- Overlap with exercise-induced anaphylaxis (EIA)—pruritis, urticaria, angioedema, respiratory distress.
- Sometimes associated with food sensitivity (allergen specific or non-allergen specific)—shrimp, shellfish, chicken, wheat (gliadins), nuts.

Treatment
- Antihistamines prior to exercise (H1 and/or H2 blockers).
- Avoidance of precipitating food allergen and exercise for 1–6h after eating.
- Severe cases may require corticosteroids.

Differential diagnosis
- Other types of urticaria—i.e. contact urticaria—IgE mediated (insect venoms, animal danders, and/or saliva, latex products).
- Drug-related urticaria (NSAIDs, aspirin).
- Other causes of physical urticaria (pressure, sunlight, vibration, cold).
- Clinical thyroid disease or underlying infection.

Cold-related injuries

Frostnip

Description
- Involves the superficial layer of skin only (first degree frostbite).
- May appear flushed or have rosy cheeks.
- Affects nose, cheeks, and ears most often.
- Will usually result in flaking of epidermis.

Risk factors
- Outdoor sports.
- Winter sports.

Prevention
- Cover all exposed skin when conditions are poor.
- Petroleum jelly or zinc oxide for protection of face and ears.

Treatment
- Treat symptomatically.
- Prevention is the best treatment.

Differential diagnosis
Viral exanthum.

Frostbite

Description
- Extended exposure to freezing temperatures.
- Results in a freezing injury to the blood vessels, nerves, and soft tissue.
- May cause first, second, or third degree injuries.
- First and second degree injuries most commonly seen in athletes.
- Most often affects the ears, penis, feet and hands.

Risk factors
- Extreme cold, wetness, wind-chill, tight and insufficient clothing.
- Vasospastic conditions, including exposure to nicotine.

Prevention
- Recognition and avoidance of unsafe conditions.
- Proper dress (non-absorbant layers, polypropylene underwear and socks, mitts with wool liner, leather outer shell).
- Keep whole body (core) warm.
- Roomy footwear, thick non-conductive sole.

Treatment
- Rapid rewarming with warm water immersion. Use caution if coexisting hypothermia. Avoid thawing and refreezing.
- Treat like burns. Protect damaged tissue from physical trauma.

Chilblains (Pernio)

Description
- Chronic exposure of extremities to sub-freezing temperatures.
- Results in breakdown of the dermis with resultant irritation and discomfort.
- Predisposes to future cold intolerance.

Treatment
- Protection from further trauma and cold.
- May require antibiotics.

Prevention
- Recognition and avoidance of unsafe conditions.
- Proper dress and hygiene.

Cold-induced urticaria

Description
- Blancheable, erythematous, edematous papules or 'wheals'.
- 'Hives' occurring with exposure to cold, or exercise in the cold.
- Caused by release of histamine from mast cells.
- Can be local or generalized, congenital or acquired.
- Can have fatigue, headache, dyspnoea.
- Intensive exposure to cold (e.g. contact with cold water) can cause cardiovascular symptoms, hypotension, collapse, even shock.
- Can be associated with cold agglutinins or cryoglobulinaemia.

Treatment
- Avoidance of exposure of extremities to cold.
- Diagnose with ice-cube 'challenge test'.
- Warn against swimming in cold water.

Differential diagnosis
- 'Angioedema': well demarcated swelling, within deep skin structures or in subcutaneous tissue, caused mainly by bradykinin production.
- Can also occur in conjunction with urticaria.

Fungal infections

Tinea pedis (athlete's foot)

Description
- Erythematous, often scaling eruptions on the plantar surface of the foot and between the toes.
- Caused by a variety of dermatophytes and yeasts. Most commonly caused by *Trichophyton rubrum, T. mentagraphytes*, and *Epidermophyton floccusum*. Sometimes *Candida*.
- Yeasts do not respond to some over-the-counter preparations.
- Diagnose using skin scrapings, clinical presentation, or fungal cultures.

Risk factors
- Chronically wet feet.
- Locker rooms and public showers.
- Diabetes.
- Immune system failure.

Treatment
- Over-the-counter preparations.
- Prescription antifungal topical preparations: are effective against both fungi, are once daily preparations, and may deliver cure within a week.
- Difficult cases may require oral antifungal agents.

Prevention
- Remove wet socks and use breathable shoes.
- Use sandals or 'flip-flops' in communal shower areas, swimming pools.
- Keep feet clean and dry.
- Drying powders (20% aluminum chloride—Drysol)
- Wash with benzoyl peroxide bar.

Differential diagnosis
- Pitted keratolysis, psoriasis.

Tinea cruris (jock itch)

Description
- Begins in the moist, warm crural folds and spreads out to become fan-shaped as it spreads to the thighs.
- Rarely involves the scrotum (see Erythrasma, p. 343).
- Reddened scaly patches with sharp margins.
- May be painful, pruritic, and weeping.
- Similar organisms as tinea pedis. Most commonly caused by *Trichophyton rubrum, T. mentagraphytes*, and *Epidermophyton floccusum*. Sometimes *Candida*.
- May be spread by contamination from infected feet.

Risk factors
- Shared undergarments.
- Tight-fitting synthetic garments.
- Prolonged maceration.

Treatment
- Similar to tinea corporis.
- Topical preparations are effective against fungi.
- Difficult cases may require oral antifungal agents.
- Antihistamine or low potency steroid creams may control itch.

Prevention
- Loose fitting absorbent undergarments.
- Change and shower soon after workout.
- Powders to keep dry. Avoid corn starch due to its conversion to sugars that may act as a growth media.

Differential diagnosis
- Intertrigo, psoriasis.

Tinea corporis (ringworm, tinea gladiatorum, scrum pox)

Description
- Presents as an itchy red rash on the trunk, leg, arm, or neck.
- Consists of small red scaling papules with raised borders, or blisters, and scales.
- Caused by the dermatophytes *Trichophyton tonsurans*, *Microsporum*, and *Epidermophyton*.
- Usually seen on hairless portions of skin.
- Usually more tissue reaction at the advancing borders of infection—accounts for the ring-like appearance.
- May be spread from mats, equipment, and clothing.

Risk factors
- Sweating, heat, and physical exertion contribute to fungal growth.
- Sports with close skin contact or communal mats (i.e. wrestling, martial arts, gymnastics).

Treatment
- Similar to tinea pedis.
- Topical antifungal preparations are effective against both fungi.
- To prevent transmission, cover with occlusive dressing for contact sports.

Prevention
- Proper treatment of mats and equipment with fungicidal cleaners after each practice/meet.
- Showering thoroughly after practices and competitions.
- Use of antibacterial soap and selenium shampoo.
- Washing practice clothes daily, no sharing of uniforms.
- Wearing headgear, washing headgear and knee pads twice a week.
- Enforcement of skin infection rules (i.e. NCAA in USA).
- Prompt treatment and isolation.

Differential diagnosis
- Contact dermatitis, atopic dermatitis.

Tinea versicolor (pityriasis versicolor)

Description
- Common fungal infection of the skin.
- Most commonly noted as macular hypopigmented or hyperpigmented lesions on the nape of the neck extending onto the trunk and arms.
- Pathogens include *Pityrosporum orbiculare* and *P. ovale* (both were previously called *Malassezia furfur*).
- Usually painless and does not itch.
- Diagnosis is by scrapings, and pathopneumonic spaghetti and meatball appearance.

Risk factor
- May affect any athlete. High recurrence rate (80% after 2yrs).

Treatment
- Treatment consists of topical antifungal or selenium based over-the-counter 'dandruff' shampoo on the skin and hair, or topical antifungal medication.
- Application prior to workouts may increase skin concentrations.
- Oral antifungal agents may be needed in the more difficult cases.
- Hypopigmented regions may take 6–8 weeks to resolve, and may be more susceptible to sun exposure.

Prevention
- Good hygiene with showering immediately after workouts, clean dry undershirts, and use of selenium-based or antifungal shampoo daily

Differential diagnosis
- Vitiligo, guttate psoriasis, nummular eczema.

Onychomycosis (tinea unguium)

Description
- Fungal infection of the nails of the fingers or more commonly the toes.
- Pathogens include many dermatophytes most commonly *Trichophyton rubrum* and *Candida*.
- May cause disfiguring thickening, and discoloration of the nails.
- Predispose to hang nails and secondary bacterial infections.

Risk factors
- Poor circulation.
- Diabetes.
- Poor hygiene.

Treatment
- Very refractory to treatment.
- Oral antifungal agents have been shown to have the best cure rates.
- May require removal of the nail for cure.

Differential diagnosis
- Psoriasis, Reiter's syndrome, nail dystrophy, nail injury.

Intertrigo

Description
- Red, macerated, half-mooned shaped plaques found in the moist body folds.
- Caused by moist irritation allowing mixed infections of dermatophytes, bacteria, and yeast to infect the superficial layer of skin.

Risk factors
- Obesity, sweating, poor hygiene.

Treatment
- Similar to tinea cruris.
- Avoid corn starch due to its conversion to sugars that act as a growth media.

Prevention
- Weight loss and good hygiene.

Differential diagnosis
- Tinea infections.

Swimmers' itch (cercarial dermatitis)

Description
- Caused by penetration of skin by 'non-human' schistosomes.
- Found in waters where molluscs (snails) and waterfowl co-habitate.
- Cercarial shedding peaks during bright, warm days.
- Cercariae that penetrate human skin die before penetrating dermal blood vessels, foreign protein causes allergic response.
- Prickling sensation at the time of penetration, red macules may be seen.
- Quiescent period followed by secondary stage of itchy red edematous papules, may get secondary infection.
- Post-inflammatory browning of skin may persist for months.

Treatment
- Systemic antihistamines.
- Topical antipruritics such as calamine lotion.
- Cold packs, topical corticosteroids.
- Hygiene to prevent secondary infection.

Prevention
- Avoidance of infested waters.

Bacterial infections

Acne vulgaris

Description
- Typical infections consist of papules, pustules, comedones, nodules, and cysts.
- Located primarily on the face, back, shoulders, and chest.
- Caused by a variety of bacteria.

Risk factors
- 70–80% of adolescents have some degree of acne.
- Worsened by sweat and occlusion from equipment that irritates skin.
- Commonly seen under helmets, chin straps, shoulder pads, jock straps.

Treatment
- Topical antibiotics (erythromycin, clindamycin), tretinoin, benzoyl peroxide.
- Oral antibiotics when severe.
- Retinoic acid (ensure that females are using contraception).

Prevention
- Good hygiene.
- Bathe immediately after workouts.
- Avoid over drying or scrubbing the skin.
- Protect from equipment.
- Properly fitted equipment.

Differential diagnosis
- Folliculitis, rosacea.

Furuncle (boil, carbuncle, abscess)

Description
- Usually begins as a *Staphylococcus* infection of the hair follicle then invading the surrounding tissues causing a collection of pus.
- Usually located on the upper extremity, buttocks, groin, axilla, neck, waist, or chest.
- Boils on the face are of particular concern because of venous access to the brain.
- Multiple boils is called furunculosis and if they interconnect, a carbuncle.

Treatment
- Boils will usually rupture on their own.
- If persistent, large, painful, or signs of sepsis, they should be lanced and appropriate antibiotics started.

Risk factors
- Diabetes mellitus, obesity, poor hygiene.

Differential diagnosis
- Epidermoid or pilar cyst, hidradenitis suppurativa.

Folliculitis

Description
- Common infection of the hair follicles often by *Staphylococcus aureus* or other skin bacteria.
- May present as macules, papules, pustules, or sometimes crusted lesions at the base of the hair shaft that may produce boils or carbuncles.
- Often seen on the back, thighs, or buttocks.
- May be due to friction from pads or shaving.
- Tend to be worse in the summer and with spandex clothing.
- Hot tub folliculitis caused by *Pseudomonas aeruginosa* infection from exposure to infected water in hot tub or whirlpool. Generally affects the axillae, breast, and pubic area, but occasionally the trunk. Usually resolves on own after 7–10 days.
- Steroid folliculitis is associated with use of anabolic steroids. Usually affects the trunk, and occasionally the neck and face. Treatments are with cessation of steroids and treat like folliculitis.

Risk factors
- Sports that require/promote shaving of the body.
- Running sports, wrestling, football, swimming.

Treatment
- Usually resolve on their own once the irritating source is removed.
- Use of antibacterial soaps or topical antibacterial ointment.
- Benzoyl peroxide.
- Refractory cases may need oral antibiotics (tetracycline or erythromycin).

Prevention
- Shower immediately after workouts.
- Keep areas clean and dry.
- Shave in the direction of hair growth.
- Application of alcohol-based aftershave after shaving.

Differential diagnosis
Acne vulgaris, rosacea, hydradenitis suppurativa.

Impetigo (ecthyma)

Description
- Highly contagious *Streptococcus* or *Staphylococcus* infection of the skin (abrasions may become secondarily impetiginized).
- *Bullous impetigo*: intact bullae may be clear or turbid, break easily.
- *Crusted impetigo*: characterized by small vesicles that form pustules and eventually become honey-coloured weeping crustations.
- Transmitted by direct contact of infected skin, towels, or equipment.
- May cause problems with the kidney (nephritis), not rheumatic fever.
- Should be treated immediately.

Risk factors
- Close contact sports such as martial arts, wrestling, rugby, etc.

Treatment
- Topical antibiotics may be sufficient, best to do culture and sensitivity.
- If in difficult areas to treat topically or if extensive, may treat with oral antibiotics (cloxicillin for bullous impetigo, penicillin V for crusted impetigo; erthyromycins or cepahalosporins are good alternatives).
- Carriage of *Staph. aureus* in anterior nares or perineum can cause recurrent infections especially in team settings—culture and treat with bacitracin ointment

Prevention
- Same as tinea corporis.

Differential diagnosis
- Seborrhoeic dermatitis, contact dermatitis, herpes simplex, scabies, bullous pemphigoid.

Cellulitis (erysipelas, Ludwig's angina, etc.)

Description
- Infection of the dermis and subcutaneous tissue by group A *Streptococcus* and *Staphylococcus aureus*.
- May be life-threatening if it involves the face, airway, or leads to sepsis.

Risk factors
- Any skin condition that may allow a portal of entry for infection.

Treatment
- Should be treated immediately with appropriate antibiotics, warm compresses, pain medication, and if extensive, irrigation and drainage.

Differential diagnosis
- Deep venous thrombosis, contact dermatitis, gout, peripheral vascular disease, insect bite.

Community acquired methicillin-resistant *Staph. aureus* (CA-MRSA)

Description
- Strain of *Staph. aureus* resistant to β-lactam antibiotics, including penicillins and cephalosporins; resistance to other classes of antibiotics, such as fluoroquiniolones and tetracylclines is increasing.
- Initially presents similar to other bacterial infections with furuncles, carbuncles and abscesses.
- Begins as small pustules, athlete may give history of 'spider bite'.
- Highly contagious, may progress rapidly to systemic symptoms.

Risk factors
- Football, wrestling, fencing.

Treatment
- Prompt recognition, immediate isolation from other team members.
- Individual treatment guided by local susceptibility data.
- High level of suspicion by physician and other health professionals.
- Strict guidelines for return-to-play. Cannot cover active lesions to allow participation.

Onychocryptosis (in-grown toenail, felon, paronychia)

Description
- Infection of the subcutaneous tissue beneath the toe nail.
- Usually caused by *Streptococcus* species and *Staph. aureus*.

Risk factors
- Improper trimming of the nails.

Treatment
- Should be treated immediately with appropriate antibiotics, warm compresses, pain medication, and if extensive or very painful, toe nail removal.

Prevention
- Proper trimming of nails.

Differential diagnosis
- Onychomycosis.

Pitted keratolysis (stinky foot, tennis shoe foot)

Description
- Characterized by many circular or longitudinal, punched-out depressions on the sole of the foot.
- Most cases are asymptomatic, but painful, plaque-like lesions may occur.
- *Dermatophilus congolensis* and *M. sedentarius* produce and excrete exoenzymes (keratinase) that are able to degrade keratin and produce pitting in the stratum corneum.

Risk factors
- Hyperhidrosis, moist socks, or immersion of the feet favors its development.

Treatment
- Treatment consists of promoting dryness.
- Socks should be changed frequently.
- Rapid clearing occurs with application of 20% aluminum chloride twice a day.
- Application twice a day of alcohol-based benzoyl peroxide (Panoxyl 5) may also be useful.
- Treatment with topical erythromycin is also curative.

Prevention
- Keep feet clean and dry.

Differential diagnosis
- Tinea pedis.

Erythrasma

Description
- Bacterial infection (*C. minutissimum*) may be confused with tinea cruris because of the similar, half moon-shaped plaque.
- Non-inflammatory, it is uniformly brown and scaly, it has no advancing border, and it fluoresces coral-red with the Wood's light.

Risk factors
- Occlusive clothing/shoes, obesity, hyperhidrosis.

Treatment
- Responds equally well to erythromycin orally 250mg qid for 2 weeks or topically bd for 2 weeks.
- The topical erythromycins contain alcohol and may be irritating when applied to the groin.

Differential diagnosis
- Dermatophytosis, pitted keratolysis, seborrhoea.

Viral infections

Verruca vulgaris (warts)

Description
- Due to a viral infection of the epidermis.
- May occur anywhere on the body.
- Presents as a rough hyperkeratotic area that may become quite large.

Diagnosis
- Importantly, they lack normal skin lines and can be differentiated from other lesions by this fact.
- May have black dots in the centre from the ruptured blood vessels present there.

Risk factors
- Skin to skin contact, immune-compromise.

Treatment
- Usually will regress spontaneously.
- May treat with cryotherapy, topical abrasives, laser, or immunotherapy.
- Should be covered to reduce the low risk of transmission.

Differential diagnosis
- Molluscum contagiosum, actinic keratosis.

Verruca plantaris (plantar wart)

Description
- Caused by a viral infection of the plantar surface of the foot.
- May be painful and cause gait abnormalities.

Diagnosis
- Similar to warts.

Differential diagnosis
- Public showers and locker rooms.

Treatment
- Treat early, rather than late.
- May use a doughnut-shaped pad during the season and definitively treat at the end of the season.
- Topical over-the-counter preparations may take weeks for cure.
- Can be treated with liquid nitrogen or 40% salicylic acid.
- Duofilm with 17% salicylic acid nightly can be used during the season.

Differential diagnosis
- Corns, calluses.

Condyloma acuminatum (genital warts)

Description
- Caused by human papilloma virus (HPV).
- May cause cervical cancer in females.

Diagnosis
- May go unnoticed in females, may be diagnosed on cervical smears.
- Diagnosed by appearance and location as well as sexual activity.

Risk factors
- Unprotected sex, multiple sexual partners.

Treatment
- Prevented by use of condoms.
- Can be treated with topical salicylic acid, cryotherapy, or laser.
- Treatment is imperative to prevent transmission.

Differential diagnosis
- Skin tags, moles, seborrhea, molluscum contagiosum, folliculitis

Molluscum contagiosum (water warts)

Description
- The viral pathogen is more infectious than normal warts, thus its name.
- Transmission is through close physical contact or auto-inoculation.
- Presents as flesh or yellowish colored papular lesions with a collapsed centre especially on the hands, face, and upper body.
- In non-immunosuppressed people—usually a benign, self-resolving infection, but can persist.

Diagnosis
- Typical appearance.
- Usually do not give a history of contact with infected person.

Risk factors
- Exposure to virus, skin to skin contact.
- More prevalent in contact sports such as wrestling, boxing, and rugby.
- Atopic dermatitis increases risk.

Treatment
- Usually resolve spontaneously after 6–9 months.
- Cryotherapy, topical salicylic acid, or even excision (curettage).
- Prevent spread by meticulous attention to hygiene after exposure to another athlete's skin secretions or inanimate objects like towels, gym equipment, wrestling mats.

Differential diagnosis
- Flat wart, condyloma acuminatum, syringoma.

Varicella (chicken pox)

Description
- Vesicular lesions that begin as papules, evolve to vesicles, and rapidly evolve to pustules and crusts.
- Spread by respiratory secretions and contact with weeping lesions.
- Preventable with new immunization.

Diagnosis
- Made by clinical history and typical lesions that begin on the face and scalp and spread to the trunk and extremities.
- Lack of exposure or immunization.

Risk factors
- Lack of immunization or disease history, exposure.

Treatment
- Symptomatic treatment with isolation until all lesions are crusted over.

Differential diagnosis
- Disseminated HSV, eczema, Enterovirus infection.

Herpes zoster (shingles)

Description
- Reinfection by Varicella zoster virus (VZV).
- Virus lies dormant within the ganglion cells and may be reactivated at any time.
- Unilateral dermatomal development of papules (24h), to vesicles. (48h), to pustules (96h), to crusts (7–10 days).
- New lesions may continue to develop for up to 7 days.
- Prevalent in the elderly.
- May be very painful and appear in any dermatome (most commonly on the thorax).

Risk factors
- Previous infection of chicken pox, immune-compromise, age.

Treatment
- Pain management.
- Prevent viral transmission (previously unexposed individual can contract chicken pox from exposure to person with shingles).
- Prevent secondary infections.
- Antiviral treatment (acyclovir, valacyclovir, famcyclovir).

Herpes simplex virus (HSV)

Description
- Caused by herpes simplex virus (HSV).
- Vesicles, pustules, erosions, and crusts.
- Regional adenopathy and systemic symptoms of fever, malaise, anorexia, and weight loss common in primary HSV infections.
- Can get intra-oral lesions, stomatitis, pharyngitis, or can just present as typical 'cold sore' (Herpes labialis).
- Often have prodromic symptoms—headache, tingling, burning, or itching of the skin at the site of recurrence.

Diagnosis
- Typical lesion and clinical presentation—oral, genital.
- Tzanck smear, viral culture, antigen detection.

Risk factors
- Altered immune status (other infection).
- Stress, sun exposure.

Treatment
- Oral therapy (acyclovir, valacyclovir, famcyclovir).
- Topical medications not very useful.
- Lower dose prophylactic therapy for recurrent cases.
- Ophthalmological consultation for slit-lamp examination and management in cases of suspected herpetic keratitis (dendritic ulcers).

Herpes gladiatorum (traumatic herpes)

Description
- Caused by HSV.
- HSV is directly inoculated onto the skin or may recur in cervical and lumbosacral dermatomes.
- Present as blisters that rupture to form a crusted surface.
- May be preceded by an itching or burning sensation.
- Maximally contagious for 5 days after blisters rupture.
- May last for 1–2 weeks.
- Infectious until lesions are crusted over.
- Seen in close contact sports such as wrestling and rugby.

Diagnosis
- Typical lesion and clinical presentation.
- Tzanck smear, viral culture, antigen detection.

Risk factors
- Exposure to virus.
- Skin to skin contact.
- Rugby (scrum pox), wrestling, and other martial arts, football.

Treatment
- Prevention of skin to skin contact to prevent transmission.
- Daily disinfection of mats and shared equipment.
- Oral therapy (acyclovir, valacyclovir, famcyclovir).
- Prophylaxis may prevent recurrence.

Chapter 13

Women

Menstrual cycle *352*
Menarche *353*
Primary amenorrhoea *353*
Menstrual irregularities *354*
Amenorrhoea *355*
Progression of menstrual changes due to strenuous exercise *355*
Dysmenorrhoea *355*
Premenstrual syndrome *356*
Contraception *356*
Treatment of menstrual irregularities *357*
Manipulation of menstrual cycle *357*
Athletic triad *358*
Pregnancy and exercise *362*
Pelvic pain *366*
Gender verification *368*
Injuries *370*

Menstrual cycle

- The normal cycle lasts from 21–36 days. The first day of menstruation is day 1 of the cycle.
- The cycle usually consists of 3–5 days of menstruation. Follicular phase is from last day of menstruation to ovulation which occurs at approximately 14 days, and the luteal phase lasts from ovulation to menstruation, which is approximately 15–28 days.
- A cycle lasting fewer than 21 days is polymenorrhoea and longer than 36 days is oligomenorrhoea. Secondary amenorrhoea is defined as having had no periods for 3–6 months.

Hormonal changes that occur during the menstrual cycle

Gonadotrophin-releasing hormone (GnRH) causes the synthesis, storage, and the activation release of follicle-stimulating hormone (FSH) and luteinizing hormone (LH).

During the follicular phase, levels of oestrogen increase so that both LH and oestrogen peak just before ovulation. Oestrogen then falls and rises again during the luteal phase. Progesterone is secreted by the corpus luteum during the luteal phase, and both oestrogen and progesterone levels fall if fertilization does not take place. Hormone levels should normally be tested after the 21st day of the cycle, during the luteal phase.

Physical exercise produces marked changes in the post-exercise pulsatile, secretion of LH, FSH, oestrogen, and progesterone, and cortisol. The more intense and longer the duration of exercise the greater the effect, resulting in marked changes in the menstrual cycle. Factors associated with changes to the normal menstrual cycle include:

- Psychological stress.
- Physical exercise.
- Seasonal rhythms.
- Circadian rhythms.
- Strenuous exercise causes an increase in dopamine, which inhibits GnRH, beta endorphins, catecholamines, oestrogens.
- Beta endorphins stimulate dopamine and combine with noradrenaline receptors in the hypothalamus, which inhibit stimulation of GnRH.

Menarche

The average age for menarche in Europe is 12–13.4yrs and in the USA, for Caucasians, it is 12.8yrs. Failure to menstruate after 16yrs of age is considered to be late menarche and the cause should be investigated. Tall thin girls tend to have a later menarche than small larger girls. In some cases, bone age may be below the chronological age due to illness or inadequate nutrition. To determine this, X-ray the carpal bones of the left hand. These can be compared with standards established by Greulich and Pyle, Tanner and Fels. To overcome X-ray exposure, there have been more recent efforts to standardize using MRI.

Later menarche tends to occur in gymnasts, ballet dancers, and athletes who start high intensity training early. Other factors which may delay menarche include low caloric intake, low body fat and high emotional stress.

Primary amenorrhoea

Any girl, who by the age of 13, has not developed any secondary sexual characteristics, or who has not menstruated by the age of 16 should be evaluated and examined. This should include a detailed medical, family, and nutritional history and, in an athlete, a record of her training and competition. Physical findings will direct the appropriate investigations and may indicate referral to a gynaecologist. The preliminary tests should include hormone levels (FSH, LH, oestrogen, progesterone, testosterone, prolactin, and thyroid function tests), US of the pelvis, and investigation for chromosomal abnormalities. Treatment for delay of menarche is advised at 18yrs because of the risk of osteopenia.

Menstrual irregularities

Menstrual irregularities tend to occur in the athletes with the most intense training schedules or in those who have participated or competed for the longest period of time.
- Polycystic ovary syndrome (PCOS) is a common and congenital cause of menstrual disorders, and can lead to a slight increase in testosterone production. Polycystic ovaries—part of PCOS, were more common amongst elite Olympic athletes (37%), than amongst women on average (20%).
- Vegetarians and people with a low caloric intake have the highest incidence of *oligomenorrhoea* and amenorrhoea.
- Menstrual irregularities are reported in 7% of recreational runners, 12% of swimmers, and 25% of distance runners.
- The incidence depends on how the menstrual irregularities are assessed and vary in studies by questionnaire or measured hormone levels.

About one-third of athletes believe that menstruation affects performance, but medals have been won during all phases of the menstrual cycle. There are no medical contraindications to exercise while menstruating. The effects of menstruation on performance appear to be sports related.

Athletes with menstrual problems often had them prior to training. Many 'normal' cycles show abnormal serum hormone levels after 21st day of cycle. Non-athletes also have problems. A mother's attitude to menstruation is often reflected in the daughter.

Multifactoral causes of all menstrual irregularities
- Stress, both psychological and physical. Severe emotional stress acts above hypothalamic-pituitary axis.
- Sudden increases in the quantity and intensity of training or increase in the number of competitions.
- Late menarche, irregular cycle prior to sports participation, intense training prior to menarche, and an immature pituitary axis.
- Inadequate nutrition, weight loss. Decreased caloric intake, and a low protein, high fibre diet results in a high serum sex hormone-binding globulin and low oestrogen, which predispose to amenorrhoea.

Amenorrhoea

- Higher incidence of musculoskeletal problems and stress fractures in amenorrhoeic athletes, particularly those with irregular menstrual cycles. Amenorrhoeic athletes with hyperprolactinaemia have an associated low bone mineral density.
- Cannot assume an amenorrhoeic athlete is infertile.
- Must rule out pregnancy and other causes of amenorrhoea.

Progression of menstrual changes due to strenuous exercise

- *Stage 1:* normal follicular, normal luteal phase.
- *Stage 2:* prolonged follicular and a shortened luteal phase results in luteal phase defects, which is associated with infertility and premenstrual tension.
- *Stage 3:* euoestrogenic anovulatory oligomenorrhoea, possibility of endometrial hyperplasia adenocarcinoma if this phase persists
- *Stage 4:* hypo-oestrogenic—amenorrhoea leads to osteoporosis and genital atrophy.

Dysmenorrhoea

- Dysmenorrhoea is due to the release of prostaglandins and is limited to an ovulatory cycle.
- Exercise has a beneficial effect and dysmenorrhoea is rare in an athlete.
- If dysmenorrhoea is present, look for pathology, e.g. fibroid or ovarian cysts, polycystic ovarian syndrome, or endometriosis.

Premenstrual syndrome

- Premenstrual syndrome (PMS) in athletes may cause problems in sports that require fine judgement; women are more accident prone, and more intolerant to alcohol. It results in irritability, mood swings, and fluid retention.
- Patients with premenstrual tension should not scuba dive. Judgement is poor and they are more accident prone.
- Diuretics should not be prescribed in athletes. Reduce training. (It is better to reduce training intensity than to over-medicate in a case of PMS, but there may be situations where mild diuretics are indicated and, as long as hydration is adequate for performance, they can be used safely and effectively. *Remember* the rules on doping, where appropriate)

Treatment

Low dose oral contraceptive pill (OCP). It is important not to start the pill just before a major competition, but ideally several cycles before the competition if possible.

Contraception

Barrier methods include condoms, either on their own or in conjunction with barrier creams, i.e. spermicidal cream or gel. Diaphragm, if correctly fitted, can be worn during exercise with hardly any side effects. Intrauterine devices may cause increased pain and bleeding. Barrier methods are not as reliable as the pill, but have fewer side effects.

It is important to start treatment with the pill, combined or progesterone only, well in advance of any competition due to individual variations in reactions to the pill. Depot- Provera should not be given to young athletes between 16-20 years, when 60% of their bone will be laid down. Depot-Provera affects bone accrual, particularly if there are other risk factors. DXA should be performed before each injection, if there is no alternative. Bone mineral density should be monitored by DEXA to study the effect on bone growth. Particularly common in the teens and early twenties.

- The oral contraceptive pill can be prescribed safely from 16yrs or 3yrs post-menarche.
- Low dose oral contraceptive pill, which consists of a combination of oestrogen and progestogens, can regulate the cycle, control the pain of dysmenorrhoea, and prevent early osteoporosis.
- Progesterone only oral contraceptive pill inhibits ovulation, but it is not as effective at reducing pain.

Treatment of menstrual irregularities

The team approach should include the athlete, physician, physiotherapist, nutritionist, physiologist, and psychologist.
- Identify cause.
- Dietary advice, increase caloric intake if necessary.
- Reduce training intensity.
- Monitor hormone levels.
- DEXA scan.
- Low dose pill.
- Monophasic pill or bi- or triphasic hormone replacement therapy (HRT).
- US of pelvis.
- Referral to gynaecologist.

Manipulation of menstrual cycle

In an athlete where menstrual problems may affect performance (e.g. PMS, dysmenorrhoea) it may be possible to manipulate the menstrual cycle.

If taking the OCP the athlete may stop taking the pill 10 days before sporting event, which will result in a withdrawal bleed. Restart a new packet of OCP at the end of menstruation, or after the sporting event. Barrier methods of contraception will be necessary until 2 weeks after commencing the pill again. Alternatively, the athlete may continue to take an oral contraceptive pill throughout the period of the sporting event. A monophasic pill is simpler to use if the athlete wishes to manipulate their cycle.

If not taking the oral contraceptive pill, menstruation may be induced 10 days before the event, by giving a progesterone derivative (e.g. progestogen only, norethisterone), for 10 days duration, then stopping the course 10 days before the event when menstruation will occur.

Athletic triad

- Amenorrhoea.
- An eating disorder.
- Osteoporosis or osteopenia (Low bone mineral density).

Each of these conditions can occur on their own or in combination.

Eating disorders or eating distress

Anorexia and bulimia may occur singly or together. There has been a marked increase in the prevalence of eating disorders in the last decade, in both the general public and among athletes. The female athlete is at risk during adolescence and young adulthood. This may be due to psychological, biological, or social pressures at this time. Other factors include poor training programmes, too many competitions, and inappropriate goals (a 'win at all costs' approach by athlete, coaches, or parents).

There is an increased incidence in sports with an emphasis on leanness, e.g. gymnastics, ballet, long distance running, synchronized swimming, skating, and in weight category sports, e.g. judo, lightweight rowing, but it can occur in any sport.

It is essential to take an accurate and detailed social, medical, and menstrual history. If there is a history of irregular periods or amenorrhoea, it is essential to do hormone levels and a DEXA scan to out rule osteopenia or osteoporosis. The result of the scan should be explained to the individual and if bone density is low, the patient must be told that it is due to loss of oestrogen because of inadequate calorie intake and that the only way to prevent fractures is for them to take control. Athletes must restore their hormone levels by increasing their body weight and take either HRT or the OCP until the bone density has improved.

Osteoporosis

Osteoporosis is characterized by a decrease in bone mass and mineral density and a deterioration in micro-architecture, which results in loss in bone strength and a greater risk of fracture.

Osteoporosis, or in a larger number of cases osteopenia, is associated with low levels of oestrogen, increased bone loss, hypercortisolaemia, low T3 syndrome, and a deficiency in IGF-1. It is a silent disease that can occur at any age.

Bone is a living tissue, which is constantly removed and replaced. The rate of turnover is determined by hormonal and local factors. It depends on the balance between Rank Ligand, which increases osteoclastic activity and bone loss, and osteoprogerin (OPG), which increase bone formation

60% of bone is laid down during the growth spurt at puberty. Peak bone mass occurs around 20yrs. Bone mass plateaus until the age of 40 and then declines at menopause. Peak bone mass is affected by genetic and environmental factors, mechanical strain, hormones, chronological age, skeletal age, and the stage of sexual maturation.

Weight-bearing activity during adolescence and early adulthood is a more important predictor of peak bone mass than calcium intake.

Young women who participate regularly in sports at school demonstrate higher bone mass than those who do not.

Bone requires normal sex hormone levels, adequate nutrition including 1000mg calcium, 800IU of vitamin D, and regular weight bearing exercise, particularly during the growth spurt. Oestrogen decline affects calcium metabolism and results in increased bone loss—low peak bone mass—and, in younger female low bone mass and osteopenia.

Low oestrogen affects vitamin D formation and, as a result, there may be an increase in PTH and bone loss. Vitamin D insufficiency is now a worldwide problem, this is due to many factors. Low levels of vitamin D may occur in all age groups, who do not get sufficient vitamin D from sunlight; this may be due to lack of exposure, or using a moisturizer containing sun block or too high sun block . In older women there is a lower amount of vitamin D precursor 7dehydrocholesterol in the skin and less efficient synthesis of vitamin D in the skin,

Vitamin D insufficiency may be due to poor nutrition, low Vitamin D intake, or poor absorption due to GI disorders, particularly gluten intolerance. The exact cause of the insufficiency must be identified and treated

Vitamin D endocrine system, is not only important for bone and muscle health, preventing falls, but it also influences many other tissues, such as the immune system, the cardiovascular/metabolic system, cell proliferation, and cancer. The greatest risk for bone and several major diseases and preventable health conditions are associated with 25(OH)D levels below 50 nmol /L.

Dietary intake, is a minor source of vitamin D, providing ≤100IU/day, Vitamin D is rare in foods other than fatty fish, eggs, and supplemented dairy products. Vitamin D can be supplied as calcium and vitamin D preparations, multivitamins, and supplements. Supplements containing vitamin D alone are not readily available, Patient compliance with supplementation therapy is poor

Mechanical stress exerts a positive effect on bone. It increases blood supply and lays down bone. Muscle action is the main stimulus for bone formation. Exercise should be weight bearing, and produce dynamic not static strains. Greater loads with fewer repetitions of a load will result in greater gains in bone mass. Lower loads repeated a greater number of times result in lower gains. The effect of exercise reflects the strains imposed at individual sites.

Bone mass

Peak height velocity for girls is between 10.5 and 13yrs and the peak height velocity for boys is between 12.5 and 15yrs.

The rate of bone turnover is determined by hormonal and local factors. Osteogenesis is induced by dynamic not static strains. The osteogenic response to mechanical loading is site-specific, so that professional tennis players, for example, have 30% greater bone density in their dominant forearm.

There is a 7–8% gain in bone mass per year during childhood and early adolescence. Daily physical exercise has a positive effect on bone. Weight training should be done for 30min at least three times a week. Weight-bearing aerobic exercise should be for 30min daily and this can be divided up into smaller time segments. Weight-bearing exercise should be continued throughout the life cycle.

Intensive endurance training and amenorrhoea may be associated with decreased trabecular bone density in young females. Those who have been running for the longest period of time have the highest incidence of oligomenorrhoea and amenorrhoea.

The best predictor of BMD of the lumbar spine in women in their thirties and forties (premenopausal) are the years of regular menstruation. The best predictor of BMD of the hip is the number of years of amenorrhoea.

Pregnancy and exercise

Exercise is now an integral part of life and many women wish to continue during pregnancy. Fit women tend to have fewer problems, regain their figure earlier, and feel better. They are less likely to be depressed. Exercise helps prevent excessive weight gain, maintains aerobic fitness, and helps sleep.

Musculoskeletal system

The anterior enlarging uterus results in a shift of the centre of gravity posteriorly, resulting in a progressive lordosis and rotation of the pelvis. Relaxin, a hormone produced during pregnancy, causes laxity of the ligaments with increased stress on the lumbar spine and ligaments. Back pain occurs in approximately 50% of pregnancies and is more common in the older age group and with increased parity. This may be due to sacroiliac strain or unilateral lumbarization or unilateral sacralization. The increased anterior flexion of the lumbar spine and slumping of the shoulder predisposes to paraesthesia in the distribution of the median or ulnar nerves.

Cardiovascular changes

There is a 30% increase in maternal blood volume during early pregnancy, which peaks at mid-pregnancy, so there is a reduced cardiac reserve during strenuous exercise. There is an increase in cardiac output due to an increase in HR and SV. There is a decrease in peripheral resistance due to the vasodilation of vessels in the skin, breast, uterus, GI tract, and kidneys.

Respiratory changes

Pulmonary hyperventilation changes include an increase in vital capacity, increased expansion of the lower ribs, a decrease in residual expiratory reserve, a decrease in $PaCO_2$, and elevation of the diaphragm. There is a reduction in pulmonary reserve in late pregnancy.

Other changes

Additional energy requirements during pregnancy

- 150 calories a day during the first trimester, 350 calories a day during the second, and 300 extra calories needed daily during the third trimester.
- Because of the greater utilization of carbohydrate, there is a greater risk of hypoglycaemia.
- Hyporesponsive to insulin due to somatomammotrophin.
- Hypoglycaemia occurs if the exercise is prolonged or strenuous.
- Higher risk of dehydration.

Placental hormones

During the first 3 months of pregnancy the hormones are produced by the corpus luteum, and during the second and third trimester by the placenta. Placental hormones include oestriol, progesterone, chorionic gonadotrophins, and somatomammotrophin, which antagonizes insulin.

Exercise increases the catecholamines, prolactin, endorphins, and glucagon. There is a decrease in insulin due to the gonadotrophins.

The placenta metabolizes amines so that only 10–15% of maternal catecholamines reach the foetus. Excess catecholamines have an adverse effect on the foetal circulation by reduced foetal breathing and reduced foetal movements.

During exercise there is a major redistribution of blood flow from the uterus to the exercising muscles. There is an increase in foetal heart rate within minutes. However, 50% of the uterine blood flow must be diverted before foetal hypoxia occurs. Signs of foetal distress include foetal tachycardia or foetal bradycardia.

Foetal heart rate usually returns to normal 15min after stopping mild or moderate maternal exercise, but it may take 30min after strenuous exercise.

Temperature changes

Maternal body temperature is increased due to foetal and placental metabolism. Under resting conditions, the foetal temperature is 0.5°C above the maternal. Trained athletes have a lower resting core temperature, and a more efficient temperature control. Not all women respond to heat stress in the same way.

During exercise there is an increase in maternal temperature followed by a rise in foetal temperature. Maternal temperature should not exceed 38°C; heart rate should not exceed 140beats/min. A core increase of 1–1.5°C in the non-pregnant woman may easily exceed 2–2.5°C, resulting in an increase of 2.5–3°C in the foetus. Heat production and heat loss depends on the intensity, duration, and efficiency of exercise, and environmental factors, such as ambient temperature, humidity, and physiological adaptation. In animals a temperature of 39°C has a tetrogenic effect on the neural tube in the foetus during the first trimester. Moderate or strenuous exercise in adverse conditions can increase the maternal temperature above 39°C. The risk of dehydration during exercise is increased in pregnant women.

Type of exercise

The type of exercise depends on their medical and obstetrical history and stage of pregnancy. Recommended exercises include: walking, running, cycling, water aerobics. Swimming can be done throughout the pregnancy. Racquet sports such as tennis, badminton, and squash are suitable provided they do not result in too great an increase in temperature. Sports to be avoided are water skiing, scuba diving, contact sports, and horse riding. The amount and type of exercise depends on a large number of factors, and recommendations must be individually based.

Contraindications to exercise

- Acute infection.
- Placenta praevia.
- Toxaemia of pregnancy.
- Hydramnios.
- Threatened abortion.
- Premature labour.
- Incompetent cervix.

Warning signs to stop exercise
- Bleeding PV
- Shortness of breath.
- Dizziness.
- Chest pain.
- Headache.
- Muscle pain.
- Decrease in foetal movement.
- Leakage of amniotic fluid.

Maternal exercise
An individualized exercise programme that is closely monitored can improve fitness and help to ensure the safety of the individual.

The intensity and amount depends on the level of fitness of the individual. If they have not exercised for some time they should start slowly, at a low intensity:
- Always warm up and cool down for at least 5min.
- Ensure adequate fluid intake to avoid dehydration.
- Use correct equipment and clothing in a well-ventilated room.
- Get up slowly from the floor to prevent postural hypotension.

Regular aerobic exercise lasting 20–40min is preferable to occasional bursts of intense exercise. Exercise should use large muscle groups. Strenuous exercise should not exceed 15min (60–90% of maximum heart rate or 50–85% of VO_2 max. Maternal heart rate should not exceed 140beats/min. Maternal core temperature should not exceed 38°C. No exercise should be performed in supine position after the fourth month. Vigorous exercise should not be performed in hot humid conditions. Ballistic movements should be avoided. Exercises that involve the Valsalva manoeuvre should be avoided.

Adequate caloric intake to meet extra needs of pregnancy and exercise involved.

The first trimester
Exercise is contraindicated in the first trimester in women with a history of spontaneous abortion. This is often associated with a luteal phase defect due to low levels of progesterone. When the placenta takes over the production of hormones, they may be able to exercise, but must be closely monitored.

Fitness can be improved during pregnancy. Pregnant women who do not normally exercise are advised to do so and can start to exercise for the first time (walking, cycling, swimming, etc.). It helps prevent excessive weight gain. Women who normally train may continue and may be monitored using HR monitors. The level and intensity must be individually prescribed. A patient with known obstetrical problems should consult an obstetrician.

The second trimester
Enlarging uterus causes the centre of gravity to be displaced posteriorly. Lumbar lordosis increases, resulting in stress on the sacroiliac joint, lumbar vertebrae, and ligaments. No exercise should be carried out in the supine position after the fourth month, as the uterus may fall back

and compresses the aorta and IVC, restricting the arterial blood flow and venous return.

The third trimester
Alterations in neck posture may result in neck pain. Fluid retention may cause carpal tunnel syndrome.

During exercise, the noradrenaline produced increases the frequency and amplitude of uterine contractions. Women with multiple pregnancies should avoid strenuous exercise. Dyspnoea may be due to displacement of the diaphragm causing a reduction in pulmonary reserve which limits exercise. Excessive exercise may cause foetal distress, intra-uterine growth retardation, or prematurity.

Pregnant women with a poor obstetrical history should consult an obstetrician. Exercise or sport may normally be resumed a few weeks after a normal delivery, depending on the individual, the sport, and type of delivery. They should all do core stability exercises to improve abdominal and gluteal muscles the day after delivery. This may be restricted, if they had a Caesarean section. Walking should start straight away; it takes approximately 6 weeks for the ligaments to recover, so sports such as golf or tennis that involve rotary movements should be avoided during this period. Any sport should be started slowly and the amount and intensity should be gradually increased.

Pelvic pain

Pelvis pain is a generic term that covers many causes, some of which may be gynaecological. It may be due to a local cause or referred. It may be acute or chronic. Local causes include the bladder, ureter, uterus, (body or cervix), broad ligament, uterine tube, ovaries, rectum, vagina, or a pelvic appendix.

It is essential to take a detailed history of the pain to include the quality, type, radiation, factors that relieve or aggravate, its relationship to menstrual cycle (to rule out an ectopic pregnancy or pain due to ovulation), associated symptoms, such as nausea, vomiting, and diarrhoea. Infection should be investigated. Routine abdominal and gynaecological examination including a PV/PR combined bimanual. Referral may be appropriate for further investigation including pelvic ultrasound. The pain may be of musculoskeletal origin.

Gender verification

Gender testing is no longer required by the IOC and was not carried out at the last three summer Olympic Games. Routine sex tests carried out at the previous Olympic Games were not appropriate, and only differentiated between females who had two XX chromosomes and a positive Barr body in the cell from a buccal smear. Individuals with only one X chromosome had no Barr body and were not considered female. The normal male chromosomal count is 46XY, normal female is 46XX.

Gender testing should not be confused with genetic sex as determined by chromosomal tests.

Eight criteria determine a person's sexual status:
- Sex chromosome constitution.
- Sex hormonal pattern.
- Gonadal sex (ovaries or testes).
- Internal sex organs.
- External genitalia.
- Secondary sex characteristics.
- Apparent sex, role in which person was reared.
- Psychological sex or gender identity.

Gender testing for sports only considers the sex chromosome pattern.

Chromosomal test discloses the Y fluorescent long arm in males or the second X (Barr body) in a buccal smear in females. If a laboratory test is abnormal, a gynaecological examination is performed.

Disorders of sex chromosomes

- *Turner's syndrome 45 XO:* is a female who has a negative buccal smear. It consists of gonadal dysgenesis, primary amenorrhoea, and immature secondary sex characteristics. There may be a mixture or mosaicism, some cells having 46XX.
- *Disorders of gonadal sex:* the chromosomal sex is normal, but the differentiation of the gonads is abnormal.
- *Pure gonadal dysgenesis:* the individual has an immature female phenotype with bilateral streak gonads, with a normal 46XX or 46XY chromosomal complement.
- *XXX triple X female:* has a tendency to secondary amenorrhoea.

Disorders of phenotypic sex

Intersex or disorders of sex development (DSD) are complicated. The phenotypic sex is ambiguous or is completely opposite to the chromosomal and gonadal sex. The clinical spectrum is very varied depending on the mixture of testicular or ovarian tissue present; they usually have ambiguous external genitalia.

Female

Congenital adrenal hyperplasia. One-half to two-thirds have XX karyotype, there may also be mosaics of, e.g. XO, XY, XYY, it is the most common form of virilization in a new born female. The incidence is 1:300–1000, there is an increased formation of dehydroepiandrosterone.

Congenital adrenal hyperplasia 44+ XX, (adrenogenital syndrome) chromatin positive nuclei, ovaries, excessive production of androgens by the adrenal glands, cause external genitalia to develop in a male direction, extent varies from enlargement of the clitoris to almost male genitalia, this is due to abnormal steroid metabolism in the foetal adrenal cortex. Congenital adrenal hyperplasia is associated with an inherited deficiency of 21-hydroxylase enzyme. Mild forms of congenital adrenal hyperplasia may only manifest as increased muscular strength in a female and a positive buccal smear.

Feminized male defective virilization of the 44XY

Androgen insensitivity syndrome (testicular feminization), normal testes develops, but Fallopian tubes, uterus, and ovaries are absent, and only the lower quarter of the vagina is present. There is a lack of testosterone receptors in the target tissues and the body is insensitive to testosterone. They produce more testosterone than a genetic XX female, but normal genetic male XY would produce much more. The testes should be removed after puberty as they are more prone to malignant change.

Testicular enzyme defects; failure of one or more enzymes that produce testosterone in the testes may result. It is similar to androgen insensitivity, but the difference is made at puberty as both oestrogen and testosterone can be blocked and no secondary sex characteristics develop.

Androgen excess in women may be due to drugs, e.g. androgens, anabolic steroids, androgenic progestagens hyperprolactinaemia. Ovarian causes include polycystic ovarian syndrome, tumours, hyperthecosis.

Adrenal causes

- Congenital adrenal hyperplasia.
- Classical or late onset, Cushing's syndrome.
- Tumours: hyperprolactinaemia.

There have been rare cases of athletes who have competed as one gender and undergone sex reassignment in later life. This has increased in the last decade

New rules permit transsexual athletes to compete in the Olympics after having completed sex reassignment surgery, being legally recognized a member of the target sex, They have undergone 2 years of hormonal therapy (unless they changed gender before puberty).

Injuries

Women develop similar injuries as men as a result of training errors, but may be more prone to certain injuries because of anatomical differences.

Injuries to knee and ankle are common, but injuries to breast are rare. There is a higher incidence of anterior cruciate ligament tears in females due to the narrow intercondylar notch of the femur and subluxation of the patella due to genu valgum. Back pain in females may be due to gynaecological causes including ovarian cysts, endometriosis, or fibroids. Water-skiing injuries during take-off, failure to rise from sitting position results in retrograde douching, which may result in haematoma of the vulva or laceration of vaginal wall. Female athletes who have recurrent stress fractures should have a biomechanical assessment, a DEXA scan and hormone levels after 21st day of cycle to determine oestrogen, progesterone, prolactin, cortisol levels, and thyroid function tests. If bone density is low, other causes of bone loss must be ruled out.

Chapter 14

Older people

Exercise and successful ageing *372*
Evidence for adopting exercise in older age *372*
Exercise as primary prevention in older age *373*
Exercise as secondary prevention in older age *373*
Recommendations for aerobic exercise in older age *374*
Recommendations for resistance exercise in older age *375*
Recommendations for flexibility/balance exercise in older age *376*
Fitness deterioration with age *378*
Exercise testing in older people *380*

Exercise and successful ageing

Successful chronological ageing is the most important medical and societal challenge of our time. We can delay some of the effects of biological ageing. The trajectory is influenced by physical activity and prescriptive exercise. Exercise means fewer chronic diseases of older age, delayed infirmity and functional vitality. An artificially imposed definition of older age has been used (over 65yrs) for simplicity, but these recommendations are relevant across the lifespan.

Active lifestyle preserves and enhances muscle strength and endurance, flexibility, cardiorespiratory fitness, and body composition, potentially reducing the risk of chronic disease associated with ageing.

Evidence for adopting exercise in older age

- Regular aerobic exercise has an inverse dose–dependent relationship with the prevalence of major chronic diseases of ageing including: coronary heart disease, osteoarthritis, type 2 diabetes, depression, some cancers, dementia, disability, falls, and loss of function.
- Regular aerobic exercise is beneficial to older adults because it increases cardiorespiratory fitness which itself is an independent risk factor for morbidity and mortality.
- Regular strength training is especially important in older adults as it is essential for the maintenance or improvement in muscle mass, muscle quality, mobility, and bone mineral density.
- Combined exercise modalities are likely more beneficial to older adults and individualized prescriptions are best.
- Stretching or low intensity exercise (Tai Chi or Medical Qigong) are unproven alone, but may contribute to improve flexibility and balance.
- Balance training should be recommended as part of an exercise intervention to prevent falls.
- Increasing physical activity in middle and older age may reduce the risk of cognitive decline in older adults.
- Despite the evidence, exercise recommendations have been poorly adopted—particularly in older age.

Exercise as primary prevention in older age

Primary prevention refers to the prevention of disease among otherwise healthy individuals. Higher fitness, achieved over 10yrs of regular exercise training in older adults, is associated with reduction in metabolic risk factors for cardiovascular disease, risk of cognitive decline, osteoporotic fractures, and greater functional independence.

Exercise as secondary prevention in older age

Secondary prevention refers to the prevention of disease among people who already have evidence of disease.
- Behavioural inertia is greater than for primary prevention. For example, patients with diabetes are less likely to be active or adopt healthy exercise habits than non-diabetics.
- Clinical inertia may be due to an incorrect belief that physical exertion is associated with an increased risk for cardiac events. Evidence now supports clinical guidelines that recommend moderate exercise for the treatment and management of established chronic diseases (including coronary heart disease, hypertension, peripheral vascular disease, type 2 diabetes, obesity, dyslipidaemia, stroke, osteoporosis, osteoarthritis, claudication, and COPD effectively reduces secondary risk.
- Older patients starting exercise training as secondary prevention should be referred to a facility experienced in exercise for older adults. They may require clinical assessment including, when appropriate, exercise stress testing. This may identify previously undiagnosed heart disease and/or help determine an appropriate exercise training prescription.

Recommendations for aerobic exercise in older age

- Older adults should participate in moderate-intensity aerobic activity for a total of 150min/week, or in vigorous-intensity activity for a total of 90min/week.
- Moderate- and vigorous-intensity activities are defined as approximately 50% and 60–70% of maximal aerobic capacity, respectively.
- Intensity can be determined from either submaximal or maximal exercise testing. Screening exercise stress testing should be considered in those patients who are new to exercise training or quite deconditioned, have known cardiovascular risk factors, a positive family history, or based on clinical presentation in consultation with the patient.
- There are some risks, but it is important to avoid discourageing older people from being active.

Exercise prescription

- *Frequency:* for moderate-intensity activities, accumulate at least 30 or up to 60 (for greater benefit) min/day. This may be made up of bouts of at least 10min each to total 150–300min/week or at least.
- 20–30min/day or more of vigorous-intensity activities to total 75–150min/week.
- *Intensity:* on a scale of 0–10 for level of physical exertion, 5–6 for moderate-intensity and 7–8 for vigorous intensity.
- *Duration:* for moderate-intensity activities, accumulate at least 30min/day in bouts of at least 10min each or at least 20min/day of continuous activity for vigorous-intensity activities.
- *Type:* any modality that does not impose excessive orthopedic stress—walking is the most common type of activity. Aquatic exercise, low impact dancing, and stationary cycle exercise may be advantageous for those with limited tolerance for weight.
- Some clinical benefits (fitness, BP, weight, blood glucose) can be seen as early as 8–10 weeks. Starting at a low level, exercise may be adjusted (~10%) every 3 months until exercise targets are achieved. A gradual increase helps encourage adherence.
- Behavioural change should be supported.
- Physical rehabilitation interventions in long-term care residents help reduce disability with few adverse events (*NB* See special considerations below).

Recommendations for resistance exercise in older age

- Older adults should undertake resistance exercises on at least 2 days/week.
- Resistance exercise should involve the major muscle groups of the body (including the upper and lower extremities and core), and should consist of 8–12 repetitions at >60% of 1 RM.
- Formal equipment is not required. Initial supervision is advised to ensure appropriate technique and safety.

Exercise prescription

- *Frequency:* at least 2 days/week.
- *Intensity:* between moderate (5–6) and vigorous (7–8) intensity on a scale of 0–10.
- *Type:* progressive weight training programme or weight-bearing calisthenics (8–10 exercises involving the major muscle groups of 8–12 repetitions each), stair climbing, and other strengthening activities that use the major muscle groups.
- For bone and muscle health including osteoarthritis, high-intensity, low-volume resistance exercise of at least 24 weeks has clinical benefit.

Recommendations for flexibility/balance exercise in older age

- Flexibility/balance at least 2–4 times a week (as warm-up/cool-down to resistance exercise sessions) but preferably daily.
- Multimodal exercise including Tai Chi, or Medical Qigong have been shown to be effective in reducing the risk falls.

Exercise prescription

- *Frequency:* at least 2 days/week.
- *Intensity:* moderate (5–6) intensity on a scale of 0–10.
- *Type:* any activities that maintain or increase flexibility using sustained stretches for each major muscle group and static rather than ballistic movements.
- *Balance exercise for frequent fallers or individuals with mobility problems, such as long-term care residents. Because of a lack of adequate research evidence, there are currently no specific recommendations regarding specific frequency, intensity, or type of balance exercises for older adults. However, it is recommended that activities could include the following:
  - Progressively difficult postures that gradually reduce the base of support (two-legged stand, semi-tandem stand, tandem stand, one-legged stand).
  - Dynamic movements that perturb the center of gravity (tandem walk, circle turns).
  - Stressing postural muscle groups (heel stands, toe stands).
  - Reducing sensory input (standing with eyes closed).

Special considerations

- The intensity and duration of physical activity should be low at the outset for those who are highly deconditioned, functionally limited, or have chronic conditions that affect their ability to perform physical tasks.
- The progression of activities should be individual and tailored to tolerance and preference.
- A conservative approach may be necessary for the most deconditioned and physically limited older adults.
- Muscle strengthening activities and/or balance training may need to precede aerobic training activities among very frail individuals.
- Older adults should exercise above the minimum recommended level if they wish to improve their fitness.
- If chronic conditions preclude activity at the recommended minimum amount, older adults should perform physical activities as tolerated so as to avoid being sedentary.

NB Running, rowing, and steppers are not recommended. Rest days are important because the elderly recover more slowly from exercise than younger people.

Prescribe exercise intensity using HRR, %HR max or RPE. Individuals with low initial exercise capacity may benefit from multiple daily sessions of short (5–6min) duration because the aerobic effect is cumulative. Initial intensity low (40–60% HRR) increasing every 2–3 weeks, as tolerated until desired total volume/intensity is reached.

Current ACSM-AHA recommendation is 8–10 different exercises for 10–15 reps on at least 2 non-consecutive days per week. Moderate effort is 5 or 6 and vigorous effort is 7 or 8 on a 10-point perceived exertion scale. Free weights can be used if supervised, caution—stability problems in the elderly, elastic bands can be used instead for RT. Ensure correct breathing, avoid Valsalva manoeuvre which can reduce venous return and increase blood pressure. Allow at least 48h between RT sessions for optimal recovery. In healthy sedentary individuals VO_2 peak can increase 10–15% with moderate intensity training (<70% HRR), increases of >30% are reported with vigorous intensity training (75 to 85% HRR) on 3–5 days per week for 30–45min per session.

Elderly individuals demonstrate adaptations to resistance training; the magnitude of the adaptation depends on frequency, volume, mode, type, and initial training state. RT programmes (8–52 weeks) can increase muscle strength and muscle mass regardless of age or gender. WBV programs (26 to 52 weeks) can increase muscle mass, strength, BMD and BMC in the elderly.

Aerobic training also improves insulin sensitivity and glucose control. Elderly volunteers exercising at 70% VO_2 peak for 60min for 7 days recorded increased insulin action and skeletal muscle GLUT4 concentration, inferring that exercise may reduce risk of type 2 diabetes or alternatively help in glucose homeostasis. An increase in mitochondrial function and content with aerobic training may also enhance insulin action.

Fitness deterioration with age

In most humans there is a physiological decline in performance from the mid to late 30s onwards. Exceptional performance is still possible, however, in later years; men and women over 80 have run marathons in under 5h.

Stature
Stature declines by approximately 1cm per decade after 40yrs. This is partly due to degenerative changes in intervertebral discs, and partly loss of vertebral bone height.

Body fat
Body fat percentage rises steadily to 23–25% in men and 32–40% in women by age 60–70yrs, while lean body mass steadily declines in both genders.

Skin
The rete pegs anchoring the epidermis to the dermis become shorter with age, leading to a greater propensity to blister formation and skin tearing. Melanocytes disappear at the rate of 2% per year and the cutaneous inflammatory response diminishes. Older people are, therefore, more susceptible to sun burn, and yet show less of the acute effects of sunburn than the young.

Muscle
In comparison with performance-matched younger athletes, the muscle of elderly athletes tends towards a predominance of slow twitch type fibres, with greater muscle capillarization. This is thought to be due to re-innervation of muscle by type 1 nerve following type 2 nerve degeneration.

Ageing also causes a decrease in myosin ATPase concentration and size and number of mitochondria. Between the ages of 60–90yrs there is greater loss in muscle power than muscle strength, 3.5 vs. 1.8% per year respectively.

Reduced strength is not usually apparent until age 40yrs, with concentric force production lost more rapidly than eccentric. Over 40yr; loss is approximately 25% by age 65, with a further proportionate drop after 65. In women, strength loss is further accentuated by the menopause.

However, these changes may be reduced or delayed. A doubling of force development with 6–8 weeks of initiation of strength training programs in those aged 56–70yr is well documented. The ability to increase strength with training is important for mobility, balance, and independence.

Respiratory
Lung connective tissue elasticity decreases, alveolar size increases, and the number of pulmonary capillaries decreases. These changes lead to an increase in the work of ventilation and decreased perfusion quality.

Cardiovascular
HR max declines with age due to decreased sympathetic tone, marked reduction in SA nodal cells, and decreased sarcoplasmic uptake of Ca^{2+}. Age-related cardiac hypertrophy can paradoxically reduce SV due to decreased chamber size.

Aerobic performance

Oxygen uptake decreases due to the cardiorespiratory factors mentioned previously. From age 20yrs the mean VO_2 max of untrained male decreases by 7.5mL/kg/min per decade. The same decrements apply to the trained male, but due to a higher starting aerobic capacity their VO_2 max data remain consistently higher than the untrained, and are 20mL/kg/min higher at 40yrs and 10mL/kg/min at 70yrs.

Response to training

Older people respond to training and, despite the decrements above, older people can improve their VO_2 max by 15% and training load by 80% after 3 months of aerobic training. There are also similar changes seen in TLac and anaerobic performance indices with appropriate training.

Exercise testing in older people

The elderly population is growing; by 2030 over 20% of USA population will be >65, the average life expectancy is approximately 84yrs.

Prevalence of chronic disease and functional impairment increases with age. In 2004 over 50% of elderly in USA had at least one type of disability (physical or non-physical) and multiple chronic diseases are common.

The decline in health and reduced mobility negatively affects the ability to perform ADLs. Rate of physical inactivity increases with age, notably <25% of elderly in USA participate in PA (4 or 5 times per week for >30min).

Physiological changes of ageing
- Cardiovascular.
- At rest, decreased HR and increased BP.
- At maximal exercise, decreased HR, decreased CO, decreased a–vO_2 difference, decreased VO_2 max, decreased cardiac and vascular response to adrenergic stimulation and no detectable change in SV.

Respiratory
At maximal exercise, decreased V_E, decreased TV, decreased Rf, decreased VC and increased RV.

Other changes
- Decreased muscle mass and strength.
- Decreased elasticity in connective tissue.
- Decreased balance and co-ordination.
- Decreased BMC and BMD.
- Decreased glucose tolerance.
- Decreased insulin action.
- Decreased metabolic rate.
- Decreased thirst sensation.
- Decreased skin blood flow.
- Decreased sweat production.

Elderly individuals have a tendency to fall, are frail, and frequently have limited ability to perform ADLs. Assessing agility, balance, gait, and co-ordination may to identify those at risk. In addition, mental (depression), and intellectual impairment (dementia, Alzheimer's) can affect ability to perform appropriate exercise and effect training compliance.

Contraindications to exercise testing include resting systolic pressure >200mmHg, diastolic pressure >115mmHg, electrolyte abnormalities, neuromuscular, musculoskeletal or rheumatoid disorders, uncontrolled metabolic diseases, moderate valvular heart disease, ventricular aneurysm, and complex ventricular ectopy.

Walking is sufficient for most. If using a handrail for balance assistance, this may artificially elevate maximal attained MET. Cycling is better for individuals with balance or gait disorders. Perform testing in the morning as many elderly are fatigued in early afternoon/evening.

Maximal attained level <7 MET, use low intensity protocol increasing by 1 to 2 MET per stage (Balke protocol).

Cycling
Initial load 25W, increase by 25W per stage, peak HR, SV, CO, and VO_2 max are lower in the elderly compared to younger people. Potential mechanisms include cardiac receptor down-regulation, PA and skeletal muscle morphological changes. Pmax is lower and, at any absolute sub-maximal load, an elderly person is closer to their anaerobic threshold, CO is generally 20–30% lower when compared with younger individuals.

Chapter 15

Head and face

Sports concussion *384*
Management of sports concussion *388*
The Standardized Concussion Assessment Tool 2 card cognitive screen in concussion *390*
Glasgow Coma Scale *392*
Traumatic brain injury *395*
The management of traumatic brain injury *396*
Traumatic intracerebral haematomas/contusion *400*
Subdural haematoma *401*
Extradural haematoma *402*
Traumatic subarachnoid haemorrhage *403*
Diffuse cerebral swelling *404*
Head injury advice card *405*
Mouthguards *406*
Helmets and head protectors *407*
Other means of preventing sports concussion *407*
Epilepsy and sport *408*
Post-traumatic headache *410*
Headaches and sport *412*
Boxing and head injury *416*
The post-concussion syndrome *418*
Fractures *420*
Eye injuries *421*

Sports concussion

- Impairment of brain function caused by trauma. May be due to direct blow or impulsive (whiplash) force.
- Transient neurological symptoms that may or may not involve loss of consciousness.
- Normal neuroimaging studies.
- Incidence 0.25–5/1000 player hours of exposure for most sports.
- Professional jumps jockeys have the highest concussion rate of any sport.
- The pathophysiology is unknown. Speculated to affect the permeability and function of cell membranes within specific parts of brain or brainstem, which results in transient functional disruption.

Subtypes

There is no scientifically valid classification of concussion at the present time.

The majority (90–95%) of sports concussions recover in 7–10 days if managed appropriately. A small group of patients take longer to recover or have persistent symptoms and need expert multi-disciplinary management. In this chapter, these will be described as "complex" concussions.

Diagnosis is based on the presence of acute signs, symptoms, and cognitive impairment.

Symptoms

For symptoms of sports concussion, see Table 15.1.

Table 15.1 Symptoms of sports concussion

Symptoms	Signs	Cognitive
Headache	Loss of consciousness	Disorientation
Dizziness	Poor balance	Confusion
Nausea	Concussive convulsion	Amnesia
Unsteadiness	Vomiting	Easily distracted
'Foggy' or 'dazed'	Slurred speech	Poor concentration
Ringing in the ears	Personality changes	Slow to answer questions
Double vision	Inappropriate playing behaviour	

History and examination

Key features on history include: time and place of injury, mechanism of injury (eyewitness or video), presence, or duration of loss of consciousness (LOC), post-injury behaviour, presence of convulsions post-injury, past medical history, medication use, drug, and alcohol history.

Physical exam centres on the exclusion of intracranial pathology (e.g. haemorrhage) by neurological examination. A baseline GCS should be recorded. In sports concussion, there may be balance abnormalities within the first 72h of injury otherwise the physical exam is usually normal.

Key symptoms to flag
These signs and symptoms may indicate an intra-cerebral injury requiring urgent medical assessment. Err on the side of caution—'If in doubt, check it out'.
- A deterioration in the level of consciousness following injury.
- Skull fracture.
- Penetrating skull trauma.
- Focal neurological symptoms or signs.
- Loss of consciousness >5min.
- Persistent vomiting or headache after injury.
- Difficulty in assessing the patient due to alcohol, drugs, epilepsy, etc.
- Other high-risk medical conditions (e.g. haemophilia).
- The lack of a responsible adult to supervise the athlete post-injury.
- More than one concussion in a match or training session.
- Head injuries in children.

Diagnostic tests

Brain CT (or where available MR brain scan) contributes little to concussion evaluation, but should be employed if you suspect an intra-cerebral structural lesion.

Genetic testing

ApoE4 is one of a number of proposed genetic risk factors for adverse outcome following all levels of brain injury. The significance of *ApoE4* in the risk of sports concussion or injury outcome is unclear.

Pre-participation physical examination

A detailed concussion and head injury (e.g. facial fractures) history is of value, but many athletes will not recognize or remember all concussions suffered in the past.

Convulsive and motor phenomena

A variety of acute motor phenomena (e.g. tonic posturing) or convulsive movements may accompany a concussion. Although dramatic, these clinical features are generally benign and require no specific management beyond the standard treatment for the underlying concussive injury. Because of the unusual and infrequent nature of this complication, it is recommended that they be managed as for a 'complex' concussion.

Second impact syndrome

Diffuse cerebral swelling is a rare but well recognized complication of mild traumatic brain injury that occurs predominantly in children and teenagers. Although repeated concussive injuries are proposed as the basis for this syndrome, a single impact of any severity may cause this rare complication.

Prevention of head injury

There is no clinical evidence that currently available protective equipment will prevent concussion. Protective equipment may prevent other forms of head injury, which may be important for those sports. However, remember the concept of *risk compensation*. This is where protective equipment results in behavioural change, including more dangerous playing techniques, with a paradoxical increase in injury rate.

Education
Athletes and their health care providers must be aware how to detect concussion, its clinical features, assessment techniques, and principles of safe return to play. Athletes particularly need to understand the significance and importance of concussion symptoms, and be able to discuss these with their doctor in a team environment, where there is no pressure to return to play prematurely.

Long-term problems
Other than the longstanding research of professional boxers and chronic brain injury, there are a number of lines of research highlighting concern over long-term sequelae of concussion in professional athletes. At this time, the incidence, risk factors, and prognosis for such problems is unknown.

Recent case reports have described the pathological findings of three cases of chronic traumatic encephalopathy (CTE) in retired professional American footballers and in a further line of epidemiological research looking at neurological problems in retired athletes, data suggests that the incidence of amyotrophic lateral sclerosis may be increased in association with head injury. There may be an as yet unknown genetic basis for this risk.

A separate cross-sectional study of 2552 retired professional NFL American footballers has identified an association between recurrent concussion and clinically diagnosed mild cognitive impairment, as well as self-reported significant memory impairments. In the same cohort, the authors found that 11.1% of all respondents reported having clinical depression. There was an association between recurrent concussion and diagnosis of lifetime depression, suggesting that the prevalence increases with increasing concussion history.

What is becoming increasingly clear from a number of diverse lines of research is that a small percentage of athletes seem to disproportionately suffer chronic or long-term sequelae from sports-related head injury. Interestingly, this does not seem to be confined to the brain, but affects the spinal cord and other parts of the nervous system. At this stage, very little is known about what type, frequency, or amount of trauma is necessary to induce the accumulation of these pathological tau proteins and more importantly why only a small number of athletes are at risk for CTE.

Management of sports concussion

Acute concussion management

When a player shows *any* symptoms or signs of a concussion:
- The player should not be allowed to return to play in the current game or practice.
- The player should not be left alone; and regular monitoring for deterioration is essential over the initial few hours following injury.
- The player should be medically evaluated following the injury.
- Return to play must follow a medically supervised stepwise process.

A player should never return to play or training while symptomatic. 'When in doubt, sit them out!'

Sideline evaluation

Sideline evaluation of cognitive function is an essential component in the assessment of this injury. Brief neuropsychological test batteries such as the Maddocks questions, Standardized Concussion Assessment Tool 2 (SCAT2) or the Standardized Assessment of Concussion (SAC) have been validated in this setting. Internationally, the SCAT2 tool is the most widely used medical assessment tool and was developed at the 2009 Zurich expert consensus conference. The SCAT2 also has the Maddocks questions, GCS and SAC embedded within the tool. There is also a 'Pocket SCAT2' version for lay or non-medical assessment.

Standard orientation questions (e.g. time, place, person) are unreliable in the sporting situation compared with memory assessment.

Maddocks questions

The Maddocks questions are a validated brief assessment paradigm that can be easily administered on a sporting field or on the sidelines. They are also included in the SCAT2 tool. Failure to answer all questions correctly should raise suspicion of a concussive injury.
- Which ground are we at?
- Which team are we playing today?
- Who is your opponent at present?
- Which quarter is it?
- How far into the quarter is it?
- Which side scored the last goal?
- Which team did we play last week?
- Did we win last week?

Sideline assessment of cervical spine injury

Think cervical spine injury, always! If an alert patient complains of neck pain, has evidence of neck tenderness or deformity, or has neurological signs suggestive of a spinal injury, then neck bracing and transport on a suitable spinal frame is essential. If the patient is unconscious, then a cervical injury should be assumed until proven otherwise. Airway protection takes precedence over any potential spinal injury. In this situation, the removal of helmets or other head protectors should only be performed by individuals trained in this aspect of trauma management.

Concussion injury severity grading

International expert consensus has abandoned anecdotal grading scales in favour of combined measures (clinical symptoms, physical exam, cognitive assessment) of recovery in order to determine injury severity and, hence, guide return to play decisions. There is limited published evidence that concussion injury severity correlates with the number and duration of acute concussion signs and symptoms and/or degree of impairment on neuropsychological testing.

Neuropsychological assessment post-concussion

Neuropsychological (NP) testing in concussion is of value and continues to contribute significant information in concussion evaluation. NP assessment should not, however, be the sole influence on the decision to return to play, but is an aid to clinical decision making. NP test batteries are most useful with baseline pre-injury testing and serial follow-up post-injury. NP assessment is problematic in under 15 years of age due to changing baselines reflecting cognitive maturation. In this age group, paediatric NP expertise may be required in some cases for a full assessment.

Post-concussion balance assessment

Balance testing, either with computerized platforms or clinical assessment (e.g. BESS scale), may offer additional important information particularly in the first 72h following injury. A balance assessment is incorporated in the SCAT2.

Return to play (RTP) protocol

The vast majority of injuries are uncomplicated or simple concussions that recover spontaneously over 7–10 days and an athlete usually proceeds rapidly through the stepwise return to play strategy. During the first few days following an injury, it is important to emphasize to the athlete that physical *and* cognitive rest is required. Activities that require concentration and attention (such as videogames) may exacerbate the cognitive symptoms and as a result delay recovery.

Return to play follows a stepwise process:
- *Step 1:* no activity, complete rest. Once asymptomatic, proceed to next level.
- *Step 2:* light aerobic exercise, such as walking or stationary cycling, no resistance training.
- *Step 3:* sport-specific training (e.g. skating in hockey, running in soccer), progressive addition of resistance training at steps 3 or 4.
- *Step 4:* non-contact training drills.
- *Step 5:* full contact training after medical clearance.
- *Step 6:* game play.

If any post-concussion symptoms occur, the patient should drop back to the previous asymptomatic level and try to progress again after 24h. In cases with persistent symptoms beyond 10 days, the rehabilitation will be more prolonged and return to play advice will be more circumspect. Such complex cases should be managed by physicians with specific expertise usually in a multidisciplinary setting.

Concussed athletes should not only be symptom free, but should not be taking any pharmacological agents/medications that may affect or modify the symptoms of concussion prior to consideration of RTP.

The Standardized Concussion Assessment Tool 2 card cognitive screen in concussion

The SCAT is a medical assessment card that may be used in the assessment of concussed athletes. The original version was developed in 2005 and then revised (called the SCAT2) following scientific studies at the 2009 Zurich international consensus meeting. In addition to symptom assessment, cognition and physical exam, the tool incorporates the Maddocks questions, GCS, and the SAC, and is designed to be used by medical staff.

A shorter version designed to be used by lay or non-medical personnel (called the 'PocketSCAT2') was developed at the same time and enables the user to suspect the diagnosis of concussion and refer the patient for medical assessment.

Glasgow Coma Scale

The most widely used traumatic brain injury severity scale throughout the world is the Glasgow Coma Scale (GCS). It is useful in categorizing the acute injury, mild, moderate, and severe injuries, and performed serially to monitor progress over time. Deterioration in the GCS score may herald intracranial complications requiring neurosurgical or neuro-intensive care intervention (see Table 15.2).

Table 15.2 The Glasgow Coma Scale

Category	Response	Score
Eye opening response (E)	Spontaneous	4
	To speech	3
	To pain	2
	No response	1
Verbal response (V)	Orientated	5
	Confused, disorientated	4
	Inappropriate words	3
	Incomprehensible sounds	2
	No response	1
Motor response (M)	Obeys commands	6
	Localizes	5
	Withdraws (flexion)	4
	Abnormal flexion (posturing)	3
	Extension (posturing)	2
	No response	1

Reproduced from Teasdale, G. and Jennett, B., *Lancet*, **304**: 7872 (1974), with kind permission from Elsevier

Flow chart

The flowchart (Fig. 15.1) is a conceptual management approach to provide advice regarding return to work and sport. At least 7 days should have passed in order to detect resolution of symptoms. In the first 7 days there are currently no prognostic means of separating simple and complex concussive injury. There is still, therefore, an important role for physician discretion in neuroimaging and/or neuropsychological assessment in this early period. This management algorithm provides general guidance only. The letters in parentheses correspond to the flowchart:
- (A) This refers to athletes with no evidence of previous concussion and no history of behavioural, neurological, psychological problems, or learning disorder. Any return to sport also presumes that the athlete is

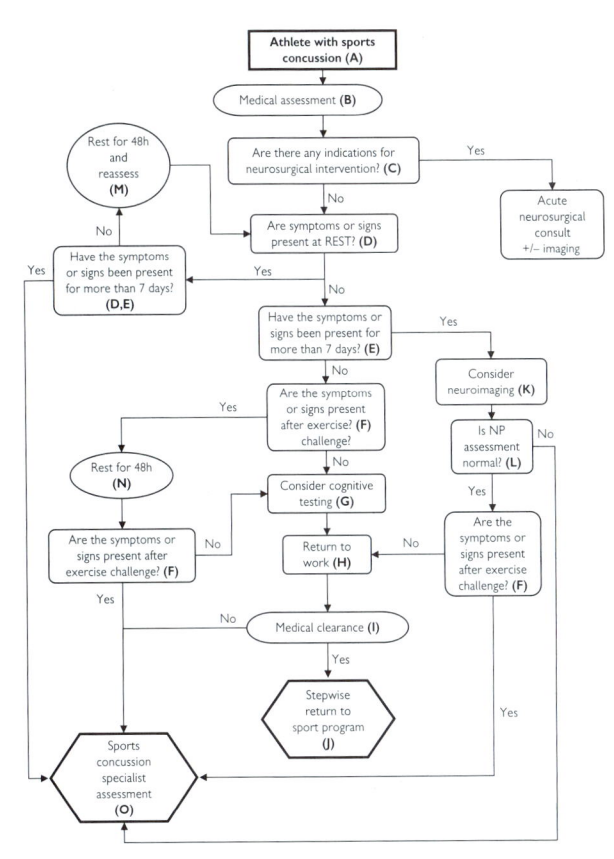

Fig. 15.1 Sports concussion algorithm.

- free of any drugs, alcohol, or medication that may mask symptoms or interfere with cognitive performance.
- (B) Initial medical assessment involves history, neurological exam, physical exam including examination of face, skull, and cervical spine and SCAT card assessment.
- (C) Indications for neurosurgical intervention are detailed elsewhere.
- (D) Symptoms and signs of concussion are presented in Table 15.1.
- (E) The Prague guidelines allow 7–10 days for symptoms and signs of simple concussion to resolve. Until this timeframe is formally validated in athletes, we recommend 7 days, although recognize that physician discretion should apply.

- *(F)* An exercise challenge requires the athlete to exercise until heart rate is greater than 60% of maximum predicted heart rate (MPHR). MPHR = 220 – age in years. As a simple 'rule of thumb' this corresponds to a heart rate of >120beats/min.
- *(G)* Formal neuropsychological testing is not required for simple concussion. However, the athlete must be able to score normally on the SCAT card mental status assessment. If this assessment is abnormal then more formal neuropsychological assessment may be warranted.
- *(H)* Return to work or school is dependent upon complete resolution of symptoms, signs, and cognitive function both at rest and after exercise. Athletes should be medically reassessed after return to work or school to ensure functional recovery before proceeding to the stepwise return to play guideline. When considering return to school, it would be prudent for the teachers and parents to be aware of potential problems that may arise at this stage.
- *(I)* Medical clearance involves an assessment of symptom recurrence after return to school and documentation that the athlete has completed all steps appropriately in the management plan and in particular, is asymptomatic at rest and following exercise challenge.
- *(J)* Stepwise return to sport programme under the return to play recommendations. All 6 steps must be completed, as described in the text and we would emphasize the important role of physician clearance at this stage.
- *(K)* Athletes with symptoms/signs lasting ≥7 days may require brain CT or MRI.
- *(L)* NP assessment is recommended in all athletes with complex concussion.
- *(M)* At 48h the athlete should be reassessed. Obviously, if there are any persistent symptoms or signs, the rest period will be greater than 48h. Once 7 days is reached and the patient is still symptomatic then the athlete would follow the complex concussion protocol and be assessed by a concussion specialist.
- *(N)* At this stage in the flowchart, the athlete is asymptomatic at rest, but symptomatic after exercise. Therefore, the athlete must return to complete rest for another 48h before repeating the exercise challenge.
- *(O)* A 'sports concussion specialist' is a neurologist, neurosurgeon, or sports medicine physician, with specific expertise in managing sport-related concussion and who has access to specialized formal neuropsychological assessment and generally works in a multi-disciplinary management setting.

Traumatic brain injury

Traumatic brain injury (TBI) is an injury to the brain or central nervous system and incorporates injuries to other structures of the head (skull bones, soft tissues, and vascular structures of the head and neck).

The crude incidence for all traumatic brain injuries varies between countries and is approximately 300/100,000 per year with 80% of those injuries being mild. Males are more than twice as likely as females to suffer a traumatic brain injury. Sporting injuries contribute approximately 10% of all cases of TBI.

General management

The major priorities at this early stage are the basic principles of first aid. The simple mnemonic DR ABC may be a useful aide-memoire (Table 15.3).

Only once these basic aspects of care have been achieved and the patient stabilized, consider moving the patient from the field to an appropriate facility. Before moving the patient, carefully assess for a cervical spine or other injury.

When in doubt, refer

Indications for urgent referral to hospital

Any player who has or develops the following:
- Fractured skull.
- Penetrating skull trauma.
- Deterioration in conscious state following injury.
- Focal neurological signs.
- Confusion or impairment of consciousness >30min.
- Loss of consciousness >5min.
- Persistent vomiting or increasing headache post-injury.
- Any convulsive movements.
- More than one episode of concussive injury in a session.
- Where there is assessment difficulty (e.g. an intoxicated patient).
- Children with head injuries.
- High risk patients (e.g. haemophilia, anticoagulant use).
- Inadequate post-injury supervision.
- High-risk injury mechanism (e.g. high velocity impact).

Table 15.3 Initial on-field assessment of concussion

D	Danger immediate environmental	Ensuring that there are no dangers which may potentially injure the patient or treatment team. This may involve stopping play in a football match or marshalling cars on a motor racetrack.
R	Response	Is the patient conscious? Can he/she talk?
A	Airway	Ensuring a clear and unobstructed airway. Removing any mouth guard or dental device which may be present.
B	Breathing	Ensure the patient is breathing adequately
C	Circulation	Ensure an adequate circulation

The management of traumatic brain injury

Acute management of sporting TBI

- An eyewitness account or, in the case of professional sport, videotape analysis may be available.
- Vital signs must be recorded be following all injuries. Abnormalities may reflect brain stem dysfunction and are important as a baseline measure.
- An acute rise in intracranial pressure (ICP) with central herniation usually manifests by rising BP and falling pulse rate (the Cushing response).
- Hypotension is rarely due to brain injury, except as a terminal event, and alternate sources for the drop in BP should be aggressively sought and treated. (Cerebral hypotension and hypoxia are the main determinants of outcome following brain injury and are treatable).
- A detailed neurological exam should performed including measurement of the GCS. It serves as a reference to which other repeated neurological examinations may be compared. Record your findings. Skull palpation should be a key component of every physical exam in head trauma. It is important to check for any evidence of CSF leakage through the nose and/or ears.

When time permits, a more thorough physical exam should be performed to exclude co-existent injuries and/or to detect signs of skull injury (e.g. Battle sign—bruising at the mastoid). Restlessness is a frequent accompaniment of brain injury or cerebral hypoxia, and may be confused with a belligerent patient who is presumably intoxicated. If the patient is unconscious, but restless, attention should be given to the possibility of increased cerebral hypoxia, a distended bladder, painful wounds, or other sources of pain. Only when one is certain that these have been ruled out may drug therapy be considered in consultation with a neurotrauma expert.

Investigations in head trauma

Indications for emergent cranial CT imaging in the initial evaluation of the head-injured patient include the following:

Indications for emergent neuroimaging

- History of loss of consciousness.
- Depressed level of consciousness.
- Focal neurological deficit.
- Deteriorating neurological status.
- Skull fracture.
- Progressive/severe headache.
- Persistent nausea/vomiting.
- Post-traumatic seizure.
- Mechanism of injury suggesting high risk of intracranial haemorrhage.
- Examination obscured by alcohol, drugs, metabolic derangement, or postictal state.
- Patient inaccessibility for serial neurologic examinations.
- Coagulopathy and other high-risk medical conditions.

CT evaluation as soon as the patient is haemodynamically stable and immediately life-threatening injuries have been addressed. Any subsequent deterioration in the neurological examination warrants prompt evaluation by CT, even if a previous study was normal.

Compared with CT, MR is time-consuming, expensive, and less sensitive to acute brain haemorrhage. Moreover, access to critically ill patients is restricted during lengthy periods of image acquisition, and the strong magnetic fields generated by the scanner necessitate the use of non-ferromagnetic resuscitative equipment. Presently, MR imaging is best suited for electively defining associated parenchymal injuries following the acute event.

Plain skull radiographs are inexpensive and easily obtained, and often demonstrate fractures in patients with extradural haemorrhage. However, the predictive value of such films is poor. Other, more traditional, diagnostic tools have largely been supplanted by cranial CT in the initial assessment of the head-injured patient.

Management of post-traumatic seizures

Impact seizures or concussive convulsions are a well-recognized sequelae of head impact. These are not epileptic, terminate spontaneously, and require no specific management beyond the treatment of the underlying concussive injury.

Post-traumatic epilepsy may also occur and is more common with increasing severity of brain injury. In this setting, a convulsing patient is at increased risk of hypoxia with resultant exacerbation of the underlying brain injury. Maintenance of cerebral oxygenation and perfusion pressure (BP) is critical in the overall management of such patients.

Because convulsions may cause a dramatic increase in intracranial pressure, they should be prevented during the recovery phase of acute head injury. Phenytoin (or fosphenytoin) is usually the drug of choice because a loading dose can be administered intravenously to rapidly achieve therapeutic concentrations and because phenytoin does not impair consciousness. Benzodiazepines (e.g. lorazepam, clonazepam, diazepam) can be used for the acute treatment of post-traumatic seizures but they produce at least transient impairment of consciousness and airway management may be required. Neither phenytoin, any of the benzodiazepines, nor any other anti-epileptic drug has been shown to be effective for preventing the development of late post-traumatic epilepsy.

Post-traumatic epilepsy should then be managed in the same manner as symptomatic partial epilepsy. Carbamazepine, phenytoin, and valproate are the drugs of choice for the initial management of secondarily generalized convulsions. Carbamazepine and phenytoin are drugs of choice for complex partial seizures, but valproate is also effective. New agents, such as gabapentin, lamotrigine, and topiramate, are also effective in the management of partial seizures and generalized convulsions. Treatments do change and it is important to keep up to date.

Non-brain head injury

Various soft tissue, bony, ocular, and other injuries may occur to the head. Scalp wounds, although dramatic in appearance, usually heal well with good wound management. Blood loss from scalp wounds may be extensive, particularly in children, but rarely causes shock. Use the usual precautions against blood-borne infections such as hepatitis B and C and HIV infection. If large vessels are severed (e.g. superficial temporal artery), the arterial bleeder should be located, clamped, and ligated. One should always inspect the wound carefully and palpate using a sterile glove inside the laceration for signs of skull fracture. A depressed skull fracture can be palpated, although a subgaleal haematoma may confuse the findings. All open fractures or depressed skull fractures should have neurosurgical consultation. Inspection of the wound will also detect CSF leaks.

The wound should be irrigated with copious amounts of saline before closing and any debris, including hair, must be removed from the wound. Bony fragments should not be removed until surgery. Primary repair should be accomplished using a sterile technique and the area immediately around the laceration should be well shaved. The galea aponeurotica should be closed first using interrupted sutures and then the superficial layer of the scalp is sutured.

Traumatic intracerebral haematomas/contusion

Subtypes/aetiology
Traumatic intracerebral haematomas are divided into acute or delayed types. Delayed traumatic intracerebral haemorrhages, which are more common, may occur from as early as 6h after injury to as long as several weeks.

Presentation
Clinical signs and symptoms depend on the size and location of the intracerebral haematoma, as well as the rapidity of its development. In most cases, there is a brief period of confusion or loss of consciousness. Only one-third of the patients remain lucid throughout their course. Impaired alertness is found frequently on initial examination.

The prime aim is to reduce post-traumatic oedema and ischaemia. Treatment includes adequate circulation and ventilation, aggressive monitoring and control of intracranial hypertension to ensure adequate cerebral perfusion pressures, close intensive care monitoring, correction of any coagulopathies or electrolyte abnormalities, and seizure prophylaxis. Interventions to control elevated intracranial pressure include mechanical hyperventilation, osmotic diuresis, and emergency ventriculostomies.

Head-injured patients should be monitored for coagulopathy for at least 24–48h after injury.

Prognosis
The overall cognitive impairment and the speed and quality of recovery are strongly related to the associated diffuse axonal injury. When occurring in isolation and when the volume is less than 30cm^3, an intracerebral haematoma is compatible with a favourable recovery. Brainstem compression and loss of consciousness significantly worsen prognosis regardless of treatment. Overall, mortality rates are in the range of 25–30%.

Subdural haematoma

Subdural haematomas can be the result of either non-penetrating or penetrating trauma to the head. There is bleeding into the subdural space due to stretching, and subsequent rupture of bridging cerebral veins. These injuries are typically seen following falls on hard surfaces or assaults with non-deformable objects, rather than low velocity injuries. In most cases, there is a brief period of confusion or loss of consciousness.

There is frequently impaired cognitive function and/or attention on initial examination. Soft tissue injuries are seen at the site of impact. Other signs of significant head trauma, which can result in subdural haematomas, include peri-orbital and post-auricular echymoses, haemotympanum, CSF otorrhoea/rhinorrhea, and facial fractures. The focal neurologic deficits depend on the location and size of the lesion. Enlargement of the haematoma or an increase in oedema surrounding the haematoma produces additional mass effect, with further depression of the patient's level of consciousness, increases in motor or speech deficit, and eventually ipsilateral compression of the third nerve and midbrain.

The impact that produces acute subdural haematoma frequently causes severe injury to the cerebral parenchyma. This co-existing severe brain injury explains, in large part, the better outcome in extradural haematomas compared with acute subdural haematomas. Indeed, in most cases of acute subdural haematoma, it is likely that the extra-axial collection is less important in determining outcome than the parenchymal injury sustained at the time of impact.

Extradural haematoma

A direct blow to the head is essential for extradural haematoma formation. As the skull is deformed by the impact and the adherent dura forcefully detached, haemorrhage may occur into the pre-formed extradural space. This injury is most commonly seen in children due to flexibility of the skull. The source of bleeding may be arterial, venous, or both. In the supratentorial compartment, haemorrhage from the middle meningeal artery contributes to at least 50% of extradural haematomas; bleeding from the middle meningeal veins accounts for an additional 33%. Haemorrhage from a fracture line may also accumulate to create a mass lesion in the extradural space.

Presentation

There is remarkable clinical variability with extradural haemorrhage. Extradural haematomas may, rarely, be asymptomatic. Most, however, present with non-specific signs and symptoms referable to an intracranial mass lesion. The mode of presentation may be correlated with the size and site of the haematoma, the rate of expansion, and the presence of associated intradural pathology. Extradural haematomas involving the temporal lobe may cause a more precipitous decline than those at other sites, due to their proximity to the brainstem.

Alteration in consciousness can be quite variable in extent and duration. The so-called 'lucid interval' occurs in less than one-third of patients, and thus is not a sensitive diagnostic discriminant.

Treatment

If a large traumatic extradural haematoma is unrecognized and/or untreated, there is progressive neurologic dysfunction due to the expanding mass lesion, ultimately resulting in transtentorial or uncal herniation, brainstem compression and ischaemia, and death. Rapid diagnosis and prompt surgical evacuation offer the best chance of a good outcome. If treatment is instituted prior to obtundation, pupillary dysfunction, and/or vegetative motor posturing, the probability of full functional recovery is high.

Prognosis

The expanding extradural lesion only partially accounts for the neurologic morbidity observed with extradural haematomas. Coincident intradural pathology is encountered in up to 50% of cases and is associated with lower admission GCS, more substantial and prolonged intracranial pressure elevation, and higher mortality. In general, it is the sequelae of these lesions that dictate the degree of residual functional impairment in patients who survive extradural haematoma.

Traumatic subarachnoid haemorrhage

Traumatic subarachnoid haemorrhage is usually classified according to the site of arterial rupture and bleeding. It is usually due to vertebral artery injury—either a tear or dissection, although it may also be due to tearing of meningeal vessels. Sub-arachnoid bleeding typically presents with florid meningeal symptoms, such as headache, neck stiffness, and photophobia.

The most common initial symptoms are neck pain and occipital headache that may precede the onset of neurological symptoms from seconds to weeks. Clinical symptoms and signs often develop with a 'stuttering' onset over days or weeks following the original injury.

Headache symptoms in most cases are ipsilateral to the vascular injury and the pain usually radiates to the temporal region, frontal area, eye, or ear. None of the reported cases of vertebral arterial rupture had cervical tenderness or objective restriction of neck movement, although a subjective exacerbation of pain did occur with neck movement.

Treatment

Medical management of subarachnoid haemorrhage (SAH) is the same as for intracerebral haematomas with intracerebral monitoring and control of intracranial pressure (ICP). Vasoactive substances released by the haematoma may promote further ischaemia, and the calcium channel blocker, Nimodipine, is used to prevent vasospasm. Operative treatment is directed toward control of IP or treatment of hydrocephalus. The prognosis is variable and many cases result in fatal outcome.

Diffuse cerebral swelling

Diffuse cerebral swelling or second impact syndrome?
Diffuse cerebral swelling (DCS) is a rare but well-recognized complication of mild traumatic brain injury in sport that occurs predominantly in children and teenagers. It is likely that a single impact of any severity may result in this rare complication; however, participation in sport often draws attention to concussive injuries in this setting.

Pathophysiology
The injured brain swells within the cranial cavity. This increase in brain volume will eventually increase ICP. In the first few hours and days following severe head injury, ICP is often raised due to increased cerebral blood flow. Later brain swelling is due to an increase in brain tissue water content. Anecdotal evidence suggests massive traumatic cerebral oedema, documented on CT scanning, occurs within 20min of cerebral injury.

Post-injury DCS can occur within minutes or be delayed for days or even weeks. Because of this theoretical risk, no athlete with a concussive injury should be allowed to return to playing or training until *all* clinical symptoms have fully resolved and cognitive function has returned to normal.

Downward displacement of the cerebrum due to increased ICP results in compression of the diencephalon and midbrain through the tentorial notch. During this process, the ipsilateral third cranial nerve and the posterior cerebral artery are compressed by the uncus and edge of the tentorium. Herniation can also compress the posterior cerebral artery to cause occipital lobe ischaemia.

Prognosis
In cases of cerebral herniation complicated by ischaemia, patients may suffer permanent neurologic sequelae if coma duration is 6h or longer. Most patients with a maximum ICP increase of less than 30mmHg experience good recovery.

Head injury advice card

All patients, whether athletes or not, should be given a head injury card following their discharge from medical care. An example is shown in Box 15.1.

Box 15.1 Head injury advice

This patient has received an injury to the head. A careful medical examination has been carried out and no sign of any serious complications has been found.

It is expected that recovery will be rapid, but in such cases it is not possible to be quite certain.

If you notice any change in behaviour, vomiting, dizziness, headache, double vision, or excessive drowsiness, please telephone

……………………………………………………………

or the nearest hospital emergency department immediately.

Other important points
No alcohol
No analgesics or pain killers
No driving
Patient's name……………………………………………..
Date and time of injury……………………………………...
Date of medical review……………………………………...
Treating physician…………………………………………..
Clinic phone number ………………………………………..

Mouthguards

There is no published evidence that mouthguards will prevent concussion, but they should be mandatory to prevent oro-facial injuries.

Types of mouthguard

- 'Stock' mouthguards that may be purchased from sporting goods stores.
- 'Mouth-formed' or 'boil and bite' guards, which are heated and immediately worn by the athlete allowing some adaptation to the dentition to occur.
- 'Custom-made' guards, which come in several types, but all require an impression cast of the patients' dentition as the initial step and the guard is made on this cast.

A custom-fitted design is necessary to ensure retention of the mouthguard in collision or contact sports, and minimize the risk of oro-facial injury. These need to be made and fitted by a dentist or dental technician. The simper designs (e.g. boil and bite) do not afford much protection, tend to fit poorly, often interfere with breathing and speech, and may obstruct the airway in an unconscious patient. They are, however, cheap, available, and used widely.

There are no acceptable international standards for mouthguards, which makes the comparison difficult, but intuitively one would expect a laminated custom-fitted guard to offer more protection, at least to the teeth.

The evidence that correctly fitting mouthguards reduce the rate of cerebral injuries is largely theoretical and no protective effect against concussion has been seen in randomized controlled trials.

Helmets and head protectors

Helmets theoretically reduce the risk of brain injury. There is published evidence for the effectiveness of sport-specific helmets in reducing head injuries in sports with high speed collisions, missile injuries (e.g. baseball) and falls onto hard surfaces (e.g. gridiron, ice hockey).

No sport-specific helmets have been shown to be of proven benefit in reducing head injury in sports such as soccer, Australian football, and rugby. Most commercially available soft helmets fail to meet impact-testing criteria that would be typical of sport-related concussion and randomized controlled trials in various football codes have failed to show a protective effect against concussion.

Other means of preventing sports concussion

Rule changes may be appropriate where there is a clear-cut mechanism of injury in a particular sport. Rule changes, such as banning spear tackles in American football appear to have reduced the incidence of catastrophic neck injury. In football (soccer) banning elbow/arm contact to the opponents head in heading contests has reduced the rate of concussions at the elite level by 50%.

Neck muscle conditioning may be of value in reducing impact forces transmitted to the brain. In theory, the energy from an impacting object is dispersed over the greater mass of an athlete if the head is held rigidly, but there is no scientific evidence that this can be effective

On-field recognition of concussive injury is a priority and application of appropriate validated guidelines in returning athletes to sport.

Epilepsy and sport

See Table 15.4 for a summary of some types of seizure and their likely aetiology.

Specific syndromes

Concussive convulsions
Defined as a convulsive episode that begins within 2s of impact associated with concussive brain injury. Following impact, there is typically a phase of brief tonic stiffening followed by myoclonic jerking. The convulsive movements may be transient but can last up to 3min in some cases. These episodes are not associated with structural or permanent brain injury and are a non-epileptic phenomenon.

Post-traumatic epilepsy
Seizures are common after severe head injury and account for 2% of the total cases of epilepsy. Post-traumatic epilepsy is categorized into immediate (within 24h of injury), early (within 1 week), and late (after 1 week) subtypes. Risk factors are prolonged unconsciousness, skull fracture, intracerebral haematomas, haemorrhagic cerebral contusion, and focal neurological signs. In addition, children have almost three times the risk of early post-traumatic epilepsy than adults for the same severity of brain injury.

Idiopathic epilepsy
One of the peaks of incidence of epilepsy is in the late teens and early twenties, the time when many sportsmen and women are actively involved in athletic pursuits. Exercise does not increase seizure frequency, affect anti-epileptic drug levels or induce epileptiform electroencephalogram (EEG) changes. There is no evidence that epileptics are more prone to seizures after head injury or that epileptics are more prone to injury than other athletes.

Other less common causes of convulsions in sport

- *Syncope:* patients who faint often have convulsive movements of the extremities, which are thought to be due to a brainstem reflex phenomenon.
- *Cardiac rhythm disturbances:* an anoxic convulsion may occur with a transient arrhythmia.
- *Movement disorders:* episodic involuntary movement disorders may be precipitated by movement or exercise.
- *Metabolic disturbances:* convulsive activity, dystonia, and syncope may occur secondary to hypoglycaemia, hyponatraemia, hypocalcaemia, and hypomagnesaemia, all conditions recognized in sports—particularly endurance running and ultra-marathons.
- Illicit drug use/alcohol.
- Pseudoseizures.

Table 15.4

	Timing of event	Type of seizure	Likely aetiology
Immediate	Seconds to hours post-injury	Generalized/myoclonic	Non epileptic
Early	Hours to 7 days post-injury	Focal	Epileptic
Late	>7 days post-injury	Generalized	Epileptic

Post-traumatic headache

Post-traumatic headache generally has a good prognosis for recovery, although some patients may remain affected for considerable periods of time.

Paradoxically, headaches may occur more often and be of longer duration in patients with concussive injury than in patients with more severe traumatic brain injury.

Classification of post-traumatic headache (International Headache Society (IHS) criteria)

- *Post-traumatic (or trauma-triggered) migraine*: in sports such as soccer, where repetitive heading of the ball gives rise to the term 'footballer's migraine'. Even mild head trauma may induce migraine.
- *Extracranial 'vascular' headache*: periodic headaches at the site of head or scalp trauma.
- *Dysautonomic cephalgia*: an unusual consequence of trauma to the anterior part of the neck, triggering autonomic symptoms from local injury to the sympathetic trunk and adjacent ganglia. This entity may be successfully treated with propranolol.
- *Headache overlap syndrome*: persistent low grade occipital headache.

Diagnostic work-up

The rate of significant neuropathological injury is between 1 and 3% in patients with headache, and the typical headaches found, even in life-threatening conditions, were non-specific in nature.

Post-traumatic headaches are generally treated in the same fashion as primary headache syndromes. Analgesic-rebound headache can complicate a post-traumatic headache disorder.

For post-traumatic migraine, aspirin and NSAIDs can be used with mild episodes and ergot preparations, and sumatriptan can be used to treat severe attacks.

Chronic post-traumatic migraine or recurrent episodes requiring prophylactic agents may be treated with amitriptyline or propranolol if no contraindications exist. Alternative agents include nadolol, timolol, amitriptyline, nortriptyline, doxepin, verapamil, non-steroidal anti-inflammatory drugs, valproic acid, methergine, methysergide, fluoxetine, or phenelzine.

Prognosis

Acute post-traumatic headache has a good prognosis and, in most cases, symptoms resolve within 1–3 months. Education and support can help patients deal with transient cognitive difficulties associated with headaches. The chronic post-traumatic syndrome with prolonged disability is difficult to treat and generally requires specialist intervention.

Headaches and sport

Classification of exercise-related headache
The IHS in conjunction with the World Health Organization (WHO).

Clinical approach to headache
- Exclude possible intracranial causes on history and physical exam. If intracranial pathology is suspected then an urgent workup is required, which may include neuroimaging studies and laboratory investigations.
- Exclude headaches associated with viral or other infective illness.
- Exclude a drug-induced headache (see 'Drugs commonly causing headache', below) or headache related to alcohol and/or substance abuse.
- Consider an exercise (or sex-related) headache syndrome.
- Differentiate between vascular, tension, cervicogenic, or other cause of headache.

Many commonly used drugs can provoke headaches. Some of these drugs such as NSAIDs are in widespread use by athletes. If not recognized, this may be the reason for treatment failure.

Drugs commonly causing headache
- Alcohol.
- Anabolic steroids.
- Analgesics.
- Antibiotics.
- Anti-hypertensives.
- Caffeine.
- Corticosteroids.
- Dipyridamole.
- Nicotine.
- Nitrazepam.
- NSAIDs.
- Oral contraceptives.
- Sympathomimetics.
- Theophylline.
- Vasodilator agents.

Clinical factors
- Age of onset of the headaches.
- Frequency and duration.
- Time of onset of headache.
- Mode of onset.
- Site of pain and radiation.
- Headache quality.
- Associated symptoms.
- Precipitating factors.
- Aggravating and relieving factors.
- Previous treatments.
- General health.
- Past medical history.
- Family history.
- Social and occupational history.
- Drug and medication use.

A full neurological and general physical examination is required with particular attention to the cervical spine as a potential source of headache: general appearance (including skin lesions such as rashes), vital signs (pulse, BP, and temperature), mental status and speech, gait, balance and co-ordination, cranial nerve and long tract examination, visual fields, acuity and ophthalmoscopic fundus exam, and skull palpation.

Key symptoms to flag

Certain symptoms may indicate the presence of more serious pathology, such as a mass lesion or infective process, and require urgent neurological assessment. These are:
- Sudden onset of severe headache.
- Headache increasing over a few days.
- New or unaccustomed headache.
- Persistently unilateral headaches.
- Chronic headache with localized pain.
- Stiff neck or other signs of meningism.
- Focal neurological symptoms or signs.
- Atypical headache/change in the usual pattern of headache.
- Headaches that wake the patient during the night or early morning.
- Local extracranial symptoms (e.g. sinus, ear, or eye disease).
- Systemic symptoms (e.g. weight loss, fever, and malaise).

Specific common headache syndromes

Migraine
Migraine is an episodic headache that is usually accompanied by nausea and photophobia, and may be preceded by focal neurological symptoms with a prevalence of 12–18% in community populations.

In elite athletes, there are specific management considerations related to the use of 'banned' drugs. Many conventional headache medications (such as beta-blockers, caffeine, codeine-containing preparations, dextropropoxyphene, narcotics, and opioids, etc.) are banned agents and their use, if detected, may result in severe penalties for the athlete concerned.

Tension-type headache
Tension-type headache results in a constant tight or pressing sensation that may initially be episodic and related to stress, but can recur almost daily in its chronic form without regard to any obvious psychological factors.

Cervicogenic headache
Abnormalities of the neck including synovial joints, the intervertebral discs, ligaments, muscles, nerve roots, and the vertebral artery. Cervicogenic headache shares many of the clinical features of chronic tension-type headache. It is usually occipital in onset and may radiate to the anterior aspect of the skull and face. The headache is usually constant in nature, lasts for days to weeks and has a definite association with movement or manipulation of cervical structures.

Benign exertional headache (BEH)
The formal criteria for BEH include:
- The headache is specifically brought on by physical exercise.
- The headache is bilateral, throbbing in nature at onset, and may develop migrainous features in those patients susceptible to migraine.
- Lasts from 5min to 24h.
- Is prevented by avoiding excessive exertion.
- Is not associated with any systemic or intracranial disorder.

The major differential diagnosis is a subarachnoid haemorrhage. Exertional headache may be due to dilatation of pain-sensitive venous sinuses at the base of the brain as a result of increased cerebral arterial pressure. A similar type of vascular headache is described in relation to sexual activity, and has been termed benign sex headache or orgasmic cephalgia.

Treatment strategies include NSAIDs such as indomethacin at a dose of 25mg 3 times per day. Other pharmacological strategies that have anecdotal support include the prophylactic use of ergotamine tartrate, methysergide, or propranolol pre-exercise. These headaches tend to recur over weeks to months and then slowly resolve, although some cases may be lifelong. In the recovery period, a graduated symptom-limited weightlifting programme is appropriate.

Effort headache
Effort headaches differ from the exertional headaches in that they are not necessarily associated with a power or straining type exercise and occur in a variety of sports. The clinical features include:
- Onset of mild to severe headache with aerobic type exercise.
- More frequent in hot weather.
- Vascular type headache (i.e. throbbing).
- Short duration of headache (4–6h).
- Provoking exercise may be maximal or submaximal.
- Patient may have prodromal 'migrainous' symptoms.
- Headache tends to recur in individuals with exercise.
- Athlete may have a past history of migraine.
- Normal neurological exam and investigations.

Boxing and head injury

Boxing-related neurological injury

In amateur boxing, the rate of acute head injury (in contested bouts) varies between 0.14 and 0.4 injuries per 1000 exposures, whereas in professional boxing the rate is up to 40 per 1000 exposures. The risk of such events is relatively low when compared with other sports. No studies have been reported to suggest that female boxers are at increased risk.

Few prospective studies enable a true estimate of the incidence or prevalence of chronic boxing-related neurological injury in either amateur or professional boxing.

The 'punch drunk' syndrome

In 1928, Harrison Martland anecdotally described a syndrome in prizefighters that was known in lay boxing circles as the '*punch drunk*' or '*slug nutty*' state, although he did not actually examine any boxer with this condition. It was later labelled dementia pugilistica, traumatic encephalopathy, or chronic traumatic encephalopathy of boxers.

In the early stages, the clinical syndrome is mixed due to lesions affecting the pyramidal, cerebellar and extra-pyramidal systems. In the latter stages, cognitive impairment becomes the major neurological feature. Throughout the course of the condition, various neuropsychiatric and behavioural symptoms may occur. Compared with professionals, amateur boxers show milder neurophysiological and neuroimaging evidence of chronic traumatic encephalopathy. There are many differing symptoms with variable degrees of severity. Neuroradiological imaging techniques have not shown any systematic evidence of brain injury in boxers.

Neurophysiological studies show variable results. EEG abnormalities may occur in one-third to one-half of punch drunk professional boxers, and consist of diffuse slowing or flat, low-voltage records.

There is indirect evidence of compromise of the blood-brain barrier as revealed by increases in creatine kinase isoenzyme BB from astrocytes during the first 9min after a boxing match, and as suggested by increased CSF protein. Similar changes are noted with creatine kinase and neuron-specific enolase with elevations following a single bout of amateur boxing. Surprisingly few detailed reports of neuropathological changes in ex-boxers have been performed.

Risk factors for chronic boxing-related neurological injury

The putative risk factors fall into two broad areas—exposure and genotype. Chronic boxing-related neurological injury is described in boxers who began fighting at a young age, had had several hundred professional fights and a long (>10yrs) career. In addition, the *ApoE4* phenotype has been associated with an increased risk of chronic boxing-related neurological injury in boxers. The concept that punch-drunk boxers were mostly nonscientific 'sluggers' known for taking a punch has passed into medical folklore despite the lack of scientific support.

Prevention

There are no scientifically validated means by which chronic boxing-related neurological injury may be prevented and neuroradiological studies are not useful as a sole screening tool:

- *Monitoring of bout frequency:* high exposure (>20 bouts) correlates with risk of chronic boxing-related neurological injury. A boxing 'passport is recommended.
- Regular, preferably annual, neuropsychological and neurobehavioral assessment.
- Regular, preferably annual, neurological examinations are recommended focusing on the cerebellar, pyramidal, extra-pyramidal systems, and gait, rather than simply being a generic neurological exam.
- An initial MR scan at first registration to exclude boxers with pre-existing CNS abnormalities and to serve as a baseline for future comparison.
- Ideally, a boxer's *ApoE4* genotype should be performed at the outset of his or her career with genetic counselling to discuss the implications of a positive finding.

A boxer's career should be terminated by the development of neurological signs.

Ideally, *ApoE4* genotype should be performed at the outset of his or her career with genetic counseling to discuss the implications of a positive finding.

A 'high risk' notification system is to be encouraged:
- Boxers who have had >20 fights (including amateur fights).
- Boxers who have had >6 losses/knockdowns.
- Active boxers >35yrs.
- Boxers who have an *ApoE4* genotype.
- Active boxing career >10yrs.
- Boxers experiencing neurological symptoms post-bout.

Screening alone will not lead to injury reduction. Injury prevention, appropriate medical advice and remedial programmes, where indicated, must be implemented. Unless boxers, medical staff, trainers, and boxing officials act on the deficits discovered during the screening process, pre-participation screening will act solely as a predictor of injury, rather than as a preventive measure.

The post-concussion syndrome

The post-concussive syndrome (PCS) remains as controversial today as when it was first proposed in the 19th century. Symptoms may include headache, vertigo, dizziness, nausea, memory complaints, blurred vision, noise and light sensitivity, difficulty concentrating, fatigue, depression, sleep disturbance, loss of appetite, anxiety, loss of co-ordination, and hallucinations. These symptoms are not the same as the acute symptoms of concussion that typically resolve over several days. The investigation of PCS is in the exclusion of other causes of ongoing symptoms. No specific treatment is available for this condition beyond general advice and reassurance.

Fractures

Skull fracture
Athletes with a cranial fracture usually have a headache, and may or may not have symptoms of an underlying brain injury. Local soft tissue swelling may also indicate an underlying fracture, and palpation of the skull should be a mandatory part of the clinical assessment of all head injuries. Percussion of the skull may result in a characteristic 'cracked pot' sound. Rhinorrhoea and otorrhoea are classic signs of skull fracture with torn dural membranes. If a glucose stick test of nasal or ear fluid leak is positive, the fluid is CSF.

In all cases of skull fracture, especially if a CSF leak is present, an urgent neurosurgical consultation is required. When a skull fracture is suspected, the patient should always be hospitalized for observation and neurosurgical evaluation. The physician should cover the injured area of an open cranial fracture with a sterile dressing.

Nasal fractures
Nasal fractures are diagnosed radiographically, using lateral images.

The patient should be referred to a facio-maxillary, or ear, nose, and throat specialist. Septum haematoma must be evacuated. Closed nasal bone reposition is the most common treatment. This should be done either immediately after the injury or 3–7 days later, when the swelling is reduced. The patient should wear a protective splint or face mask for 4 weeks when participating in training or competition.

Mandibular fractures
Mandibular fractures are the second most common group (13–45%) of sport-related facial injuries and are usually caused by a blow to the lower jaw, such as may occur in combat and team sports, or in a fall where the lower jaw or the chin hits a hard surface. Symptoms include swelling and haematoma, problems with occlusion, mucous membrane tears, differences in the level of the tooth row, mobility in the area of the fracture, and hypoesthesia with nerve damage in the mental nerve area. The standard radiographic examination is an orthopantomogram.

Most lower jaw fractures should be treated by a specialist. If proper occlusion is achieved after the operation, the prognosis is good.

Zygomatic fracture
Typical cheekbone fractures involve the zygomatico-maxillary complex: the infra-orbital rim, the orbital floor, and the lateral orbital rim. Cheekbone fractures are the third most common sport injury to the face. The clinical presentation is a flattening of the prominence of the cheekbone. If the cheekbone is pressed inward, it may be difficult for the patient to open the mouth wide. Double vision and nerve injury corresponding to the infra-orbital nerve are symptoms of a fracture in the orbital floor. A CT scan with axial and coronal views provides the best imaging.

Eye injuries

Contusion of the eyeball
Contusion of the eyeball may be caused by direct blows to the eye (boxing), a ball in the eye (squash), crashing into a hard object, and falling accidents. Tearing, light sensitivity, and blepharospasm (cramps of the eyelid) are signs and symptoms of contusion of the eyeball. Look out for swelling and bleeding in the eyelid, subconjunctival bleeding, corneal oedema, corneal damage, bleeding in the anterior chamber (hyphema), separation of the iris (iridodialysis), traumatic paresis of the pupil (mydriasis, oval pupil), accommodation paresis, lens damage, or dislocation, bleeding in the vitreous, retinal damage (bleeding or oedema), or damage to the optic nerve. Visual acuity *must* be assessed in every eye injury and threshold for referral to an ophthalmologist should be low.

Perforation of the eyeball
Ski poles in the eye, bow and arrow shooting accidents, and accidents with other sharp objects frequently cause eye perforation. Ruptures of the eye may also be caused by powerful blunt contusion trauma. In that case, the eye ruptures at the weak points (along the limbus and the optic nerve). Visual acuity *must* be assessed in every eye injury. If perforation is suspected, the patient should be sent to the nearest ophthalmology department urgently.

Chapter 16

Spine

History *424*
Examination *426*
Special tests *429*
Investigations *430*
Acute spinal injury *432*
Acute injuries of the back in sport *433*
Management of musculoligamentous injuries of the back *433*
Disc disease *434*
Pars interarticularis and spondylolysis *438*
Pars interarticularis and spondylolisthesis *442*
Scheuermann's disease *446*
Sacro-iliac joint *447*
Ankylosing spondylitis *448*
Conditions affecting the spine in children and adolescents *452*

History

Question the athlete and witnesses of injury. Study the videotape if available in acute injury.

Understand the demands of sport, exercise, and occupation.

Pain
- Character.
- Location and radiation.
- Relationship to exercise or activity.
- Alleviating or relieving factors.

Neurological symptoms
- Numbness, pins and needles.
- Weakness.

Past history
- Spinal problems.
- Orthopaedic problems.

Family history
- Spinal problems.

Some signposts to the aetiology include: medical (insidious and persistent, worse in morning), mechanical (intermittent and associated with activity), disc herniation and nerve impingement (radiates to lower leg or foot), tumour (night pain), relief from aspirin (osteoid osteoma).

Problems that show familial predisposition: disc disease, ankylolising spondylitis, Reiter's syndrome, other spondylolarthropathies.

Red flags in history of patient with back pain
Require consideration of pathology that might be life-threatening or require urgent intervention:
- Less than 10yrs of age.
- First episode of back pain and over 60yrs old.
- Unexplained weight loss.
- Chronic cough.
- Night pain.
- Inter-menstrual bleeding.
- Altered bowel function.
- Altered bladder control.
- Visual disturbance, balance problems, upper limb dysaesthesias.
- Past history of cancer or corticosteroid use.
- Bilateral weakness of lower extremities.

Examination

Inspection

With patient standing
- *From behind:* check level of shoulders, lateral curvature/scoliosis, normal alignment, lengths of lower limbs (level of posterior superior iliac spines), or hair tufts over spine.
- *From side:* check increased kyphosis, decreased lordosis.

NB Scoliosis may be due to unilateral muscle spasm, or nerve root irritation due to disc herniation.

Palpation

Palpate each spinous process, sacroiliac joints, facet joints for tenderness, muscle spasm, and consider the anatomy (Figs. 16.1 and 16.2).

Active and passive movement

Restriction of spinal movement may be due to muscle spasm as a result of pathology in one or more functional unit. Note pain during any of the movements tested.
- Lumbar flexion (normal 40° to 60°) occurs by reversing the lordosis. During re-extension the lumbar lordosis is regained in the final 45°. NB Toe touching with straight legs is influenced by hip mobility, hamstring tightness—so not useful. However, this may be confirmed by measuring the increased distance between marked points over the spinous processes with flexion (Schrober's test).
- Lumbar extension (normal 20–30°) is painful with facet joint or pars interarticularis pathology—called 'posterior element pain'. This can be due to posterior disc pathology or closing of the foramen of nerve roots.
- Lumbar lateral flexion (normal 20°) is painful with ipsilateral facet joint pathology or lateral disc protrusion (radicular pain), but is often a non-specific sign.
- Lumbar rotation occurs with thoracic rotation (normal 90°) and is assessed with pelvis and hips fixed (held by examiner or sitting).

Neurological examination

- *Sensory:* light touch over back and abdomen, legs, perianal sensation.
- *Lower limb reflexes (L4 knee, S1 ankle), superficial anal reflex:* touching perianal skin causes contraction of sphincter and external anal muscles (S2, S3, and S4).
- *Motor:* squat and return to standing, walk on heels (weak ankle dorsiflexors exposed—L4) and then toes (weak triceps sura exposed—L5). Muscle strength testing for nerve root assessment (L1—hip flexion, L2—hip flexion, L3—knee extension, L4—foot dorsiflexion, L5—hallus extension, foot eversion, S1—knee flexion and foot plantar flexion). Sphincter tone and contractility.

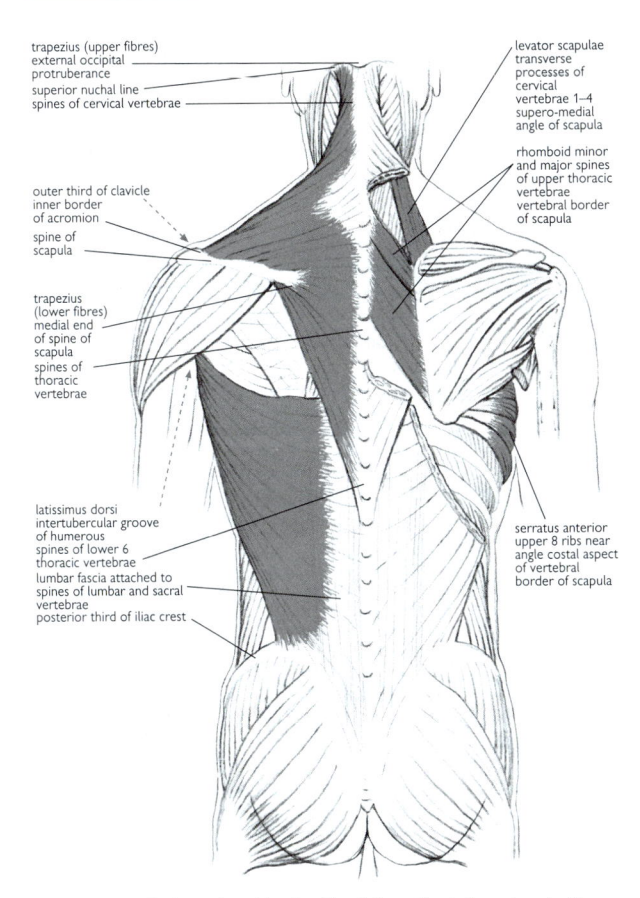

Fig. 16.1 Superficial muscles of the shoulder girdle and back. Reproduced with permission from MacKinnon P and Morris J (2005). *Oxford Textbook of Functional Anatomy* Vol 1. Oxford University Press, Oxford. © 2005.

428 CHAPTER 16 **Spine**

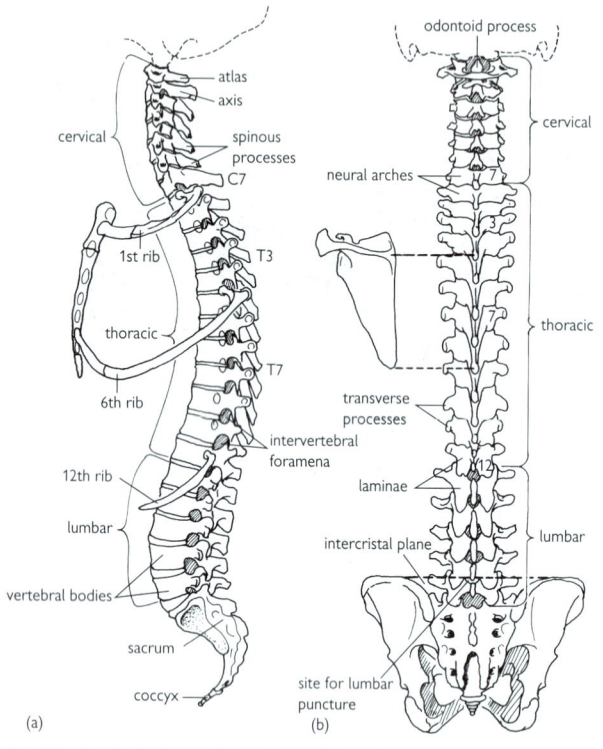

Fig. 16.2 Vertebral column: (a) lateral view; (b) posterior view. Reproduced with permission from MacKinnon P and Morris J (2005). *Oxford Textbook of Functional Anatomy* Vol 1. Oxford University Press, Oxford. © 2005.

Special tests

Sciatic and femoral nerve tension tests

Principle
Stretching the dura and nerve root to produce leg pain. Positive will produce the patient's radicular symptoms.

Sciatic nerve tests
Straight leg raise.
- *Lasegue test:* patient supine with hips flexed to 90°. Knee slowly extended.
- *Bowstring sign:* examiner presses in popliteal fossa and causes increased pain in leg.
- *Slump test:* patient sits 'slumped'. Progressive increase in tension by flexing neck, extending knee, and dorsiflexing foot.

Notes
- Ankle dorsiflexion and neck flexion should aggravate radicular pain or decrease angle of straight leg raise.
- *False positive:* pain with less than 30° of straight leg raise (SLR), production of back pain with no leg pain.

Femoral nerve test
Prone
- Knee flexed to 90° and hip extended—a positive test is recorded if there is pain in the thigh with hip extension.

One-legged hyperextension and Fitch test

In those with posterior element pathology, pain is reproduced in the back when the patient hyperextends, while standing on one leg. The Fitch test includes rotation, as well as one-legged hyperextension and may be more sensitive.

Gillet test of sacro-iliac joint

Examiner places thumb on PSIS and the other thumb on the midline of sacrum at similar level in standing patient. They observe the relative movements of the thumbs as the patient flexes the hip more than 90°. The inominate bone is expected to rotate posteriorly and, hence, the thumb on PSIS should move caudally. The contralateral inominate movement can also be assessed and should not move caudally.

Schrober's Test

A mark is made at the level of the posterior iliac spine on the vertebral column (level of L5). The examiner places one finger 5cm below this mark and another finger 10cm above the mark. The patient is then instructed to touch his toes. If the increase in distance between the two fingers on the patients spine is less than 5cm then this indicates restricted lumbar flexion.

Investigations

Guided by history and examination
General problem—degenerative changes appear in asymptomatic from early age.

X-rays
Routine AP and lateral specialized oblique.
- Advantages cheap, low radiation dose, define bones.
- Disadvantages do not define soft tissues.
- AP—check spinous process, 2 transverse processes, 2 pedicles, 2 laminae, and 2 facet joints (vertical in lumbar spine) at each level, assess alignment.
- Lateral—see bodies of vertebrae, disc spacing increasing from L1–L4, lumbar intervertebral foraminae alignment will give smooth curve of posterior aspects of the bodies forming the lumbar lordosis.
- Oblique—for facets joints and pars interarticularis.
- See 'Scottie Dog'—neck is pars, nose is transverse process, eye is pedicle, ear is superior articular process, front legs are inferior articular process. Collar = spondylolysis.

Bone scan
Technetium-labelled injection is taken up in areas of increased osteoblastic activity demonstrating increased metabolic activity in bone. Detected by gamma camera. Reveals stress fractures (i.e. spondylolysis), but also epiphyses and metaphyseal bone plates of young.
- *Advantage:* high sensitivity.
- *Disadvantage:* low specificity, radiation dose.

Single photon emission computer tomography (SPECT)
- Gives more precise anatomical localization of 'hot spot' than bone scan.
- Use to locate spondylolysis.

Computer tomography
Allows visualization of bony configuration and good visualization of paraspinal soft tissues.
- *Advantage:* good to detect fractures and impingement of spinal canal, evaluate spinal tumours.
- *Disadvantages:* radiation dose, slices may miss pathology.

Myelography
An injection of radio-opaque dye into the spinal canal reveals an outline of the spinal cord and nerve roots on subsequent plain X-rays. This can reveal nerve root compression, though not its cause (i.e. prolapsed disc, osteophyte or tumour).

CT myelography
Myelography is combined with CT technology for even greater detail.

Magnetic resonance imaging
- Provides excellent visualization of soft tissues—including discs.
- Can assess impingement of nerve roots.
- May see haemorrhage from ligamentous injury.
- Can detect atrophy in paraspinal muscles.
- Detects changes in the spinal cord, such as syringomyelia.
  - *Advantage*—no radiation.
  - *Disadvantage*—cost.

Discography
Injection of radiopaque dye into the disc space under pressure—pain response assessed.

Acute spinal injury

History and examination
Consider forces involved and take history from the patient and witnesses. Review video if available.

Examine carefully to exclude injuries that could produce instability (threaten neurological structures).

Immobilizing the spine
Though 'airway' is a priority in an unconscious player, the cervical spine should be protected by employing a jaw thrust in preference to the head tilt-chin lift maneouvre. Inadequate immobilization in transporting player from pitch could worsen clinical condition!

When to immobilize?
- Pain in spine secondary to high velocity injury.
- Any neurological signs.
- Severe spinal pain (for comfort).

Transportation should be on a spinal board by trained personnel to ensure immobilization in position athlete was found. In general, equipment such as helmets should only be removed by those trained to do so.

Cervical spine injury and potential instability should be presumed in anyone who is unconscious after head injury. The cervical spine will need assessment by cervical spine X-ray and CT of entire neck.

Acute injuries of the back in sport

- Muscular strains (see Fig 16.1).
- Ligamentous sprains.
- Contusions.
- *Fractures:* transverse processes, ribs (*NB* beware renal injury with injury at costovertebral angle—assess abdominal tenderness and haematuria and consider intravenous pyelogram or renal ultrasound) posterior elements—generally stable and not associated with neurological damage.
- *Compression fractures of the vertebral bodies:* unless trauma was extreme, are usually pathological (i.e. often osteoporotic in elderly athletes).
- *Fracture dislocations:* high-energy injuries (e.g. diving, car racing) with high risk of spinal cord injury.
- *Thoracic disc herniation:* occurs occasionally in athletes, as in the general population (1.6 per 1000), but is not associated with athletic activities—lateral herniation presents with chest wall pain in dermatomal pattern and central herniation with lower extremity spasticity and paraparesis.
- Lumbar disc disease.

Management of musculoligamentous injuries of the back

Sprains and strains of the back are common. They do not require radiological evaluation if the clinical findings do not indicate other causes. Cold therapy should be used for 48–72h and muscle spasm may be controlled by anti-spasmodics. Rehabilitation is important and aims to restore normal muscle strength and firing patterns. Tight muscles, typically hamstrings and hip flexors, may need to be stretched to prevent recurrence.

Disc disease

Disc disease is a continuum from degeneration to herniation. There is a loss of water content with age and this permits more stress to be transferred to the annulus fibrosis, which may develop radial tears. These have the potential for herniation,

Disc degeneration
A desiccated disc with tears may give local pain.

History
- Pain often precedes activity, but may be aggravated by it.
- Findings may be similar to central musculoligamentous injuries.

Investigations
Not indicated in most minor cases. However:
- Plain radiographs may show loss of disc height in advanced cases and there may be associated facet joint arthrosis.
- MRI reveals loss of disc water content, small disc bulges, and annular tears.

Treatment
- *Medication:* adequate analgesia and anti-spasmodics.
- *Ice:* provides an analgesic effect.
- *Heat:* improved mobility.
- Rehabilitation to improve muscle strength and firing to decrease the load on the disc.
- Address hamstring or hip flexor tightness

Intradiscal electrothermal annuloplasty (IDET)—if tears are apparent in the disc, thermal coagulation has been achieved by a probe inserted into the disc. The benefits of this treatment are not yet proven.

Disc herniation

In disc herniation (or 'slipped disc'), the nucleus pulposis extrudes through a tear in the annulus fibrosis most commonly at L4/L5 and L5/S1. They occur most often in the 5th decade of life, although up to 2% occur in those under 18yrs. Such herniation may press on the nerve root causing leg pain (called 'sciatica'), numbness and weakness. Pain may also be generated by the release of inflammatory molecules (e.g. tumour necrosis factor-alpha) and is known as 'chemical radiculitis'.

Cervical disc herniation occurs most often in the lower cervical spine and is a cause of pain in neck, arm, or head. Numbness and weakness may occur. Thoracic disc herniation is rare, but may be a cause of chest or abdominal pain.

History
- Initially symptoms suggestive of disc degeneration, then a 'pop' in the back with more acute intense back pain.
- Buttock and leg pain develops over the next 48h.
- Leg pain aggravated by sitting.
- Leg pain improved by lying.
- Leg pain worsened by coughing, sneezing, lifting, and straining.
- Leg numbness and weakness, tingling or numbness

Examination
- Patients may stand with a list away from the side of the leg pain.
- Flex asymmetrically away from side with leg pain with active lumbar movement.
- Muscle weakness. (Signs depend on level of herniation.)
- Sensory (numbness) loss. (Signs depend on level of herniation.)
- Diminished or absent reflexes. (Signs depend on level of herniation.)
- Sciatic or femoral nerve tension signs:
  - Reduced SLR.
  - Lasegue positive.
  - Bowstring positive.
  - Slump test positive.

Investigations
MRI is the investigation of choice, though CT and CT myelography have previously been useful. MRI can demonstrate the four stages of disc herniation:
- Degeneration.
- Protrusion.
- Extrusion.
- Sequestration.

Proximity of disc bulge to neural structures can be assessed.

Treatment
- *Medication:* analgesia and anti-spasmodics.
- Bed rest when severe pain significantly restricts movement.
- Generally encourage activity as soon as the patient can cope with it.
- Back extension exercises may be useful.
- Epidural injections may help with pain control, but do not improve neurological deficit.
- Rehabilitation of flexibility and strength must be complete before return to sport

Prognosis
Most improve significantly with conservative management over 6 weeks.

Persistent cases of radiculopathy (e.g. pain below knee or into anterior thigh for upper lumbar herniations) might consider surgical options although studies suggest the long term results are no better than with continued conservative management:
- Discectomy or microdiscectomy.
- Laminectomy or hemilaminectomy.
- Artificial disc replacement.
- Lumbar fusion for recurrent herniation.
- Chemonucleolysis: an injection of a proteolytic enzyme chymopapain to dissolve the extruded disc material.

Cauda equina syndrome
Cauda equina syndrome occurs with a central disc herniation.

History
- Bilateral leg pain.
- Numbness: 'saddle anaesthesia'.
- Faecal incontinence.
- Urinary retention.

Examination
- Loss of perianal, scrotal sensation.
- Loss of anal sphincter tone.

Requires early surgical decompression—refer urgently to neurosurgical team.

Pars interarticularis and spondylolysis

Definitions
- *Pars interarticularis*: bridge of bone between inferior and superior articular process of vertebra (also called 'isthmus').
- *Spondylolysis*: separation in the pars interarticularis of the posterior elements of the spine.

Posterior element injury
The pars interarticularis is vulnerable to stress fracture in those engaging in repeated hyperextension, rotation, and side flexion of the spine. This occurs in many sports but, because of the nature of the sport, occurs particularly in fast bowlers in cricket and in gymnasts. The injured pars interarticularis tends to be contralateral to the bowling arm in cricketers,[1] but spondylolysis are often painless in gymnasts. Imaging with bone scan and CT reveals a continuum of mild stress reaction to complete fracture with potential for non-union. The lower three lumbar vertebra are most at risk (see Fig. 16.3). The term spondylolysis covers separations in the pars interarticularis, but separations have also been described in the pedicle and other posterior elements of the spine.

History
Posterior element pain is characterized by pain on spinal extension. The pain of spondylolysis may be of bone stress injury with pain building during repeated activity and resolving with rest.

Examination
- *Stork test:* one legged hyperextension—pain when the ipsilateral foot to the side of the pars lesion is on the ground.
- *Fitch test:* stork test with rotation towards the affected side is more sensitive of a bone stress lesion.

Investigations
- *Plain radiography:* oblique view shows a 'collar' on the Scottie dog—poor sensitivity.
- *Triple phase bone scan with SPECT:* excellent localization of 'hot spots' in the posterior elements indicating possible sites of spondylolysis. Used to target reverse gantry computerised tomography (rg-CT).[2]
- *Reverse gantry CT:* excellent at delineating pathoanatomy. However, combination with SPECT subjects patient to significant radiation.
- MRI is increasingly being used, but does not pose radiation risks. Shows bone stress as oedema and spondylolysis as cortical separation. Sometimes used to target rg-CT. (See Fig. 19.3)

---

[1] Gregory PL, Batt ME, Kerslake RW. (2004.) Comparing spondylolysis in cricketers and soccer players. *Br J Sports Med* **38**: 737–42.
[2] Gregory PL, Batt ME, Kerslake RW, Scammell BE, Webb JF. (2004). The value of combining single photon emission computerized tomography and computerized tomography in the investigation of spondylolysis. *Eur Spine J* **13**(6): 503–9.

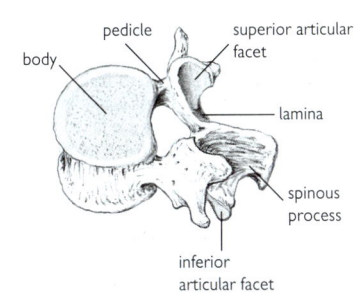

Fig. 16.3 Typical lumbar vertebra (L4) from above and side. Reproduced with permission from MacKinnon P and Morris J (2005). *Oxford Textbook of Functional Anatomy* Vol 1. Oxford University Press, Oxford. © 2005.

Prognosis
Six weeks rest may be sufficient for those with early bone stress reaction, but 12 months may be required to allow healing of established stress fractures. Established spondylolysis with wide sclerotic bone margins and negative bone scan are unlikely to heal, even with rest.

Management
- *Rest*: increased uptake on bone scan, SPECT or bone oedema on MRI indicates bone stress and treatment should include rest from pain-provoking activities, which is usually sport. A thoracolumbar corset may be used to prevent hyperextension. 6 weeks rest may be sufficient for those with early bone stress reaction, but 12 months may be required to allow healing of established stress fractures.
- *Rehabilitation* of the spinal and abdominal musculature is necessary after the period of rest and before a return to sport.
- *Surgery*: stabilization of spondylolisthesis (e.g. Buck fusion—pedicle screws and bone graft) may be considered for those with persistent pain despite adequate conservative treatment.[3] A local anaesthetic 'lysis' block may give useful information regarding the potential benefit of treating the lysis surgically Though most achieve pain control, few reach elite sporting levels after surgery.
- *Return to sport*: imaging is not useful in predicting time to return to sport. It is wise to wait until the athlete is pain free throughout a progressive rehabilitation programme before attempting this.
- In established spondylolysis (wide bone margins with no uptake on bone scan or SPECT) management is designed to allow pain to settle and then rehabilitation to provide dynamic stability through exercises and an earlier (less cautious) return to sport may be attempted. Pain preventing successful return to sport could be treated by surgical stabilization.

[3] Debnath UK, Freeman BJC, Gregory P, *et al.* (2003). Clinical outcome and return to sport following surgi-cal treatment of spondylolysis in young athletes. *J Bone Jt Surg [Br]* **85-B:** 224–9.

Prevention

The prevalence of spondylolysis in some sports has been so high and the proportion of players lost from the sport so high that governing bodies have tried to find ways to prevent this stress injury. In cricket, fast bowlers are susceptible and the following measures are taken to protect them:
- Until aged 19yrs the number of overs bowled per day in matches or balls bowled in practice are restricted. The number increases towards 19 when skeletal maturity is presumed and hence the bones thought to be less vulnerable.
- Coaches are made aware of bowling techniques which are thought to predispose to spondylolysis. These are 'mixed' techniques which involved more counter-rotation of shoulders on hips.
- Coaches are encouraged to coach young fast bowlers to use a safer technique (side-on, front-on or mid-way).
- Coaches are involved in the rehabilitation of fast bowlers with spondylolysis and will try to mould a technique that does not involve a mixed action.

Further reading

Standaert CJ, Herring SA. (2000). Spondylolysis: a critical review. *Br J Sports Med* **34**(6): 415–22.

Pars interarticularis and spondylolisthesis

Definition
Spondylolisthesis: anterior displacement of one vertebral body on another.

Classification of spondylolisthesis
Classified in 1976 by Wiltse et al.:[1]
- Dysplastic.
- Isthmic (lytic or elongated).
- Degenerative.
- Traumatic (fractures).
- Pathological.

Staging of spondylolisthesis
By displacement of vertebral body and relative to the body anteroposterior diameter, classified in 1932 by Meyerding:[2]
- *Stage 1:* <25%.
- *Stage 2:* 25–50%.
- *Stage 3:* 50–75%.
- *Stage 4:* >75%.

Asymptomatic spondylolisthesis is present in about 5% of the skeletally mature general population. More than 90% of such lesions are at L5. They are not present in the newborn, but have been seen in 6yr-olds.

Spondylolisthesis: clinical

Examination
- A step in the spine.
- Hamstrings are often tight (differentiate from sciatic nerve tension).

Investigations
- Lateral plain X-rays.
- MRI provides information on nerve root foraminae and disc quality, which may be compromised in spondylolisthesis.

Prognosis
Spondylolisthesis may progress in the skeletally immature. However, sporting involvement does not appear to be a risk factor and therefore there is no evidence to bar an athlete from participation. Nevertheless it may be wise to avoid gymnastics and weightlifting if at stage 2 or 3. Surgery may be considered for those at Stage 3 or those with nerve root entrapment.

---

[1] Wiltse LL, Newman PH, Macnab I. (1976). Classification of spondylolisis and spondylolisthesis. *Clin Orthop* **117:** 23–9.
[2] Meyerding HW. (1932). Spondylolisthesis. *Surg Gynecol Obstet* **54:** 371–7.

Spondylolysis and spondylolisthesis in the young athlete

- This stress fracture or defect of the pars interarticularis appears to be caused often by activities that require excessive lumbar extension and rotation, e.g. gymnastics, bowling in cricket, and serving in tennis.
- Some children may also have a genetic weakness in the pars interarticularis that predisposes to this condition.
- Most common at L5 (85–95%) and L4 (5–15%), but occasionally occurs at a higher level.
- Can be unilateral or bilateral.
- If the pars defect is bilateral, slippage can occur—spondylolisthesis (vertebra slips forward on the one below) and is graded according to amount of slippage.
- Progression of spondylolisthesis is uncommon, but is most likely to occur during the time of peak height velocity.

History
- May be asymptomatic. Do not assume that back pain is due to a radiologically proven spondylolysis or spondylolisthesis unless the clinical picture is consistent.
- Symptomatic pars stress fractures present with an insidious onset of unilateral or bilateral pain in the lumbar region (most commonly at the level of the belt) which may then radiate to the buttocks and leg.
- Pain is worse with activities requiring lumbar extension.

Examination
- May have increased lumbar lordosis.
- Lumbar tenderness maximal over facet joint at the affected level.
- Pain reproduced by lumbar extension, which is often worse when standing on the leg of the affected side.
- No neurological signs in the lower limbs.

Investigation
- X-ray including oblique view. This gives the classic 'Scottie dog' appearance when a pars defect is present. However, if recent onset the X-ray is often normal. Lateral view is useful to diagnose and grade spondylolisthesis.
- A bone scan including SPECT views is most sensitive for recent stress fractures. A 'hot spot' at the site of the defect suggests that the fracture is recent and active. If no hot spot (therefore no increased osteoblastic reaction) then no active remodelling is occurring. However, bone scan changes often remain positive for many months and are not useful as a means of timing return to sport.
- CT scanning is useful for staging fractures.

Treatment
- Avoid lumbar extension activities.
- Brace to prevent lumbar extension (e.g. modified Boston brace), especially if the child has pain with activities of daily living. This may remind child not to play sport. Use of a brace has not been shown to increase the rate of fracture healing.

- *Physiotherapy:*
  - Abdominal strengthening programme.
  - Postural retraining to address excessive lumbar lordosis and anterior pelvic tilt.
  - Improve hamstring and gluteal flexibility.
- Return to sport, which usually occurs within 3–6 months, should be based on symptom resolution, absence of clinical signs, and good core trunk strength.

Prognosis
- Fractures treated in the early phase appear to have a good prognosis, especially if they are unilateral.
- Early and progressive stage fractures have a 40–80% chance of fracture healing.
- Terminal stage fractures rarely unite.
- Nevertheless, excellent clinical outcomes can be achieved in the absence of fracture healing.

Management of spondylolisthesis
- Monitor for slip progression during the growing years, as progression may require surgical stabilization.
- Refer to a spinal surgeon—these children should avoid sports requiring lumbar extension and contact:
  - Persistent pain despite appropriate rehabilitation.
  - Those with a grade 3 or 4 spondylolisthesis (>50% slip).
  - Slip is progressing.

Further reading
Morita T, Ikata T, Katoh S, Miyake R. (1995.) Lumbar spondylolysis in children and adolescents. *J Bone Jt Surg (Br)* **77B**: 620–5.

Scheuermann's disease

Scheuermann's disease is osteochondrosis affecting the growth plates of the vertebral bodies in the thoracolumbar spine of young adults and sometimes adolescents and is a cause of kyphosis. The 7th to 10th thoracic vertebrae are most commonly affected.

Scheuermann's disease may be a co-incidental radiographic diagnosis or the cause of non-specific low back pain in an active adolescent or young adult.

History
- Mid-thoracic pain with activity.
- Deformity: rounding of upper back, poor posture—may be painless.

Examination
- Kyphosis.
- Axial tenderness.
- Paraspinal muscle spasm.
- Excessive lumbar lordosis.
- Tightness of hamstrings and thoracolumbar fascia.

Investigations
- *Plain radiographs:*
  - Diagnosed on finding wedging of >5° in three or more consecutive vertebrae on lateral X-ray is diagnostic.
  - Vertebral body wedging.
  - Schmorl's nodes (irregular ossification in the cartilage end plates) due to herniation of nucleus pulposus—also occur in Wilson's disease, sickle cell anaemia and spinal stenosis.
- MRI detects decreased water content and loss of disc height.

Prognosis
- Scheuermann's disease is generally benign with complications rare (e.g. myelopathy or cardiothoracic compromise) and for most the associated pain is self-limiting, stopping with skeletal maturity.

Treatment
NB Exercises will not correct deformity.

Initial treatment
- Analgesia.
- Physiotherapy:
  - Flexibility (hamstrings and thoraco-lumbar fascia).
  - Strengthening (back extensors and abdominals).
- Bracing considered for severe pain not controlled by analgesia and exercises symptoms.
- Sport permitted if pain is not aggravated.
- Kyphosis greater than 50° in the skeletally immature: bracing (e.g. a Milwaukee brace).
- Kyphosis greater than 75° and progressing despite bracing and exercises—consider posterior instrumentation and surgical fusion. Contact sports are prohibited after surgery.

Sacro-iliac joint

Movements of the sacroiliac joint are subtle, but during running the ilium rotates posteriorly from foot contact to midstance, when it rotates anteriorly until toe off.

Sacroiliitis is usually a manifestation of seronegative arthritidies, such as ankylosing spondylitis or Reiter's syndrome. Pain from the sacroiliac joint may also come from trauma or overuse injury.

Factors that might predispose to over-use type injury of sacro-iliac joint
- Ligamentous laxity due to hormonal changes of pregnancy.
- Excessive side-to-side movement of pelvis in running.
- Forced extension of hip in gymnastics.
- Decreased hip rotation, e.g. due to degenerative joint disease.
- Leg length discrepancy.
- Running on uneven terrain or cambered road.
- Shoes or orthotics.

History
- Pain in low back and or buttock often in relation to activity.
- Pain radiates to posterior thigh, but rarely to knee.
- Unilateral low back pain, e.g. on hopping.
- Aching rest pain, especially after prolonged sitting.

Examination
- Local pain over joint line (posterior inferior iliac spine).
- Pain on compression or distraction of the iliac crests.
- Pain on flexion abduction external rotation (FABER) leverage test.
- Asymmetric movements of malleoli on long sit-up.
- Asymmetric movements of PSIS on active lumbar flexion (standing or sitting).
- Gillet test.

Investigation
- Plain radiographs may show sclerosis, joint narrowing, and osteophytes in chronic cases.
- Bone scan may be hot at sacroiliac joint (sacro-iliitis, raising possibility of systemic disorder.
- HLAB27 may be positive in those with ankylosing spondylitis.

Treatment
- Address biomechanical factors, such as leg length discrepancy, hip rotation restriction, footwear, training factors.
- *Analgesia:* NSAIDs, paracetamol, or codeine.
- Ice.
- For sacro-iliac dysfunction consider chiropractic corrections or osteopathic manipulations.
- Second line treatment might include corticosteroid or sclerosant injections.
- If sacro-iliitis—will need to treat underlying systemic disorder (consider referral to rheumatologist).

Ankylosing spondylitis

- A chronic inflammatory arthritis: TNF α and IL-1 are implicated.
- Affects spine and sacroiliac joints sometimes leading to fusion of the spine. Complete fusion results in a spinal rigidity ('bamboo spine').
- An autoimmune disease: although autoantibodies specific for ankylosing spondylitis (AS) have not been identified.
- One of the spondyloarthropathies with a strong genetic predisposition (other spondyloarthropathies: Reiter's syndrome (reactive arthritis) and those associated with ulcerative colitis, Crohn's disease, psoriasis). About 90% of the patients express the HLA-B27 genotype. Other genetic association: ARTS1 and IL23R.[1]

History

- Young adult (e.g. aged 18–30) when symptoms first arise.
- Chronic pain and stiffness in the lower or sometimes entire spine.
- Sacroiliac joint pain: referred to buttock or posterior thigh.
- Men to women 3:1 and often worse in men.
- Pain is often severe on rest, improves with physical activity (not all).

Associations

- 40% have eye problems: iridocyclitis or uveitis (redness and pain of eye, vision loss, floaters, photophobia).
- Fatigue and nausea.
- Onycholysis: lifting of the nails.
- Swelling of large limb joints (e.g. knee, ankles) especially in younger patients.
- Pain in ankles and feet.
- Enthesitis (e.g. insertional Achilles tendinopathy, lateral epicondylitis, calcaneal spurs).
- Other seronegative spondyloarthropathies (e.g. Reiter's syndrome (reactive arthritis) and those associated with ulcerative colitis, Crohn's disease, psoriasis).
- Rarely—aortitis, apical lung fibrosis, and ectasia of the sacral nerve root sheaths.

Examination

- Assess posture and curvature or spine.
- Schober's test: clinical measure of flexion of the lumbar spine.
- See Sacro-iliac joint examination.
- Measure chest expansion with respiration.
- Examine other joints and entheses.
- Inspect nails.
- Auscultate heart.
- Inspect eyes.

---

[1] Brionez TF, Reveille JD. (2008). The contribution of genes outside the major histocompatibility complex to susceptibility to ankylosing spondylitis. *Curr Opin Rheumatol* **20**(4): 384–91.

ANKYLOSING SPONDYLITIS

Investigations
- *Lateral lumbar spine X-ray:* bamboo spine, but X-ray changes may take 10yrs to appear after onset.
- *Magnetic resonance images of sacroiliac joints:* reliability not known.
- *CT sacroiliac joints:* reliability not known.
- CRP and an increase in the ESR may increase during acute inflammatory periods—not diagnostic.
- *HLA-B27:* higher risk than the general population of developing the disorder—but is not diagnostic in a person with back pain. Over 95% of people that have been diagnosed with AS are HLA-B27 positive, although this varies (50% of African American patients with AS possess HLA-B27, 80% among AS patients from Mediterranean countries).

Diagnosis
The Bath Ankylosing Spondylitis Disease Activity Index (BASDAI) is an index designed to detect the inflammatory burden of active disease.[2] The BASDAI helps diagnose AS in the presence of other factors such as:
- HLA-B27 positivity.
- Persistent buttock pain which resolves with exercise.
- X-ray or MRI evident involvement of the sacroiliac joints.

Management

Aim
No cure is known for AS, so treatments intend to reduce symptoms and pain.
- Medication to reduce inflammation (NSAIDs and COX-2 inhibitors) and pain (paracetamol or opioids).
- *Physical therapy:*
  - Movements diminish pain and stiffness, frequent changes of position or activity may be helpful.
  - Occupations and sport may be impossible.
  - Maintenance of good posture is a worthy goal, but the patient may still lose this despite best efforts.
  - Swimming preferred exercise—involves all muscles and joints in a low gravity environment.
  - Stretching in yoga, tai chi, Pilates, etc.
  - Moderate-to-high impact exercises (e.g. jogging) may worsen symptoms.
- *Second line medication to achieve immunosuppression with DMARDs:*
  - Ciclosporin.
  - Methotrexate.
  - Sulfasalazine.
  - Corticosteroids.
- Use BASDAI[2] to assess need to move from NSAIDs to Biologics (score 4/10 is cut off). Biologics or TNFα antagonists are promising though expensive.
  - Etanercept.
  - Infliximab.
  - Adalimumab.

---

[2] Garrett S, Jenkinson T, Kennedy L, Whitelock H, Gaisford P, Calin A. (1994). A new approach to defining disease status in ankylosing spondylitis: the Bath Ankylosing Spondylitis Disease Activity Index. J Rheumatol 21 (12): 2286–91

NB Risk of infection—TB screen prior to treatment, avoid others known to have infections (even common cold) and stop if develop infections such as sore throat.

Use Bath Ankylosing Spondylitis Functional Index (BASFI) to assess patient's functional impairment due to the disease as well as response to therapy.[3]

Surgery

Usually last resort can be considered for:
- Joint replacements, e.g. knees and hips.
- Correction of severe flexion deformities, e.g. of the neck or other spine—high risk procedures.

Beware anaesthesetic complications:
- Changes in the upper airway cause intubation problems.
- Spinal and epidural anaesthesia difficult due to calcification of ligaments.
- Stiffness of ribs results in diaphragmatic ventilation and decreased pulmonary function.
- Aortic regurgitation.

Prognosis

- Ranges from mild to debilitating.
- Some respond well to medical management others refractive.
- Some have episodic course—relapses and remissions.
- Others persistent unremitting.
- Complicated by:
  - Dactylitis or enthesitis.
  - Syndesmophytes and spinal osteophytes.
  - Fusion of the vertebrae occurs.
  - Spine may become osteopenic or osteoporosis and lead to compression fractures and further deformity and pain.
  - Paresthesia may result from inflammation of tissue surrounding nerves.
  - Other organs may be involved heart (aortic regurgitation, AV node block), lungs (lung fibrosis), eyes, colon, and kidneys.
  - Amyloidosis.
  - Very rarely cauda equina syndrome.
- Some have shown success in sports at a high level despite suffering AS, e.g. Mike Atherton and Michael Slater (cricket), Rico Brogna (Baseball), Ian Woosnam (golf).

---

[3] Calin A, Garrett S, Whitelock H, Kennedy L, O'Hea J, Mallorie P, Jenkinson T. (1994). A new approach to defining functional ability in ankylosing spondylitis: the development of the Bath Ankylosing Spondylitis Functional Index. *J Rheumatol* **21** (12): 2281–5.

Conditions affecting the spine in children and adolescents

Spondylolysis and spondylolisthesis

Aetiology
- This stress fracture or defect of the pars interarticularis is often associated with activities that require excessive lumbar extension and rotation, e.g. gymnastics, bowling in cricket and serving in tennis.
- Some children may also have a genetic weakness in the pars interarticularis that predisposes to this condition.
- Most common at L5 (85–95%) and L4 (5–15%), but occasionally occurs at a higher level.
- Can be unilateral or bilateral.
- If the pars defect is bilateral, slippage can occur. This is referred to as a spondylolisthesis (where a vertebra slips forward on the one below) and is graded according to amount of slippage.
- Progression of spondylolisthesis is uncommon, but is most likely to occur during the time of peak height velocity.

Clinical features
- May be asymptomatic. Do not assume that back pain is due to a radiologically proven spondylolysis or spondylolisthesis unless the clinical picture is consistent.
- Symptomatic pars stress fractures present with an insidious onset of unilateral or bilateral pain in the lumbar region (most commonly at the level of the belt) which may then radiate to the buttocks.
- Pain is worse with activities requiring lumbar extension ± rotation.

Physical examination
- May have increased lumbar lordosis.
- Tenderness over spinous process or facet joint region at affected level.
- Pain reproduced by lumbar extension, which is often worse when standing on the leg of the affected side.
- No neurological signs in the lower limbs.

Investigations
- X-ray including oblique view. This gives the classic 'Scottie dog' appearance when a pars defect is present.
- Lateral view is also useful to determine whether a spondylolisthesis exists, and its severity.
- Spondylolisthesis is graded 1–4 according to the degree of slip; grade 1: 25%, grade 2: 25–50%, grade 3: 50–75%, grade 4 >75%.
- With recent symptom onset the X-ray is often normal.
- A bone scan including SPECT views is very sensitive for recent stress fractures. A 'hot spot' at the site of the defect suggests that the fracture is recent and active. If no hot spot (i.e. no osteoblastic reaction) is seen, active remodelling is not occurring.
- Bone scan changes often remain positive for many months and are not useful as a means of assessing healing or timing of return to sport.
- CT scanning is useful for staging fractures.

- In view of the ionizing radiation involved in the combination of bone scanning and CT in this adolescent population, MRI imaging can be used instead of bone scan and CT with only a small loss in sensitivity.

Management of spondylolysis
- Avoid lumbar extension activities.
- Some clinicians recommend the use of a brace to prevent lumbar extension (e.g. modified Boston brace), especially if the child has pain with activities of daily living.
- Use of brace has not been shown to increase rate of fracture healing.
- Physiotherapy should include an abdominal strengthening programme and postural retraining to address excessive lumbar lordosis and anterior pelvic tilt.
- A flexibility programme to improve hamstring and gluteal flexibility should also be included.

Return to sport
- Return to sport, which usually occurs within 3–6 months, should be based on symptom resolution, absence of clinical signs and good core trunk strength.

Prognosis
- Fractures treated in the early phase appear to have a good prognosis, especially if they are unilateral.
- Early and progressive stage fractures have a 40–80% chance of fracture healing.
- Terminal stage fractures rarely unite.
- Excellent clinical outcomes can be achieved even in the absence of radiological fracture healing.

Management of spondylolisthesis
- Monitor for slip progression during the adolescent growth spurt, as progression may (rarely) require surgical stabilization.
- If persistent pain despite appropriate rehabilitation and in those with a grade 3 or 4 spondylolisthesis (>50% slip) or where the slip is progressing, referral to a specialist is indicated. These children should avoid sports involving lumbar extension and contact.

Scheuermann's disease

Pathology
- Osteochondrosis affecting growth plates (ring epiphysis) of vertebral bodies.
- Compressive forces cause anterior wedging deformity of the vertebral bodies, resulting in a thoracic kyphosis.
- Affects thoracic spine predominantly, but can occur in the lumbar spine or at the thoracolumbar junction.
- Commonest cause of adolescent kyphosis.

Clinical features
- Commonly presents in active adolescent.
- May have mid-thoracic pain with activity.
- May present as a painless thoracic kyphosis in late teens or 20s.
- Tightness of hamstrings and thoracolumbar fascia is common.
- Excessive lumbar lordosis often present.

Diagnosis
- Wedging of >5° in three or more consecutive vertebrae on lateral X-ray is diagnostic.
- Schmorl's nodes (irregularities in the cartilage end-plate causing irregular ossification) commonly present.

Treatment
- Aim of treatment is to resolve pain and stop progression of deformity.
- A high level of evidence does not exist for any of the current treatments used in Scheuermann's disease.
- Physical therapy involving hamstrings and thoracolumbar fascia stretches and strengthening of the spinal extensors.
- If symptoms severe or kyphosis is progressing, an extension brace (e.g. a Milwaukee brace) may be required although these are cumbersome and compliance is generally poor.
- Rarely, surgery is required to prevent progression of kyphosis or when pain and deformity is severe.

Prognosis
- Exercises will ↓ symptoms, but will not correct existing deformity.
- Use of brace before skeletal maturity may improve kyphosis.
- Pain usually self-limiting and resolves with skeletal maturity unless kyphosis is severe.

Limbus vertebra

Pathology
- Small, corticated, osseous density adjacent to vertebral body.
- Thought to be vertebral ring apophysis that has failed to fuse due to acute or repetitive trauma.
- Contrast injected into the nucleus pulposis at the affected level surrounds the limbus fragment suggesting that it results from herniation of disc material.
- Majority affect the anterosuperior corner of the vertebral body, but can less commonly be postero-inferior.
- Usually occur in mid-lumbar spine.

Clinical features
- Antero-inferior lesions may present with pain or stiffness, but are usually asymptomatic.
- Postero-inferior lesions may present with radicular pain 2° to nerve root compression.

Treatment
- No specific treatment is indicated for anterosuperior limbus vertebrae.
- Postero-inferior limbus vertebrae with associated nerve root compression may require surgical decompression.

Chapter 17

Shoulder

Anatomy *456*
History *460*
Examination *462*
Special tests *464*
Nerves *470*
Shoulder disorders *471*
Acute traumatic causes *472*
Conservative management of shoulder dislocation *474*
Rehabilitation after shoulder dislocation *475*
Example of final pitch-based rehabilitation *482*
Acromioclavicular joint separations *484*
Sternoclavicular joint separations *485*
Glenoid labrum tears *486*
Biceps tendon dislocation *488*
Fractures of the shoulder *489*
Chronic over-use disorders *490*
Atraumatic causes *498*

Anatomy

Important areas of shoulder anatomy
See Fig. 17.1.
- Musculotendinous units of the rotator cuff and biceps.
- Bony landmarks of the humerus, scapula, and clavicle.
- Four joints of the shoulder.

Rotator cuff
The rotator cuff comprises the tendons of four muscles.
- The subscapularis is located anteriorly on the scapula.
- The supraspinatus, infraspinatus, and the teres minor are located posteriorly on the scapula.
- All are closely associated with the glenohumeral capsule, as is the biceps tendon.
- Primary function of the rotator cuff is to position the humeral head in the glenoid allowing larger muscles to provide necessary power.

Humerus
Important bony landmarks of the shoulder.
- Greater tuberosity of the humerus:
  - Insertion site of the supraspinatus, infraspinatus, and teres minor tendons.
  - This prominence is often associated with impingement.
  - When testing for impingement on physical exam most tests attempt to force the greater tuberosity under and against the acromion and the coraco-acromial ligament, thus catching or 'impinging' the subacromial structures.
- The bicipital groove is a palpable indentation immediately medial and anterior to the greater tuberosity of the humerus:
  - It houses the tendon of the long head of the biceps.
  - It is easily identified if the humerus is alternately internally and externally rotated, while palpating this area.
  - There is a retinaculum that holds the biceps tendon in place.
- On the anterior and inferior border of this groove is the lesser tuberosity, the insertion site of the subscapularis.

Articulations
There are three true joints of the shoulder (Fig. 17.2):
- The glenohumeral, acromioclavicular, and the sternoclavicular joints:
  - The latter two may have a fibrocartilagenous disc present within the articulation.
  - As with all true joints, they are susceptible to various arthritides and trauma.

The fourth joint, the scapulothoracic joint, is a physiological joint, and may be associated with pain syndromes, bursitis, and neuropathies.

The clavicle and its attachments with the sternum, acromion, and coracoid processes are the only bony attachments of the shoulder to the thorax. These connections absorb a large portion of traumatic stresses to the upper extremity and are therefore more susceptible to injuries.

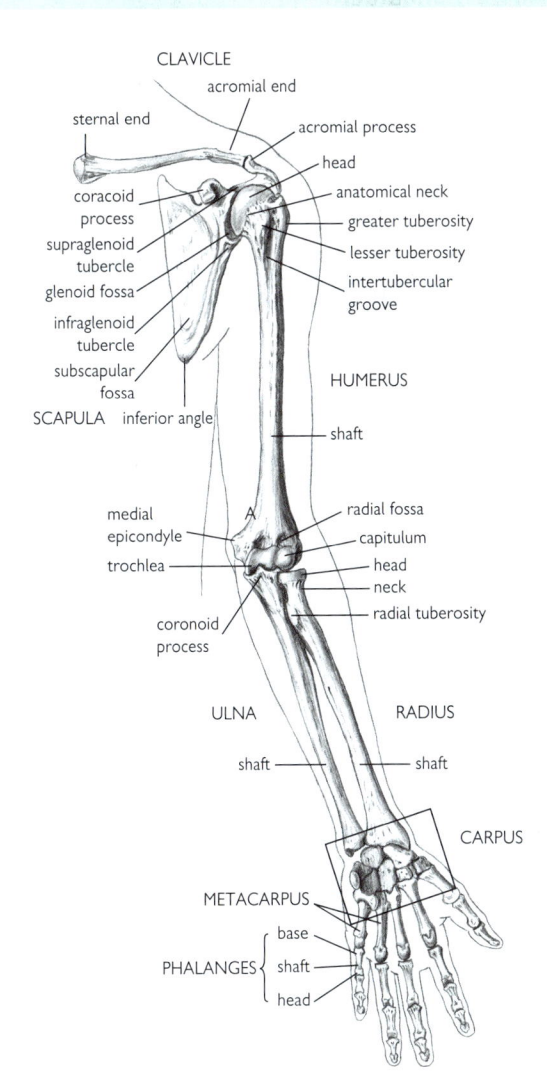

Fig. 17.1 Bones of shoulder girdle and upper limb; anterior view. Reproduced with permission from MacKinnon P and Morris J (2005). *Oxford Textbook of Functional Anatomy*, Vol. 1. Oxford University Press, Oxford. © 2005.

Glenohumeral joint
- The glenohumeral joint sacrifices the bony and ligamentous stability of other joints for increased range of motion.
- The primary stabilizers of the joint are the musculotendinous complex of the rotator cuff and joint capsule, including the labrum.

Bursae

There are 4 important bursae in the shoulder:
- *The subacromial bursa:*
  - Located immediately inferior to the acromioclavicular joint and superior to the glenohumeral joint.
  - It is often involved in impingement syndrome.
  - Injection of local anesthetic into this bursa with eradication of symptoms is the basis of the impingement test.
- The subdeltoid bursa: located inferior to the deltoid tendon on the lateral shaft of the humerus.
- The subscapular bursa: located between the joint capsule and the tendon of the subscapularis muscle.
- The subcoracoid bursa: located between the joint capsule and the coracoid process of the scapula.

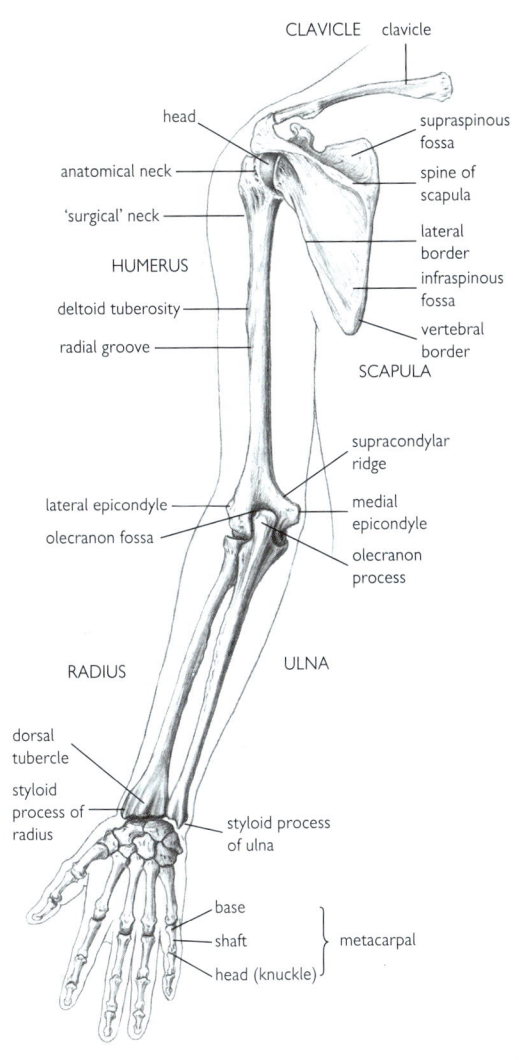

Fig. 17.2 Bones of shoulder girdle and upper limb; posterior view. Reproduced with permission from MacKinnon P and Morris J (2005). *Oxford Textbook of Functional Anatomy* Vol. 1. Oxford University Press, Oxford. © 2005.

History

The key to effective differential diagnosis is a thorough history. Key questions in the evaluation are:

- What is/are the predominant symptom(s)?
- Chief complaints may range from pain to instability to weakness. If pain is the predominant symptom, ask the patient to describe the quality of the pain, its location, and quantify the severity of the pain on a scale from 1 to 10. This helps you assess the results of treatment.
- How long have the symptoms been present? How have they developed or how have they changed? Have you had similar symptoms in the past? Was there any history of trauma (recent or remote)?

These questions help to determine whether the problem is chronic or acute in nature. If trauma was involved, the exact mechanism may help to determine the diagnosis. A history of chronic dislocation or recurrent subluxations may be a clue to instability. Persistent pain with overhead activities may be due to impingement.

- Where did the pain begin and has it changed in its location? Does the shoulder hurt at night? What position do you normally sleep in? Are there certain positions or activities that bother it more than others?

These questions attempt to localize the problem. Night pain or pain with overhead activities may signify impingement and/or rotator cuff tear; while pain with lifting, pushing open a car door, or carrying luggage may be due to underlying instability.

- What is your job? What are your hobbies or sports activities?
- Injuries due to over-use are often seen in workers who have to work overhead frequently. They are especially susceptible to impingement syndrome, subacromial bursitis, and acromioclavicular problems. Certain sports have an increased incidence of shoulder injuries, especially volleyball, swimming, the overhead throwing sports, racquet sports, hockey, wrestling, weightlifting and body-building.
- What has been done so far for treatment? Have there been any prior injuries or surgery to either of the shoulders?

These are important to know because they may alter the examination, or the comparison with the opposite shoulder.

- Do you have any problems with neck pain? Is there any pain radiating into the shoulder or down the upper extremity? Do you have any associated abdominal pain, or chest pain? Is there a history of weight loss, fatigue, or fevers?

Determining whether pain is referred from the cervical spine, abdomen, or chest wall may prevent an expensive and inappropriate work-up. Constitutional signs of malignancy or a septic arthritis are rare, but may be helpful in the diagnostic process.

Examination

Inspection
- *Exposure (including shoulder blades):* women may use bra and/or tie gown around upper chest with arms out.
- *Muscle atrophy:*
  - Biceps atrophy may be due to musculocutaneous nerve injury.
  - Scapular winging may be due to long thoracic nerve injury.
- *Asymmetry:*
  - A pronounced biceps may be due to rupture of the long head of the biceps tendon, giving a 'Popeye' defect.
  - Prominence of the scapular spine may be due to nerve palsy in young patients, or a long-standing rotator cuff tear in older patients.
- *Screen for referred pain:*
  - Cervical spine.
  - Cardiopulmonary.
  - Abdominal.

Palpation
Localize the point of maximum tenderness (Table 17.1) only after the remainder of the exam is complete. Discomfort felt by the patient initially in the examination may cause guarding to the point of missing an important examination finding or making the examination significantly less useful.

Active and passive movements
- There are nine movements described in the shoulder:
  - Abduction (normal 180°).
  - Adduction (normal 45°).
  - Flexion (normal 180°).
  - Extension (normal 45°).
  - Internal rotation (IR, normal 70°).
  - External rotation (ER, normal 75°).
  - Protraction, retraction, and elevation.
- Assess smoothness of the scapulohumeral and scapulothoracic movement, and test for a 'painful arc' which may suggest impingement, rotator cuff problems, or labral tears.
- Impingement pain is usually from 90–120° of abduction.
- Restricted or painful IR at 90° of abduction may also signify shoulder impingement.
- IR is best observed with Apley's (behind the back) scratch test: at least 55° of IR is required to perform this manoeuvre, and range of motion can be quantitated according to the level of the thoracic or lumbar spine that they can reach (T7 is at the inferior angle of the scapula) for comparison after treatment.

Table 17.1 Palpation points

Bony palpation	Palpation of the soft tissues
Suprasternal notch	Rotator cuff muscles
Sternoclavicular joint	Subacromial/subdeltoid bursae
Clavicle	Axilla
Coracoid process	Major muscles of the shoulder
Acromioclavicular joint	
Acromion	
Greater tuberosity of the humerus	
Bicipital groove	
Lesser tuberosity of humerus	
Spine of the scapula	
Medial border of the scapula	

Special tests

The special manoeuvres for evaluation of the shoulder are presented below as described in the literature, and organized according to the problem they evaluate. The reader may have been taught varying or different techniques for the tests presented here. Be cautious in modifying the test, as validity testing will no longer be applicable. A literature review of these manoeuvres is summarized in Table 17.2, but you should be aware that additional well-designed studies are needed in many cases.

Glenohumeral joint stability

Anterior apprehension test

With the scapula stabilized (or in the supine position), the arm is passively moved out to 90° of abduction and gently externally rotated until there is apprehension and the patient resists further ER. The feeling that the joint is going to dislocate (apprehension) constitutes a positive test. Pain alone does not necessarily signify instability. Caution should always be exercised not to completely dislocate the joint with this manoeuvre.

Relocation test

The patient is supine with the arm held in the apprehension position as described above. With a positive test, a posterior force placed on the anterior humerus will relieve the apprehension. Further ER may then be possible. If the posterior force is removed, apprehension returns. This is sometimes called the 'surprise test'.

Augmentation test (fulcrum test)

To define an occult instability, examiner should place hand underneath the humeral head posteriorly, while the patient is supine and in the apprehension position. This may elicit a positive apprehension test.

Load and shift test

While stabilizing the scapula, the humeral head is loaded medially against the glenoid while in the neutral position. A posterior and anterior stress is applied to the humeral head, as if to shift it anteriorly and posteriorly. Translation of up to 50% of the width of the humeral head is considered normal. Movement to the rim of the glenoid is considered subluxation.

Posterior apprehension

The shoulder is passively moved to 90° of abduction and gently internally rotated until the patient is apprehensive and resists further attempts at IR. A posteriorly directed force placed upon the humeral shaft may intensify the feeling of instability.

Sulcus sign

The arm is passively at the side in the standing or sitting position. The humerus is distracted inferiorly. The sulcus sign is an indentation seen immediately inferior to the acromioclavicular joint and signifies an inferior instability. Normal is less than 1cm. Some patients are able to do this spontaneously as a 'party trick'. Look for generalized hyperlaxity.

Table 17.2 Shoulder (glenohumeral) joint: movements, principal muscles, and their innervation[1]

Movement	Principal muscles	Peripheral nerve	Spinal root origin
Flexion	Pectoralis major (clavicular part)	Pectoral nerve (medial and lateral)	C 5, 6
	Deltoid (clavicular part)	Axillary nerve	C 5, 6
Extension	Latissimus dorsi	Nerve to latissimus dorsi (thoracodorsal nerve)	C 5, 6, 7, 8
Abduction	Supraspinatus (initial 20°)	Suprascapular nerve	C 5, 6
	Deltoid	Axillary nerve	C 5, 6
Adduction	Pectoralis major	Pectoral nerves (medial and lateral)	C 5, 6
	Latissimus dorsi	Nerve to latissimus dorsi	C 5, 6, 7, 8
Medial (internal) rotation	Pectoralis major	Pectoral nerves (medial and lateral)	C 5, 6
	Latissimuss dorsi	Nerve to latissimuss dorsi	C 5, 6, 7, 8
	Subscapularis	Subscapular nerves (upper and lower)	C 5, 6
	Teres major	Lower subscapular nerve	C 5, 6
Lateral (external) rotation	Infraspinatus	Suprascapular nerve	C 5, 6
	Teres minor	Axillary nerve	C 5, 6
	Deltoid (posterior fibers)	Axillary nerve	C 5, 6
Circumduction	Combinations of the above		

[1] Reproduced with permission from MacKinnon P, Morris J (2005). *Oxford Textbook of Functional Anatomy Vol 1.* Oxford: Oxford University Press, ©2005.

Impingement syndrome

Neer's sign (impingement sign)

This test attempts to force the greater trochanter under the acromioclavicular joint to compress the bursa, rotator cuff, and biceps tendon. The arm is placed into maximum forward flexion and IR, while stabilizing the scapula. The test is positive if pain is experienced.

Hawkin's sign
With the elbow flexed at 90° and the shoulder forward flexed at 90° the humerus is progressively internally rotated in order to grind the proximal humerus against the acromioclavicular joint. The test is positive if pain is experienced.

Impingement test
The impingement test involves the injection of 10cm^3 of a 1% lidocaine solution into the subacromial space. Greater than 80% resolution of the pain with repeat testing for impingement signs is a positive test suggesting impingement syndrome.

Posterior impingement sign
Executed with the patient supine. The arm is placed in 90–110° of abduction and in slight extension (10–15°). The shoulder is rotated into maximum ER. Recreating symptoms marked by complaints of pain deep within the posterior aspect of the shoulder is indicative of a positive test for posterosuperior glenoid impingement.

Rotator cuff

Drop arm test
With the arm straight, shoulder abducted past 90°, and then forward flexed to 30° the patient is asked to slowly lower it to the side. With a supraspinatus tear he/she is unable to lower the arm slowly and the arm drops to the side.

Jobe's manoeuvre (empty can test)
With the arm straight, and the shoulder abducted to 90° and horizontally adducted to 30°, the humerus is internally rotated to 45° (as if emptying a beverage can). With a supraspinatus tear, the patient is unable to maintain the position against resistance. The shoulder must be compared with the opposite side. In a recent study, the position of supination (the 'full' can position) provided improved isolation of the supraspinatus. It is therefore recommended that both pronation and supination be utilized.

Gerber's lift off test (lift off test)
With the dorsum of the hand placed over the sacrum, the patient is asked to push away from the back against resistance. With subscapularis weakness or tear, there is weakness on the affected side compared with the contralateral side.

Belly-press test
If the patient is unable to reach the hand behind the back because of restricted range of motion, then it can be placed on the belly instead. The examiner attempts to pull the hand out/away as the patient resists.

External rotator test
With the elbows down at the side and at 90° of flexion, and the humerus in 45° of IR, the patient is asked to externally rotate the humerus against resistance. With infraspinatus weakness there is weakness on the affected side as compared to the contralateral side.

ER lag sign
This tests the integrity of the infraspinatus and supraspinatus. The patient is seated with his/her back to the examiner. The elbow is passively flexed to 90°, with the shoulder held at 20° of abduction in near maximal ER (maximal ER minus 5° to avoid elastic recoil). The patient is then instructed to maintain this position while the examiner releases the arm, supporting only the elbow. The sign is positive if a >10° lag or an angular drop is seen.

The drop sign
This tests mainly the infraspinatus integrity. The patient is seated with his/her back to the examiner. The affected arm is held at 90° of abduction and at almost full ER with the elbow flexed at 90°. The patient is then asked to maintain this position while the examiner releases the hand and supports the arm only at the elbow. The sign is positive if a >10° lag occurs.

The IR lag sign
This tests mainly the subscapularis integrity. The patient is seated with his/her back to the examiner. The affected arm is held behind the back. The elbow is flexed to 90° and the shoulder held at 20° of abduction and 20° of extension. The patient's hand is then pulled away from the back until it is in almost maximal IR. The patient is then asked to maintain this position as the examiner releases the hand and supports the arm only at the elbow. The sign is positive if a >10° lag occurs.

Acromioclavicular joint
Crossover test ('scarf' sign)
With the elbow extended, the arm is brought across the chest stressing the acromioclavicular joint. Tenderness is felt in the superior and lateral shoulder if the test is positive.

Biceps
Yergason's test
With the elbow at 90° and the wrist held in pronation the patient will experience pain if attempting to supinate the wrist against resistance.

Speed's test
With the elbow flexed at 30°, the shoulder at 60° of flexion and the wrist supinated, the patient will experience pain if attempting to flex the arm against resistance.

Labral tears
Biceps load test II
With the patient in the supine position the examiner holds the patient's wrist and elbow with the shoulder in 120° of abduction and maximally externally rotated. The elbow is placed in 90° of flexion and the forearm supinated. The patient is asked to flex the elbow against the examiner's resistance. The test is considered positive for a labral lesion if there are increased complaints of pain with resisted elbow flexion.

Anterior slide test (Kibler)
The patient is examined either in a standing or sitting position, hands on the hips and thumbs pointing posteriorly. One of the examiner's hands is placed across the top of the shoulder from the posterior direction, with the index finger over the anterior acromion. With the other hand, the examiner applies a forward and slightly superiorly directed force to the elbow and upper arm. The patient is asked to push back against this force. Pain localized to the front of the shoulder under the examiner's hand and/ or a pop or click in the same area, is considered a positive test.

Clunk test
While applying gentle axial pressure to the humerus with the elbow at 90°, the humerus is rotated internally and externally while simultaneously abducting the arm. If the examiner's opposite hand is placed underneath the humeral head, a clunk, pop, or snap may be felt if a labral tear is present.

Crank test
With the patient in the sitting or standing position, the arm is elevated to 160° in the scapular plane. An axial load is applied to the humerus, while simultaneously internally and externally rotating the humerus in the glenoid fossa. Pain or reproduction of the patient's symptoms (usually pain or catching) is considered a positive test.

O'Brien test
Performed with the patient in the sitting position, the shoulder is abducted to 90° with the elbow in full extension. The forearm is then pronated with the thumb pointing down. A downward force is placed on the arm by the examiner. The force is repeated with the forearm in the supinated position with the thumb pointing upwards. Pain or clicking inside the shoulder joint is considered a positive test for a labral lesion. Pain more superficially, over the acromioclavicular joint indicates pathology in that joint.

Thoracic outlet syndrome

Adson's manoeuvre
While feeling the radial pulse the arm is passively abducted, extended, and externally rotated (simultaneous abduction and ER of the arm compresses the brachial plexus against the scalene muscles). The head is extended and turned to the side of the lesion, while the patient holds his/her breath. Loss of or a diminished radial pulse is a positive test.

Wright's manoeuvre (hyperabduction manoeuvre)
Similar to Adson's manoeuvre, but the arm is hyperabducted over the head, while externally rotated and extended (this simulates compression of the neurovascular bundle beneath the pectoralis tendon). Loss of or a diminished radial pulse is a positive test.

Costoclavicular manoeuvre (military brace position)
The patient sits upright and thrusts the shoulders backward, while the hands rest on the thighs. This narrows the space between the clavicle and the first rib. This may reproduce the symptoms if a 'backpacker's neuropathy' is present.

Roos test (overhead exercise test)
The arms are abducted to 90°, shoulders externally rotated, and the elbows flexed to 90°. The hands are opened and closed for 3min to reproduce the symptoms. This may be positive in baseball pitchers with symptoms while in the cocking phase (though this mechanism may also represent an anterior instability). In extreme cases, there may also be blanching of the affected hand(s) with this test.

Subscapular bursa
- Located between the scapula and the thoracic wall.
- May be multiple small bursae.
- May become inflamed with over-use, causing 'snapping scapula'.
- Often difficult to diagnose.
- May need to managed surgically if persistent symptoms.

Nerves

The brachial plexus is a complex array of roots, trunks, divisions, cords, and branches.
- Any of these areas may be injured with compression or stretching of the brachial plexus.
- Because of the high incidence of anterior shoulder dislocations, the most likely peripheral nerve to be damaged is the axillary nerve.
- Other peripheral nerves that are likely to be damaged include the suprascapular, musculocutaneous, and the long thoracic nerves.

Shoulder disorders

Epidemiology
- Shoulder pain is the second most common musculoskeletal complaint seen by practitioners: 1.2–2.5% of attendances in primary care.
- Rotator cuff lesions (65%).
- Pericapsular soft tissue pain (11%).
- Acromioclavicular joint pain (10%).

Factors related to early recovery
- Mild trauma.
- Acute onset.
- Over-use problems.
- Early presentation.

Problems that are related to prolonged recovery
- Diabetes mellitus.
- Cervical spondylolysis.
- Radicular symptoms.
- Advancing age.
- Involvement of the dominant extremity.

Causes
Causes of increased susceptibility to injury include:
- An inherently less stable joint.
- The fact that we 'abuse' the joint with repetitive work activities and participate in sports that push the limits of the joint.

Differential diagnosis
Acute problems with rapid onset over days to a few weeks include:
- Trauma.
- Acute over-use.
- Cervical nerve root compression.

Age of the patient and history may narrow the differential diagnosis:
- Patients below the age of 45 often have a biomechanical cause to their problem, such as instability or tendinopathy..
- Those older than 45 are more likely to have degenerative conditions, such as osteoarthritis or rotator cuff tears.
- Evaluate the patient for adhesive capsulitis if there is a history of diabetes mellitus, progressive pain, and loss of motion.

Acute traumatic causes

Anterior glenohumeral instability
- From grade I, with less than 50% subluxation of the humeral head beyond the glenoid fossa, to grade IV, which is a complete dislocation.

Anterior dislocation
- If a patient lands on the posterior aspect of the shoulder during a fall forcing the humeral head anteriorly on the glenoid or if there is forced ER, while the upper extremity is abducted.
- The pressure of the anterior glenoid on the posterior humerus during dislocation may cause a small compression fracture or divot on the posterior humeral head known as a Hill–Sach's lesion.
- While the humeral head is being forced anteriorly, the anterior capsule may tear the labral cartilage away from the underlying glenoid, termed a Bankart lesion, worsening the anterior instability.

History and examination
- Patients usually present with pain in the anterior and lateral shoulder.
- They will often complain of an inability to move the shoulder without significant pain and, in many cases, 'know' it is dislocated.
- With an acute anterior dislocation, the acromioclavicular joint may be prominent on exam, and the shoulder appears 'sunken'.
- Patients will hold the arm in a partially abducted and externally rotated position.
- If the shoulder has relocated, they may have signs of instability on examination, or a positive Speed's test or apprehension test.

Investigation
- Diagnosis of dislocation is usually obvious on inspection.
- May be identified by X-ray evaluation, particularly the scapular Y view.
- A thorough neurovascular exam should be documented in all cases.

Treatment
- Immediate reduction preferably after evaluation by X-ray.
- Surgical intervention after the first dislocation is unusual, but may be appropriate in:
  - High performance athlete at risk for repeated dislocations (football, hockey, or other collision sport).
  - Worsening symptoms of instability despite conservative treatment.
- Consider a rotator cuff tear in the first time dislocater who is older than 45 years of age.
- There is a trend now towards immobilization in ER for a period of time, to allow tissues to heal in a more physiologic position.
- Followed by appropriate physiotherapy.

Posterior glenohumeral dislocation
Posterior dislocations account for only 4% of dislocations. Posterior dislocations generally require great force and are often seen after motor vehicle accidents, seizure activity, repetitive weight lifting, or in football linemen. The mechanism is usually a force applied to the forward flexed upper extremity at 90°, forcing the humerus posteriorly. It may also occur

after an anterior blow to the shoulder. A small avulsion of the posterior glenoid labrum may occur resulting in a reverse Bankart lesion.

History and examination
- Patients with posterior dislocations will present with the arm in IR, and held close to the thorax.
- They are generally unable to abduct or externally rotate the shoulder.
- The coracoid may be prominent and the humeral head difficult to palpate.

Investigations
- Routine shoulder films may miss this injury: only axillary or scapular Y views demonstrate this well.

Treatment
Treatment is reduction.

Inferior glenohumeral dislocation
Inferior glenohumeral dislocations are unusual because of the protection given by the acromion. This may represent a generalized laxity and be associated with multidirectional instability. The mechanism is usually a forced abduction injury aided by caudal pressure on the proximal upper arm. The acromion acts as a fulcrum and forces the humeral head inferiorly. Also called 'luxatio erecta' because of the shoulder position.

History and examination
- With chronic instability there is pain while the arm is down by the side or overhead.
- These patients may also complain of easy fatigability while carrying loads.
- On inspection the acromion may be prominent.
- There may be a positive sulcus sign.
- Forced abduction may cause pain or apprehension.

Investigations
Scapular Y views demonstrate this dislocation well.

Treatment
- Treatment is by immediate reduction with both pre- and post-reduction films.
- Rehabilitation.
- Surgical stabilization may be possible even if multidirectional instability is present.

Conservative management of shoulder dislocation

For the elite athlete, or in cases of reoccurrence, a surgical stabilization may be the treatment of choice. For most athletes, however, the first time dislocation will be managed conservatively. Estimated time to return to sport with conservative management: 3 months.

During all rehabilitation programmes following shoulder dislocation, it is important to ensure the appropriate balance and restoration of scapulo-thoracic stabilization, glenohumeral stabilization and humeral control, and the various neuromuscular mechanisms involved in their modulation.

Rehabilitation after shoulder dislocation

Immobilization stage

Initially, this will involve immobilization in a sling for 2–4 weeks. Longer periods of immobilization may be reserved for younger athletes.

Aims during immobilization
- Minimize atrophy of the shoulder muscles.
- Maintain elbow mobility and strength.
- Maintain wrist mobility and strength.

Treatment
- Electrical muscle stimulation.
- Isometric strengthening exercises:
  - Elbow—flexion and extension.
  - Grip strengthening.
- Active/assisted shoulder mobilizations within the limits of pain.

Post-immobilization: weeks 1–3 (early stage)

Aims
- Begin to assess and manage underlying risk factors.
- Begin strengthening of the rotator cuff complex.
- Begin joint approximation and neuromuscular exercises.
- Gain full passive ROM.
- Enhance static and dynamic control of shoulder complex.
- Improve shoulder complex positional awareness.

Assess risk factors
Some athletes are predisposed to shoulder dislocation. Internal risk factors interact with an inciting event (e.g. fall on an outstretched arm) or in certain cases extrinsic risk factors (e.g. poor underfoot conditions), to cause the injury. Highlighting risk factors and implementing an appropriate rehabilitation programme can greatly decrease the chance of reoccurrence.

NB Adolescent athletes run a high risk of re-dislocating their shoulder, if they are managed conservatively. This should be clarified at the early stages of rehabilitation.

Common intrinsic risk factors
- Mechanical instability/hypermobility.
- Functional instability/decreased joint positional sense.
- Muscle weakness of:
  - The rotator cuff complex.
  - Lower trapezius.
  - Rhomboids.
  - Serratus anterior.
- Poor scapulo-humeral rhythm.
- Poor technique, e.g. tackling in contact sports.
- Inappropriate training drills.
- Poor general conditioning.

- Previous injury.
- Injury from inciting event, e.g. Bankart lesion, Hills–Sachs lesion, glenoid labrum damage.

General exercises

Mobility
- Active assisted exercises up to full shoulder elevation through the scapular plane.

Shoulder complex strengthening
- *Postural correction:*
  - Athlete focuses on finding and maintaining a good postural (neutral) position of the shoulder complex in a prone position, progressing to supine, sitting and standing.
  - Athletes are then encouraged to maintain a good (neutral) shoulder complex posture and move the arm actively into the scapular plane.
- *Scapulo-thoracic training:*
  - Shoulder blade squeezes—athlete is instructed to pull shoulder blades together and downwards with arm in neutral position. This can be progressed by repeating this movement with arms in 45° abduction.
  - Pillow squeezes—athlete places a pillow in their axilla, they then adduct their arm to squeeze it against their body.
  - Serratus anterior training—in supine lying, athletes straighten their arm into end position for bench press, they are then encouraged to reach further towards the ceiling by protracting their scapula.
- *Joint approximation/positional sense training:* in a prone position with both forearms in contact with the ground, the athlete gently transfers weight over to the injured side. *NB* both forearms remain in contact with the ground at all times. Athlete must aim to prevent shoulder blade protraction/winging.
- *Isometric strengthening exercises:* This should be performed in a neutral shoulder position with the flexed elbow resting on a table or similar surface. Using their unaffected limb, the athlete adds resistance to the affected side (5–10s hold × 8 reps × 3 sets). After 2 weeks, the athlete should perform these exercises in various positions of elevation within the scapular plane. Shoulder movements strengthened should include:
  - Flexion.
  - Extension.
  - IR.
  - ER.
  - Abduction.
  - Adduction.
- *Dynamic strengthening exercises:* these should be initiated in side lying, before progressing to standing. Movements should include:
  - *IR*—from neutral to full IR.
  - *ER*—from full IR to neutral.
  - *IR*—from full ER to full IR.
  - *ER*—from full IR to full ER.
  - *Flexion*—neutral to 30°.
  - *Abduction*—neutral to 30°.

See Fig. 17.3.

Post-immobilization:.weeks 4–10 (middle stage)

Aims
- Progress strengthening.
- Increase neuromuscular control.

General exercises
- Neuromuscular exercises in the middle stages of rehabilitation should incorporate progressive weight-bearing (axial loading) of the shoulder joint. Initially, the hand should be placed on a fixed stable base of support, progressing to a moveable surface:
  - In a four point kneeling (hands and knees) position, keeping knees and hands in contact with the floor, gently transfer weight to each corner of support. *To progress:* Lift the uninjured arm from the floor; lift uninjured arm and contralateral hip from the floor.
- Push-ups.
  - *Pushups plus*: at the end of each press-up, keeping the elbows straight, protract shoulder as far as possible; ensure movement happens in straight line and that the thoracic spine does not excessively flex; keep head in neutral position; try to keep shoulder blades flat against back.
  - *Step press ups*: athlete performs press ups with one arm on a small step, and the other on the ground; alternate leading arms.
- *To progress*: increase the speed of the movements; use dynamic surface, e.g. a press up with hands resting on a Wobble board or with feet resting on a balance pad.

Rhythmic stabilization exercises
These are short, fast, oscillatory movements at the shoulder joint used to develop muscle activation, endurance, and neuromuscular control. Rehabilitation tools such as a body blade may be useful adjuncts at this stage of rehabilitation. Typical progressions may be as follows:
- Oscillate the body blade as quickly as possible ensuring that movement occurs through rotation of the glenohumeral joint *not* wrist, elbow, or shoulder girdle movement (Fig. 17.3).
- *To progress*, perform in the following positions:
  - Neutral with elbow bent to 90°.
  - 45° abduction side with elbow bent to 90°.
  - 90° abduction side with elbow bent to 90°.
  - Arm above head.
  - Throwing position.
  - All fours with affected arm raised in front.

Strengthening
Once the athlete has gained a good baseline of shoulder control and strength in a neutral position, strengthening through range is essential and should progress to include a rotatory component. The following shoulder strengthening exercises may be included:
- IR.
- ER.
- *Scaption exercises*: shoulder abduction with IR (empty can) using theraband or light dumbbell.

- Horizontal abduction using cable.
- Horizontal abduction using theraband or light dumbbell.
- Seated row using cable pulley or theraband.

More functional or sports specific strength training can be undertaken using combined movements. For most sports these should focus on diagonal, multiplanar shoulder movements. For example a Sword draw exercise, which involves moving from shoulder IR/adduction/extension to ER/abduction/flexion with an extended elbow.

In other sports it may be important to introduce a flight/plyometric phase at this stage. This might be initiated as follows:
- Stand in front of wall with shoulder in 90° flexion.
- Slowly fall forwards against wall onto outstretched hand.
- Push backwards off wall using protraction of shoulder—*not* elbow or wrist movement.
- Progress by standing further away from wall

Post-immobilization:.weeks 10–12 (end stage)

Aims
- Advanced neuromuscular control.
- Increase strength and power
- Focus on sports-specific rehabilitation.

Neuromuscular progressions

For most sports, end stage rehabilitation should incorporate unstable surfaces and rotational, multi-directional exercises. These may include:
- *Axial compression with rotation (closed chain rotation)*: the athlete adopts a press up position with hands on a slide board or other low friction surface. Keeping both hands in contact with the surface, they must perform alternative rotational movements at the arm (as if they were polishing the surface). To progress: increase the size and speed of the movements.
- *Press up to rotate*: in full elbow extension the athlete lifts the uninjured arm, and brings it into abduction, whilst maintaining single arm support and control with the weight-bearing injured arm.
- *Gym ball walk outs*: the athlete starts in a press up position with both their thighs resting on a gym ball and their hands on the floor in front; they must walk forwards and backwards on their hands, allowing the gym ball to roll under their body. To progress: place hands onto other labile surfaces, e.g. balance pad, medicine ball, or add time constraints.
- *Clap press ups*: advanced exercises could also involve a clap press up undertaken on a dynamic surface, e.g. medicine ball, Wobble cushion, gym ball.

Eccentric external rotator strength

Essential for safe return to throwing activities. Eccentric external rotator strengthening should be carried out only when the athlete has adequate control and stability to do so. High load eccentric training should be introduced gradually at first to avoid significant muscle soreness and associated reduction in upper limb control.

- Eccentric ER can be trained initially using the following exercises:
  - Sit with arm in 90° abduction, use unaffected arm to position shoulder in ER. Theraband can be used in the early stages to provide resistance. Slowly and in a controlled manner, internally rotate the shoulder.
  - This can be progressed by using a cable pulley system or dumbbell.
  - Further progression is introduced by removing any support for the elbow and moving further into a functional throwing position, and by gradually increasing the speed of movement.
- More advanced eccentric ER training may be undertaken using a modified dumbbell that has weight applied to only one end:
  - Athlete holds the end where there is no weight and, with the shoulder in the correct position, forcefully internally rotates the shoulder as quickly as possible.
  - The external rotators must eccentrically contract to brake the movement. Begin with 3 sets of 4 reps progressing to sets of 12 reps.

Strength and conditioning

Initially, the athlete should carry out each activity using dumb bells. Form and fatigue can be compared with the uninjured side.

A typical circuit might include:
- Chest press.
- Shoulder press.
- Chin ups.
- Upright rows.
- Bicep curls.
- Triceps extensions.

On successful completion of a dumbbell strengthening programme, the athlete may progress back into Olympic lifting drills. Technical drills should be used initially before increasing weight and resistance.

Athletes returning to contact sports may have a higher risk of reoccurrence, therefore other higher demanding conditioning drills may be of benefit in the later stages of rehabilitation, and these include:
- Single arm cleans.
- Pec fly/alternate pec fly.
- Eccentric dumbbell catch: this should involve high speed ER rotation training, at 90° of shoulder abduction.
- Medicine ball throws:
  - These should begin with two hands using: chest pass; overhead—forwards and back; and lateral throw at waist height/shoulder height/in elevation.
  - Progress to single arm: throwing forwards from 90° abduction; and these can be carried out lying on a gym ball or standing and throwing the ball against a wall.
- Overhead squat or other advanced Olympic lifting drills, such as wide arm shoulder press, or snatch balance.

Return to play

Prior to a safe return to play, the athlete must have achieved the following:
- Full pain-free ROM.
- Negative shoulder apprehension test
- Regained/improved static and dynamic control of the shoulder complex through all resisted movements/weight bearing movements.
- Strength equal to uninjured side—in particular through IR and ER. An isokinetic measurement of IR and ER in 90° of abduction may be the most challenging and functional test of strength.
- Full participation in strength and conditioning.
- Negative apprehension/sound technique during higher risk sporting activity, e.g. front- or side-on tackling in rugby football.

Example of final pitch-based rehabilitation

For example rugby, football.

The very nature of contact/collision sports increase the risk of shoulder injury, therefore prior to a full return to training, athletes must be strong enough and confident enough to perform every potential match scenario that may involve direct or indirect shoulder contact.

Note that in each of these drills, the athlete should be technically and tactically proficient; therefore, the lead rehabilitation therapist may require input and advice from coaching staff.

- *Down and ups*: in these drills the athlete must drop onto the ground before quickly pushing back onto their feet. Variations include:
  - Dropping onto front.
  - Dropping onto R/L side.
  - Dropping to retrieve a ball.
- *Contact drills:*
  - Side contacts (athlete makes side on body contact with a tackle pad/bag or player using the injured shoulder, with his/her arm remaining in minimal abduction).
  - Athlete performs a rugby hand off, with increasing running speed, and at various angles.
  - *Taking tackles*: initially, this can be performed at walking pace and progressed to include a game related skill such as presenting the ball/passing the ball out of the tackle.
  - *Making tackles*: initially the target (tackle bag/pad/player) should be static. Tackle difficultly should be progressed from making a front on tackle, to a side on tackle. Further progression should be made through increase of speed/strength of hit/intensity of the session, tackling a dynamic target, adding tactical decision making.

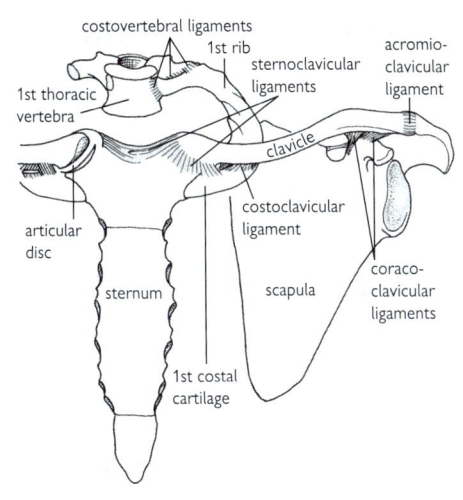

Fig. 17.3 Bones and ligaments of the shoulder girdle. Reproduced with permission from MacKinnon P and Morris J (2005). *Oxford Textbook of Functional Anatomy*, Vol. 1. Oxford University Press, Oxford © 2005.

Acromioclavicular joint separations

Acute acromioclavicular sprains or separations are a common traumatic injury, usually resulting from a fall onto the lateral shoulder.
- Grade I is a mild sprain to the acromioclavicular ligaments. There is no separation of the acromioclavicular joint compared with the unaffected side.
- Grade II involves rupture of the acromioclavicular ligament, but the coracoclavicular ligament is intact. There is less than 1cm displacement of the acromion from the clavicle.
- Grade III involves complete rupture of both acromioclavicular and coracoclavicular ligaments.
- Grades IV, V, and VI injuries are also described, and will usually require referral, but these are rare.

History and examination
- Patients will usually present with pain in the lateral shoulder. Sometimes over the distal trapezius with radiation to the proximal humerus. There may be swelling and/or bruising in anterior shoulder.
- Motion is usually intact, but limited by pain.
- Palpation over the acromioclavicular joint may be tender.
- The patient may not feel pain if there is a Grade III separation and may only sense instability.
- The cross-over test may be positive.

Investigations
- The diagnosis is usually made on examination.
- Grading of sprains relies on radiological examination with comparison with the opposite shoulder.
- Weighted films to overcome splinting due to pain have not been shown to be necessary. (These were previously done to distinguish Grade II from Grade III sprains, to make decisions regarding surgery; but there is no advantage to operative fixation of Grade III sprains.)

Treatment
- Treatment is primarily symptomatic.
- The shoulder should be immobilized for a short period of time (1–2 days for a Grade I, and 5–7 days for a Grade III).
- Braces and long-term use of slings are not recommended.
- Range of motion exercises should be started as soon as tolerated.
- Surgical stabilization is usually not necessary. Only indicated for chronic pain, instability, or for aesthetic reasons. In cases of aesthetics, the patient may only be 'trading a bump for a scar'.

Sternoclavicular joint separations

Sternoclavicular joint separations are much less common than acromioclavicular separations. Anterior and/or superior subluxations are seen more frequently than posterior subluxations. The injury involves disruption of both the sternoclavicular and costoclavicular ligaments. They are graded as first, second, or third degree injuries depending on the degree of associated capsular disruption. The most common mechanism is a fall onto the lateral or posterolateral shoulder, often with a concurrent force applied to the opposite shoulder. This may be seen in a takedown in wrestling or a pile-up in football or rugby. Less commonly, a posteriorly-directed force directly over the sternoclavicular joint may occur, which can result in a posterior dislocation.

History and examination
While elevating the shoulder there may be a visually or palpably obvious subluxation accompanied by a pop or click.

Investigations
- The dislocation is more easily seen on the serendipity view during plain film examination.
- If suspicion is high, but not obvious on plain film there may be a role for CT scan or MRI in the diagnosis.
- The proximal clavicular epiphysis does not fuse until the patient is in the early 20's, therefore there is possibility of fracture through this.

Treatment
- Treatment consists of rest, ice, and NSAIDs.
- Third degree injuries are rare, but serious if present because of the possibility of superior mediastinal injury and injury to the great vessels. These cases must be reduced immediately.
- *On-the-field technique:* can put a sandbag underneath shoulder-blades with the patient supine, traction to abducted arm in line with clavicle. Sometimes need to use a towel clip to grab onto clavicle.
- If unable to reduce this way, have to proceed to the operating room.
- Chronic subluxations can occur in overhead sports, such as volleyball, and can be troublesome to manage. In sports such as rowing, it may be possible to have the athlete switch sides, or switch to sculling.

Glenoid labrum tears

Glenoid labrum tears are most often seen after a glenohumeral dislocation. These patients typically have fallen onto an outstretched arm or have an over-use injury, such as in throwing athletes. During an anterior dislocation, the humeral head may tear the anterior and inferior labrum off the underlying glenoid. This may result in a Bankart lesion. If the lesion is present in the superior labrum extending anteriorly to posteriorly beneath the biceps tendon it is termed a superior labrum anterior to posterior (SLAP) lesion. SLAP lesions are associated with marked anterior instability, Bankart lesions, and rotator cuff tears.

Labral lesions are graded as follows:
- *Type 1:* fraying of the superior labrum.
- *Type 2:* fraying plus separation from glenoid.
- *Type 3:* bucket-handle tear of the superior labrum.
- *Type 4:* bucket-handle tear extending into the biceps tendon.

Posterior impingement

Partial tear of the posterior superior glenoid labrum, which may lead to impingement of the rotator cuff. Seen in throwing athletes. The tear itself may be due to traction of the biceps tendon on the superior labrum and posterior rotator cuff weakness. This leads to anterior and superior humeral translation and pinching of the posterior inferior structures during the cocking phase of throwing or in overhead activities.

History and examination
- Glenoid labrum tears are often seen in throwers with pain during the cocking, release, and/or follow-through phases of the throw.
- The pain is usually present in the posterior shoulder.
- Popping, clicking, and snapping are also common complaints.
- They may notice that they cannot throw as hard or for as long as they could previously.
- On examination, patients with labral tears often have a positive Speed's test and often have positive labral tests.
- They may be tender to palpation around the anterior and posterior glenohumeral capsule.
- Signs of anterior instability may also be present.

Investigations
- Routine X-rays are usually normal unless a bony Bankart or Hill–Sachs lesion is seen.
- Diagnosis is usually based on MRI or CT evaluation. (Double contrast CT scans may elucidate labral pathology, but not as well as MRI. An MRI arthrogram may delineate labral lesions best, but with newer higher resolution MRI machines, this may not be necessary.)

Treatment
If a labral tear is suspected, referral is appropriate because of the chronic nature of the injury, instability, and impingement symptoms.

Biceps tendon rupture

Complete disruption of the tendinous fibres of the biceps occurs most often within the bicipital groove. Occasionally, it presents at the distal tendinous pole. Rupture occurs during a forceful flexion of the elbow, often during weight-lifting or catching a heavy object.

History and examination
- The patient has immediate pain either in the shoulder and proximal biceps, or in the distal biceps.
- Occasionally, there is swelling and ecchymosis.
- They may feel a pop or snap during the initial injury.
- On examination they usually have an obvious bulging defect in the biceps, caused by the retraction of the muscle belly, and referred to as the 'Popeye defect'.
- They may have mild weakness to resisted flexion of the elbow and supination of the forearm if there is a proximal rupture. This may be quite pronounced if there is a distal rupture.

Investigations
- Plain films are usually normal.
- Diagnostic US may be useful.
- An MRI is only necessary if the diagnosis is uncertain.

Treatment
- Treatment of proximal biceps ruptures is conservative, with good results especially in the elderly. The defect generally remains.
- Surgery is indicated if there is a distal tendon rupture at the elbow or a complete tear of the tendons of both the short and long heads of the proximal biceps.
- With single proximal tendon tears, there may only be a surgical indication for heavy manual workers, certain athletes, or for cosmetic reasons.

Biceps tendon dislocation

Biceps tendon dislocation occurs because of retinacular incompetence allowing the long head of the biceps to separate from the bicipital groove of the humeral head. This is often seen in conjunction with a rotator cuff tear or in impingement syndrome.

History and examination
- The patient will present with pain in the anterior shoulder sometimes associated with a snapping or clicking sensation.
- These symptoms may be more pronounced with overhead activities, or with internal and ER.
- On examination they usually have a positive Speed's and Yergason's test.
- They may also have signs of a rotator cuff injury or impingement.

Investigations
- Diagnosis is by history and clinical exam.
- MRI is not usually indicated, but dynamic diagnostic US may be extremely helpful to visualize subluxation/dislocation of tendon.

Treatment
- Conservative treatment if there is an isolated biceps tendon dislocation.
- If the patient fails conservative treatment, surgical stabilization may be attempted.
- Associated rotator cuff tears and impingement should be treated as indicated.

Fractures of the shoulder

Clavicle fractures

History and examination
- Clavicle fractures are very common, and usually follow a fall or a direct blow to the clavicle.
- There is immediate pain and, if there is an associated pneumothorax, there may be shortness of breath or signs of a tension pneumothorax.
- With severe displacement, the brachial plexus may be damaged.
- Evaluate the patient for swelling and deformity of the clavicle, any subcutaneous crepitation, pneumothorax, or neurovascular deficits of the upper extremity.
- X-ray should include clavicular views and a chest film.

Treatment
- Even significantly displaced fractures of the middle third of the clavicle will heal well functionally.
- Management of uncomplicated clavicular fractures includes a sling or figure of eight brace until comfortable, followed by range of motion exercises.
- Referral is necessary with comminuted fractures.
- Treatment of very proximal and very distal fractures is controversial, and referral may be appropriate. There is a tendency at the present time towards operative fixation with a reconstruction or dynamic compression plate, particularly in athletes such as rowers, in whom it is necessary that the healed clavicle be out to length.

Scapular fractures
- Fractures of the scapula are rare.
- Because of the severe trauma required to fracture the scapula, always assess for trauma to other areas. If the fracture is through the scapular notch, there may be associated nerve compression from haematoma.
- The treatment of most scapular fractures involves immobilization in a sling for two to three weeks accompanied by early range of motion exercises as tolerated.
- Significantly displaced scapular fractures or those that involve the glenoid, neck, acromion, or coracoid require orthopaedic referral.

Fractures of the proximal humerus
- Most proximal humeral fractures can be treated by immobilization in a sling for 1–3 weeks.
- The patient should start range of motion exercises as soon as tolerated.
- In about 20% of fractures there is displacement of the humeral head, the lesser or greater tuberosity, or the humeral shaft. Fractures of the anatomic neck, epiphyseal plate, greater tuberosity avulsion fractures, or fractures involving the humeral head also need to be referred.
- Avulsion fractures of the greater tuberosity at the insertion of the supraspinatus can be managed conservatively.

Chronic over-use disorders

Instability of the glenohumeral joint

History and examination
- Some patients may present with pain, but no history of trauma. This is often seen with repetitive throwing and overhead work, which can cause small labral or capsule tears, and place extra stress upon the rotator cuff muscles. Recurrent microtrauma may lead to impingement syndrome or osteoarthritis.
- Those with anterior instability typically have a positive apprehension sign, relocation test, and possibly an anterior load and shift test.
- In posterior instability there may be a positive posterior apprehension sign, and perhaps a positive posterior load and shift test.
- Having the patient do a push-up against the wall may reproduce symptoms.
- Inferior instability may show upon examination as a positive sulcus sign.
- Carrying weights or suitcases may reproduce symptoms.
- Multidirectional instability may have signs of anterior, posterior, and/or inferior instability. These patients may have generalized joint laxity (assess the knees and elbows for hyperextensibility, the ability to abduct the thumb to the forearm when the wrist is flexed, or extension of the metacarpophalangeal joints past 90°).

Investigation
- Routine X-rays may show signs of chronic subluxation, such as erosion of the glenoid rim, Hill–Sachs lesions, and lesser tuberosity fractures. X-ray can also show a Bankart lesion.
- An MRI may be useful in diagnosing small labral tears and demonstrate a rotator cuff tear, if suspected.

Treatment
- 80–90% of non-traumatic instabilities respond well to physical therapy, but do poorly with surgical intervention.
- If the initial dislocation occurred before the age of 30, only about one-third need operative treatment.
- If a Hill–Sach's lesion, attenuated ligaments, or a torn labrum are present, if recurrent dislocations occur after rehabilitation or if the patient plateaus at an unacceptable level, physical therapy will probably not resolve the problem, and the patient may benefit from a stabilizing procedure.

Impingement syndrome and tendinopathy of the rotator cuff muscles (supraspinatus, infraspinatus, subscapularis)

Impingement syndrome is an over-use injury with impingement of the rotator cuff muscles between the greater tuberosity of the humerus and the acromion, coracoid, and/or coracoacromial ligament (Figs. 17.4 and 17.5). The rotator cuff, biceps tendon, and the subacromial bursa may all be affected. It occurs with over-use of the shoulder or in chronic instability. It is more accurately described as tendinopathy of the affected tendon(s), as it has been demonstrated that there is little to no inflammation in the tissue (i.e. not 'tendonitis'), only degenerative changes.

The supraspinatus and biceps tendons are at particular risk because of their position under the coraco-acromial arch. If the humeral head moves superiorly due to the laxity, the resulting instability may accentuate impingement symptoms. Increased mechanical irritation of the bursa and rotator cuff muscles over time can result in increased fibrosis and partial thickness rotator cuff tears and/or partial thickness biceps tendon tears. Eventually, this may lead to full thickness rotator cuff and biceps tendon tears. The combination of laxity and impingement is often seen in swimmers and overhead throwers. Impingement syndrome may also result from direct trauma (such as a fall onto an elbow or an outstretched hand), muscular imbalances, posterior capsule tightness, or anatomical overgrowth of the acromion process. Impingement is rarely seen in patients less than 40 years of age, unless there is trauma involved or they are a pitcher. Sports at particular risk are pitching, swimming, tennis, weight lifting, and golf, especially if the patient is overtraining or has poor technique.

History and examination
- The onset of pain is usually gradual and may be present for weeks or months. It is usually located in the lateral deltoid just distal to the tip of the acromion. It may also present with pain in the biceps radiating down to the elbow.
- Pain is usually worsened with overhead activities and when lying on the involved side, and may be worse at night.
- The patient may complain of popping, snapping, or grinding.
- On examination, there may be pain between 90–120° of abduction (painful arc).
- There may be tenderness with internal and ER while the shoulder is at 90° of abduction.
- Hawkin's and Neer's tests may be positive.
- The impingement test is usually positive.
- There may be signs of rotator cuff and biceps tendon irritation as well as frank weakness due to pain. This must be re-evaluated after treatment to rule out a complete or partial tear of these tendons.

Investigation
- Radiographic evaluation is usually normal unless there is acromial overgrowth or degenerative joint disease.
- Radiological evidence of calcification suggests calcific tendonitis (see Calcific tendinopathy of the hip, p. 608).

Treatment
- Treatment is with rest, range of motion exercises, and strengthening exercises of the scapular stabilizing muscles and thorax.
- Injection of steroids across (but not into) the superior aspect of the rotator cuff may be of benefit to some patients.
- More recently, injection of platelet-rich plasma (PRP) into partial rotator cuff tears is being tried (under US guidance). Although there is little to no evidence for this, anecdotally it appears to help.
- If conservative measures fail after 6 weeks or if partial or complete tears are present surgical intervention should be obtained.
- Prevention is by avoidance of improper techniques used in overhead sport activities and minimizing offending activities.

Rotator cuff tears

Rotator cuff tears occur when there is a complete separation of the tendinopathic fibres. Most cases are seen in patients over 40 years of age and most have longstanding impingement symptoms. This may be due to age, vascular changes, trauma, attrition, or impingement. If acute trauma is involved, it is usually due to a fall onto an abducted arm or a direct blow to the lateral shoulder. The most likely tendon to be affected is the supraspinatus (Fig. 17.4). The tear may then extend to the infraspinatus, and in severe cases, it may involve the teres minor and biceps tendon. The subscapularis (Fig. 17.5) is rarely involved.

History and examination
- The patient usually presents with weakness and poorly localized pain that may radiate to the humerus.
- Pain is worsened with overhead activities.
- Approximately 50% associate their pain with a specific trauma.
- Inspection may demonstrate wasting of the supraspinatus and infraspinatus if the problem has been longstanding.
- The rotator cuff may be tender to palpation or there may be crepitus in the subacromial bursa.
- Direct testing of the muscles of the rotator cuff will demonstrate weakness when compared with the unaffected side (Jobe's test and Gerber's manoeuvre).
- The strength of the external rotators may be affected in extensive tears due to the involvement of the infraspinatus.
- Patients usually have less tenderness with passive than active range of motion.
- Most patients will have one or more of the lag signs present, and possibly a positive drop arm test.
- Tests for impingement are often positive including the Hawkin's, Neer's, and the impingement test.

Investigation
- Plain films may only show acromial overgrowth.
- The gold standard had been the arthrogram, but it is less reliable in diagnosing partial thickness tears and unreliable in determining the size and extent of tears.
- MRI (and sometimes diagnostic US) is now used more often as a non-invasive replacement that can differentiate complete and partial tears and visualize other shoulder conditions, such as articular cartilage damage or tears of the glenoid labrum.
- Unless a complete rotator cuff tear is suspected, an MRI or CT need not be obtained unless the patient has failed 6–8 weeks of conservative therapy. An arthrogram or MRI adds little information unless surgical intervention is planned. Diagnostic US is less expensive, and may be less sensitive and specific but specificity and sensitivity are highly reliant on technician expertise.

CHRONIC OVER-USE DISORDERS 493

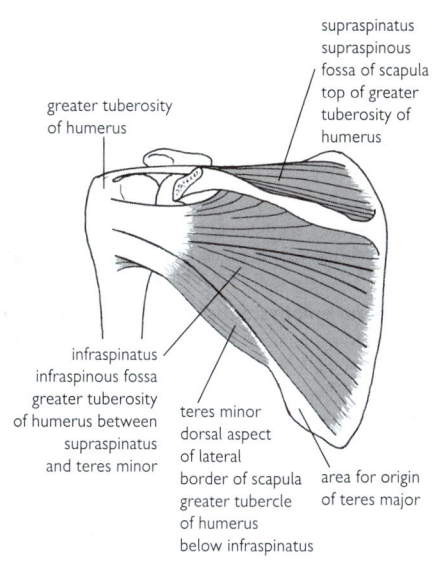

Fig. 17.4 Supraspinatus, infraspinatus, teres minor; acromion removed. Reproduced with permission from MacKinnon P and Morris J (2005). *Oxford Textbook of Functional Anatomy*, Vol. 1. Oxford University Press, Oxford. ©2005.

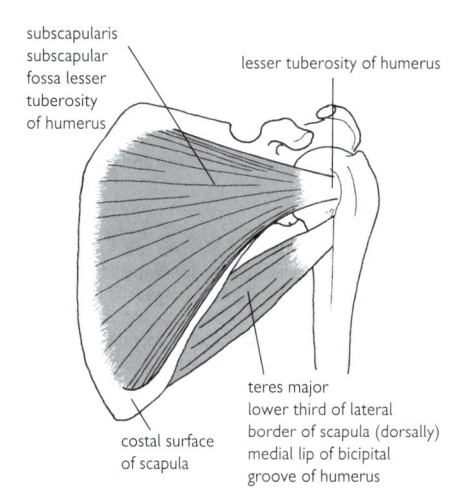

Fig. 17.5 Subscapularis and teres major. Reproduced with permission from MacKinnon P and Morris J (2005). *Oxford Textbook of Functional Anatomy*, Vol. 1. Oxford University Press, Oxford. ©2005.

Treatment
- Treatment is usually with rest, and protection and avoidance of all overhead activities.
- Physical therapy.
- Subacromial injections are recommended by some experts but the evidence from randomized controlled trials is equivocal and there is some suggestion that they may impede tendon repair. Use in patients over 40 with caution.
- If symptoms persist for more than 6–8 weeks, or if there are high demands by the patient, they should be referred to orthopaedic assessment for debridement of partial thickness tears or repair of full thickness tears. Mostly done arthroscopically now.

Proximal humeral epiphysiolitis (Little Leaguer's shoulder)

Stress injury to proximal humeral physis to shear forces associated with repetitive throwing and pitching. May be the first stage of a continuum to a physeal stress fracture.

History and examination
- Usually presents in adolescence with shoulder pain on throwing.
- No history of specific injury.
- Usually full ROM.
- Swelling uncommon.

Investigation
- AP X-ray in ER demonstrates widening of proximal humeral physis. May need to be compared with other side.

Treatment
- Rest from throwing (usually >2 months required).
- Graduated return to throwing when asymptomatic.
- Adhere to age guidelines regarding pitching limits and correct throwing technique (if needed) to prevent recurrence.

Prognosis
- Usually good.
- Small risk of premature growth plate closure and subsequent humeral length discrepancy.

Biceps tendinopathy

Biceps tendinopathy is characterized by pain and sometimes inflammation of the long head of the biceps tendon within the bicipital groove. These patients are usually young or middle aged. This condition is often due to repetitive elbow flexion or supination, and in particular activities that require reaching, and overhead lifting; recreational activities, such as tennis, swimming, golf, or throwing sports. It is often associated with impingement syndrome and/or rotator cuff tears.

History and examination
- The patient will present with diffuse pain in the anterior shoulder.
- The pain is usually worse during and directly after activity and improves with rest.
- There is usually no pain at night.

- Symptoms may be present for a variable length of time.
- On examination there is tenderness with resisted flexion of the elbow and supination of the wrist.
- There may be tenderness to palpation within the bicipital groove and along the long head of the biceps tendon.
- There may also be limitation of the extremes of abduction, IR, and ER.
- Speed's and Yergason's test are typically positive for pain.
- There may be biceps weakness secondary to pain.

Investigations
- X-rays are usually normal.
- MRI is usually not warranted unless a repairable biceps or rotator cuff tear is suspected. Diagnostic US will sometimes show fluid in the biceps tendon sheath.

Treatment
- Rest, ice, local heat, and protection.
- Gentle stretching and exercise.
- The patient may benefit from a formal physical therapy programme if a quick return to activities is important.
- Oral anti-inflammatories may be of benefit.
- While injection of the tendon with corticosteroids directly is not recommended, subacromial injection or US-guided injection into the biceps tendon sheath may be of benefit.

Calcific tendonitis

With degeneration of the collagen fibres of the rotator cuff tendons, calcium salts may infiltrate the substance of the tendon and cause inflammation. This may be associated with acute or chronic symptoms, and may secondarily involve the bursa. The most common site is the supraspinatus tendon, but it may also occur in/around the biceps tendon, infraspinatus, or subscapularis tendons.

History and examination
- There may be severe pain affecting sleep.
- If calcification is chronic, the patient may have symptoms more like an impingement syndrome.
- On examination, the patient may hold the arm splinted against the body, and be in such pain that examination is not possible.
- Any palpation over the affected area produces significant tenderness.
- The tenderness may affect range of motion.
- A globally tender shoulder that the patient is unwilling to move.

Investigations
- X-ray examination of the shoulder may show calcifications.
- AP views in ER and IR will show the rotator cuff best.
- Bicipital groove views show biceps tendon calcifications.
- Diagnostic US is useful for diagnosis and treatment.

Treatment
- Treatment by injection of a lidocaine and steroid preparation may be effective and provide dramatic relief. Protect biceps movement for 2 weeks after such an injection.
- Oral anti-inflammatories rarely provide as significant an improvement.
- Physical therapy.
- Surgical intervention is rarely required.

Acromioclavicular degenerative joint disease

Degenerative joint disease of the acromioclavicular joint is common and develops much earlier than that of the glenohumeral or sternoclavicular joint.

History and examination
- The patient usually complains of intermittent pain, gradual in onset, but may present after trauma.
- There may be intermittent swelling, popping, clicking, or grinding.
- On examination the patient is usually tender over the superior and anterior aspect of the acromioclavicular joint.
- There may be a prominence to the acromioclavicular joint on inspection.
- The cross-over test is usually positive.

Investigations
- X-ray.
- Diagnosis can be verified by injection of lidocaine into the joint, and resolution of the pain supports the diagnosis.

Treatment
- Treatment is usually symptomatic.
- Injection with a steroid may be of benefit.
- Surgical intervention consists of resection of the distal clavicle and removal of the intra-articular disc, if present, but is unusual.

Adhesive capsulitis (frozen shoulder)

Adhesive capsulitis may be due to prolonged immobilization or disuse due to pain, reflex sympathetic dystrophy, or idiopathy. The pathophysiology is unclear. Patients with diabetes mellitus are more at risk. The patient is often female with involvement of the non-dominant arm.

History and examination
- The pain is usually gradual in onset and located over the insertion of the deltoids.
- Patients may report difficulty sleeping on the affected side.
- On examination, active and passive range of motion to abduction, IR, and ER, are limited by adhesions in the capsule.
- There is no specific point tenderness, but often a diffuse tenderness exists especially with movement.

Treatment
- Treatment is by intensive physical therapy.
- Cortisosteroid injection into the glenohumeral joint can also be tried.

- It may take years to completely resolve, and the disease can recur later in the opposite shoulder.
- Surgical manipulation under anesthesia may be required.

Osteolysis of the distal clavicle

Often caused by chronic over-use, but may also be initiated by an acute traumatic injury. Weight-lifters appear to be more prone. Osteolysis of the distal clavicle usually presents with chronic pain in the lateral superior shoulder lasting longer than four months.

History and examination
- Pain is usually a dull ache over the acromioclavicular joint. There may be weakness and pain with flexion and adduction.

Investigation
- Diagnosis is usually by plain X-ray, which may show osteopenia with tapering of the distal clavicle, and associated osteophytes, subchondral erosions, and cysts. There is a typical 'moth-eaten' appearance to the joint. Early disease can be diagnosed with a bone scan. Can be bilateral.

Treatment
- Injection of corticosteroids into the joint can be useful.
- Treatment is usually by surgical resection of the distal end of the clavicle (Mumford procedure), if the pain is unacceptable.

Atraumatic causes

Thoracic outlet syndrome
There are four areas of potential compression:
- Compression of the subclavian vein between the anterior scalene, clavicle, and first rib.
- Compression of the brachial plexus and subclavian artery between the anterior scalene, middle scalene, and first rib.
- Compression of the neurovascular bundle between the clavicle and the first rib.
- Compression of the neurovascular bundle as it passes under the tendinous portion of the pectoralis minor.

Cervical ribs are the most common bony anomaly seen with thoracic outlet syndrome. 10% of these, however, are asymptomatic. Trauma, as a precipitating factor, is not uncommon.

History and examination
- Patients may complain of neurologic, vascular, or combined symptoms.
- Neurological symptoms consist of pain, often sharp, but sometimes aching, that radiates from the neck or shoulder into the forearm or hand, often following an ulnar nerve distribution.
- Paresthesias and hyperaesthesias may also be present.
- Symptoms may be exacerbated by overhead activity.
- Vascular symptoms that originate from the subclavian artery may cause pain over the supraclavicular space.
- There may be associated pale, cold, or numb fingers.
- Activities that involve elevation or abduction of the arm may worsen such symptoms.
- Compression of the subclavian vein may cause pain over the supraclavicular space or the feeling of pressure in the extremity.
- On examination, the extremity may appear dusky, swollen, mottled, or blue, or it may appear entirely normal.
- The patient may have a positive Wright's manoeuvre, Roos manoeuvre, and/or Adson's test.

Investigations
- X-ray evaluation of the cervical spine and chest.
- If vascular compromise, Doppler studies will usually define the area of concern. Angiograms are usually necessary if there are abnormalities seen on Doppler.
- Electrodiagnostic studies may be needed if neurologic compromise is suspected.

Treatment
- Shoulder strengthening exercises concentrating on posterior scapular stabilization, if the patient's symptoms are not disabling or consistent with vascular compromise.
- If there is vascular compromise, or conservative treatment fails, surgical intervention usually consists of resection of the first rib.

Reflex sympathetic dystrophy (shoulder-hand syndrome)

History and examination
- Shoulder involvement is common in reflex sympathetic dystrophy.
- Clinically, it presents as pain and limitation of motion with dystrophic skin changes of the ipsilateral hand and arm.
- There may be pain and swelling in the distal extremity.
- It is bilateral in 25–30% of cases.
- Risk factors include cardiovascular disease, recent myocardial infarction, cervical disc disease, and shoulder, arm, or neck trauma.
- No obvious inciting event is present in at least 25% of the patients.

Investigations
- Abnormal resting sweat output (RSO) studies in combination with quantitative sudomotor axon reflex tests (QSART) are thought to correlate strongly with the diagnosis of reflex sympathetic dystrophy.
- Technetium pyrophosphate bone scan is a sensitive tool and demonstrates increased blood flow to the involved extremity and mild synovitis.
- X-rays may show peri-articular osteoporosis, and erosions.

Treatment
- Treatment with a short course of steroids and active, assisted range of motion of the hand, elbow, and shoulder provides adequate treatment in most patients.
- Sympathetic blockade or surgical sympathectomy may be needed for patients with persistent symptoms.

Septic arthritis

Septic arthritis of the shoulder is rare. It is most frequently seen in infants and children 2 years of age or younger, but may be seen at any age. It represents a surgical emergency. If left untreated it could lead to septic shock, arthritis, or a fused joint. There is an increased incidence in those patients with diabetes mellitus, cancer, hypogammaglobulinaemia, or chronic liver disease, and in those receiving corticosteroid or immunosuppressive drugs. The more common organisms to infect the joint are Staph. aureus (most common in adults), N. gonorrhoeae, Strep. pneumoniae, Strep. pyogenese, H. influenza (most common in neonates), and Gram negative bacilli.

History and examination
- The patient usually presents with pain, swelling, and loss of range of motion of the joint with no apparent portal of entry.
- Occasionally, they may present following an aspiration or injection procedure of the joint.

Investigations and treatment
- Diagnosis is by aspiration of joint fluid.
- If frank pus is present, immediate incision and drainage should be performed and the patient started on IV antibiotics.
- If the clinical suspicion is high and the joint fluid appears normal or equivocal the patient should be started on IV antibiotics until the cultures return.

Osteonecrosis (ischaemic necrosis or avascular necrosis)
- Ischaemia of the humeral head is typically referred to as avascular necrosis (AVN) of the humeral head.
- It is associated with haemoglobinopathies, pancreatitis, alcoholism, and connective tissue disease. It has also been documented in gout, osteoarthritis, burns, Gaucher's disease, prolonged immobilization, pregnancy, hyperparathyroidism, and cytotoxic treatments.
- The patient will usually present with chronic shoulder pain and limited range of motion.
- X-ray changes are not seen until several months after the onset of pain.
- Technetium pyrophosphate bone scanning is useful in detecting early ischaemic necrosis as is MRI.
- Treatment is limited to supportive care, but in cases of severe pain total joint arthroplasty may be necessary.

Cervical radiculopathy
- Always consider the cervical spine in any evaluation of shoulder pain.
- Cervical radiculopathy causes deep burning pain that radiates from the shoulder to the fingertips and may be associated with paresthesias.
- It is often relieved by forward shoulder elevation or repositioning/gentle traction of the neck.
- Range of motion of the cervical spine should be tested.
- Spurling's manoeuvre and an atlanto-occipital axial compression test should be performed.
- Motor function should be evaluated in the upper extremity, arm, and hand. Fine movements of the hand should be evaluated.
- Deep tendon reflexes should be tested in the upper extremity, as well as a sensory exam.
- An appropriate cervical work-up should precede a shoulder work-up if any abnormalities are found.
- It is not uncommon for patients with shoulder disorders to have concomitant cervical spondylitis and/or degenerative disc disease.
- It is frequently helpful to do X-rays of the cervical spine prior to referral to physical therapy for shoulder pathology, so it can be treated too.

Tumours of the shoulder
- The most common malignant bony tumours of the humerus are Ewing's sarcoma and osteosarcoma. These tend to occur in adolescence.
- Chondrosarcomas, although rare, tend to occur during the 3rd to 7th decade. Most cases in adults, however, represent metastatic lesions (especially hypernephroma) or multiple myeloma.
- Other lesions seen include osteochondromas, chondroblastomas,
- giant cell tumours, aneurysmal bone cysts, and Pancoast tumours of the lung.
- Tumours may present with pain that is worse at night and, in some cases, may be significantly improved with NSAIDs.
- Plain radiographs may identify the lesions, but MRI is usually needed for clarification.

Referred pain from the chest and abdomen
- The phrenic nerve arises from the 4th cervical nerve, but also receives branches from the 3rd and 5th nerves. It begins at the posterior scalene muscle, descends the chest in the lateral part of the pericardium and ends at the diaphragm. Branches of this nerve provide sensory innervation to the mediastinal and diaphragmatic pleura, diaphragmatic peritoneum, and probably the liver, gall bladder, and inferior vena cava. Irritation of the diaphragm or the innervated areas of the pleura or peritoneum will stimulate the phrenic nerve.
- Since these nerves also innervate the skin of the neck, supraclavicular area, and shoulder, pain may be referred to these areas.
- Pneumonia, pulmonary infarction, empyema, neoplasm, hepatobiliary disease, subphrenic abscess, splenic injury, or a pseudocyst of the pancreas can all produce shoulder pain.

Chapter 18

Elbow and forearm

History *504*
Examination *504*
Special tests *506*
Medial collateral ligament injury *507*
Medial collateral ligament instability in children *508*
Traction apophysitis medial humeral epicondyle
 ('Little Leaguer's elbow') *509*
Lateral epicondylitis *510*
Medial epicondylitis *512*
Osteochondritis dissecans of the capitellum or radial head *514*
Panner's disease *515*
Acute injuries *516*
Chronic elbow injuries *522*

History

- Onset, mechanisms, previous injuries.
- Symptoms including pain site(s), radiation, and temporal pattern, provocative factors/movements, swelling, locking, tingling, numbness, vascular changes, clicking.
- Are there neck, forearm, or hand symptoms?

Examination

Inspection

See Fig. 18.1 for the anatomy of the elbow joint.
- Look at soft tissue contour for evidence of wasting or asymmetry of muscle bulk, muscle fasciculation, scars, deformities, and alignment. Over-development of the dominant arm is common.
- Look for swelling and soft tissue masses in the antecubital fossa.
- Estimate the carrying angle with the arm extended.
- Inspect posteriorly for dislocation, olecranon bursa, effusion, and triceps tendon tear (excessively bony prominence, with a gap just above).
- Inspect laterally for synovitis or effusion which may be evident in the triangular space between the lateral epicondyle, the head of the radius, and the tip of the olecranon.

Palpation

- Examine the bony landmarks with the arm flexed at 90°.
- Tenderness in the area of the medial collateral ligament (MCL) indicates injury.
- Palpate the radial head for tenderness (fracture, synovitis, osteoarthritis, dislocation). Palpate the radiocapitellar joint during pronation/supination (degenerative change, synovitis).
- Check the biceps tendon (tenderness) and brachial pulse in the cubital fossa.
- Palpate the lateral collateral ligament and the lateral epicondyle.
- Palpate the ulnar nerve posterior to the medial epicondyle for thickening and/or irritability. Anterior subluxation of the ulnar nerve is often evident with flexion and reduced with extension and can be associated with a click during movement.
- The flexor-pronator muscle group may be tender (and even swollen) at its origin with medial epicondylitis.

Movements

Assess passive and active range of motion and movement against resistance (for specific muscle groups) and compare sides.

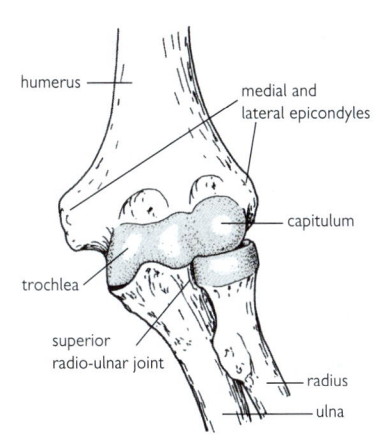

Fig. 18.1 Articular surfaces of elbow joint (anterior aspect). Reproduced with permission from MacKinnon P and Morris J (2005). *Oxford Textbook of Functional Anatomy*, Vol. 1. Oxford University Press, Oxford. © 2005.

Special tests

Assess MCL and LCL with elbow in 30° of flexion looking for pain and laxity.

Lateral epicondylitis
- *Prime test:* patient extends elbow, pronates the forearm and extends the fingers. The examiner applies downward force to the middle finger (extensor digitorum communis).
- Resisted wrist extension is tested with the forearm pronated and the elbow in two positions: firstly extended then flexed to 90° (extensor carpi radialis brevis).

Medial epicondylitis
- Resisted wrist flexion with the elbow flexed and forearm supinated.
- Resisted forearm pronation with the forearm extended and in neutral rotation.

Distal biceps tendon
- Remember to test by resisted supination with elbow in 90° flexion.

Neurovascular status
- *Tests of ulnar nerve entrapment:* Tinel's test, and sustained elbow flexion test (same principle to Phalen's test at wrist).
- *Ulnar nerve instability:* repeated flexion/extension of the elbow reproduces ulnar nerve symptoms and nerve subluxation.

Medial collateral ligament injury

History and examination
Acute or chronic medial collateral ligament (MCL) injury in adults is due to repetitive valgus extension overload which occurs usually in throwers, but can occur with direct trauma. MCL instability and a wedging effect of the olecranon into the olecranon fossa may cause a posterior osteophyte which can irritate the ulnar nerve. A sudden onset of pain during throwing, with an associated 'pop' or 'snap' may indicate an acute injury. In chronic cases there is progressive medial elbow pain that is functionally limiting and worse during the acceleration phase of throwing.

On examination there is swelling, local MCL tenderness and instability. Flexion contractures and cubitus valgus deformities are common in throwers. Posteromedial osteophytes may be palpable. Olecranon tenderness is worsened by bringing the arm into valgus and extension.

Investigations
Plain X-rays may be normal. In chronic cases there may be ectopic bone formation in the MCL, posteromedial osteophyte formation at the olecranon and conoid tubercle, and loose bodies. Stress films may confirm medial instability. MRI allows assessment of the MCL.

Treatment
Aim to settle the acute symptoms where present and to restore normal range of motion with relative rest, ice, analgesics, and NSAIDs. PRP injection may be considered in lower grade injuries. Commence passive and active range of motion exercises early, with a strengthening regime. Throwing activities are resumed when there is full range of motion. Surgery is considered with chronic instability and impairment. Excision of osteophytes and local debridement or a straight osteotomy, 1cm proximal to the tip of the olecranon may be considered in those with impingement. For instability, reconstruction using a tendon graft; repair may be performed in the acute rupture.

Prevention of the condition is important through adequate conditioning, warm-up, stretching, and appropriate technique.

Medial collateral ligament instability in children

History and examination
This usually occurs in relation to throwing or racket sports. Medial apophysitis is a true epicondylitis due to traction and inflammation of the growth plate at the medial epicondyle. 'Little Leaguer's elbow' is due to a variable combination of a medial apophysitis, MCL injury, and instability, compressive changes at the radiocapitellar joint and osteochondrosis. There is usually gradual onset of an aching pain at the medial elbow and there may be weakness of grip and paraesthesiae in the distribution of the ulnar nerve. An acute avulsion injury at the apophysis can also occur. In the acute avulsion there is a 'pop', followed by medial swelling and weakness.

On examination, there may be swelling and tenderness at the medial epicondyle, and perhaps bruising and flexion contracture. Pain is exacerbated by passive extension of the elbow and wrist. With an avulsion injury, a fragment may be palpable. Stress testing may show medial instability. Lateral elbow tenderness, pain on movement and on compression of the joint indicates lateral compressive changes.

Investigations
US demonstrates the state of the ligament, avulsion fragments, degree of separation, local fluid collection. MRI also may demonstrate bone bruising and state of growth plates. Plain X-rays may be normal or may show widening of the physis, fragmentation or avulsion of the apophysis, in comparison to the other side. Gravity valgus stress views may be considered.

Treatment
Relative rest, analgesics, ice, stretching. Healing can be prolonged. When avulsion has occurred, treat according to degree of displacement. Immobilize for 2 weeks with mild displacement followed by progressive rehabilitation. With large or rotated fragments, consider open reduction and fixation.

Traction apophysitis medial humeral epicondyle ('Little Leaguers' elbow')

Causes
This condition is commonly seen in the young throwing athlete. The valgus force imparted to the elbow when throwing causes compression of lateral elbow structures and stretching of medial elbow structures. This results in traction of the wrist flexors on the medial epicondylar apophysis.

Clinical features
- Insidious onset of pain over the medial epicondyle (common flexor origin), exacerbated by pitching, bowling, and throwing long distances.
- May have difficulty fully extending the elbow.
- Focal tenderness ± swelling over the common flexor origin.
- Pain is reproduced by passive dorsiflexion of the wrist with the elbow in the extended position and with resisted wrist flexion.

Diagnosis
- Usually clinical.
- If onset of pain is acute, X-ray may be warranted to exclude an avulsion fracture of the medial epicondylar apophysis.

Treatment
- Rest from throwing activities until pain resolves.
- Stretching program for wrist flexors.
- As pain improves, a strengthening program should be instituted to avoid further injury on resumption of throwing.
- Return to sport should begin with throwing short distances at reduced pace and gradually increasing throwing distance and pace if asymptomatic.
- Full recovery can be expected.

Lateral epicondylitis

History and examination

This is a tendinopathy of the common extensor—supinator tendon rather than epicondylitis. Degenerative micro-tears (due to repetitive mechanical overload) are found in the common extensor—supinator tendon, with the origin of extensor carpi radialis brevis (ECRB) most commonly affected.

There is often a history of overuse, involving repetitive flexion-extension or pronation-supination activity. There is acute or chronic lateral epicondylar pain and tenderness worse with gripping. Among tennis players, the backhand stroke is commonly implicated and those players with a faulty technique are most likely to be injured. Equipment factors include a racquet that may be too heavy or too light, a grip that is too big, string tension that is too tight, and the use of heavy or wet tennis balls. 13% of elite players and up to 50% of non-elite tennis players have symptoms suggestive of lateral epicondylitis and approximately half of these have symptoms for an average duration of 2½ years. It may occur in other sports (e.g. golf—where it is more common than 'golfers elbow'). It particularly affects those aged 40–60yrs.

On examination there is tenderness over the ECRB origin at the lateral epicondyle. The tenderness may be diffuse, over the origins of extensor digitorum communis (EDC) and/or extensor carpi radialis longus (ECRL). One or more provocation tests may be positive. Look for other possible causes of lateral elbow pain including the neck. Examine the equipment and assess technique.

Investigations

US can be considered an extension of the clinical examination. It shows decreased echogenicity, inhomogeneity, and thickening of the tendon, and a local fluid collection may be seen. Micro-tears, typically on the deep surface, may be evident. Neovascularization, representing disordered repair, local calcification at the tendon insertion and irregularity of the bone surface may all be noted. Other imaging studies are not routinely performed unless other pathologies are suspected. A plain radiograph may help to evaluate for OA of the radiocapitellar joint. On MRI there may be increased signal intensity of the extensor tendons close to their insertion on the lateral epicondyle, and the surrounding anatomy can also be evaluated, either by plain MR or with the assistance of contrast. CT is best for bony anatomy (e.g. small osteophytes/loose bodies).

Treatment

Relative rest, ice (10min every hour in the acute stages), analgesia, and NSAIDs (topical NSAIDs are preferable). Compression straps or counter-force braces applied distal to the bulk of the extensor mass may help. The brace is tightened to a comfortable degree of tension with the forearm muscles relaxed, so that a maximum contraction is limited. Constant use of the brace not advised.

Stretching of the forearm extensors and range of motion exercises at the elbow and wrist should start early. Progressive rehabilitation for strength and endurance of the forearm extensor-supinator group as soon as pain allows, progressing according to symptoms. Use ice after early rehabilitation sessions to limit an excessive inflammatory response. In chronic cases, NO patches, US-guided platelet rich plasma injection(s), and/or extracorporeal shock wave therapy may be considered. (NO (nitric oxide) releasing patches, also known as glyceryl trinitrate (GTN) patches, have been advocated in the treatment and repair of tendinopathies, primarily on the basis of enhancing tenocyte function. Low dose patches (e.g. ¼ Deponit 5 patch/24h) are used. Headaches and skin sensitivity may occur).

Corticosteroid injections are no longer commonly recommended. There may be short-term pain relief, but there is no evidence of benefit over placebo in the longer term, and there are risks: SC atrophy, tendon rupture, and others.

Address the cause. In tennis players, technique and equipment factors must be addressed. Evaluation of technique with the help of a coach may prove beneficial. Improvements may be noted by avoidance of the leading elbow during backhand, ensuring that the forearm is only partially pronated, the forward shoulder is lowered, and the trunk is leaning forward. The patient should also consider a change in racquet (different weight, shock absorbency, grip size) reducing string tension to 2–3 pounds less than the manufacturers' recommendations (i.e. 50–55 pounds), using slower, lighter tennis balls, and playing on slower courts.

Surgery is reserved for those patients with disabling symptoms who fail to respond to all the above measures over some months. Options include repair of the extensor origin after excision of the torn tendon, granulation tissue and local drilling of the subchondral bone of the lateral epicondyle, with an aim to increasing blood supply. The elbow is placed in a posterior plaster splint for a week, then in a lighter splint for 2 weeks, with the elbow in 90° flexion and in neutral rotation. Range of motion exercises are commenced thereafter, with a progressive strengthening regime. Light activities can be recommenced at 3 months, but the patient can expect to wear a counterforce brace initially.

Other surgical options include reduction of the tension on the common extensor origin by fasciotomy, direct release of the extensor origin or lengthening of the ECRB tendon distally. Fasciotomy and complete extensor tendon release can result in loss of strength, and lengthening of ECRB distally appears to be effective only in the minority of cases. Whilst intra-articular procedures such as synovectomy and division of the orbicular ligament have been suggested, these seem inappropriate for an extra-articular condition. Some surgeons advocate decompression of the radial or posterior interosseous nerves on the basis that posterior interosseous nerve (PIN) entrapment is contributing to—or is the primary cause of—chronic symptoms.

Medial epicondylitis

History and examination

This is not a true epicondylitis, but an overuse injury of the common tendinous origin of the flexor-pronator muscle group. It commonly occurs with repetitive flexion and pronation, less commonly with valgus stresses, and is seen in throwing and racket sports and in golfers ('golfer's elbow'). See Figs. 18.2 and 18.3.

It causes an acute/chronic aching pain at the medial elbow and proximal flexor musculature of the forearm. There may be weakness of grip. Some patients have paraesthesiae in the ring and little fingers suggestive of an ulnar neuropathy.

On examination there is tenderness at the medial epicondyle and there may be reduced range of motion at the elbow, due to pain on stretching of the flexor-pronator group with full extension. Other causes of medial elbow pain should be considered including radiation from the neck. One or more of the provocation tests may be positive.

Investigations

US shows decreased echogenicity, inhomogeneity, and thickening of the tendon. Neovascularization, representing disordered repair, local calcification at the tendon insertion and irregularity of the bone surface may all be noted. A local fluid collection may be present.

Treatment

Relative rest, ice, analgesics, NSAIDs, and a reverse counterforce brace. Aim to commence rehabilitation, including early stretching of the wrist and elbow and a progressive strengthening regime of the wrist flexors and forearm pronators. Return to activities when there is full pain free range of movement and strength of grip, forearm pronation, and wrist flexion has returned to at least 80% of normal. In chronic cases, NO patches, US-guided platelet rich plasma injection(s) and or extracorporeal shock wave therapy may be considered. Corticosteroid injections are rarely necessary and care must be taken because of the proximity of the ulnar nerve.

Prevention includes adequate conditioning of the forearm, attention to technique, and adequate warm-up, stretching, and cool down. Reduce the causes through proper sporting technique and equipment.

Surgery is rarely required. Standard approaches include release of the tendinous origin of pronator teres, and usually a portion of flexor carpi radialis (FCR), debridement, and decompression of the ulnar nerve distal to the medial epicondyle. Post-operative rehabilitation is continued for 6 months before a return to full activities. Complications of surgery include loss of full elbow extension (up to 5°) in 1% of cases, superficial infection (in less than 1%), and damage to the ulnar nerve and MCL.

Osteochondritis dissecans of the capitellum or radial head

Pathology
- Focal area of avascular necrosis affecting the subchondral bone of the capitellum, or less commonly, the radial head.
- Thought to result from compression of lateral elbow structures, leading to vascular compromise and softening of the articular cartilage, followed by fragmentation of the subchondral bone and, later, loose body formation.

Causes and risk factors
- Usually occurs in young athletes involved in throwing sports or sports requiring upper limb weight bearing such as gymnastics.
- The child is usually between the ages of 10 and 16, and presents with pain and swelling in the dominant elbow in throwers.

Clinical features
- Pain exacerbated by throwing or upper-limb weight bearing.
- May have difficulty fully straightening the elbow.
- May describe locking sensation secondary to loose body formation.

Signs
- Elbow effusion and loss of full extension.
- Tenderness localized to the capitellum or radial head.

Investigations
- X-rays may show flattening of the capitellum ± fragmentation and loose body formation.
- In early stages may be necessary to X-ray other side for comparison to detect subtle changes.
- MRI is useful for detecting loose bodies and early stages of osteochondritis dissicans (OCD), which may be difficult to visualize on X-ray.

Treatment
- Early recognition is important.
- Rest from aggravating activities.
- Local physiotherapy to reduce swelling and restore range of movement.
- Exercise program to improve forearm strength should follow.
- If loose bodies present, a surgical opinion should be sought.

Return to sport
- When there is resolution of symptoms and effusion and restoration of a full pain-free range of motion.

Prevention
- Guidelines regarding pitching should not be exceeded and activity should stop if symptoms recur.

Prognosis
- Early diagnosis will improve prognosis.
- With disruption of the joint surfaces and loose body formation, long-term disability and osteoarthritis can result.

Panner's disease

Pathology
- An elbow condition of 8–10yr-olds similar to Perthes' disease of the hip.
- Microvasculature disruption → fragmentation of the entire capitellar ossification centre.

Clinical features
- Usually presents in a manner similar to that of OCD capitellum, but in a younger age group (<10yrs).
- Child with Panner's disease may not have a history of elbow overuse.

Investigations
- X-rays demonstrate diffuse changes in the capitellar epiphysis.
- MRI may be required to detect subtle changes.

Treatment
- Rest from aggravating activities.
- Local physiotherapy and range of motion exercises.

Prognosis
- Panner's disease has a better prognosis than that of osteochondritis dissecans capitellum. Loose body formation does not occur and it is rare to have any long-term sequelae.

Acute injuries

Tear or rupture of the distal biceps

History and examination

This may occur with trauma, usually with the elbow in 90° flexion. There is typically a sudden tearing pain in the antecubital fossa followed by a deep aching discomfort, with bruising and weakness of supination and flexion and grip strength. It is more common with anabolic steroid use.

On examination, there is a palpable gap, a bulbous swelling in the arm, and weakness. A partial tear of the tendon produces pain and there may be swelling and local crepitus on supination and pronation.

Investigation
- US and/or MRI. Note imaging evaluation of these injuries can be challenging. Liaise closely with radiologist where necessary.

Treatment
- Management of rupture is early surgical repair.
- Management of tears depends upon the size of the tear and the level of disability. In less severe cases, may be possible to proceed as for chronic tendinopathy.

Triceps tear/rupture

History and examination

Triceps rupture is usually an avulsion injury at the tendo-osseous junction. Patients may describe a sudden tear or pop, pain, swelling, and weakness of elbow extension. Partial ruptures, usually in the central third of the tendon, can also occur. Other injuries may occur simultaneously, including fracture of the radial head. The injury usually occurs after a fall onto the outstretched hand, but can occur after a direct blow. If there is spontaneous rupture, consider anabolic steroid use. On examination there is swelling, a palpable gap, and weakness of elbow extension.

Investigations
- US will confirm tendon tear/rupture, avulsed segment, and degree of separation.
- A lateral plain X-ray will usually show flecks of avulsed bone proximal to the olecranon.
- Exclude a fracture of the head of the radius.

Treatment
- Tendon reattachment is usually recommended with acute rupture.
- Reconstruction may be considered if there is delay or if there is underlying tendon disease.

Elbow dislocation

History and examination

These may be complicated (with fracture) or simple (without). Displacement is usually posterior or posterolateral and there is considerable soft tissue injury. They usually occur after a fall onto the outstretched hand with the elbow in extension. On examination there is pain, swelling,

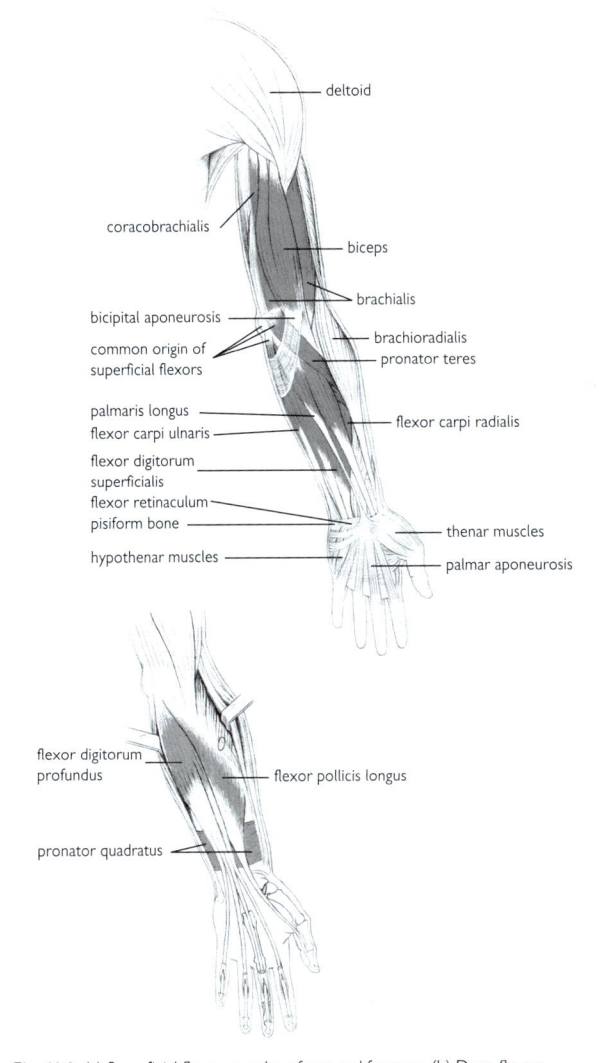

Fig. 18.2 (a) Superficial flexor muscles of arm and forearm. (b) Deep flexor muscles of the forearm. Reproduced with permission from MacKinnon P, Morris J. (2005). *Oxford Textbook of Functional Anatomy*, Vol. 1. Oxford: Oxford University Press, ©2005.

deformity, and possible neurovascular symptoms. It is important to assess neurovascular status.

Investigation
- X-ray confirmation looking closely for fractures, especially of the radial head and olecranon process.

Treatment
- Analgesia and relaxants.
- Early reduction is often possible.
- Apply longitudinal traction with one hand and with the other apply pressure to relocate the olecranon back onto the trochlea.
- Assess neurovascular status and elbow stability (extent of soft tissue damage) afterwards.
- In some, closed reduction may be necessary under general anaesthetic.
- Splint and sling after relocation, for approx. 1–3 weeks (time frame dependent upon instability), then gentle, slow rehabilitation.

Supracondylar fractures

History and examination
These usually occur in children and often with a fall onto outstretched hand with elbow pushed into extension. On examination there is pain, swelling, and S-deformity of elbow. Most are displaced so it is essential to check neurovascular status (15% have a neurological injury).

Investigation
- X-ray to confirm.

Treatment
- With an undisplaced, place in a collar and cuff for 3 weeks, and monitor serially to assess for displacement.
- Displaced fractures and most adults require a closed reduction and, if necessary, fixation.

Lateral condylar fractures

History and examination
Separation can occur at growth plate especially aged 4–10yrs and this may cause long-term growth plate damage. Patients describe lateral elbow pain, swelling, dysfunction.

Investigation
- Confirm on X-ray.

Treatment
- Splint an undisplaced separation in a backslab at 90°.
- If displaced, reduction and fixation is necessary.

Radial head and neck fractures

History and examination
Radial head fractures usually occur in adults and radial neck injuries in children. They occur after a fall onto an outstretched hand, with the elbow pushed into valgus. On examination there is tenderness, swelling, and there may be limitation in supination/pronation.

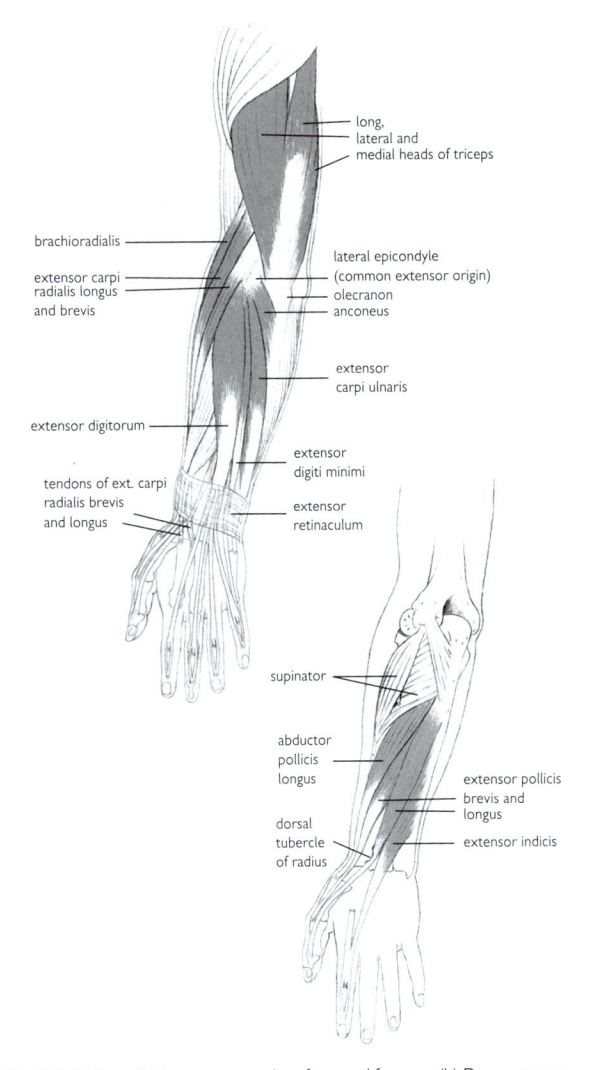

Fig 18.3 (a) Superficial extensor muscles of arm and forearm. (b) Deep extensor muscles of the forearm. Reproduced with permission from MacKinnon P and Morris J. (2005). *Oxford Textbook of Functional Anatomy*, Vol 1. Oxford University Press, Oxford. © 2005.

Investigation
- X-ray.

Treatment
- An undisplaced fracture of the radial head in adults is treated in a backslab.
- A displaced fracture requires open reduction and fixation or if comminuted, excision may be necessary.
- In children, where the fracture is of the radial neck, closed or open, reduction is needed if there is angulation beyond 20° of radial tilt.

Monteggia fractures (ulna fracture with radial head dislocation, in children)

History and examination
This usually occurs after a fall onto an outstretched hand. There is diffuse elbow pain, swelling, and there may be global limitation.

Investigation
- On X-ray, the line through the middle of the radial shaft should bisect the radial head in all views. This fracture can be missed.

Treatment
- Closed reduction and immobilization.
- Monitor for displacement on X-ray.

Chronic elbow injuries

Distal biceps tendinopathy
Tendinosis of the distal end of biceps brachii can occur with repetitive supination and pronation activities. Pain is felt in the antecubital fossa and local swelling and tenderness may be noted. Pain is worse with resisted supination. Treatment includes relative rest, ice, NSAIDs, and modification of activities, progressive rehabilitation. Use of NO patches, PRP injections can be considered.

Ulnar neuropathy

History and examination
The ulnar nerve is vulnerable along its path through the cubital tunnel posterior to the medial epicondyle and particularly if there is a shallow ulnar groove within the tunnel, hypermobility, or laxity of the soft tissue constraints of the nerve in the tunnel. Those who perform repetitive throwing or flexion activities are particularly vulnerable to dislocation or subluxation of the nerve. Recurrent dislocation of the ulnar nerve occurs in 16% of the normal population. The nerve is at risk of direct trauma. The nerve can also be compressed by hypertrophied forearm musculature, by the aponeurosis of flexor carpi ulnaris, a ganglion situated in the cubital tunnel, local bony anomalies, or by adhesions within the cubital tunnel. The ulnar nerve may be injured with fractures or dislocations, in progressive valgus deformity after ulnar collateral ligament (UCL) injury, or lateral epicondylar fracture. There may be entrapment between the two heads of flexor carpi ulnaris (FCU), distal to the medial epicondyle. At the wrist injury may occur through compression, OA, pressure against bicycle handlebars, tumours, haemorrhage, and the usual causes of mononeuritis (diabetes, vasculitides, sarcoid, amyloid, RA, SLE, malignancy).

There may be a sharp deep aching pain at medial elbow and proximal forearm, which may radiate proximally or distally and may be noted only during flexion and valgus stresses. Neurological disturbances including paraesthesia, dysaesthesia, and anaesthesia in the ulnar one-and-a-half digits are noted early in the condition. Whilst clumsiness is frequently reported, true motor weakness is rare. Recurrent dislocation or subluxation of the nerve can cause a 'popping' or 'snapping' sensation with elbow flexion and extension.

On examination, look for valgus deformity of the elbow, a mild flexion contracture and MCL instability, soft tissue swelling at the ulnar groove, with tenderness and thickening of the nerve. There may be wasting of the small muscles of the hand and hypothenar eminence, but sensory changes occur late. Elbow flexion and Tinels tests are insensitive. Those with ulnar nerve subluxation may be able to demonstrate the phenomenon and it may be possible to dislocate the nerve from the groove. A Martin Gruber anastomosis, where there is communication between the median and ulnar nerves in the forearm, occurs in 15% of people and may confuse clinical findings. Examine the cervical spine and look for hypermobility syndrome. May be mistaken for a common flexor origin (CFO) tendinopathy.

Investigations
- US may demonstrate thickening of the nerve, instability, and surrounding structures (especially UCL and CFO tendon).
- Nerve conduction studies may show reduced conduction velocity by more than 33% across the site of compression compared to the unaffected arm.
- An X-ray will show bony abnormalities (in particular, osteophytes).

Treatment
- Relative rest and protection; splinting the elbow at 30° of flexion may provide symptomatic relief.
- Ice, NSAIDs, and simple analgesics are often unhelpful.
- NO patches.
- Gentle range of motion exercises are commenced as soon as tolerated.
- Return to normal activities can commence after full strength is regained with a progressive strengthening regime of forearm musculature and correction of faulty technique/instability where appropriate.
- Surgical decompression, transposition and correction of instability/other pathology may be necessary.
- All potential sources of compression of the nerve should be explored, even when a specific site of compression has been indicated by electro diagnostic studies, since more than one site of compression can exist.

The pronator syndrome

History and examination
Median nerve compression at the elbow and proximal forearm is known as the pronator syndrome. It causes a vague aching pain at the proximal, volar surface of the forearm. There is often a history of repetitive strenuous use of the forearm. There may be dysaesthesias in the distribution of the median nerve in the hand. If compression occurs at the ligament of Struthers (a band between the medial epicondyle and the supracondylar process), symptoms are worse with flexion of the elbow against resistance between 120° and 135° flexion. Compression at the bicipital aponeurosis can cause indentation of the pronator muscle mass below the medial epicondyle and symptoms are increased by active and passive forearm pronation. Compression can also occur within the pronator teres due to hypertrophy or tightness of the muscle, when symptoms are worse with resisted pronation of forearm with the wrist in flexion (to relax flexor digitorum superficialis (FDS)) or at FDS, when the symptoms are aggravated by resisted flexion of FDS of the middle finger, and with passive stretching of finger and wrist flexors. If there is weakness of pinch grip, the condition should be differentiated from anterior interosseous syndrome.

Investigation
- Electrodiagnostic studies help to confirm median nerve latency, but may not localize the lesion to the forearm.
- US may (rarely) demonstrate a site of compression.

Treatment
- Passive stretching of the forearm musculature, relative rest, NSAIDs, and elbow splinting in neutral rotation.

- Symptoms may take 2–3 months to improve.
- Surgical intervention is avoided where possible, but is indicated with significant/progressive neurophysiological deficit. It involves exploration of the nerve from 5cm proximal to the elbow and in the forearm, at potential sites of compression.

Anterior interosseous syndrome

History and examination
This occurs with lifting heavy weights and where there is cumulative trauma. Compression of the anterior interosseous nerve results in a pure motor paralysis of flexor policis longus (FPL) and the index flexor digitorum profundus. There may be weakness of pronator quadratus. Those patients with a Martin Gruber anastamosis may experience weakness of the ulnar intrinsic muscles and/or weakness of flexor profundus to other fingers. Patients may describe a short episode of pain, which subsides to leave motor weakness. On examination there is weakness of pinch grip.

Investigation
- After 2–3 weeks, EMG studies will show signs of denervation of affected muscles.

Treatment
- NSAIDs and relative rest for 8–12 weeks.
- Those who remain symptomatic are considered for surgery, which involves a similar approach to pronator syndrome.

Radial nerve lesions

History and examination
Depending upon which portion of the nerve is affected, symptoms may be motor (PIN), sensory (superficial radial nerve), or both. Posterior interosseous nerve entrapment occurs at 5 sites, but most commonly at the arcade of Frohse at the proximal edge of supinator, deep to extensor carpi radialis longus. Nerve compression can also occur due to synovitis at the radiocapitellar joint, fractures, ganglia tumours, vascular anomalies, or other local masses. The superficial radial nerve can be entrapped alone or in combination with the posterior interosseous branch. The radial nerve can also be entrapped above the level of the elbow, due to a lateral intermuscular septum, although this is rare.

The injury occurs with repetitive rotary movements, e.g. discus throwing and racquet sports. There is aching pain in the belly of the extensor muscles, of insidious onset, worse with forearm pronation and wrist flexion. Pain may be more diffuse over the extensor forearm; there may be exacerbation after exertion and pain at night. Patient may have been diagnosed with 'resistant tennis elbow'. On examination there is tenderness to palpation over the course of the PIN, deep to the extensor muscle belly and just distal to the radial head. Pain may be reproduced with resisted extension of the middle finger with the elbow extended, and on resisted supination of the extended forearm.

Investigation
- Neurophysiology studies are frequently normal.
- There may be a decrease in motor conduction velocity in the radial nerve across the entrapment site, and changes in the muscles innervated distal to the entrapment site.
- US and/or MRI to identify causes of compression.

Treatment
- Stretching and activity modification.
- In resistant cases, exploration of the nerve is necessary.
- Surgical procedures used in the treatment of lateral epicondylitis may be followed.

Forearm compartment syndrome

History and examination

This may occur acutely after trauma or may present with chronic symptoms. It is less common than in the lower legs and is associated with lifting heavy weights and, in particular, activities that involve elbow and wrist flexion (see Table 18.1). Anabolic steroid use can be a factor. It causes exertional forearm pain and there may be paraesthesiae in the forearm and hand. The symptoms gradually resolve with cessation of activity. On examination, there may be little to find at rest, although the forearm is usually muscular.

Investigation

- The diagnosis may be confirmed by intracompartmental pressure monitoring before and after exercise (normal range 0–8mmHg), although diagnostic levels for forearm compartment syndrome have not been set.
- Sustained compartment oedema post exercise on MRI may help in making the diagnosis.

Treatment

- Fasciotomy.

Radial head bursitis and other causes of lateral elbow pain

Radial head bursitis can occur with repetitive pronation/supination and may be confused with distal biceps tendinitis. There is local pain and tenderness in the antecubital fossa and there may be fullness or swelling in this area. Pain is worse with pronation. US confirms the diagnosis. Treatment is symptomatic with modification of activities, ice, and NSAIDs. Aspiration and injection of corticosteroid in rare cases under guidance may be necessary.

Other causes of lateral elbow pain include articular disorders: arthropathies, osteochondritis dissecans, and osteochondrosis of the humeral capitellum, synovitis of the radiohumeral head, and fractures.

Olecrannon bursitis

History and examination

Bursitis usually occurs as a result of trauma; a direct blow or repetitive friction. It may be acute or chronic, septic, or aseptic and caused by trauma, sepsis, crystals, inflammatory arthritis, uraemia, or calcific deposits. Septic bursitis (most commonly *Staph. aureus*) can arise due to direct inoculation through local skin. Steroid injections precede infections in up to 10% of cases.

On examination there is discrete swelling at the posterior elbow, representing thickened bursa and/or bursal fluid. In sepsis or crystal induced bursitis the patient may be systemically unwell with a fever, cellulitis, and local lymphadenopathy.

Investigation
- US confirms the diagnosis and identifies other local pathology that can cause posterior elbow pain, e.g. synovitis in the elbow joint proper, triceps tendinosis, etc.
- Inflammatory markers (ESR, CRP) and white cell count may be elevated in systemic sepsis and crystal induced bursitis.
- If sepsis is suspected, blood cultures and sterile aspiration of the bursal fluid, plus analysis by Gram stain and culture and crystals is essential.

Treatment
- Most uncomplicated cases are managed symptomatically with regular ice, NSAIDs, and local protection by an elbow pad or dressing. Aspiration without injection can help to relieve pain and allows bursal fluid to be obtained for examination. Injection of hydrocortisone 10mg is rarely necessary, but may benefit persisting bursitis especially with an inflammatory arthritis/crystals. Relative rest for 5 days after aspiration is recommended.
- In acute post-traumatic bursitis, repeat sterile aspiration of blood provides symptomatic relief and should be followed by a compressive dressing, regular icing, and NSAIDs. Steroid injections have no role. Return to contact activities is permitted once the patient is asymptomatic, but a protective elbow pad should be worn initially.
- Where sepsis is confirmed in those who are systemically well and with little cellulitis, aspiration of the bursa is followed by oral broad spectrum antibiotics. Progress should be monitored and intravenous antibiotics commenced in those who fail to respond, and early in those with systemic symptoms. Open drainage and lavage may be necessary.

Table 18.1 Radio-ulnar and wrist joints: movements, principal muscles, and their innervation. Reproduced with permission from MacKinnon P and Morris J. (2005)

Movement	Principal muscles	Peripheral nerve	Spinal root origin
Supination	Biceps	Musculocutaneous nerve	C 5, 6
	Supinator	Radial nerve (deep branch)	C 5, 6, 7
Pronation	Pronator teres	Median nerve	C 5, 6, 7
	Pronator quadratus	Median nerve	C 5, 6, 7, 8
Flexion	*Common flexor origin muscles*		
	flexor carpi radialis	Median nerve	C 5, 6, 7
	flexor carpi ulnaris	Ulnar nerve	C 5, 6, 7, 8
	(palmaris longus)	Median nerve	C 5, 6, 7
	Long digital flexors	Median and ulnar nerves	C 5, 6, 7
Extension	*Common extensor origin muscles*		
	extensor carpi radialis longus and brevis	Radial nerve (trunk and deep branch*)	C 5, 6, 7
	extensor carpi ulnaris	Radial nerve (deep branch*)	C 5, 6, 7, 8
	Long digital extensors		
Abduction	Flexor carpi radialis	Median nerve	C 5, 6, 7
	Extensor carpi radialis longus and brevis	Radial nerve	C 5, 6, 7
	Abductor pollicis longus and brevis	Radial nerve (deep branch*)	C 5, 6, 7, 8
Adduction	Flexor carpi ulnaris	Ulnar nerve	C 5, 6, 7, 8
	Extensor carpi ulnaris	Radial nerve (deep branch*)	C 5, 6, 7, 8

* The deep branch of the radial nerve is also called the posterior interosseous nerve from its position in the extensor compartment posterior to the interosseous membrane.

Oxford Textbook of Functional Anatomy, Vol 1. Oxford University Press, Oxford. © 2005.

Chapter 19

Wrist and hand

Epidemiology *530*
Wrist biomechanics *531*
Fracture of the distal radius/ulna (Colles' fracture) *532*
Fracture of the scaphoid *532*
Fracture of the hamate *533*
Fracture of the pisiform *534*
Fracture of the metacarpal bones *534*
Bennett's fracture *534*
Phalangeal fractures *535*
Dislocation of the carpal bones *536*
Dislocation of the 1st metacarpophalangeal joint *536*
Dislocation of the interphalangeal joints *537*
Mallet finger *537*
Jersey finger *538*
Boutonniere deformity *538*
Boxer's knuckle *538*
Ulnar collateral ligament injuries (skier's thumb) *539*
Carpal tunnel syndrome *540*
Ulnar nerve compression *540*
Other nerve injury syndromes *541*
De Quervain's tenosynovitis *541*
Other tendinopathies *542*
Ganglion *542*
Impaction syndromes *543*
The paediatric wrist *544*

Epidemiology

- Overall, wrist and hand injuries account for between 3–9% of all sports injuries.
- Incidence varies between sports, with up to 87% of gymnasts reported to experience wrist pain during their career, due to the wrist being a weight-bearing joint in many of the activities of this sport.
- Hand injuries account for 44% of all injuries in rock climbing.
- Injuries to the hand and wrist are common in tennis and golf (especially the left hand in right-handed golfers).
- The majority of injuries are soft tissue, but a diagnosis of 'wrist sprain' should only be made by exclusion of other more serious injuries.
- Hand and wrist injuries are more common in children, and may involve the epiphyseal plates with the potential for growth disturbance.

Wrist biomechanics

See Fig. 19.1 for an anterior view of the carpal bones.
- Normal daily activities require 30° of extension, 5° flexion, 10° radial deviation, and 15° of ulnar deviation.
- Throwing requires a similar degree of extension and radio-ulnar deviation, but flexion is increased to 80–90° at the end of the acceleration phase prior to ball release.
- Studies of the golf swing have shown a flexion-extension arc of 103° in the right wrist compared with 71° in the left wrist for right handed players (advanced players show less movement at the left wrist but more at the right).
- With an intact triangular fibrocartilage complex (TFCC), the radius bears 82% and the ulna 18% of the force during axial loading of the wrist.
- This pattern of force transmission can be altered in sports such as gymnastics, where a significant load can be applied to the ulnar side of the wrist.
- Excision of the TFCC increases the load on the radius to 94%.
- Ulnar shortening (negative ulnar variance) of 2.5mm reduces the ulnar load bearing to 4%, while lengthening by 2.5mm increases it to 42%.

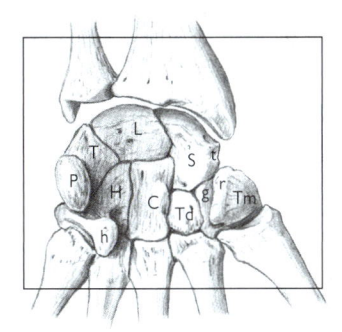

Fig. 19.1 Carpal bones; anterior view. Reproduced with permission from MacKinnon P and Morris J (2005). *Oxford Textbook of Functional Anatomy*, Vol 1. Oxford University Press, Oxford. ©2005.

Fracture of the distal radius/ulna (Colles' fracture)

History and examination
- Common in the elderly athlete (approximately 7% of all Colles' fractures occur during sport) and are caused by a fall on the outstretched hand.
- Fractures in the younger athlete may be accompanied by intra-articular injury and warrant careful assessment.
- Dorsal angulation and impaction leads to the classic 'dinner fork' deformity.
- May involve the epiphyseal plate in children (especially distal radius) and careful follow up is required to ensure that premature growth arrest does not occur (see also 📖 'The Paediatric Wrist', p. 544).

Investigation
- Diagnosis confirmed by X-ray.

Treatment
- Accurate closed reduction and cast immobilization for 6–8 weeks with regular review to ensure that a satisfactory position is being maintained. Physiotherapy to restore range of movement should be started following removal of cast.
- Any intra-articular involvement in the young athlete should be treated by open reduction and internal fixation to restore joint congruity.

Fracture of the scaphoid

History and examination
- Caused by a fall onto the outstretched hand and, therefore, common in football, basketball, hockey, and rugby. These injuries may also occur in boxing.
- Clinical findings include tenderness in the anatomical snuff box (always compare with the uninjured side) and over the palmar scaphoid.
- There will be pain when an axial load is applied to the first metacarpal.
- Common in sport and are important not to miss, as they have the potential for delayed or non-union, with subsequent avascular necrosis and long-term disability.

Investigations
- Plain X-rays may initially be normal and, therefore, if suspected, initial treatment should be immobilization in a scaphoid plaster of Paris (POP) followed by repeat X-ray in 10 days.
- MRI scan, if available, is very useful in making an early diagnosis of scaphoid fracture.

Treatment
- Fractures with a good potential to heal include incomplete, undisplaced fractures, and those involving the distal scaphoid.
- Treatment is immobilization in a scaphoid cast for a period of 8–12 weeks (average time to union $9^{1}/_{2}$ weeks). Physiotherapy should be commenced immediately post-immobilization to restore range of movement and function.
- Those requiring surgery include displaced or proximal pole fractures and those with greater than 15° of angulation.
- Non-union occurs in approximately 10–15% of cases—this complication is preventable by early recognition and appropriate treatment.
- A diagnosis of a 'sprained wrist' can only be made by exclusion, and it is much better to err on the side of caution and immobilize all cases of suspected scaphoid fracture, even if the initial X-rays are negative.

Fracture of the hamate

History and examination
- These fractures occur in racquet sports and golf, caused by the butt of the racquet or golf club forcibly impacting on the hypothenar eminence and hamate hook. In golf may be due to the club being gripped too close to the butt.
- Fractures of the hook of the hamate comprise 2–4% of all carpal fractures. Stress fractures have been described in some sports, e.g. baseball.
- Injury to the ulnar nerve may occur in this area and cause the patient to present with numbness and paraesthesia or weakness of the ulnar innervated muscles, as well as pain and tenderness to direct palpation.

Investigation
- Diagnosis is confirmed on CT scan—fractures of the hamate are difficult to see on plain X-rays.

Treatment
- Non-displaced fractures are treated conservatively with cast immobilization for 4–6 weeks.
- Displaced fractures require open reduction and internal fixation, or excision of the fractured hook.

Fracture of the pisiform

History and examination
- The pisiform may occasionally be fractured by a direct blow.

Treatment
- Treatment is excision with preservation of the flexor carpi ulnaris tendon.

Fracture of the metacarpal bones

History and examination
- Fractures of the neck of the 5th metacarpal are common in combat sports (hence, the term 'boxer's fracture').
- See Fig. 19.2 for anatomy.

Investigations
- X-ray: fractures of the metacarpal bones may be transverse, oblique, or comminuted.
- It is important to check for malrotation (best observed by asking the patient to make a clenched fist).

Treatment
- Non-displaced fractures should be treated conservatively with cast immobilization—any displacement should be managed surgically.
- Return to sport depends on the need for hand function, but can be expected after approximately 2 weeks in stable, non-displaced fractures.
- Angulation is common, but if greater than 60° then the fracture should be reduced and immobilized in a metacarpal splint.
- Shortening may occur and percutaneous pinning should be considered in the competitive boxer.

Bennett's fracture

- A fracture/dislocation of the base of the first metacarpal.
- The pull of abductor pollicis longus causes displacement of the metacarpal shaft.
- Treatment is by closed or open reduction and pinning, followed by 4–6 weeks cast immobilization.
- A further period of splinting is necessary on return to sport.

Phalangeal fractures

- It is very important to check for malrotation (most common in spiral fractures of the proximal phalynx)—ask the patient to make a clenched fist and any rotational deformity should become obvious.
- Also assess for any tendon or volar plate injury.
- Stable fractures can be managed conservatively by 'neighbour' splinting for 3–4 weeks, but careful follow up of all injuries is advised to ensure return of full function.

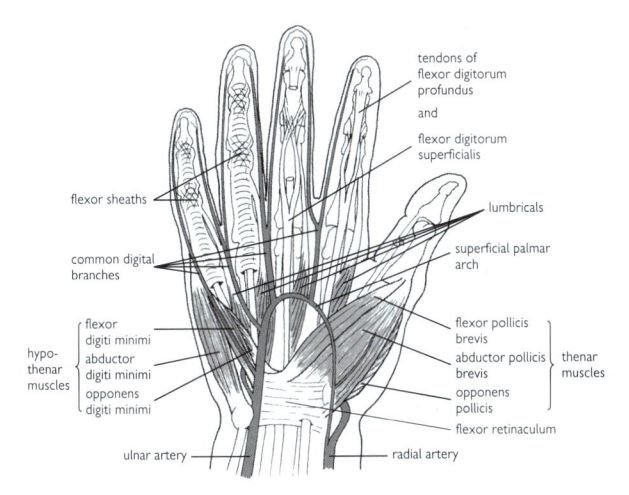

Fig. 19.2 Superficial aspect of palm. Reproduced with permission from MacKinnon P and Morris J. (2005). *Oxford Textbook of Functional Anatomy*, Vol. 1. Oxford University Press, Oxford. © 2005.

Dislocation of the carpal bones

History and examination
- Acute dislocations of the lunate may occur following a fall.
- The lunate dislocates anteriorly and may cause compression of the median nerve.
- More common than an acute dislocation is the development of scapholunate dissociation following a tear of the scapholunate ligament.
- There is tenderness over the radial side of the lunate and Watson's test will be positive (pressure over the scaphoid tuberosity as the wrist is moved from ulnar to radial deviation will result in the scaphoid being felt to sublux dorsally).

Investigation
- A clenched fist postero-anterior (PA) X-ray will demonstrate a gap between the scaphoid and the lunate in cases of scapholunate dissociation (the 'Terry Thomas' sign).

Treatment
- Treatment of lunate dislocation is by open reduction and repair of the torn ligaments followed by eight weeks cast immobilization.
- Treatment of dissociation following a tear is surgical with open reduction internal fixation (ORIF) and repair of the damaged ligament.

Dislocation of the 1st metacarpophalangeal joint

History and examination
- Rarely, the 1st MCP joint can be dislocated dorsally.

Investigation
- X-ray.

Treatment
- This requires open reduction as the metacarpal head becomes button holed between the lumbrical and long flexor tendons.
- Following reduction a splint should be worn to prevent the terminal 30° of extension at the MCP joint for 6 weeks.

Dislocation of the interphalangeal joints

History and examination
- Dislocations of the DIP joints are often caused by a ball hitting the tip of the finger, e.g. in cricket.
- Dislocations of the PIP joints are extremely common in sport and may be reduced on the field of play.

Investigations
- X-rays should be performed to exclude a volar plate injury—the more serious of which will require ORIF.
- It is important not to undertreat these injuries as residual deformity and disability can result.

Treatment
- Following successful reduction the PIP joint should be splinted for 3–4 weeks in slight flexion with a block of approximately 30° to full extension.

Mallet finger

History and examination
- Rupture of the long extensor tendon at or near its attachment to the terminal phalanx results in an inability to actively extend the tip of the finger.
- They commonly occur when the point of the finger is struck by a ball, e.g. in attempting to catch a cricket ball or football.

Investigation
- X-ray.

Treatment
- Occasionally a small avulsion fracture may be evident on X-ray and should be treated by surgical fixation to achieve the best results.
- Otherwise treatment is with a splint which holds the DIP joint in extension for a period of 8 weeks.
- It is very important that the splint is worn continuously, even in bed at night. If removed, e.g. for washing, then care should be taken to ensure that the terminal phalanx is held in full extension at all times.
- Splinting is effective even in injuries up to 3 months old.

Jersey finger

History and examination
- Avulsion of the flexor digitorum profundus tendon at its attachment to the flexor aspect of the distal phalanx results in an inability to actively flex the tip of the finger.
- As the name suggests, it is usually caused when a player tries to grab the jersey of an opponent and the finger is forcibly extended.
- The ring finger is most often involved.
- When examining for this injury, the PIP joint should be fixed in extension and the patient asked to actively flex the DIP joint.

Investigation
- X-ray.

Treatment
- Treatment is by early surgical intervention to reattach the avulsed fragment followed by a period of immobilization in a splint.

Boutonniere deformity

History and examination
- Disruption of the central slip of the extensor digitorum communis tendon at the PIP joint may result in the development of a fixed flexion deformity at the PIP joint with subsequent hyperextension at the DIP joint—the so-called Boutonniere deformity.

Investigation
- X-ray.

Treatment
- Inability to actively extend the PIP joint or the presence of an extensor lag in an acute injury should result in the finger being splinted to hold the PIP joint in full extension for a period of 6 weeks.
- Treatment in established cases is very difficult and prevention is the best policy.

Boxer's knuckle

- Direct trauma, due either to single or repetitive blows, can cause a longitudinal tear in the extensor digitorum communis tendon and joint capsule in the boxer.
- The 3rd MCP joint is most commonly affected as it is most prominent when the fist is clenched.
- Examination may reveal a palpable defect in the extensor mechanism or a lag in active extension at the MCP joint.
- Treatment is surgical repair of the defect followed by 6 weeks of immobilization and rehabilitation to regain full range of movement and strength.

Ulnar collateral ligament injuries (skier's thumb)

History and examination
- Injury to the ulnar collateral ligament of the thumb is common in skiers and results from a fall on the outstretched hand forcing the thumb into abduction and extension against the ski-pole.
- It may also occur on dry slopes when the thumb is caught between the spaces in the carpet.
- On examination there will be tenderness to palpation at the ulnar side of the thumb at the level of the 1st MCP joint.
- There will be excessive (more than 30° compared with uninjured side in a complete tear) laxity when the thumb is stressed into abduction.

Investigation
- X-ray to exclude an avulsion fracture.

Treatment
- Partial tears of the UCL (10–20° of laxity with a definite end point) can be treated conservatively with splint immobilization for a period of 6 weeks.
- Complete tears should be repaired surgically as there is a significant chance of the torn ligament becoming interposed between the adductor aponeurosis (the so-called Stener lesion) and its distal attachment, preventing healing of the ligament, and resulting in chronic instability and disability.
- Following surgery the thumb is immobilized for 6 weeks and should be protected with strapping for another 8 weeks on return to sport.
- The term 'gamekeepers thumb' is used to describe a chronic injury of the UCL—due to the gradual attenuation of the ligament over years caused by breaking rabbits' necks.
- Injuries to the radial collateral ligament of the thumb may also occur. These can generally be treated conservatively with cast immobilization as the risk of soft tissue interposition is less and good results can be expected.
- Tears of the collateral ligaments of the PIP joint can occur at any of the fingers, e.g. when attempting to catch a ball or falling onto the finger.
- Stable injuries (where the joint surfaces are exactly parallel) can be managed conservatively by neighbour strapping—unstable injuries require surgical intervention.
- Collateral ligament sprains can result in many months of discomfort and swelling.

Carpal tunnel syndrome

History and examination
- Caused by compression of the median nerve within the carpal tunnel at the wrist joint. May occur in athletes secondary to flexor tenosynovitis.
- More common in pregnant patients and those with diabetes and hypothyroidism, it can occur with repetitive overuse.
- The patient presents with pain or tingling in the distribution of the median nerve in the hand (thumb, index, middle, and radial half of the ring finger).
- Symptoms are often worse at night and in chronic cases can lead to muscle wasting of the thenar eminence.
- Tinel's sign may be positive over the median nerve at the wrist.
- Phalen's test is positive if numbness is elicited by holding the wrist in hyperflexion for 30s.
- The differential diagnosis includes cervical radiculopathy and a thorough examination of the cervical spine should be performed.

Investigation
- The clinical diagnosis may be confirmed by nerve conduction studies, although this is generally not necessary unless surgical treatment is being considered.

Treatment
- Milder cases can be treated by corticosteroid injection, while more severe cases will require surgical decompression.
- Splinting of the wrist and NSAIDs may be helpful.

Ulnar nerve compression

History and examination
- Compression of the ulnar nerve at the wrist can occur as the nerve passes through the Canal of Guyon between the pisiform and the hamate.
- This is common in cyclists and is due to pressure of the hands against the handlebars especially in the drop position.
- Symptoms can be motor (weakness of finger abduction), sensory (numbness or tingling in the ulnar 1 and 1/2 digits), or mixed, depending on the branch of the nerve affected.

Investigation
- The clinical diagnosis may be confirmed by nerve conduction studies.

Treatment
- Treatment includes the use of cycle gloves or handlebar padding and changes to the position of the hands when cycling, anti-inflammatory medication or, in severe or chronic cases, surgical decompression.

Other nerve injury syndromes

- Direct compression of the PIN (radial tunnel syndrome) can occur in gymnasts due to hyperextension of the wrist and in athletes who repetitively supinate and pronate their forearms (racquet sports, golf).
- It can mimic lateral epicondylopathy of the elbow, although the site of tenderness is distal to the common extensor origin.
- Can cause aching pain in the wrist and paraesthesia in the hand.
- Repetitive traction of the superficial branch of the radial nerve can occur and cause pain and numbness over the radial aspect of the dorsum of the hand and thumb.
- Treatment is activity modification and splinting the wrist in a dorsiflexed position.

De Quervain's tenosynovitis

History and examination
- Inflammation of the tendon sheath of *extensor pollicis brevis* (EPB) and *abductor pollicis longus* (APL) can occur as they pass through a tight fibrous tunnel at the level of the radial styloid.
- Common in racquet sports and rowers, as well as in certain occupations, for example carpenters.
- In the acute stage there will be swelling, tenderness, and occasionally palpable crepitus at the base of the thumb with pain on resisted testing.
- Finkelstein's test is performed by adducting the thumb across the palm of the hand and then placing the wrist into ulnar deviation—this manoeuvre will cause pain in affected individuals.

Investigation
- None required—this is a clinical diagnosis.

Treatment
- Treatment may include avoidance of aggravating activities, a short period of immobilization in a splint and corticosteroid injection to the tendon sheath.
- Response to corticosteroid injection is variable, with one-third of patients requiring more than one injection.
- In chronic cases the tendon sheath may become thickened and stenosed requiring surgical decompression.

Pain may arise more proximally, at the site where the tendons of APL and EPB cross over the wrist extensors. This condition is known as Intersection syndrome and occurs approximately 6–8cm from Lister's tubercle.
- Treatment is similar that used for De Quervain's tenosynovitis.
- Surgery is occasionally necessary.

Other tendinopathies

- All tendons which cross the wrist are subject to overuse and can become painful— extensor carpi ulnaris (ECU) and FCU and radialis (FCR) are particularly prone to developing problems.
- ECU tendinopathy is associated with the double handed backhand technique in tennis.
- US scanning of the affected area is useful to assess the injured tendon, and to differentiate tenosynovitis from tendinopathy or intratendinous tear.
- Acute subluxation of ECU can occur in sports such as tennis, golf, and weightlifting. Dynamic ultrasonography can be used to demonstrate this.
- If identified acutely, immobilization in pronation and radial deviation is generally successful.
- Surgical stabilization is necessary in recurrent or chronic cases.
- Patients with tendinopathy/tenosynovitis should be referred to a physiotherapist for treatment with local electrotherapeutic modalities and a programme of eccentric strengthening exercises.
- A steroid injection into the tendon sheath under US guidance may be beneficial in cases of tenosynovitis, but should not be used if a tear is present. The use of autologous blood or platelet rich plasma injections has not been studied in tendinopathies around the wrist joint.
- Stenosing tenosynovitis can affect any of the flexor tendons of the hand at the level of the MCP joint, causing a triggering effect (*trigger finger*).
- A tender thickening or nodule is felt at this level.
- A single steroid injection to the affected tendon sheath is usually curative.
- Surgery is only very rarely necessary.

Ganglion

History and examination

- A ganglion is a degenerative cyst of either a joint capsule or tendon sheath.
- They are very common at the wrist, especially at the scapholunate joint.

Treatment

- Often asymptomatic, larger ganglions may be treated by aspiration and cortisone injection.
- However, recurrence is very common—the only definitive treatment is complete surgical excision.

Impaction syndromes

History and examination
- Several impingement or impaction syndromes can occur at the wrist joint—these are especially common in gymnasts.
- Entities described include the ulnar-triquetral, scaphoid, and triquetro-lunate impaction syndrome.
- Soft tissue impingement (capsulitis) may also occur (diagnosed by excluding other causes of dorsal wrist pain, e.g. ganglion).

Investigations
- MRI scan may be helpful in showing bone stress and in excluding other causes of wrist pain.
- These conditions require rest from the impact activities which cause pain until symptoms resolve.

The paediatric wrist

Distal radial physeal stress injury

Pathology and cause
- Stress reaction at the distal radial physis.
- Occurs secondary to compressive overloading.
- Most commonly seen in gymnasts secondary to upper-limb weight-bearing.
- >80% of the compressive load is transmitted through the radius with upper limb weight-bearing, which explains why this condition affects the radial and not the ulna physis.

Clinical features
- Insidious onset of unilateral or bilateral dorsal wrist pain ± swelling
- Pain is exacerbated by upper-limb weight-bearing, e.g. hand stands, bench presses, or use of parallel or uneven bars.
- Limitation of wrist dorsiflexion often present.
- Focal tenderness over the distal radial physis.
- Forced extension of the wrist reproduces the pain.

Investigations
- Affected epiphysis appears widened, sclerotic, and irregular on X-ray.
- MRI or imaging of the asymptomatic side may be required to detect subtle changes.

Management
- As with other stress reactions, management involves unloading the injured area (i.e. avoiding upper-limb weight bearing) until the pain resolves.
- Physiotherapy is aimed at restoring full range of movement and strengthening the wrist flexors.
- If the distal radial physis appears to be closing prematurely, specialist referral is warranted.

Prognosis
- If untreated, distal radial physeal stress injury can cause premature closure of the growth plate: premature closure of the distal radial physis results in positive ulnar variance (a relative overgrowth of the ulna), which is not an uncommon finding in gymnasts.

Triangular fibro-cartilage complex tears

The triangular fibrocartilage complex is composed of triangular fibrocartilage and ligaments on the ulnar side of the wrist between the ulna and the carpus.

Mechanism of Injury
- Can be torn with activities involving wrist extension and ulnar deviation, e.g. gymnastics and tennis

Clinical features
- Present with ulnar wrist pain ± swelling exacerbated by wrist dorsiflexion and ulnar deviation.
- Clicking sensation may be present.

THE PAEDIATRIC WRIST

- Grip strength is commonly reduced.
- May have a previous history of distal radial physeal stress injury

Investigations
- X-ray may reveal positive ulnar variance, but MRI is diagnostic.
- When MRI is not available, arthrography can be used to determine the presence of a tear.

Treatment
- Conservative treatment involves rest from provocative activities and splinting or taping to prevent excessive dorsiflexion and ulnar deviation.
- Local physiotherapy can reduce pain and swelling.
- If symptoms do not settle with conservative treatment, orthopaedic referral is required for wrist arthroscopy, removal of the torn cartilage and sometimes an ulnar osteotomy to correct positive ulnar variance.
- Symptoms are likely to recur when associated with positive ulnar variance and when provocative activities are continued.

Kienbock's disease

Pathology
- Avascular necrosis affecting the lunate of unknown aetiology.
- Often associated with repeated minor wrist trauma.

Clinical features
- Commonly presents in adolescence or later with a restricted range of movement in the wrist and loss of grip strength.
- Dorsal wrist pain is exacerbated by loading the extended wrist
- Often a history of recurrent loading of the wrist, e.g. racquet sports, repetitive falls.

Investigations
- X-ray may be normal in the early phases, but later demonstrates sclerosis and flattening of the lunate.
- May be associated with negative ulnar variance.
- Bone scan and MRI will be positive in the early stages.

Treatment and prognosis
- If diagnosed in the early stages before significant X-ray changes have occurred, rest from exacerbating activities, and bracing or cast immobilization may prevent compression.
- If compression of the lunate has occurred, orthopaedic referral is required.
- In cases of chronic pain where conservative treatment has failed, wrist arthrodesis may be required.
- Long-term disability is common after compressive changes have occurred.

Chapter 20

Abdomen

Abdominal injury *548*
Splenic bleeding *549*
Liver damage *549*
Pancreatic damage *549*
Renal trauma *550*
Ureteric avulsion *551*
Bladder rupture *551*
Urethral rupture *551*
Injuries of the scrotum and testes *551*
Bowel rupture *552*
Diarrhoea (runner's trots) *553*
Renal physiology and exercise *554*
Side strain *557*

Abdominal injury

Abdominal viscera are vulnerable in contact sport and, although the ribs and pelvis provide some protection, the main protection is by the abdominal musculature. In addition, superficial structures such as skin, subcutaneous tissues, and muscle may be injured. Diagnosis is usually obvious, and management is as for skin and SC wounds elsewhere in the body. Nevertheless, rectus abdominus muscle rupture with damage of epigastric artery may produce a large haematoma. The swelling may first be thought of as arising from an abdominal organ, but the later bluish discoloration gives a clue that it does not. The swelling will not cross the midline or extend beyond the lateral border of the muscle. It is relatively immovable due to the rectus sheath. US or MRI will confirm if required.

The winded athlete

A blow to the solar plexus, with abdominal muscles relaxed, leaves the athlete temporarily unable to breathe. This is frightening for the athlete and the pitch side doctor should provide confident reassurance, ensure the airway is open and clear, loosen any restrictive clothing or equipment, and encourage a slight flexion of the trunk. After the episode has passed, the doctor should consider visceral and rib injury.

History

Location of pathology may be obscure as pain can be referred:
- To shoulder from diaphragm (liver).
- To shoulder blade from gall bladder.
- To left chest from spleen.
- To umbilicus from appendix or pancreas.
- To testis from ureter and groin.

Examination

Signs of serious intra-abdominal injury
- Absence of normal respiratory movements of abdomen.
- Guarding.
- Rebound pain.
- Absence of normal bowel sounds.
- Referred pain to shoulder or back.
- Falling BP, increased pulse rate.

Delayed or slow haemorrhage from abdominal trauma is possible and so reassessment over several days is warranted.

Immediate management of any abdominal trauma will be assessment and appropriate treatment of haemodynamic shock.

Splenic bleeding

The spleen lies on the 9th to 11th ribs on the posterior wall of the abdomen and thus is unusually injured in sport unless enlarged. US is the most convenient means to assess splenic enlargement beyond clinical examination. The most common cause of splenomegaly in athletes is glandular fever (infectious mononucleosis), and this causes the spleen to be vulnerable in blows to the left upper quadrant. Consequently, athletes should be advised against contact sport whilst the spleen is enlarged. The exact time period following the onset of glandular fever is controversial, although 5 weeks is the minimum. FBC, liver enzymes, and abdominal examination should have normalized. Some practitioners recommend 6 months off contact sport and, even then, athletes should be warned to report any abdominal discomfort for thorough assessment.

The spleen may also be ruptured by a fractured rib. The athlete will have persistent aching in the left flank following the initial acute pain. Sometimes there is an intervening period with no pain. Some have referred pain to the shoulder.

Clinicians should be alert to splenic bleeds. CT scan can confirm the diagnosis. Though minor splenic injuries can be treated conservatively and with ongoing observation, rapid blood loss demands splenectomy.

Liver damage

Lacerations of the liver are rare in sport, although subcapsular haemorrhage may occur and give rise to right upper quadrant pain and tenderness. US or CT scan may confirm the diagnosis.

Pancreatic damage

The pancreas lies deep at the back of the abdomen and is rarely injured in sport. Epigastric pain radiating to the back after severe blunt trauma, with midline tenderness, distension, and loss of bowel sounds due to reflex ileus, should lead the clinician to consider pancreatic damage. Serum amylase will be elevated and CT will confirm the diagnosis.

Renal trauma

The kidneys have some protection from blunt trauma from the 11th and 12th ribs, psoas muscle, and surrounding fat. However, renal contusions do occur, particularly in the young where the relative size of the kidney is larger. The kidneys are the most commonly injured abdominal organ in sport and result in many hospitalizations. The kidneys are vulnerable when the abdominal muscles are relaxed, and typically this might occur when leaping high and reaching for a ball, whilst taking a blow from another athlete, e.g. during basketball or at the rugby line-out.

Grading of renal injury
- *Grade I:* cortical lacerations without extravasation.
- *Grade II:* deep cortical laceration.
- *Grade III:* calix laceration.
- *Grade IV:* vascular pedicle rupture.

History
- *Flank pain:* although this may refer anteriorly.
- *Haematuria:* the amount of blood in the urine does not correlate to the seriousness of the injury. *NB* There may not be frank haematuria following a vascular pedicle injury.

Examination
- Microscopic haematuria.
- Dropping BP (<90mmHg systolic).
- Palpable mass.

Investigations
- Intravenous pyelogram (IVP).
- *CT scan:* provides additional information about other abdominal viscera that might be injured.

Management
Depends on extent of injury. Few (<10%) require surgery though indications are:
- Persistent retroperitoneal bleeding.
- Urinary extravasation.
- Non-viable renal tissue.
- Renal vascular pedicle injury.

Return to Sport
Even for Grade I injuries, return to strenuous sport should be delayed 4 weeks to reduce the risk of re-bleeding (maximum at 15–21 days). Contact sport should be avoided for at least 6 weeks and follow-up should be for 6 months with repeat BP and urinalysis. Hypertension and hydronephrosis are late complications.

Ureteric avulsion

Rare in sport, although described in motor vehicle and equestrian sports. Gives rise to severe back pain and peritoneal irritation. Confirmed by IVP, requires surgical management.

Bladder rupture

Bladder rupture may occur with severe trauma of abdomen or pelvis. Suprapubic tenderness and haematuria will be present with contusions, but signs of peritonism (abdominal rigidity or rebound tenderness) indicate rupture and leakage of urine. Rupture requires prompt surgical treatment.

Urethral rupture

Urethral rupture is rare in sport and tends to occur with a straddle injury, cycling, gymnastics, or equestrian, or in association with pelvic fractures. It is a more common injury in men than women and it is the bulbous urethra that is more likely to be injured than the penile, which can move more freely. There will be blood at the meatus, as well as signs of perineal trauma. Surgical repair are and a suprapubic catheter required.

Injuries of the scrotum and testes

External to the abdomen, the scrotum, and contents are vulnerable to injury from blunt trauma.

Prevention
- Some athletes wear protective equipment (cricketers and hockey goalkeepers, for example).

History and examination
- Scrotal swelling after trauma suggests a ruptured testis or ruptured pampiniform plexus of veins.
- In the case of ruptured pampiniform plexus of veins, a varicocele becomes a haematocele. A haematocele does not transluminate well, so if the testicular shadow is visible through the fluid a hydrocele is more likely.

Investigations
- US examination is effective at diagnosing the ruptured testis, which requires urgent surgery.

Return to sport
- If trauma does not result in swelling and scrotal examination is normal, the athlete may be treated by scrotal support, NSAIDs, and return to activity when pain subsides.

Bowel rupture

Rarely the bowel may be ruptured in severe blunt trauma in sport. There will be abdominal pain and blood in the peritoneum may irritate the diaphragm giving shoulder pain. Examination reveals tenderness, guarding, even abdominal rigidity and loss of bowel sounds. Shock may be indicated by clammy skin, tachycardia, and falling blood pressure. Peritoneal lavage may detect blood. Free air may be seen under the diaphragm in the upright plain abdominal X-ray. Prompt surgical treatment is required.

Diarrhoea (runner's trots)

Urgency to defecate, abdominal cramps, and diarrhoea frequently occur in long-distance runners, called 'runner's trots' and can be related to several factors:
- Athletes may have increased catecholamine levels.
- Athletes tend to have high carbohydrate diets, which can increase intestinal transit time.
- Reduced visceral flow leading to relative ischaemia of the bowel, particularly as duration of exercise increases.

Renal physiology and exercise

Renal parameters at rest
- Renal blood flow is 20% of cardiac output (1200mL/min).
- Renal plasma flow—700mL/min.
- Glomerular filtration rate (GFR)—15% of plasma flow—105mL/min.
- Smaller proteins than albumin are filtered, but then reabsorbed in proximal tubules.

Renal response to exercise
- Renal blood flow decreases.
- GFR is maintained or decreases.
- Increased filtration of macromolecules (albumin) giving rise to a 'glomerular' pattern of protein loss.
- In intense exercise, reabsorption of small proteins (microglobulins) declines giving rise to a tubular pattern of protein loss.

The decrease in renal blood flow is mediated by catecholamines and the sympathetic nervous system and is related to intensity of exercise, such that it may reduce to 25% of resting flow with strenuous activity. Plasma flow may reduce to 200mL/min in such circumstances, yet GFR is often maintained. With dehydration GFR may drop. With intense exercise ADH and aldosterone levels increase to preserve water and sodium. During such activity more red and white blood cells are found in the urine.

Athletic pseudonephritis
Described by Gardner (1956),[1] athletic pseudonephritis is the presence of red and white blood cells, haemoglobin, myoglobin, protein, and casts in the urine after exercise. This is recognized to be a benign situation and has attracted various names depending on the activity with which the findings are associated:
- Stress haematuria.
- Marathoner's haematuria.
- 10,000m haematuria.
- March haemaglobinuria.
- Jogger's nephritis.

Proteinuria
Common in contact and non-contact sports and between 70 and 100% of runners are reported to have protein in their urine. This relates to intensity and not duration of event and is maximal within 30min of exercise.

The pattern is glomerular (macroglobulins) for moderate exercise, but glomerulotubular (macro- and microglobulins) for intense exercise. This may be due to hypoxic damage to nephrons due to decreased blood flow, or efferent glomerular arteriolar constriction being greater than afferent, and so increasing filtration pressure.

---

[1] Gardner KD, Jnr. (1956). Athletic pseudonephritis; alterations of urine sediment by athletic competition. *J Am Med Ass* **161**(17): 1613–17.

There are other causes of proteinuria:
- Physiological proteinuria (<100mg/L).
- Orthostatic proteinuria.
- Glomerulonephritis (>0.2g/day).
- Nephrotic syndrome (>0.05g/kg body wt/day).
- Cystitis/pyelonephritis.
- Hypertension.
- Diabetes mellitus.

Physiological proteinuria is common in adolescents (60%) and recurs in up to 30%. It is benign.

Orthostatic proteinuria clears with recumbency and so early morning urine might be negative. Prognosis is good if normotensive and protein loss 750mg/day.

Typically, proteinuria records ++ or +++ on urinalysis corresponding to up to 300mg/L, post-exercise. With a positive urinalysis for protein following exercise and no other symptoms to indicate another cause, repeat the urinalysis after 48h of rest. The urine should be negative to protein.

Haematuria

Haematuria may be macroscopic and dramatic after exercise, and may include clots. Microscopic haematuria is almost universal and dipsticks, may detect as few as 1 million red cells/L, whereas 100 million red cells/L is more likely to indicate abnormality. Dipsticks are sensitive, detect the haem group and so show up myoglobinuria and haemoglobinuria.

Haematuria has been reported in high numbers of:
- Ice hockey players (100%).
- Swimmers (80%).
- Boxers (73%).
- US footballers (60%).
- Soccer players (50%).
- Runners (10–25%).

Proportions depend on the definitions used in the studies and on the intensity of exercise, although contact also clearly plays a part in some sports.

Early cystoscopy in females showed 'kissing' lesions, localized bladder contusions, urothelial loss, from trigone and interureteric bar leading to theories of bladder 'slapping' being a cause of haematuria in sports. However, the red cells seen in the urine of marathon runners are often dysmorphic, suggesting damage at the glomerular level. The explanation may be hypoxic damage to the nephron or increased filtration pressure (see 📖 Proteinuria, p. 554).

Other causes of haematuria:
- Acute glomerular nephritis.
- Pyelonephritis.
- Acute tubular necrosis.
- Urinary tract infection (UTI).
- Stones.
- Cancer (esp. >40yr-olds).
- Haemoglobinuria or myoglobinuria.
- Spurious.

History may include trauma, pain, fever, dysuria, and weight, or appetite loss. Examination findings may include renal tenderness, oedema, raised temperature, raised blood pressure, cachexia. If these are not present and there is a clear relationship to exercise, repeat the urinalysis after 48h rest. Consider further investigation if haematuria persists including microscopy and culture (MCS) of mid-stream sample (MSU), IVP, US examination of the renal tract and cystoscopy. Clotting studies may be performed to exclude a bleeding disorder and FBC performed to rule out anaemia.

If 'athletic haematuria' is the final diagnosis, the prognosis is good and there is no need to restrict sporting activity. Adequate hydration before and during exercise may help preserve glomerular filtration and keep the bladder reasonably full to prevent 'slapping'.

Haemoglobinuria

If the urine is positive for blood on urinalysis, but red cells are not seen on microscopy, haemoglobin from the breakdown of red cells may be present in the urine. This has been described in relation to long marches in the military and in contact sports such as karate. It is generally a benign condition.

Myoglobinuria/exercise induced rhabdomyolysis

The presence of myoglobin in the urine indicates the breakdown of muscle, 'rhabdomyolysis'. It has been recorded both in endurance sports, such as marathon running, and in contact sports, such as American football. The urine appears tea- or cola-coloured. The urinalysis is again positive for blood, but negative for red cells.

Myoglobin is broken down to haematin. Haematin is nephrotoxic and so there have been concerns that athletes with myogloinuria may go into acute renal failure. However, the risk of acute renal failure in association with sport appears to be small. Sinert proposed a nephrotoxic factor was missing in the rhabdomyolysis of sport, unlike medical causes of rhabdomyolysis.[1] Nevertheless, it is probably best to avoid myoglobinuria if possible by adequate hydration, nutrition, and conditioning.

Acute renal failure in sport

Though rare in sport, acute renal failure is associated with exercise to exhaustion in hot conditions. Those who are less fit and those who become dehydrated or hyperpyrexial are at risk. Important preventative factors include adequate hydration, nutrition, exercising in cooler environment, and not exercising to exhaustion.

Spurious causes of red urine

Medication (e.g. rifampicin, nitrofurantoin) and diet (e.g. beetroot) give rise to red urine, but urinalysis will be negative.

---

[1] Sinert R, Kohl L, Rainone T, Scalea T. (1994). Exercise-induced rhabdomyoloysis *Ann Emerg Med.* **23** (6): 1301–6.

Side strain

Sports involving strong eccentric lateral flexion of the trunk are susceptible to side strains. This involves strain of the insertions of the internal or external oblique attachments to the lower ribs.

History
- Sudden onset of pain during sporting activity (such as bowling in cricket or serving in tennis) at the costal margin.
- Inability to continue performing same activity due to pain.

Examination
- Local tenderness at the costal margin often in the axillary line.
- Aggravation of pain with cross-over sit-up.
- Pain on resisted side flexion.

Investigations
USS or MRI show haematoma and fibre disruption of insertion of oblique abdominal muscles near one of lowest four ribs or their cartilage.

Management
- Rest from causal activity.
- Ice for first 48 to 72h.
- Progressive rehabilitation according to pain level (flexibility in side flexion, core stability work to sit ups to cross over sit ups to sport specific activity).
- Cautious use of corticosteroid injection (consider Doping Regulations) in chronic cases.

Prognosis
- Most recover in 4 to 6 weeks.
- Chronic cases may be due to rib impingement on pelvic brim and surgical intervention may be useful.
- Recurrence is not unusual.

Chapter 21

Hip and pelvis

Examination 560
Special tests 566
Femur: acute injury 568
Growth plate injury 570
Femoral neck stress fracture 572
Trochanteric bursitis 574
Ilio-tibial band syndrome 576
Thigh contusion 578
Myositis ossificans 580
Osteoarthritis of the hip 582
Pubic bone stress injury (osteitis pubis) 584
Sports hernia (Gilmore's groin) 585
Groin pain 586
Rehabilitation for over-use injuries 588
Avulsions around the ilium 594
Piriformis syndrome 595
Snapping hip syndrome 596
Hamstring Injury 598
Management of hamstring injury 602
Obturator nerve entrapment 606
Dislocation and subluxation of the hip joint 607
Stress fractures of the pubic rami 608
Calcific tendinopathy of the hip 608
Acetabular labral tears 609
Femoroacetabular impingement 610
Loose bodies 611
Ischial (ischiogluteal) bursitis 612
Sacro-iliac joint disorders 613
The paediatric hip 614

Examination

The usual presenting complaints are:
- Pain.
- Limp.
- Discomfort leading to reduced walking/running distances.
- Snapping or clicking sensation of the hip.
- Stiffness/reduced range of motion.
- Deformity.

Inspection
- Examine gait:
  - Look for evidence of asymmetry or biomechanical abnormality.
  - Scars.
  - Sinuses.
  - Swellings/masses.
  - Muscle wasting.
  - Apparent limb length by measuring the distance from umbilicus to medial malleolus.
- True limb length discrepancy is noted by measuring the distance from anterior superior iliac spine (or any ipsilateral fixed bony point) to medial malleolus after squaring the pelvis (unmask the fixed abduction or adduction deformity of the affected limb so that both anterior superior iliac spine and medial malleolus are levelled, and place the normal limb in a similar position).

See Figs. 21.1, 21.2, and 21.3.

Palpation
- Skin temperature.
- Tenderness over the greater trochanter and in the groin area.
- Palpate swellings/masses if present.

Active and passive movements

The pelvis must be squared and stabilized before hip movements are measured (see Tables 21.1 and 21.2).

A normal hip has:
- Flexion range of 0–130°.
- Extension of 0–10°.
- Abduction of 0–45°.
- Adduction of 0–40°.
- IR of 0–30°.
- ER of 0–60°.

Note pain or restriction at the extremes of range of movement. IR is restricted in early osteoarthritis. In advanced osteoarthritis, there is fixed flexion deformity with absent extension, decreased abduction, adduction, and ER and IR. All movements may be associated with pain.

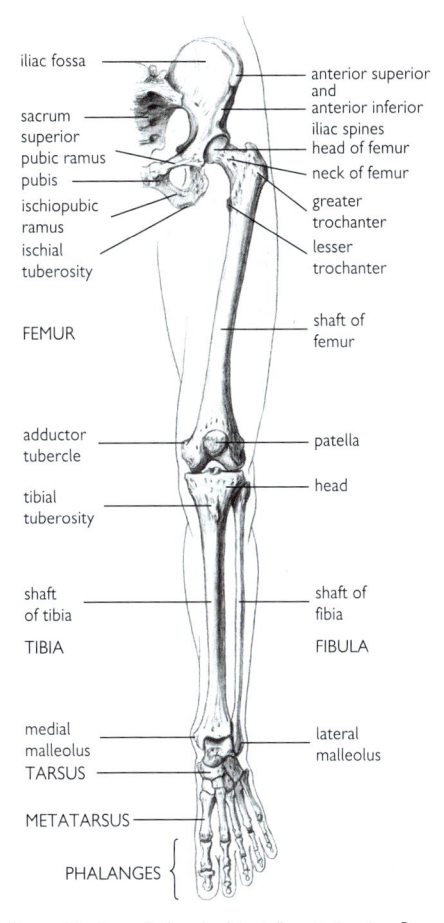

Fig. 21.1 Bones of the lower limb and pelvic girdle: anterior view. Reproduced with permission from Mackinnon P and Morris J. (2005). *Oxford Textbook of Functional Anatomy*, Vol. 1. Oxford University Press, Oxford. © 2005.

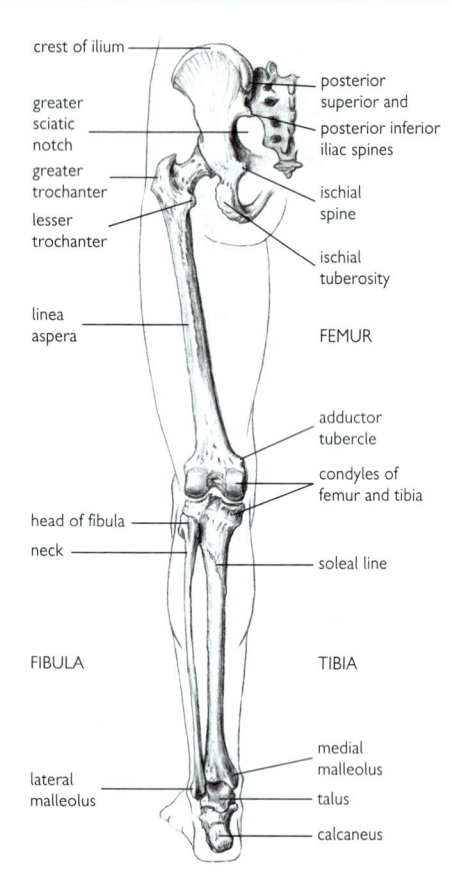

Fig. 21.2 Bones of the lower limb and pelvic girdle: posterior view. Reproduced with permission from Mackinnon P and Morris J. (2005). *Oxford Textbook of Functional Anatomy*, Vol. 1. Oxford University Press, Oxford. © 2005.

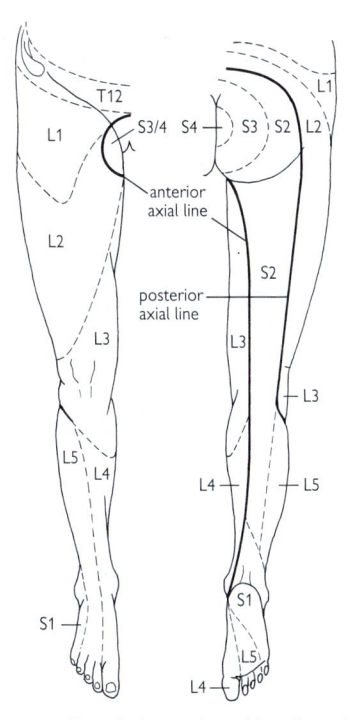

Fig. 21.3 Dermatomes of lower limb; note the axial lines. Reproduced with permission from Mackinnon P and Morris J. (2005). *Oxford Textbook of Functional Anatomy*, Vol. 1. Oxford University Press, Oxford. © 2005.

Table 21.1 Hip joint: movements, principal muscles, and their innervation. Reproduced with permission from Mackinnon P and Morris J (2005)

Movement	Principal muscles	Peripheral nerve	Spinal root origin
Flexion	Psoas major	Ventral rami of lumbar nerves	L 1, 2, 3
	Iliacus	Femoral nerve	L 2, 3
	Rectus femoris	Femoral nerve	L 2, 3, 4
	Pectineus	Femoral nerve	L 2, 3, 4
Extension	Gluteus maximus	Inferior gluteal nerve	L 5, S1, 2
	Hamstrings (semimembranosus, semitendinosus, biceps femoris (short- and long head)	Sciatic nerve (tibial component-except for the short head of biceps femoris supplied by the peroneal component)	L 4, 5, S1, 2
Adduction	Adductors longus, brevis, magnus, and gracilis	Obturator nerve	L 2, 3, 4
Abduction	Gluteus medius and minimus	Superior gluteal nerve	L 4, 5, S1
	Tensor fasciae latae	Superior gluteal nerve	L 4, 5, S1
Medial Rotation	Tensor fasciae latae	Superior gluteal nerve	L 4, 5, S1
	Gluteus medius and minimus	Superior gluteal nerve	L 4, 5, S1
	Adductor longus	Obturator nerve	L 2, 3, 4
Lateral Rotation	Obturator externus	Obturator nerve	L 2, 3, 4
	Sartorius	Femoral nerve	L 2, 3, 4
	Quadratus femoris	Sacral plexus	L 4, 5, S1
	Obturator internus	Sacral plexus	L 5, S1, 2
	Gluteus maximus	Inferior gluteal nerve	L 5, S1, 2

Oxford Textbook of Functional Anatomy, Vol. 1. Oxford University Press, Oxford. © 2005.

Table 21.2 Main spinal nerve root supplying the movements of the lower limb. Reproduced with permission from Mackinnon P and Morris J (2005)

	Movement	Main nerve roots
Hip	Flexion, adduction	L 2, 3, 4
Knee	Extension, abduction	L 4, 5, S1
	Extension	L 3,
Ankle	Flexion	L 5, S1
	Flexion (plantar flexion)	L 5
Subtalar joint	Extension (dorsiflexion)	L 5, S1
	Inversion	L 5
Toes (long muscles)	Eversion	L 5, S1
	Flexion (plantar flexion)	L 5, S1, 2
Toes (small muscles of foot)	Extension (dorsalflexion)	L 5, S1, 2, 3
		S1, 2, 3

Because of the rotation of the lower limb, extension of the knee is supplied by higher segments.

Oxford Textbook of Functional Anatomy, Vol. 1. Oxford University Press, Oxford. © 2005.

Special tests

Trendeleburg test
Helps to assess the integrity of the abductor mechanism of the hip. Patients are asked to stand on one leg, and the position of the pelvis is noted. If the pelvis drops and patients sway to loaded leg, the test is positive. Pain on weight-bearing, weakness of hip abductors, shortening of femoral neck, and dislocation or subluxation of the hip joint result in a Trendelenburg +ve test.

Thomas' test
Fixed flexion deformity of the hip can be masked by the increased pelvic tilt and exaggerated lumbar lordosis. This test helps unmask a fixed flexion deformity of the hip and identify the limitation in the range of hip flexion.

With the patient supine, both hips are flexed until the lumbar lordosis is obliterated (confirmed by examiner's hand). The normal (or contralateral) hip is kept flexed, and the affected hip is lowered to the maximum possible extent. The angle between couch and the lower limb is the fixed flexion deformity angle.

Tests for suspected labral tears
- Pain on flexion, adduction, and IR of the hip joint occurs with anterior superior tears.
- Pain on passive hyperextension, abduction, and ER occurs with posterior tears.
- Pain moving the hip from a position of full flexion of the hip with ER and full abduction, to extension, abduction, and IR occurs with anterior tears.
- Pain moving the hip from extension, abduction, and ER to flexion, adduction, and IR occurs with posterior tears.

The above movements may also be accompanied by a clicking and/or locking sensation.

Complete the examination by performing neurovascular examination of the lower limb, and examining the contralateral hip and ipsilateral knee, and spine.

Faber test
The manoeuvre is performed with the patient in supine position with the affected leg flexed and the foot on the opposite knee (flexion abduction ER of the hip). The patient's pelvis is stabilized by placing a hand on the iliac crest of the opposite side. The examiner presses down on the flexed knee. The test is positive if there is pain at the hip or sacral joint, or if the leg cannot be placed parallel to the opposite leg. Pain in the groin area suggests a hip pathology, while pain in the sacro-iliac area indicates a sacro-iliac joint (SIJ) pathology.

Piriformis test
The patient lies on the unaffected side or supine. The affected leg is in 60° of hip flexion. The knee should be bent and relaxed with the foot on the unaffected leg. The examiner places one hand on the hip for stabilization

and exerts a downward pressure on the knee with the other hand, while rotating the hip internally. The test is positive if there is pain or tightness. If the sciatic nerve is compressed (piriformis syndrome), the patient experiences radicular-like symptoms.

Ober's test (ilio-tibial band)
The patient lies on the unaffected side with the hip flexed. The examiner passively extends and abducts the hip. If the leg remains in the abducted position, it indicates a positive test (contracture of the ilio-tibial band). If the leg adducts, the test is considered negative. Localized pain over the greater trochanter during the Ober's test may indicate an underlying trochanteric bursitis.

Investigation
- Plain radiographs, CT, MR, and bone scan, and arthroscopy are helpful to confirm clinical diagnoses.

Femur: acute injury

Femoral shaft fractures, while unusual in most sports, are an emergency and associated injuries must be ruled out. Follow advanced trauma life support (ATLS) guidelines (airway with cervical spine control, breathing, circulation, disability assessment, and exposure) when managing such injuries. A secondary survey will help identify associated injuries.

Fractures are usually closed, and if open, are often within-out injuries. The mechanism is usually a torsional stress causing a spiral fracture that may extend into the proximal or distal metaphysis. A direct force causes transverse or oblique fractures. Severe trauma results in comminuted/segmental fractures. There are often other injuries associated with femoral shaft fractures so, look out for ipsilateral fractures of the neck of the femur and/or the posterior wall of the acetabulum.

Fractures can be classified on the basis of the site of injury, the extent of fracture, the configuration, the relationship of fracture fragments to each other and the relationship to the external environment, with important influence on the prognosis. The AO Classification is widely accepted.

History and examination
- Severe pain, with obvious swelling and deformity.
- Unable to move the limb.
- Beware of hypovolaemic shock; up to 1.5L of blood may be lost into the thigh.
- Check and document the presence of distal pulses and the neurological status of the affected limb.

Investigation
- Radiographs to include both hip and knee joints. The incidence of ipsilateral femoral shaft and femoral neck fractures is 3%.
- CT scan or MRI can provide additional information, especially in complex fractures.

Treatment
- *Manage shock*:
  - Two wide bore venous cannulae (brown- or grey-coloured).
  - Hartmann's solution is preferred.
  - Urinary catherization.
  - Cross-match 2–4units of blood.
- Analgesia.
- Adequate splint (Thomas splint).
- Femoral fractures generally require a surgical treatment, with different techniques according to the type of fracture and patient characteristics.
- Gold standard is early closed intramedullary nailing for closed fractures (<24h).
- Fix femoral neck first, if present.
- Open fractures need emergency debridement and stabilization.
- Paediatric femoral shaft fractures can be managed with traction.

Complications
- Fat embolism.
- Infection.
- Delayed union requiring dynamization of interlocking nail.
- Non-union may need reamed exchange nailing.
- Malunion (may need corrective surgery).

Growth plate injury

The growth plate (physis) can be injured in many ways. The most common cause is trauma. Less common causes include disuse, infection, tumour, vascular impairment, neural involvement, metabolic abnormalities, radiation, laser injury, electrical injury, burns, frostbite, chronic stress, and iatrogenic or surgical insults.[1]

Physeal fractures

The physis is the weakest structure near a paediatric joint. They occur in a male:female ratio of 2:1. In males, the peak incidence is at 14yrs, and in females it is at 11–12yrs. (The most common sites of injury are the phalanges of fingers (37%) followed by the distal radius (18%).) Children present with pain, inability to use the limb, and, less commonly, deformity. AP and lateral radiographs of the affected part usually confirm the diagnosis. Occasionally, stress views, tomograms, CT scans, MR scan, or a US scan can help detect growth plate injury.

Classification

The Salter–Harris classification of the physeal injuries is widely used:
- Separation of the epiphysis from the metaphysis with disruption of the complete physis.
- Separation of part of the physis, with a portion of metaphysis attached to the epiphysis (Thurston–Holland sign).
- Fracture of the epiphysis extending into the physis.
- The fracture traverses metaphysis, physis, epiphysis and the articular cartilage.
- This injury is end-on crush of the physis. Diagnosis is retrospective as radiographs are normal at initial presentation. MRI can be useful for the diagnosis.

Treatment

- Immediate anatomical reduction either by gentle closed or open methods, and adequate fixation (conservative or surgical) aid restoration of function and normal growth.

Complications

- If the entire physis is affected, bone growth and, therefore, length is retarded. If a part of physis is affected, angular deformity may result.

---

1 Peterson HA. (2001). Physeal injuries and growth arrest. In: Beaty JH, Kasser JR. (eds), *Fracture in Children* (pp. 91–138) Philadelphia: Lippincott Williams & Wilkins.

Femoral neck stress fracture

Stress fractures of the femoral neck or pubic rami may cause hip and groin pain. These fractures usually result either from abnormal forces acting on normal bone, or normal forces acting on abnormal bones.

The most common stress fractures in sport are fatigue fractures, resulting from excessive stress on the bones.

Long distance runners and dancers (especially females) are more prone to femoral neck stress fractures. Predisposing factors include changes in the training programme with increase in intensity, frequency, and duration, changes in shoes, running on a different surface, nutritional deficiency, and abnormal menstrual cycles and hormonal imbalance in female athletes.

Femoral neck stress fractures are classified by Fullerton and Snowdy[1] as tension (type I—superior aspect of the femoral neck), compression (type II—inferior aspect of the femoral neck), or displaced (type III), from the mechanism of injury. This classification has an important influence on the prognosis, as the tension surface femoral neck stress fractures are at significant risk of non-union, deformity, and avascular necrosis. Compression surface femoral neck fractures usually have a good prognosis and may be treated with reduced/altered activity followed by gradual return to sport.

History and examination
- Deep aching pain in the groin that may radiate to the knee.
- Pain is progressive, occurs with activity, and resolves with rest.
- Pain becomes constant if activities are continued without modification.
- May present with a limp.
- May be no specific site of point tenderness.
- Range of motion of the hip, particularly IR, may be limited due to pain.
- Walking, static running, or hopping on the affected extremity often reproduces the pain.

The differential diagnosis includes infection, tumour, compartment syndrome, arthritis, ligamentous, or soft-tissue injuries. The history may be non-specific, but clinicians should always be alert to the possibility, especially in high risk groups.

Investigations
- Plain radiographs may be negative.
- MRI is more sensitive, specific, and accurate than a bone scan in identifying a femoral neck stress fracture.

Treatment
- Tension (type I) and displaced (type III) fractures should be referred urgently to an orthopaedic surgeon for internal fixation.
- Internal fixation aids early rehabilitation and return to sports.
- Compression (type II) can be managed conservatively with non- or partial weight-bearing depending on pain and analgesia. The patient may start non-impact activities once pain-free.

Complications
- Avascular necrosis.
- Non-union (with conservative management).
- Varus deformity (with conservative management).
- Displacement (with conservative management).

Prognosis
- Any of the above complications may lead to inability to return to pre-injury performance levels.

Prevention
- A gradual progression in the intensity and duration of all conditioning activities is crucial in the prevention of stress fractures.
- A useful rule of thumb is that an increase in training volume (distance) or intensity should not exceed 10% per week.

Trochanteric bursitis

Inflammation of the greater trochanteric bursa. This bursa minimizes the friction between the greater trochanter and the ilio-tibial band, which passes over the bursa. Bursal inflammation may be caused by several conditions, such chronic microtrauma, arthritis, regional muscle dysfunction, over-use, or acute injuries.

Predisposing factors include a broad pelvis (female runners), training on banked surfaces or roads with a slope, and a recent increase in mileage, duration, or intensity of training.

There are many bursae in the hip and groin region, but the most commonly involved sites are the trochanter, the ischial and iliopectineal bursae.

History and examination
- Lateral hip pain, occasionally radiating along the distal lateral thigh.
- May be associated with snapping or clicking sensation.
- Point tenderness over the greater trochanter may be associated with crepitus on hip flexion and extension.
- Pain at the extremes of hip rotation, abduction, or adduction (trochanteric)
- Pain of contraction of hip abductors against resistance (trochanteric).
- *Pseudoradiculopathy*: pain radiating down the lateral aspect of the thigh (trochanteric).
- While diagnostic criteria have been proposed, their sensitivity, specificity, and predictive value have not been established.[1]
- These criteria propose that lateral hip pain and tenderness around the greater trochanter must be present in combination with 1 of the following:
  - Pain at the extremes of rotation, abduction, or adduction.
  - Pain of contraction of the hip abductors against resistance.
  - Pseudoradiculopathy: pain radiating down the lateral aspect of the thigh.

Provocative positions include ER and adduction.
The differential diagnosis includes:
- Stress fractures.
- Gluteus medius tendinopathy (dancers).
- Lumbosacral radiculopathy.
- Avascular necrosis.
- Osteoarthritis.
- Septic bursitis

Investigations
Diagnosis is usually made by clinical examination:
- Radiographs may help rule out other conditions.
- The role of US and MRI is unclear.

---

1 Alvarez-Nemegyei J, Canoso JJ. (2004). Evidence-based soft tissue rheumatology: III: trochanteric bursitis. *J Clin Rheumatol.* **10:** 123–4.

Treatment

Most patients improve with conservative management, which includes:
- Rest.
- Ilio-tibial band and tensor fascia lata stretching.
- Gluteal muscle strengthening.
- Anti-inflammatory drugs.
- Iontophoresis.
- US.
- Injection of local anaesthetic (5mL of 1% lignocaine 10mg/mL) into the point of maximal tenderness.

If surgery is required, the ilio-tibial band is released by a cruciform incision with or without debridement of the trochanteric bursa. The ilio-tibial band may also be Z-lengthened or an ellipse of tissue can be excised. Recently soft tissue endoscopy has been used to excise the bursa.

Treatment of septic bursitis

Uncomplicated superficial septic bursitis responds well to aspiration and appropriate antibiotic therapy. Repeat aspiration may be indicated if swelling, tenderness, and erythema recur. If there are comorbidities or the patient is systemically unwell, IV therapy is recommended. The duration of antibiotic administration may range from 1 to 4 weeks depending on individual response.

Surgical lavage and debridement is indicated if aspiration has not adequately drained the bursa, if an abscess is present, or if a sinus has formed.

Ilio-tibial band syndrome

The ilio-tibial band is a strong tendinous structure originating from the tensor fasciae latae and the gluteus maximus muscle, with insertion on the fibular head and the lateral patellar retinaculum.

The ilio-tibial band syndrome (ITBS) is an over-use injury, characterized by pain on the outer aspect of the knee due to irritation and inflammation of the distal portion of the ilio-tibial band as it crosses the lateral femoral epicondyle. This is seen in long-distance runners, cyclists, and other endurance athletes.

Friction (or impingement) occurs predominantly in the stance phase, between the posterior edge of the ilio-tibial band and the underlying lateral femoral epicondyle. Downhill running predisposes the runner to ilio-tibial band friction syndrome because the knee flexion angle at footstrike is reduced.

History and examination

Pain is usually poorly localized over the lateral aspect of the knee, is aggravated by running long distances or excessive striding, and is more severe running downhill. Pain may be relieved by walking with a stiff or a straight knee.

Point tenderness about 2cm above the joint line when the knee is flexed at 30° and palpated over the lateral femoral epicondyle.
- Flexion and extension of the knee may produce a crepitus.
- Pain is worse during weight-bearing flexion and extension. Pain is typically worse at the 30° while flexion is occurring.

The differential diagnosis includes knee pathologies including meniscal tears, ligament injuries, and loose bodies.

Investigations

Diagnosis is usually clinical. Investigations including radiographs and MRI scan help rule out other pathologies, but cannot positively confirm ITBS. An MRI may show bone oedema at the lateral femoral epicondyle

Treatment

Conservative treatment is effective in most cases. It includes:
- Reduction of activity.
- Oral anti-inflammatories.
- Ice, heat, US, and/or electrical stimulation.
- Stretching exercises to address any excessive ITB tightness.
- The optimum treatment is physiotherapy in combination with analgesic/anti-inflammatory medication.
- Local anaesthetic and corticosteroid injections repeated twice at two weekly intervals may be helpful in resistant cases

Surgery may be offered to patients who are resistant to conservative management. It is performed with the knee held in 30° of flexion and consists of cruciform incision of the ilio-tibial band or a limited resection of a small triangular piece at the posterior part of the ilio-tibial band covering the lateral femoral epicondyle. Prognosis is good with low morbidity, and quick return to sports.

Thigh contusion

Proximal thigh contusions are common athletic injuries, particularly as a result of direct trauma in contact sports. The muscle is compressed between the external force and the femur below. Severe injuries result in large haematomas that limit range of motion. See Fig. 21.4.

There is often significant haemorrhage and swelling.

History and examination

Classification: ROM assessed at 12–24h after the event.
- *Mild thigh contusions:* active ROM of the knee >90°.
- *Moderate thigh contusions:* active ROM of the knee 45–90°.
- *Severe thigh contusions:* active ROM of the knee <45°.

Treatment

The initial management of an anterior thigh contusion is rest, immobilization with knee in flexion, ice, and compression to maintain motion and minimize haematoma formation.
- Weight-bearing should be limited until the patient regains good quadriceps muscle control and 90° of pain-free knee motion.
- Functional rehabilitation and non-impact sports are allowed when the range of motion has reached 120°, and there is no residual muscle atrophy.
- *Return to full activity:* normal strength and range of motion (3 weeks). More severe injuries may have a longer recovery time.

Average disability time is 13 days for mild contusions, 19 days for moderate contusions, and 21 days for severe contusions.

If there is a major haematoma and if an athlete struggles to regain motion, refer to an orthopaedic surgeon or a radiologist for evacuation or aspiration of the haematoma. MRI or US scan will demonstrate the size and location of the haematoma. The aspiration can be performed under ultrasound guidance with aseptic technique. Protect the involved area with padding to avoid repeat injury.

Complications

- Myositis ossificans development depends on the severity of the initial injury. It is more likely with repeated trauma. This process may appear histologically similar to osteosarcoma, but the history is usually distinct and the periphery of a myositis ossificans lesion is mature. (Myositis ossificans, p. 580).
- Loss of range of motion and loss of functional outcome.

Indomethacin may be useful for prevention of myositis.

Monitor high-energy contusions closely for thigh and gluteal compartment syndromes in acute stages. Emergency fasciotomy may be rarely required, but serial examination is an absolute requirement.

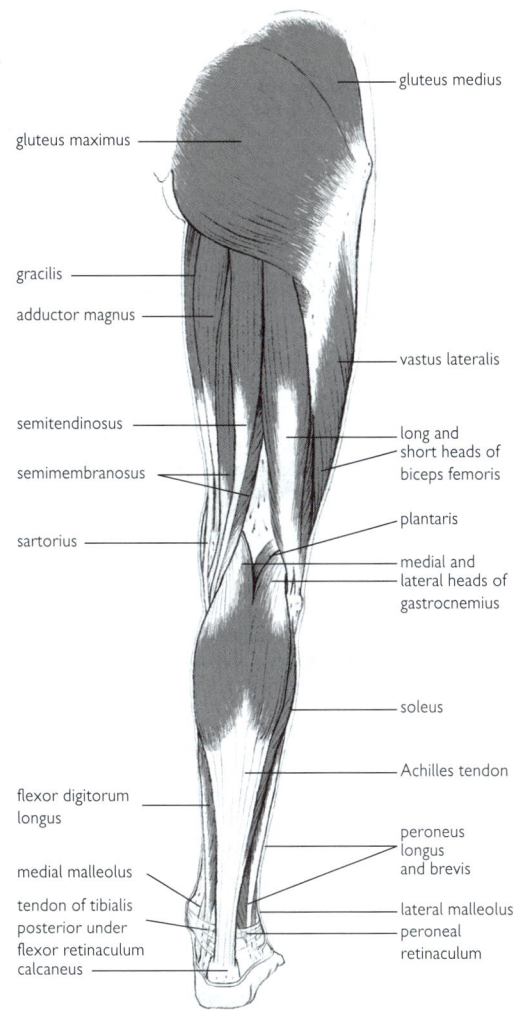

Fig. 21.4 Muscles at the back of the lower limb. Reproduced with permission from Mackinnon P, Morris J. (2005). *Oxford Textbook of Functional Anatomy*, Vol. 1. Oxford: Oxford University Press, ©2005.

Myositis ossificans

Myositis ossificans comprises two syndromes characterized by heterotopic ossification (calcification) of muscle. The first is usually a self-limiting condition in which a mass of heterotopic bone forms within the soft tissues. The term is a misnomer, as the muscle is not inflamed, and the process is not limited to muscle. Other descriptive terms include heterotopic bone formation, pseudomalignant osseous tumour of the soft tissue, extra-osseous localized non-neoplastic bone and cartilage formation, myositis ossificans circumscripta, and pseudomalignant myositis ossificans. The condition develops within 1–2 weeks of direct trauma to the area or unusual muscular exertion. Many patients cannot remember a particular trauma. It is more common in adolescents and young males. Typical sites include the thigh (quadriceps femoris and adductor muscles), elbow (flexor muscles), buttocks (gluteal muscles), the shoulder, and the calf. The proximal portion of the extremity is more frequently affected than the distal part. The pathological process includes muscle necrosis and haemorrhage after trauma. Histologically, there is marked proliferation of spindle cells with a well-recognized zoning phenomenon.

- The least differentiated tissue lies in the central zone.
- In the middle or intermediate zone, the osteoid is more organized and separated by a loose cellular stroma.
- The outer zone is the most mature consisting of well-formed bone which may form a shell around the entire lesion. Cartilage formation may also be present.

Soft tissue or bone sarcomas do not exhibit a similar zonal phenomenon.

The second condition, myositis ossificans progressiva (also referred to as fibrodysplasia ossificans progressiva), is an inherited affliction, autosomal dominant pattern, in which the ossification can occur without injury, and typically grows in a predictable pattern. Specific gene mutations have been identified in two rare inherited disorders that are clinically characterized by extensive and progressive extraskeletal bone formation-fibrodysplasia ossificans progressiva and progressive osseous heteroplasia. In fibrodysplasia ossificans progressiva, activating mutations in activin receptor type-1, a bone morphogenetic protein type I receptor, induce heterotopic endochondral ossification, which results in the development of a functional bone organ system that includes skeletal-like bone and bone marrow. In progressive osseous heteroplasia, the heterotopic ossification leads to the formation of mainly intramembranous bone tissue in response to inactivating mutations in the *GNAS* gene.

History and examination

There is usually pain, swelling, and stiffness of the surrounding joints.

On examination, there is often a red, warm swelling with soft tissue tenderness. In later stages, a hard mass is palpable.

Investigations

In the early stages, plain radiographs may be unremarkable except for non-specific soft tissue swelling. A periosteal reaction may be seen if the lesion is juxtacortical. By 2–6 weeks there is faint calcification and at

6–8 weeks, a lacy pattern of new bone forms around the periphery of the mass. Complete maturation is usual in 5–6 months.

A bone scan is highly sensitive because of the profuse osteoblastic activity and bone formation, and is non-specific, as soft tissue and bone tumours also show increased activity.

The MRI findings vary according to the stage of the disease.

The differential diagnosis includes soft tissue sarcoma and osteogenic sarcoma.

Treatment

Rest the part in a functional position until pain subsides. Gentle active movements may begin once pain improves. Oral biphosphonates, potent inhibitors of calcification are effective in modifying the process of heterotopic ossification.

Surgical resection is appropriate if the mass causes functional impairment and is best performed when the lesion has matured. Rapid recurrence occurs after resection of an immature lesion. If left alone, the mass may reduce in size with time and, in some instances, disappear.

Osteoarthritis of the hip

A progressive degenerative joint disease of the hip. (Coxarthrosis: coxa is hip, arthrosis is degeneration of a joint. Osteoarthritis is a misnomer as inflammation is not the primary pathologic process). The incidence of idiopathic hip OA increases with age. (It rarely occurs before the age of 24yrs. From 25–34yrs 2%, from 35–44yrs 4%, from 45–54yrs 16%, from 55–64yrs 31%, and 65+yrs 47%). Two million people in the UK suffer with osteoarthritis and, of those, 210,000 have moderate to severe osteoarthritis of the hips.

Ex-professional footballers had a significantly higher prevalence of OA of the hip than an age-matched group of radiographic controls. A Finnish study of international competing athletes showed increased risk OA of the hip for all athletes, but those involved in endurance sports (long distance running, cross-country skiing) were admitted to hospital care for OA at a later age than those involved in power sports (boxing, weightlifting, wrestling, throwing) or mixed sports (soccer, hockey, basketball, track).

Regular cyclical loading of joints is required to maintain normal articular cartilage composition, structure, and function. Prolonged static loading, repeated sudden excessive loading, or the absence of loading may, however, cause degradation of articular cartilage.

Repetitive joint use, under abnormal loading conditions, is a risk factor for OA. This includes:
- Participation in heavy physical activity before 50yrs of age.
- An elite level in high joint loading sports.
- Combination of heavy recreational physical activity with heavy occupational workload.
- Continued use of the joint after injury in sporting activity.

History and examination
Symptoms usually include pain, stiffness, deformity (late stages), and loss of mobility.

Clinical findings
- Muscle wasting.
- Tenderness.
- Deformity.
- Reduced range of motion (loss of IR seen in early OA, normal range is 0–40°).
- Crepitus.
- Alteration of gait.

Investigation
Plain radiographs demonstrate:
- Loss of joint space.
- Osteophyte formation.
- Subchondral cyst formation.
- Subchondral sclerosis.
- Erosion of bones, loose bodies, and subluxed joint are characteristic of advanced OA.

Treatment
- Analgesia.
- NSAIDs.
- *Physiotherapy:* strengthening exercises, range-of-motion exercises, and functional training are beneficial.
- Oral chondroitin sulphate and glucosamine sulphate may help to alleviate pain in early OA of the hip.
- Osteotomy, total hip replacement, and hip resurfacing are the surgical options.

Osteotomy, if performed in the early stages, can delay the progression of OA of the hip due to redistribution of load on the articular cartilage. Eventually, patients who undergo osteotomy may require total hip replacement.

Some factors that may suggest a poorer outcome have been identified. The most important patient-related factors are secondary osteoarthritis as the indication for surgery such as post-childhood hip disorders or AVN, female gender, smaller component sizes and older age (>65yrs for males and >55yrs for females). In addition, surgical technique (approach and cementing technique) and component design are also important determinant factors for the risk of failure.

Pubic bone stress injury (osteitis pubis)

Pubic bone stress injury (osteitis pubis) is an over-use injury caused by biomechanical overloading of the pubic symphysis and adjacent parasymphyseal bone caused imbalance in forces from the abdominal and groin musculature with resultant bony stress reaction. Clinically, it is characterized by acute and/or chronic groin pain.

It is usually secondary to over-use or trauma. It occurs typically in sports with sprinting, kicking, and sudden changes of direction, such as running, basketball, soccer, ice hockey, Australian football, and tennis. Pelvic surgery and childbirth also predispose to osteitis pubis. Other conditions like poor conditioning, exercising on hard surfaces, excessive training, and muscular imbalance can increase the risk of developing osteitis pubis.

It may occur in almost any patient population, is self-limiting and usually improves within 1yr. It is recurrent in 25% of athletes.

History and examination
- Exercise-induced pain or pubic tenderness.
- Pain may also occur while walking, radiating to the perineal, testicular, suprapubic, or inguinal region, and can also develop in the scrotum after ejaculation.
- Clicking may indicate vertical instability.

Clinical findings
- Tenderness over pubic symphysis, aggravated by pelvic compression.
- Painful hip abduction.
- Wide-based gait.

The differential diagnosis includes adductor sprains, a hernia, prostatitis in men. Sexually-acquired reactive arthritis (SARA) can manifest as osteitis pubis. Osteomyelitis of the symphysis pubis can occur concomitantly with osteitis pubis. A biopsy and culture of the affected area is necessary to rule out osteomyelitis.

Investigations
- Radiographs are negative in the early stages. They may reveal widening of symphysis pubis, irregular contour of articular surfaces, and peri-articular sclerosis in late stages.
- Flamingo views help demonstrate vertical instability of the symphysis.
- US may show superior joint capsule irregularity.
- MRI (gold standard) reveals bone oedema in early stages.
- CT scan, bone scintigraphy can confirm osteitis pubis.

Treatment
- Rest.
- Avoidance of pain producing activity.
- Analgesics.
- Strengthening and balancing exercises of muscles acting as opposing forces across the symphysis pubis (rectus abdominus, iliopsoas, adductors)
- Rarely, vertical instability of symphysis pubis can complicate osteitis pubis. This is surgically managed by arthrodesis with compression plating and bone grafting.

Sports hernia (Gilmore's groin)

Sports hernia (Gilmore's groin) is an over-use syndrome common in athletes participating in sports that require repetitive twisting and turning at speeds, e.g. field hockey, ice hockey, soccer, and tennis.

Hip abduction, adduction, and flexion-extension with the resultant pelvic motion produce a shearing force across the pubic symphysis, leading to stress on the inguinal wall musculature perpendicular to the fibres of the fascia and muscle. Pull from the adductor musculature against a fixed lower extremity can cause significant shear forces across the hemipelvis. Subsequent attenuation or tearing of the transversalis fascia or conjoined tendon can be the source of pain. Abnormalities at the insertion of the rectus abdominis muscle or avulsions of part of the internal oblique muscle fibres at the pubic tubercle, abnormalities in the external oblique muscle and aponeurosis, entrapment of the genital branches of the ilio-inguinal or genitofemoral nerves have been suggested as sources of pain.

History and examination

Unilateral groin pain of insidious onset, which occurs with exercise, and is aggravated by coughing and sneezing, may radiate laterally, across the midline, into the adductor region, scrotum, and testicles. Occasionally, athletes report a sudden tearing sensation.

Clinical findings
- Local tenderness over the conjoined tendon, pubic tubercle, and midinguinal region, or a tender, dilated superficial inguinal ring.
- Pain with resisted adduction, resisted sit-up, and reproducible with Valsalva manoeuvre.

The differential diagnosis includes osteitis pubis, adductor tendinopathy, symphyseal instability, osteoarthritis, and tumour.

Investigations
- Plain radiographs and bone scan can help rule out the above conditions.
- MRI may be useful to detect abnormalities within the muscles or pubic symphysis.

Treatment

Conservative management is occasionally effective for groin injuries, but results in a protracted clinical course. Rehabilitation involves core stabilization exercises and the maintenance of muscle control and strength around the pelvis. Surgery can be considered if conservative management fails after 6–8 weeks.

Conventional or laparoscopic herniorrhaphy is usually successful. Mesh reinforcement is often performed during these repairs. Return to sports within 6–12 weeks after specific rehabilitation targeted at abdominal strengthening, adductor muscle flexibility, and a graduated return to activity. If adductor muscle pain is present pre-operatively, adductor muscle release or recession is combined with herniorrhaphy.

Other 'minimal access' operations are used to ensure rapid return to play in professional sport. This includes the Muschaweck operation, where suture re-inforcement of the posterior inguinal wall (without hernia repair) is used to relieve pressure on the genito-femoral nerve.

Groin pain

A non-specific, descriptive syndrome which is difficult to diagnose because of the complex anatomy and the possibility of co-existing injuries (see Box 21.1).

The overall incidence of injuries causing groin pain varies, but it is prevalent (2–5%) in athletes participating in ice hockey, fencing, handball, cross-country skiing, hurdling, high jumping, and soccer (5–7% of all soccer injuries). These sports involve side-to-side cutting, quick accelerations and decelerations, and sudden directional changes. The diagnosis may be unclear in up to 30% of cases.

History and examination

Acute onset of groin pain may be due to muscle contusion, sprain, or bony injury including fractures and dislocation of the hip joint. In complete muscle tears, a gap may be palpable between the ruptured ends. In athletes with bony injuries, there is pain, swelling, deformity, and inability to bear weight on the affected limb. The history should include the onset, inciting event, and aggravating and relieving factors.

Children and adolescents presenting with groin pain and pain on weight-bearing of the affected limb should be evaluated to exclude septic arthritis, avascular necrosis of the hip, Legg-Calve-Perthes disease, and slipped capital femoral epiphysis (Box 21.2). Apophyseal avulsion fractures may present with acute groin or hip pain after an injury. Tendon lesions are rare in children and adolescents.

Clinical examination
- Adequate exposure of the groin and hip.
- Inspection of the symmetry and anatomic irregularity.
- Palpation of the affected area for tenderness.
- Assessment of the range of motion of the joints.
- Measurement for discrepancy of leg length (b 'Examination of the hip', p. 560).
- Evaluation of gait, including the performance of sprints, jumps, and activities that exacerbate the athlete's pain.
- Neurological examination may reveal areas of numbness and motor weakness.

Investigations
- Plain radiographs may show fractures, avulsion fractures in adolescents, established osteitis pubis, later stages of stress fracture and osteomyelitis, slipped femoral epiphysis, or osteoarthritis.
- A bone scan can help demonstrate osteitis pubis, stress fracture, osteomyelitis, synovitis, avascular necrosis, sacro-iliitis, tenoperiosteal lesion, or muscle tear.
- Sonograms may show a muscle tear, haematoma, inguinal hernia, or bursitis.
- Nerve conduction studies may demonstrate ilio-inguinal neuropathy or obturator neuropathy.
- CT scans and MRIs may show disc pathology, radicular lesions, osteitis pubis, and other bone and soft tissue.

Box 21.1 Common disorders producing groin pain in adults

Acute onset
- Muscle strains.
- Contusions (hip pointer).
- Acetabular labral tears and loose bodies.
- Proximal femur fractures.

Insidious onset
- Sports hernias and athletic pubalgia.
- Osteitis pubis.
- Bursitis.
- Snapping hip syndrome.
- Stress fractures.
- Osteoarthritis.

Other disorders
- Lumbar spine abnormalities.
- Compression neuropathies.

Box 21.2 Disorders producing groin pain in children and adolescents

Acute onset
- Contusions (hip pointer).
- Avulsions an apophyseal injuries.
- Proximal femur fractures.

Insidious onset
- Avascular necrosis of the hip.
- Legg–Calve–Perthes disease.
- Slipped capital femoral epiphysis.

Rehabilitation for over-use injuries

This approach is suitable for a range of over-use or stress related overload injuries around the hip and pelvis region. These include pubic stress/pubalgia, adductor tendinopathy, osteitis pubis, sports hernia. The progression of rehabilitation will depend on the longevity and severity of symptoms, the nature of sporting activity, and the number of risk factors identified.

Risk factors

This is possibly the most important aspect of managing any over-use injury. Once the risk factors are identified, rehabilitation should be started as soon as possible.

Common intrinsic risk factors
- Weakness of hip adductors.
- Weakness of gluteal muscles.
- *Decreased ROM of hip:* in particular IR, external rotation and extension.
- *Reduced flexibility of hip musculature:* in particular adductors/gluteals.
- Poor lumbopelvic control.
- Poor lower limb alignment.

Adjunctive treatment during rehabilitation

Massage
- Manual therapy usually focuses on the areas that are overactive/shortened; commonly the gluteus medius, piriformis, and adductor muscle group.
- Deep transverse friction massage on the common adductor tendon (if involved) should also be of benefit.
- *Electrotherapy:* various electrotherapeutic modalities or local icing can be used to promote healing and improve symptomatic relief.

Level 1 rehabilitation

Mobility
Adequate mobility should be gained through hip, lumbar, and pelvic areas. Stretching should be progressed from static to dynamic and from passive to active.

Introduce basic strengthening and motor control exercises
- *Exercises to enhance balance and pelvic awareness:*
  - In single leg standing athletes must maintain good pelvic and lumbar alignment (i.e. neutral position avoiding excessive lordosis, lumbar flexion, or lateral pelvic tilt) and hold for 45s × 5.
  - *Bent leg fall out*—supine lying with hips (45°) and knees (90°) in flexion and feet on floor. Throughout the exercise ensure that the pelvis stays in contact with the floor and the lumbar spine remains

in a neutral position. Drop leg outwards into ER, movement should be restricted to the hip joint.
  - *Lying on back, knees bent, back flat against floor*—slowly straighten alternate legs keeping back flat (3 × 10 repetitions).
- *Static adduction strengthening*: in all cases, the athlete should be instructed to perform a static hip adduction contraction at a pain free level. Supine, hips (45° flexion) and knees (90° flexion), feet on floor, squeeze ball between knees. (5–10s holds × 8). Repeat in supine with hips and knees in 0° extension.
- *Running man exercise*: standing on right leg, the athlete moves the left leg and arms in running motion. To progress repeat with right leg at 45° of flexion (30s × 6).
- *Mini-squats* (two legs) bend knee to 30° (3 × 20 repetitions).
- Standing on one leg, throw ball against wall and catch, progress by standing on unstable surface.

Level 2 rehabilitation

Progress motor control training and trunk strength
- Bent leg fall out exercise (as above) with theraband/manual load.
- Static adduction strengthening (as above), but progress by adding knee to chest movement during squeeze.
- *Long leg PNF exercises*: athlete starts in supine position, with hip in flexion, adduction, and IR, they then slowly move limb to finish in a position of hip extension, abduction and ER. Progress by adding manual resistance or ankle weights.
- Resisted hip adduction with pulley or theraband. Progress by adding hip rotation, and simultaneous arm swings to encourage cross limb co-ordination
- *Worm exercise*: supine, hips (45°) and knees (90°) in flexion, feet lifted approximately 15cm from the floor, arms in flexion (90°) squeeze ball between knees, slowly rotate legs and pelvis to the right, whilst moving upper limbs and torso to left, repeat in a rocking movement.

Introduce lower body conditioning and strength
- *Lunge walk*: aim to finish each lunge with thigh parallel to ground, tall spine, keep knee in alignment with 2nd toe during lunge (no weight) (20m × 5 × 3 sets).
- *Step-ups*: use approximately 30cm step (3 × 20 repetitions with no weight).
- *Mini trampoline exercises*: gently bounce for 1min × 5 on single leg. Progress to throwing and catching ball.
- *Lunge stabilization exercise*: adopt ½-lunge position, maintaining a tall spine, throw and catch a ball (1min × 3 to each leg).
- *Swiss ball ½ squat exercise*: athlete places a Swiss ball between their back and a wall, in standing position, roll down to a squat position (45–90° knee bend), hold for 2s, and up again (6 × 3 sets).

Level 3 rehabilitation

Introduce progressive running
Running must be introduced gradually and without pain, and be consistent with the ability of the athlete. Straight line running is commenced first, allowing sufficient time for gradual acceleration and deceleration. Once the athlete can run at 80% in a straight line without pain, directional changes should be introduced slowly to allow time for tissue adaptation.

Directional running may be introduced as follows:
- Long gradual curved (snake) running patterns.
- Forward/backward running to fixed point.
- Sideways running to a fixed point
- *Figure of 8 runs:* athlete runs in a figure of eight pattern. Start with long gradual curves progressing to short, sharp curves at fast speed.
- Agility drills using ladders or cones.
- *Cross overs/carioca runs:* sideways running where athletes rotate their pelvis and allow their feet to cross midline of body; this encourages cross-limb and lumbo-pelvic co-ordination
- *Sidestep/cuts:* begin with 45° side step to the affected side (i.e. stepping off unaffected limb) and progress by stepping off affected side. Once this can be performed without pain, progress to 90° cuts and eventually to 180° turns. Further progression can include stepping around cone at speed and eventually adding a dynamic target (opponent).

Kicking drills
Progressive kicking programme
Athletes should begin by kicking a ball that is moving towards them. Short distance kicks should be used initially. This can be progressed by kicking a ball that is moving in various directions, followed by kicking a ball from the hand and eventually kicking a dead ball. Focus should be on maintaining accuracy and technique. Kicking should only be carried out exercises after a progressive warm-up.

Session 1
- 20m × 10
- 30m × 5
- 40m × 5

Session 2
- 30m × 10
- 40m × 5
- 50m × 5

Session 3
- 30m × 10
- 40m × 10
- 50m × 5

Session 4
- 30m × 10
- 40m × 10
- 50m × 5
- 50m × 5

To progress kicking, increase until doing 10 repetitions at each distance and then concentrate on increasing force and speed.

When the above sessions can be completed without pain, carry out the kicking at the end of at the following drills:
- Side stepping at 45° and 90°.
- Curved running drills.
- Lateral running with sudden change of pace and direction.

Advanced strengthening and control exercises for the pelvis and hip

Advanced strengthening and control exercises for the pelvis and hip region should be introduced, some examples are:
- Exercise 1—*prone bridge* (Fig. 21.5): in a face down position, balance on the tips of your toes and elbows while attempting to maintain a straight line from heels to head. Hold for as long as you can without pain. Repeat for set of 4–3–2.
- Exercise 2—*isometric hold* (Fig. 21.6): try to maintain body in a horizontal position. Hold until onset of pain. Repeat for set of 4–3–2.
- Exercise 3—*eccentric trunk lowering* (Fig. 21.7): start in position 1 shown below, slowly and in controlled manner lower upper body to position 2. Pull self back to position 1 using arms and repeat controlled lowering (3 sets × 10 repetitions).

End stage rehab

Introduce sudden changes of pace and direction in all the above running and kicking exercises e.g. introduce sudden change from sideways running to straight sprint followed by high speed snake run and kicking a dead ball.

Once this can be done without pain, introduce competition altering the following variables as appropriate to the sport and individual:
- Distance covered.
- Pace and intensity.
- Patterns of movement (falling, direction changes, spinning, getting up, etc.).
- Space limitations.
- Feet action (quick, fast, powerful).
- Use of ball (dribbling, carrying, receiving/giving pass).

Surgery

- If all other modalities do not control symptoms, surgery may be considered. It may include debridement, excision of the tendinopathic area, tenotomy, and bone marrow stimulation of the pelvis through drilling of the pubic bone.

592 CHAPTER 21 **Hip and pelvis**

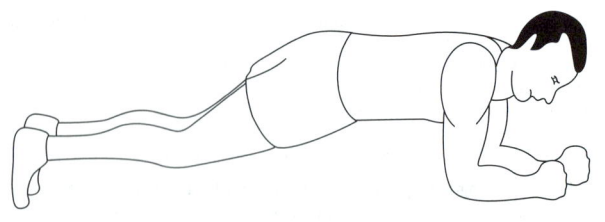

Fig. 21.5 Prone bridge.

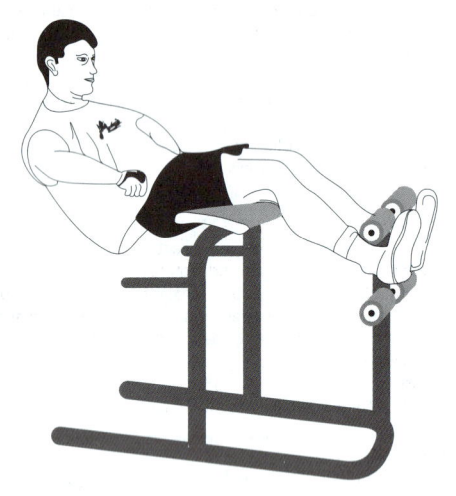

Fig. 21.6 Isometric hold.

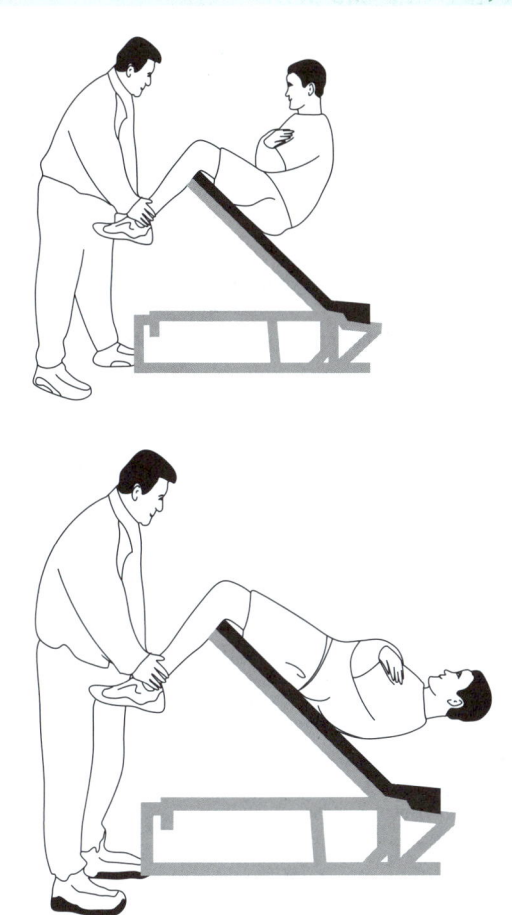

Fig. 21.7 (a), (b) Eccentric lowering.

Avulsions around the ilium

Growth plate injuries are unique to young athletes with skeletal immaturity. Two types of epiphyses are found in the extremities:
- *Traction epiphyses* (or apophyses) are located at the site of attachment of major muscle tendons to bone and are subjected primarily to tensile forces.
- *Pressure epiphyses* are situated at the end of long bones and are subjected mainly to compressive forces. The relative weakness of the growth plate at the apophysis of skeletally immature athletes predisposes them to a variety of avulsion fractures. Usually, they result from a violent eccentric muscle contraction.

Avulsion fractures of the anterior superior iliac spine (ASIS) are usually due to:
- Avulsion of the sartorius origin.
- Avulsion of the tensor fascia lata origin.

Avulsion of sartorius is usually due to sprinting. The fragment is smaller and displaced anteriorly. Tensor fascia lata avulsion is due to twisting injury. The fragment is much larger and displaced laterally.

Avulsion of anterior inferior iliac spine results from forceful flexion of the hip by the rectus femoris. Avulsion of the ischial tuberosity results from forceful contraction of the hamstrings.

History and examination
- Severe, sudden-onset, and well-localized pain over anterior superior iliac spine.
- Localized tenderness, swelling, and eventual ecchymosis.
- Posture that reduces tension on the involved muscle.
- Resisted contraction or stretch of the involved muscle worsens the pain.

Investigations
- Plain radiographs, including comparison views, can usually identify the injury if the fragment is visible.

Treatment
Conservative
- Rest.
- Analgesia.
- Comfortable positioning with protected weight-bearing and gradual return to activity.
- Strengthening is begun after full, pain-free range of motion is achieved.

The periosteum and surrounding fascia often limit severe displacement. Reported disadvantages include a reduction in strength, function, and, in some patients, the formation of a painful callus.

Surgery is preferred to conservative management if:
- The size of the fragment is large enough to hold metal work.
- Displacement of the fracture fragment is ≥2cm.

Return to play
Patients should not return to competition until full strength and motion are restored.

Piriformis syndrome

Piriformis syndrome is caused by irritation or compression of the sciatic nerve at the piriformis muscle. This syndrome is characterized by tingling, numbness, and pain along the path of the sciatic nerve in the affected leg.

Causative factors include an abnormal tenseness or spasticity of the piriformis caused either by trauma and over-use, or by muscle and nerve anomaly. In about 6% of the population, the sciatic nerve passes through the piriformis muscle. Tumours, vascular anomalies, and changes of gluteal muscles and nerves can cause piriformis syndrome. Post-traumatic piriformis syndrome may be secondary to a contusion in the gluteal area. It occurs in middle-aged recreational athletes playing tennis, running, and cross-country skiing.

History and examination
- Pain located maximally at the middle-upper part of the buttock during and after physical exercise.
- Pain radiates to posterior thigh, calf, outer leg, ankle, and heel. There may be night pain.
- The leg may be held in semiflexion and in ER.

Differential diagnosis includes entrapment of the gluteal nerves, hamstring pain from entrapment of the posterior cutaneous nerve of the thigh, sciatica.

Clinical findings
- Pinpoint tenderness on palpation at the upper middle gluteus, resisted internal–ER tests with straight leg may be positive.
- SLR test negative.
- Reflexes, motor functions, and sensations are usually normal.
- Piriformis stretching is positive.
- Local anaesthetic infiltration test positive: pain disappears.

Investigations
- MR scan demonstrates the size and thickness of piriformis muscles, side difference, and anomalies.
- Electoneuromyography (ENMG) examination may demonstrate distal radiculopathy or changes of proximal, but not lumbar nerve roots.
- Treatment.

Conservative management
- Muscle stretching.
- Pelvic posture correction, core stabilization, hip and SIJ mobilization, strengthening of the gluteal and pelvic musculature.
- Local anaesthetic and a steroid injection into the piriformis muscle can be useful if physiotherapy fails. Important to avoid sciatic nerve.

Surgical management
- Offered after failure of conservative management.
- Piriformis muscle is divided and sciatic nerve is released.
- The results are good or excellent in 50–85% of cases.

Snapping hip syndrome

Snapping hip syndrome is a benign condition where an audible snap or click occurs on flexion and extension of the hip (coxa saltans—coxa is Latin for hip, and saltans means jumping; is a term to describe the feeling of the popping or snapping hip).

- External causes include snapping of the ilio-tibial band or gluteus maximus over the greater trochanter.
- Internal causes are snapping of the iliopsoas tendon over the iliopectineal eminence, over the femoral head, or over the lesser trochanter.
- Intra-articular causes include acetabular labral tear, and intra-articular loose body.

External

History and examination

More common and occurs more often in females.

- Audible, painless snapping with a sensation of the hip jumping out of place or giving way.
- The thickened posterior border of ilio-tibial band or anterior border of gluteus maximus muscle near its insertion catch the superior margin of the greater trochanter as the hip is flexed, adducted, or internally rotated causing snapping.
- Reproducible by passive hip flexion in an adducted position with the knee in extension.

Treatment

- Reassure that the hip joint is not subluxing or dislocating.
- Conservative management with rest, analgesics, NSAIDs, ice, US, phonophoresis, iontophoresisis is usually successful.
- Stretching and strengthening exercises of ilio-tibial band.
- Refer to orthopaedic surgeon for surgical release or Z-plasty of ilio-tibial band if conservative management fails.

Internal

History and examination

Less common. Snapping sensation localized to the anterior part of the groin. May reproduce the snapping by extending and adducting the hip from a flexed and abducted position. The iliopsoas tendon shifts from lateral to medial over the iliopectineal eminence and/or the femoral head when the hip is brought from flexion into extension.

Investigation

- Ultrasonography during hip motion may demonstrate the tendon subluxation.
- MRI scan will help demonstrate thickened tendon, and fluid in the iliopsoas bursa.
- Bursography may reproduce the symptoms associated with abnormal movement of the iliopsoas tendon and is diagnostic of internal snapping hip syndrome, but is invasive. Local anaesthetic injection (5mL of 1% lignocaine 10mg/mL) into the iliopsoas bursa and/or around the tendon may be diagnostic.

Treatment
- Conservative management with rest, analgesics, NSAIDs, ice, US, phonophoresis, and iontophoresisis is usually successful.
- Stretching of the hip flexors and rotators, then strengthening and gradual return to sport.
- Symptoms refractory to physical therapy may be relieved by surgical lengthening of the iliopsoas tendon.

Intra–articular

History and examination
- Trauma, or synovial chondromatosis may predispose to intra-articular loose bodies.
- Labral tears may cause groin pain. Incidence is high in patients with dysplastic hips.

Investigation
- Plain radiographs help rule out bony pathology.
- MR arthrography can help confirm diagnosis.
- Arthroscopy of the hip joint may be both diagnostic and therapeutic in these patients, and is considered the gold standard.

Hamstring injury

The hamstring muscle group is prone to strains, which mostly occur near the proximal musculotendinous junction. Hamstring injuries account for 30–40% of lower limb injuries sustained in sports. Hamstring strain recurrence is 33%. Such injuries occur commonly in sports that require rapid active knee extension (e.g. sprinting, track and field, jumping, football, rugby) and in sports where there is muscle contraction at a position of maximal muscle lengthening (e.g. martial arts, dance, water-skiing). The mechanism of injury is usually a sudden passive stretch or a protective eccentric action (muscle develops tension while lengthening). Predisposing factors for hamstring injuries include:

Extrinsic factors
- Warm up.
- Fatigue.
- Fitness level and training modalities.

Intrinsic factors
- Eccentric strength deficits (muscle unable to develop tension).
- (Imbalance in torque > 15% between left and right; reduced Hamstring:quadriceps ratio <0.6).
- Flexibility.
- Age.
- Joint dysfunction.
- Immobilization and rehabilitation of injured muscle.

History and examination

There may be sudden onset of sharp posterior thigh pain. This may be associated with an audible pop, resulting in immediate disability.

On examination, there may be bruising on the posterior thigh localized to the site of injury, or it may be more diffuse. There is tenderness on palpation, and muscle spasm over the hamstring musculature. In complete proximal ruptures, a palpable defect is present proximally, and the muscle belly is prominent distally.

The differential diagnosis includes L5/S1 radiculopathy, that may cause posterior thigh pain resembling an hamstring injury.

Investigation
- Plain radiograph (to exclude bony avulsion from ischial tuberosity).
- US scan (dynamic method, useful for diagnosis and follow-up).
- MRI (better details).

Treatment

Conservative
- Rest the limb to prevent further injury.
- *Ice*: apply as soon as possible as it helps prevent further bleeding, swelling, and alleviates pain. Apply ice for ≤20min for every 2h for first 48–72h.

Avoid direct contact of ice with skin to prevent ice burns. Crushed ice in a plastic bag, commercial cold packs, wrapping the ice in a damp towel, or bags of frozen peas are different suggested modes of applying ice.
- Compression.
- Elevation helps reduce the haematoma formation and limits tissue damage.
- Active range of motion exercises within limits of pain tolerance after 1–5 days depending on the severity of injury.
- Mobilize using crutches until pain free.

Inflammation is essential for the process of healing. NSAIDs, by their anti-inflammatory effect, may delay healing. No additive effect on healing of acute hamstring injuries was found when meclofenate or diclofenac was added to standard physiotherapeutic modalities in a double-blind placebo-controlled trial. Therefore, NSAIDs are not recommended in the management of acute hamstring injuries.

Physiotherapy
(A complete rehabilitation programme is described later.)
- Early immobilization may accelerate the formation of a granulation tissue matrix and hasten healing.
- Prolonged complete immobilization will result in muscle atrophy, loss of strength and length, and inelastic scar formation (to be avoided).
- In the first 4 weeks following injury, physical therapy is focused on strengthening, improving range of motion (ROM), and flexibility:
  - Passive static stretching is begun.
  - Warm up the muscle tissues prior to stretching and exercising.
  - Strengthening exercises initiated by an expert therapist, within the available pain-free range of motion.
  - Later, concentric exercises with resistance, increasing gradually as tolerated.
  - The next stage is the inclusion of high-speed, low-resistance isokinetic exercises.
  - Resistance is increased gradually, while exercise speed is decreased.
  - The patient then progresses from concentric to eccentric strengthening exercises.
- After 4 weeks, stretching and strengthening exercises are continued to maintain flexibility and an adequate hamstring-to-quadriceps strength ratio. (Strength testing can be performed using isokinetic exercise equipment.)

A rehabilitation programme consisting of progressive agility and trunk stabilization exercises is more effective than a programme emphasizing isolated hamstring stretching and strengthening in promoting return to sports and preventing injury recurrence in athletes suffering an acute hamstring strain.

Surgical management
The indication for surgery in an acute hamstring strain is a complete rupture at or near the origin from the ischial tuberosity, or distally at its insertion. These should be identified clinically by a large defect or from an

ischial tuberosity bone avulsion with displacement by 2cm on radiographs. In such cases, reattachment is indicated.

In chronic cases, tendinopathy results from scarring and abnormal healing. The diagnosis is clinical and confirmed by imaging (MRI). Surgical management is by longitudinal tenotomy of the tendinopathic hamstring tendon close to the insertion. The surgical results are usually good.

Return to play
- When the strength of the injured hamstring reaches 90% of the strength of the unaffected hamstring and when the patient has a full ROM.
- At least a 50–60% hamstring-to-quadriceps ratio is desired.
- Prior to return to play, sports-specific training maximizes recovery and minimizes chances for additional injury.

Prevention
- Pre-exercise stretching.
- Adequate warm-up.
- Avoid block drills too early in the training season.
- Thermal pants may help reduce risk of recurrent hamstring injury.

Identification of the factors leading to injury and the development of appropriate preventative strategy to avoid re-injury is crucial.

Pre-season screening may identify athletes at risk due to deficits in skills, aerobic and anaerobic capability, general health, or musculoskeletal function, as these may predispose to hamstring injuries.

Management of hamstring injury

Early stage hamstring injury management is key to successful rehabilitation. Controlled mobilization should be performed within the limits of pain as soon as possible. If the early stage goals are not met, then accelerated rehabilitation may be contraindicated.

Early stage: days 1-3

Key aims
- Minimize inflammation.
- Prevent scarring.
- Minimize muscle spasm.
- Progressive loading.
- Assess risk factors.

Risk factors
Often the athlete may have one or more intrinsic risk factors, which have predisposed to hamstring injury. These should be assessed as early stage. Common risk factors include:
- Poor general conditioning.
- Hamstring weakness/fatigue.
- Poor recovery strategies.
- Poor training periodization/inappropriate training.
- Decreased lower limb flexibility.
- Decreased neural mobility—lower limb and lumbosacral plexus:
  - Poor running style
  - Running styles that place a high load on the hamstrings may cause early fatigue, overload and an increased change of injury.
- Poor lower limb alignment, e.g. anterior rotation of pelvis:
  - Tight hip flexors.
  - Decreased strength/activation gluteal muscle.
  - Over-activity of erector spinae muscles.

General exercises
- *Active knee flexion/extension:* sitting off the end of a bed, maintaining a good postural alignment (avoiding excessive pelvis rotation), the athlete actively bends and straightens the knee. This exercise should be pain free. Perform 30 repetitions × 6 times per day.
- *Slump (neural) mobilization:* sitting off the end of a bed, athlete adopts a slumped position (chin to chest, rounded shoulders and spine), the athlete actively bends and straightens the knee slowly. Again this should take place within the pain free range of movement. Perform 30 repetitions × 6 per day.
- *Massage:* Lighter techniques such as effleurage may help minimize protective muscle spasm.
- *Electrotherapy:* low-level laser therapy, electrical stimulation.
- Ice, compression, and elevation.

MANAGEMENT OF HAMSTRING INJURY

Middle stage: days 3-14

Key aims
- Optimal loading of hamstring muscle (isometric progressing to concentric muscle loading).
- Begin to address/correct risk factors.
- Begin cardiovascular conditioning.

General exercises
- *Isometrics:* in a prone position, the athlete uses the uninjured leg to resist active knee flexion. This exercise should be pain free. Begin with 10s holds × 10. Perform at the inner (>90°knee flexion) middle and outer (10–45° knee flexion) ROM.
- *Concentrics:* in a prone position, the athlete uses the uninjured leg to resist active knee flexion through the full ROM. Use the maximum amount of resistance without causing pain. To progress, use therapist resistance, ankle weights, dynabands.
- *Step-ups:* leading with the injured leg, the athlete steps up onto a height (approx knee height), holds for a few seconds, before slowly lowering down. This movement should be performed slowly, maintaining good posture throughout the movement, particularly at the lumbar pelvic region.
- *Lunges:* leading with the injured leg.
- *Gluteal exercises:*
  - Bridging—supine lying, arms crossed across the chest, hips (45°) and knees (90°) in flexion, both feet on ground. Athlete is instructed to push down through heels to lift pelvis and spine off the ground. Shoulders should remain in contact with the ground. Hold position for 3s, slowly return to prone.
  - To progress—increase distance between feet; decrease hip and knee flexion angle (e.g. hips at 30°, knees at 30°); perform a single leg bridge.
  - Kneeling hip extension/Bird dog exercise— athlete adopts a 4-point kneeling position (hands and knees). Athlete is instructed to maintain neutral pelvis and lumbar spine (i.e. avoid excessive arching or rounding of the spine), while they extends the hip and knee joint of the injured leg.
  - To progress—the contralateral shoulder is simultaneously elevated through flexion.

Cardiovascular
- Cross trainer.
- *Bike:* aim for a progressive increase up to pre injury heart rate/RPM levels.
- *Jogging:* build to 10min jogging, up to 50%.

NB Jogging should be performed at a slow steady pace. At no stage should the athlete accelerate sharply. Jogging must be stopped immediately in the event of even mild tightness or apprehension.

Late phase: days 14–28

Key aims

Increase eccentric loading (lengthening contraction)
- Progress gluteal/core training.
- Begin progressive running.

Progressive eccentric hamstring loading
- *Nordic (Norwegian) hamstring curls:*
  - These are a high load eccentric exercise. To begin with, 3 sets of 4 repetitions may be sufficient. The athlete starts in a kneeling position (knees at 90° flexion, hips in neutral). Throughout this exercise a therapist or training partner must hold their feet. Maintaining a good posture (straight back and avoiding excessive pelvic tilt), the athlete lets their trunk fall forward, hinging at the knee joint, using eccentric hamstring control to slowly lower them down into a fully prone position. Initially, most athletes need to use their upper body to cushion them onto the ground (finishing in a press up position).
  - *To progress*—athlete stops at various points through the range.
- *Hamstring flicks:* in a prone position, with the injured side in full knee flexion, the athlete quickly extends their knee; the hamstrings are used to brake the movement just prior to full knee extension (i.e. preventing locking or hyperextension at the knee).
- *Hamstring wobbles:* in a prone position, holding the knee at 90 degrees of flexion, the athlete performs small, fast oscillations into knee flexion and extension. Repeat at inner and outer ROM.
- *Leg swings*—standing on the uninjured side, the athlete flexes and extends the hip joint. This should be repeated with the knee in varying degrees of flexion.
  - *To progress*—increase the speed of movement, up to 60 repetitions/min.
- *Leg speed/technical running drills:*
  - *Hip drives*—standing on the uninjured side with the injured foot just off the ground. Maintaining good posture at the lower back/pelvic region, the athlete quickly flexes the hip of the injured side (to 90–110° hip flexion), with the knee in approximately 90° flexion and ankle in full dorsi flexion. Return slowly to a starting position.
  - *Hip extensions*—as above, except at the end of the movement, instead of slowly returning to the starting position, the athlete drives their leg back into hip extension/knee extension.
  - Walking lunges progressing to jump lunges.
  - *Single leg good mornings/arabesque*—athlete starts by standing on the injured leg, with their knee in slight flexion. They then tip their body forward (as if they are bowing), hinging at the hip joint and maintaining a straight back. To progress: increase the depth of the bow; add resistance (holding dumb bell), increase speed.

Progressive running

A coach/therapist/practitioner should be present during all running session. Any deviations from normal running gait, differences in leg cadence, or subjective complaints of apprehension or tightness are indications for immediate cessation of the running session.

All sessions should begin with a 10min warm-up:
- For most hamstring injuries, running should begin with slow jogging (short stride lengths, with increasing cadence) and backwards running
- Progressive running drills can be used to increase speed:
  - *Accelerate for 40m*—maintain speed for 20m, decelerate for 40 m, then stop. 8 repetitions.
  - *To progress*—the acceleration distance should be decreased with the maintenance distance increasing.
- *Athlete performs curved/arc runs:* progressed as above.
- *Shuttle runs:* running back and forward to a fixed point or cones.
- *Pick-ups/fartlek running:* e.g. from a 70% run, the athlete slows to 50%. On command (visual/verbal) they must then accelerate gradually back up to 70%, initially, a long acceleration distance (e.g. 30m) is used; this distance can be decreased as the athlete progresses. This can also be progressed by add defender/opposition as a cue to change speed or direction.
- *Running with a skill added:* e.g. running to catch/control or kick a ball. To progress:
  - Catches are more demanding, requiring faster reaction/greater leg speed.
  - Multidirectional.
  - Add competition/opponent.
  - Add decision making or a tactical component to the drill.

Return to play

Prior to beginning full training, the athlete must have achieved all preset rehab goals. In all cases the following objective measures should be equal to the contralateral side and/or pre-injury data.

These should include:
- Appearance/general tone.
- Slump (neural mobility tests).
- Straight leg raise.
- Lower limb (Hamstring) flexibility.
- Eccentric strength:
  - Isokinetic assessment.
  - Nordic hamstring curls.

Field-testing

- 10m/20m/30m sprints or shuttle runs.
- Agility drills.
- Vertical jump.
- Skill-related (e.g. Kicking, reaching).

Obturator nerve entrapment

History and examination
The obturator nerve (L2–4) is formed in the psoas muscle and descends within the muscle, emerging from the medial border at the brim of the pelvis. The obturator nerve divides at the obturator notch into anterior and posterior divisions in the obturator foramen. The anterior division supplies the hip joint and adductor longus, brevis, and gracilis, with a sensory branch to the medial thigh. The posterior division supplies obturator internus and adductor magnus.

Entrapment of the nerve may occur within fascia as it leaves the pelvis, or by an obturator hernia or intra-pelvic mass. There is usually pain and dysaesthesia in the medial thigh, together with weakness of the adductor group, worsened by activity. Examination is often normal although there may be reduced cutaneous sensation over an area of skin along the middle of the medial thigh and/or weakness of adductors.

Investigations
- Specialized neurophysiological tests or nerve blockade may confirm the diagnosis.

Treatment
- Surgical release of the fascia overlying the nerve in the obturator foramen will release the entrapment.
- Neurolysis along the length of the nerve from the obturator foramen to the fascia between pectineus and adductor longus is required to ensure release.

Dislocation and subluxation of the hip joint

History and examination
Dislocation of the hip occurs only with considerable trauma, but subluxation may occur in adolescents with congenital hyperlaxity syndrome (or more rarely in those with significant neuromuscular impairment). Patients may describe a clunking, snapping, or popping in the groin followed by aching. Examination may be normal although usually there is hypermobility and poor pelvic girdle muscle strength.

Diagnosis
- Plain radiography.
- MRI: haemartrosis, posterior acetabular lip fracture/labral tear and iliofemoral ligament lesion.

Treatment
- Physical therapy in rehabilitation after relocation: muscle strengthening and stability exercises.
- Surgical treatment may be required for labral tear repair, removal of loose bodies and hip stabilization.
- Thermal capsular shrinkage of the hip may be considered.

Stress fractures of the pubic rami

History and examination
Pelvic stress fractures, most frequently involving the pubic rami, account for 1–2% of stress fractures, and can be serious. Arise due to over-use (fatigue fractures) or subnormal bone strength (insufficiency fractures).

Patients usually describe severe, deeply felt pain in the groin, and possibly the perineum, of gradual onset. Symptoms may follow an increase in training load or with minimal or no trauma during a long distance race, in an osteoporotic individual. Weight-bearing is painful; pain occurs at rest and at night. Sudden worsening may indicate completion of the fracture. Advise patient to rest and urgently investigate problem.

Investigations
- As with all stress fractures, the diagnosis can usually be made by plain X-ray after 3 weeks, but earlier on technetium bone scan or MRI scan.

Management
- Rest is essential, in the expectation that the fracture will heal without complication. Patients should be non-weight-bearing with crutches, while symptoms persist.
- Athletes can participate in non-weight-bearing sports when the stress fracture has settled sufficiently to allow walking.

Calcific tendinopathy of the hip

History and examination
Calcification at the site of origin of one or more muscles of the thigh, most commonly the rectus femoris, gluteus maximus, or vastus lateralis, is rare.

There may be severe groin pain and limitation of movement (due to pain), without a history of trauma. On examination, there may be pain induced global limitation of movement and/or pain on resisted testing of affected muscle groups.

Investigation
- Confirmation on X-ray or US.

Treatment
- Relative rest.
- Analgesics or NSAIDs.
- US.
- Shock wave therapy.
- If necessary, image-guided local corticosteroid injection.

Acetabular labral tears

History and examination
The acetabular labrum is a thick rim of dense fibrous tissue, which provides extra stability. The labrum can degenerate and tear, producing a flap, which can interfere with the joint and give a deep, painful clunk during a range of activities. There is an association between labral lesions and adjacent acetabular chondral damage, and labral disruption and degenerative joint disease are frequently part of a continuum of joint pathology. On examination there may be impingement on IR.

Symptoms
- Painful episodes of anteromedial snapping or clicking.
- Intermittent hip instability and locking, or decreased IR.

Physical examination
- Reproduction of pain/clicking by bringing the hip from flexed, abducted and externally-rotated position to adducted, internally rotated, and extended position (inverse for posterior tears).

Diagnosis
- Plain radiographs are useful for differential diagnosis. Radiograph may show lateral marginal sclerosis in long-standing cases.
- MR arthrography of the hip may be helpful, particulalry with lesions of the superior labrum.
- Arthroscopy is the gold standard

Prognosis
- Good with early diagnosis and treatment (before cartilage damage).

Treatment

Conservative treatment
- Limited weight-bearing, analgesia, limitation of activity (4–6 weeks).

Surgical treatment
- Open/arthroscopic trimming/repair.

Femoroacetabular impingement

Femoroacetabular impingement (FAI) is due to abnormal contact between the proximal femur and the acetabular rim.

The impingement may be a consequence of activities requiring a high range of motion of the hip, or can be a secondary to an abnormal anatomic configuration of the hip.

There are two types of FAI: the Cam and the Pincer. Patients can commonly present a combination of both types of FAI.

The 'cam' type is characterized by an abnormal configuration of the head-neck junction in the proximal femur with an inadequate head–neck offset leading to a damage of the acetabular labrum and articular cartilage.

The 'pincer' type is characterized by an abnormal acetabular rim contacting a normal femoral head-neck junction. In this case, the consequent ossification of the acetabular rim can lead to further deepening of the acetabulum and therefore more over-coverage of the femoral head.

The first type, more common in males, usually occurs in patients affected by hip deformities, such as post-traumatic deformities, slipped capital femoral epiphysis, Perthe's disease, or avascular necrosis of the hip. The pincer impingement is more common in middle aged females, in association with condition like coxa profunda, acetabular anteversion, or retroversion and acetabular protrusion.

Symptoms
- Hip/groin pain.
- Limitation of ROM.
- Snapping or clicking sensation.
- Mechanical symptoms in presence of labral pathologies.

Physical examination
- Restricted hip range of movement (particularly IR).
- Positive impingement test: pain exacerbated by forced IR and adduction (anterior FAI) or by forced ER in full extension (posterior FAI)

Diagnosis
- *X-rays:* alteration of hip anatomy, decreased joint space, sclerosis.
- *MRI:* bony oedema, labral pathologies.

Treatment

Non-operative
- Modification of activity, avoiding excessive hip movement.
- NSAIDs.

Arthroscopy
- Debridement of labral lesions and chondral damage areas.
- Labral repair for specific tears.
- Microfracture technique for cartilage lesions.
- Osteophytes resection.

Open surgery
Hip osteoplasty, periacetabular osteotomy.

Loose bodies

Intra-articular loose bodies can cause hip pain, groin pain or hip stiffness.

The presence of intra-articular loose bodies is usually associated with other hip pathologies including synovial chondromatosis, pigmented villonodular synovitis, osteochondritis dissecans, degenerative osteoarthritis, avascular necrosis. Furthermore, they are frequently found in patients who sustain traumatic hip dislocations or lower-energy trauma (causing chondral injury and loose body formation). Intra-articular loose bodies can be ossified or non-ossified, osteochondral, chondral, fibrous, or foreign.

Symptoms
- Mechanical symptoms including catching, locking, clicking, or giving way.
- Anterior groin pain.
- Hip stiffness.
- Occasionally history of dislocation or low-energy traumas.

Clinical examination
- Limited range of motion.
- Catching.
- Grinding.

Diagnosis
- Ossified or osteochondral loose bodies are the most easily identified on plain radiographs or CT scans.
- MRI with gadolinium contrast or magnetic resonance angiography (MRA) are more useful for identifying cartilaginous loose bodies and are useful for characterizing associated synovial or soft tissue pathology.[1]

Complications
Symptomatic loose bodies within the hip can cause the destruction of hyaline cartilage with resultant degenerative arthritis.

Treatment
- Arthroscopy is the emerging gold standard for removal of loose bodies.[2]
- Open approaches provide limited visualization of the articular surface and are associated with considerable morbidity.

Ischial (ischiogluteal) bursitis

History and examination
This may occur after a direct blow to the ischial tuberosity, and cause localized pain and tenderness.

Investigation
- Confirmed with US.

Treatment
- Relative rest, ice, anti-inflammatories, and cushioning are usually effective.
- A local guided injection of corticosteroid may be necessary.
- Surgical excision of the bursa is rarely necessary.

Sacro-iliac joint disorders

History and examination
The SIJ is very stable with little joint movement. There is no single fixed axis of motion, with flexion/extension, translation, and rotation. The motions of the SIJ include the anterior or posterior tilt of both innominate bones on the sacrum, the anterior tilt of one innominate bone, while the opposite innominate bone tilts posteriorly on the sacrum, which occurs during gait, the sacral flexion or extension (respectively 'nutation' and 'counter-nutation' rocking movements), in which the motions of the sacrum occur simultaneous with motion of the ilium.

While walking and running, the SIJs and ligaments absorb and dissipate stresses developed by twisting of the pelvis from flexion of one hip and extension of the other. Loss of mobility may cause stress fractures. There is debate as to whether the SIJ causes lower back and buttock pain in the absence of a true inflammatory sacro-iliitis.

There may be joint strain or dysfunction following a direct blow to the joint, forceful torsion of the pelvis when rising from the crouched position, or sudden strong contraction of the hamstrings and/or abdominal muscles. But, beware, as 'sacro-iliac strains' are often subsequently found to be due to other pathologies. Forces on the sacro-iliac ligaments are more likely to result in injury to the lumbosacral ligaments.

Pain may be felt in the buttock, groin, or thigh with activity and, in severe cases, at rest. Stress tests may exacerbate the pain.

Investigations
- Radiographs of the SIJ are often normal in the absence of an inflammatory process.
- Bone scans can demonstrate sacro-iliitis and stress fractures at the ridges of joint surfaces.
- Where sacro-iliitis is shown, it is important to look for the cause including seronegative arthropathy or pyogenic infection.

Treatment
- Muscle imbalance affecting the muscles of the thigh and abdomen and co-existing abnormalities in the lumbar spine should be addressed.
- Manipulation may help.
- A sacro-iliac belt can provide some symptomatic relief.
- Sacroiliitis, if part of an inflammatory arthritis, should be treated with analgesics, anti-inflammatories, physiotherapy, other approaches indicated for the systemic condition, and where necessary image-guided local corticosteroid injection.

The paediatric hip

Perthes' disease
Aetiology
- Avascular necrosis of the femoral head of unknown aetiology.

Clinical features
- Presents at age 3–10yrs, most commonly at 5-6yrs.
- Boys > girls in ratio 4:1.
- May be hip, groin or sometimes knee pain, although pain is not a feature after the early stages.
- May present with a painless limp.

Investigations
- X-ray changes depend on the stage of disease.
- In early stages, widening of the joint space may be the only sign. This is followed by patchy sclerosis, flattening, fragmentation and collapse of the femoral capital epiphysis.
- Bone scanning is useful in early cases, when X-ray is normal.

Treatment
- Should be referred to a paediatric orthopaedic surgeon for management.
- Treatment varies according to the amount of the femoral head involved and the age at presentation.
- Includes modifying activity, use of braces and, in severe cases, femoral osteotomy.
- Bisphosphonates may be useful in early stages.

Prognosis
- Depends on multiple factors, including the age at presentation and amount of surface area involved.
- The younger the presentation (<5) the better the prognosis.
- Risk of osteoarthritis depends on irregularity of joint surface.

Slipped upper capital femoral epiphysis (SUCFE)
Pathology
- Displacement of the epiphysis before skeletal maturity.
- Associated with delayed maturation and growth-plate stress (secondary to obesity).
- Hormonal factors may also play a role.
- 30% of cases have bilateral involvement, not always at the same time.

Clinical features
- Boys > Girls (2:1).
- Overweight pubertal boy with pain and a limp.
- Pain localized to the hip, groin or knee.
- Onset of pain usually gradual but may be acute.
- Limitation of hip abduction, flexion and IR.

Investigations
- X-ray demonstrates slip, which is graded from 1 to 3.
- Subtle changes seen on X-ray before slip occurs, include widening and irregularity of epiphysis.

Treatment
- Orthopaedic referral for consideration of open reduction and stabilization is required.

Prognosis
- Good if condition treated promptly with surgical stabilization.
- If untreated, may result in avascular necrosis or premature osteoarthritis.

Irritable hip

Aetiology
- Unknown, but thought to be a transient synovitis, which may have viral or autoimmune precipitant.

Clinical features
- Child (usually aged 2–8yrs) presents with pain or limp lasting from a few days to 1 week.
- Restricted hip ROM due to pain.
- Hip quadrant test (adduction, IR and compression with hip and knee flexed) positive.

Diagnosis
- Diagnosis of exclusion.
- X-rays, bone scans, and MRIs are normal.
- FBC usually normal. May show mild elevation of white cell count (WCC) and ESR.
- Important to exclude other more serious conditions, such as Perthes' disease, slipped upper capital femoral epiphysis and septic arthritis.

Treatment and prognosis
- Rest and analgesia.
- Ibuprofen may shorten course of symptoms.
- May recur.
- Prognosis is good, with no known long-term complications.

Avulsion fractures

Aetiology
- Result of acute traction episode of the involved apophysis (by rectus femoris, hamstrings or iliopsoas).
- Same injury mechanism in adult would produce muscle tear.

Clinical features
- History of sudden onset of pain associated with a rapid eccentric contraction of the involved muscle-tendon unit, e.g. sprinting in the case of rectus femoris, or hurdling in the case of the hamstrings

Diagnosis
- X-ray of involved apophysis is diagnostic, although need high index of suspicion as avulsed fragment may be difficult to detect.

Treatment
- Depends on amount of separation and the site involved.
- Stretching and a graduated strengthening programme combined with local physiotherapy.
- Graduated return to sport when symptoms have resolved.
- Surgical reattachment usually not necessary unless the bony fragment is displaced more than 2cm.
- Good prognosis with adequate rehabilitation.

Traction apophysitis of the ischial tuberosity

Aetiology
- As for other traction apophysitis.
- Repetitive traction of the hamstrings tendon at its origin at the ischial tuberosity.

Clinical features
- 12–16yr-old athlete involved in activities requiring forced hip flexion, such as dancing, football, hurdling and long-jump.

Diagnosis
- Clinical.
- No tests required unless avulsion fracture suspected.

Treatment and prognosis
- Same management principles as traction apophysitis in other regions.
- Prognosis is good.

Hip dysplasia

Aetiology
- Mild hip dysplasia and congenital dislocation of the hip are thought to represent the 2 ends of the spectrum of developmental hip disorders.
- Characterized by acetabular dysplasia and under-coverage of the femoral head.
- Risk ↑ with family history.
- ↑ Risk with hypermobility.

Clinical features
- May be detected with newborn screening involving US.
- May present in childhood, adolescence or early adult life as pain in the hip or knee, or gait disturbance.

Diagnosis
- US in infancy.
- X-ray in older children.

Treatment
- Prevention and early identification is best to promote normal joint development.
- If instability detected in infancy, usually treated with abduction splinting.
- Significant hip dysplasia with instability diagnosed after onset of walking usually requires surgical management.
- Untreated hip dysplasia is thought to increase the risk of early hip OA.

Femoroacetabular impingement (FAI)

Aetiology
- Results from abnormal contact between the femoral neck and acetabulum.
- Causative factors include previous SUCFE, femoral osteotomy, or femoral neck fracture and, more recently, high level impact-loading sports participation in early life is thought to predispose to femoral head-neck pathomorphology.
- In most instances, causative factors cannot be identified.

Classification
- *Cam type*: abnormal shape of the femoral head-neck junction. This type is more common in males.
- *Pincer type*: over-coverage of the acetabulum. This type is more common in females.

Clinical features
- Groin pain exacerbated by physical activity.
- May describe locking or catching sensation consistent with labral pathology.
- IR and adduction range may be limited with pain at end of range.
- FAI impingement test (passive hip flexion to 90° with IR and adduction) reproduces pain.
- Cam type FAI often presents in male adolescents or young adults.
- Pincer type FAI usually presents later in middle age.
- Both types of impingement result in damage to the acetabular labrum and chondral surface with increased risk of hip OA.

Diagnosis
- X-ray.
- MRI: for assessing chondral damage and acetabular labral tears.

Treatment
- Conservative treatment is often not effective due to the mechanical nature of the condition, but involves limiting the extremes of movement and strengthening the hip stabilizers.
- Hip arthroscopy is useful for addressing simple labral tears and chondral lesions, and can be used to debride excess bone.
- Open arthroplasty required for inaccessible lesions.

Chapter 22

Knee

History *620*
Examination *622*
Special tests *626*
Investigation of knee injuries *628*
Medial collateral ligament *629*
Rehabilitation after medial collateral
   ligament sprain (grade 2) *630*
Lateral collateral ligament *635*
Anterior cruciate ligament *636*
Posterior cruciate ligament *638*
Meniscal injuries *639*
Articular cartilage injury *639*
Anterior knee pain *640*
Patellar dislocation *641*
Hoffa's syndrome *641*
Ilio-tibial band friction syndrome *641*
Patello-femoral pain (syndrome) *642*
Patellar tendinopathy *643*
The paediatric knee *644*

History

If acute
- *Mechanism of injury:* e.g. twisting or in contact.
- *Degree of pain and disability:* able to weight bear/continue.
- Audible 'pop' or 'crack' at time of injury.
- *Swelling:* site and speed of onset—e.g. immediate or the next day.
- Site of symptoms.
- *Symptoms since:* pain, giving way, instability, or locking.
- Referral of pain.
- Past injury history.

If insidious
- Specific location of pain.
- *Aggravating factors:* e.g. stairs or sitting for long periods.
- Night pain.
- Associated crepitus or clicking.
- Locking, swelling, or giving way.
- Past injury history.
- Past medical history.
- Any other joints affected.

Examination

Inspection

The knee consists of two joints (see Figs. 22.1 and 22.2):
- Tibio-femoral.
- Patello-femoral.

In standing

Look for evidence of asymmetry or biomechanical abnormality, e.g.:
- Leg length.
- *Scoliosis:* symmetry of body creases.
- Squinting patellae or malalignment.
- Weight held equally through both lower limbs.
- *Muscle wasting:* especially quadriceps.
- Scars or bruising.
- Loss of contour around patella, suggestive of effusion.
- Hyper-recurvatum of knees.
- Pronation/supination of feet.
- Swelling in popliteal fossa.

Functional tests

- Whilst standing, functional tests such as squatting, lunging, hopping, stepping, or eccentric exercises can be assessed in an attempt to reproduce symptoms.

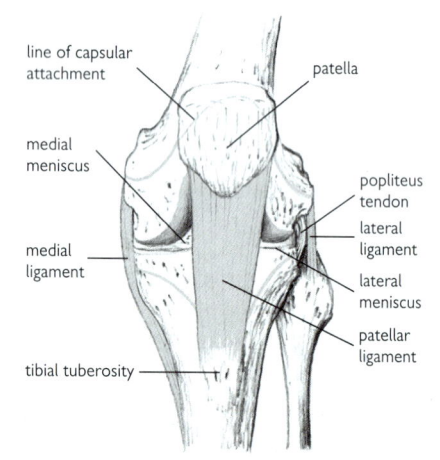

Fig. 22.1 Knee joint: anterior view showing capsule attachments and ligaments. Reproduced with permission from MacKinnon P and Morris J. (2005). *Oxford Textbook of Functional Anatomy*, Vol. 1. Oxford University Press, Oxford. © 2005.

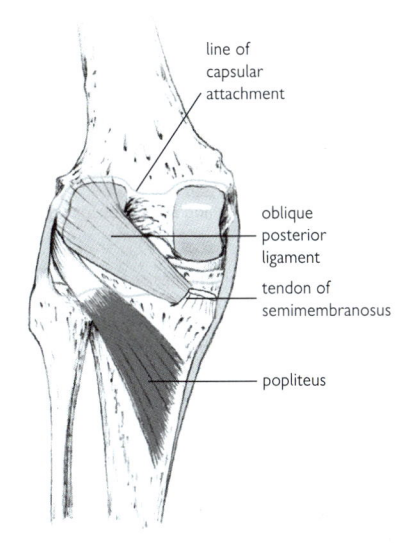

Fig. 22.2 Knee joint: posterior view showing oblique posterior ligament and attachment of popliteus. Reproduced with permission from MacKinnon P and Morris J. (2005). *Oxford Textbook of Functional Anatomy*, Vol. 1. Oxford University Press, Oxford. © 2005.

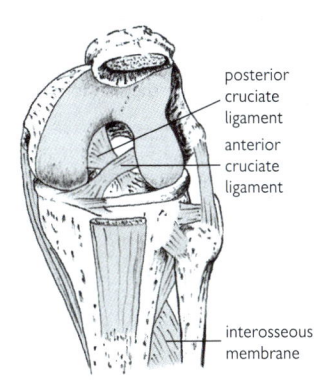

Fig. 22.3 Cruciate ligaments, anterior view. Reproduced with permission from MacKinnon P and Morris J. (2005). *Oxford Textbook of Functional Anatomy*, Vol. 1. Oxford University Press, Oxford. © 2005.

Palpation

In supine
- Assess for evidence of effusion, using fluid shift technique.
- *Patella:* assess position, angulation, freedom of movement, retropatellar crepitus, discomfort, and apprehension.
- Medial and lateral retinaculum for tenderness.
- Quadriceps muscles, tendon, and patellar tendon for tenderness or thickening.
- Tibial tubercle, check for swelling and any posterior sag compared with the other side.
- Fat pad.
- Medial and lateral tibio-femoral joint lines.
- Medial and lateral collateral ligaments.
- Lateral femoral condyle, including ilio-tibial band.
- Head of fibula and superior tibio-fibular joint.

In prone
- Hamstrings.
- Popliteal fossa for evidence of cyst.
- Medial head of gastrocnemius.

Active and passive movements
- Range of active movements should be −5° to 140° (i.e. hyperextension to full flexion).
- Apply gentle pressure at the end of range of active movement to assess joint 'end-feel' and passive joint movement. Note any hardness or unnatural springiness, as well as any discomfort.
- Assess hamstring flexibility at 90° of hip and knee flexion.
- Assess the subject's hip joints and straight leg raise to eliminate any possibility of referred pain, particularly in adolescents, where slipped upper femoral epiphysis should always be considered.
- If hyper-recurvatum of the knees is noted in standing or excessive hyperextension in supine, consider checking for more generalized hypermobility syndrome.

Resisted movements
- Check for pain and/or weakness on resisted knee extension (rectus femoris and quadriceps).
- Check for pain and/or weakness on resisted knee flexion (hamstrings).

Special tests

Medial and lateral collateral ligaments
- Resist inward (medial) and outward (lateral) movements at the knee.
- Ligaments are taut in full knee extension and are best assessed by valgus and varus forces applied by the examiner whilst the leg is supported in approximately 30° of knee flexion.

Ligament injury grading
- Grade 1 pain felt on stressing ligament, but no laxity.
- Grade 2 (partial tear) pain and some laxity at site of injury, but a solid 'end-feel' at the limit of range.
- Grade 3 (complete tear) pain and laxity with no 'end-feel' at limit of range of movement. Clinically it may be difficult to distinguish between grades 2 and 3 due to pain-induced muscle spasm.

Anterior and posterior cruciate ligaments (see Fig. 22.3)

The anterior cruciate ligament (ACL)
- Prevents the tibia from extending forward from the femur and helps control pivoting movements.
- Often injured in twisting or hyperextension movements.

The posterior cruciate ligament (PCL)
- Less commonly injured than the ACL.
- Limits backward movement of the tibia on the femur.

ACL and PCL can be assessed clinically in two ways:

Anterior and posterior draw tests
- Subject sits with knees bent at 90°.
- Posterior sag is excluded by examiner inspecting tibial tubercle from the side, to check for any loss of prominence, which may suggest a lax PCL.
- The examiner sits on the foot of the subject on the side to be tested. The hamstrings must be relaxed to allow the ACL to be stressed.
- Gentle traction is applied to the tibia forward (to assess ACL, called the anterior draw test). The tibia can then be gently pushed backwards (to assess the PCL, posterior draw test).
- Laxity and 'end-feel' are again important factors.
- If indicated, the posterior draw test can be repeated with the foot externally rotated. This will test for any evidence of posterolateral corner disruption.

Lachman's test
- A useful test as a positive result is less reliant upon the subject not having any hamstring contraction as at the time of the draw tests.
- The subject sits on the couch and the examiner holds the thigh firmly, and flexes the knee to approximately 15°. The tibia can then be drawn forward or backward to assess cruciate integrity.

Many sports people have well-developed quadriceps musculature. If the examiner finds that Lachman's test is difficult to perform because of this, then the examiner's knee can be placed under the thigh of the subject to support the knee in 15° flexion and allow the tibia to be drawn to and fro.

Pivot shift test
- The knee is held in full extension and the tibia internally rotated.
- As the knee is flexed, a valgus force is applied to the joint.
- This tests for a deficient ACL.
- A positive test will reveal a 'clunk' as the lateral femoral condyle (dislocated in internal rotation in an ACL deficient knee) relocates.

Menisci

Medial and lateral meniscal injury will often be suspected from the history. There are several methods of meniscal assessment.

McMurray's test
- A flexion-rotation test, with the knee being flexed fully and extended, whilst internal and external rotation pressure is placed upon it.
- Positive tests are obtained with pain and/or palpable internal 'clinking' felt by the examiner's hand on the joint line.

Ilio-tibial band

Can be assessed for tightness.

Ober's test
- The subject lies on their side with the lower leg flexed at the hip. The upper leg is then extended at the hip with the examiner's hand resting on the pelvis to keep that neutral. The examiner then adducts the extended hip and the subject's knee should comfortably reach the couch. If the ITB is tight, the pelvis will move out of neutral or the knee will extend before it reaches the couch.
- Tightness of the ITB can be confirmed on modified Thomas' test when the relaxed leg falls into external rotation at the hip.
- ITB friction syndrome can be diagnosed by pressure from the examiner's thumb over the subject's lateral femoral condyle, while the knee is repeatedly flexed and extended from 0 to 30°.

Investigation of knee injuries

Plain X-ray

Acute
To exclude fractures:
- Tibial plateau.
- Patellar stress.
- ACL avulsion.
- Osteochondral.

Skyline views can be obtained to assess the retro-patellar surface.

Non-acute
- Osteoarthritis (weight-bearing).

MRI scan
If suspected:
- Meniscal pathology.
- ACL/PCL tear.
- Articular cartilage damage.
- Patellar tendinpathy.

'Bone bruising' may be seen on MRI scans after significant knee injuries. Findings are sub-chondral bone oedema in the affected part.

Ultrasound
- Invaluable to assess patellar tendon pathology, particularly if degeneration (shows as areas of hypoechogenicity) or tear is suspected.
- Also useful to assess popliteal cysts or bursitis.

Arthroscopy
- Still sometimes used to confirm a clinical diagnosis, but less so since the advent of MRI.

Medial collateral ligament

History and examination
- MCL is a strong band of tissue on medial aspect of knee.
- Resists valgus strain.
- Often injured in football, rugby, and skiing.
- *Mechanism of injury:* any forceful movement of the lower leg outward at the knee or a hard blow to the outside of the lower thigh, which causes the knee to buckle.
- MCL is closely associated with the medial meniscus and the two structures are often injured in combination.
- Any forceful rotational element, in addition to a valgus strain can rupture MCL, medial meniscus, and anterior cruciate—a severe injury described as O'Donoghue's Triad.
- Symptoms include pain, mild to moderate swelling on the medial aspect of the knee, joint effusion (not immediate) and feeling of instability (like a 'wobbly' table leg).
- Injuries to MCL are graded 1 to 3 according to severity (see 📖 'Knee examination', p. 626).

Treatment
- Most MCL injuries are treated by rehabilitation after initial 'PRICE' management.
- MCL injuries that occur in association with meniscal or cruciate damage are more likely to require surgical repair.

Rehabilitation after medial collateral ligament sprain (grade 2)

Time to return to function: 4–8 weeks.

Protection stage (up to 4 weeks)
- Up to 4 weeks of protected weight-bearing may be advised depending on clinical severity. This is often undertaken with the knee supported in a brace at approximately 30° of flexion.
- Care must be taken to minimize quadriceps inhibition/weakening/atrophy during this stage.
- Static hamstring stretching: this is usually most comfortable in 10–15° knee flexion and is important to minimize the degree of secondary hamstring tightness.
- Ice, compression, and elevation can be of benefit in the acute phases.
- Electrotherapeutic modalities may be of the use in the acute and sub-acute stages, e.g. low level laser therapy and electrical stimulation.

Post protection: days 1–7

Key aims
- Increase ROM through knee flexion and extension.
- Address any quadriceps inhibition/weakening/atrophy.
- Encourage heel-toe gait pattern with full knee extension.

Mobility/stretching
- *Heel slides:* athlete flexes and extends the knee joint though the full pain free ROM.
- Static hamstring stretching should be continued through this phase if needed.

Strengthening/recruitment
- *Static quadriceps training:* with the knee straight tighten the quadriceps muscle. Simultaneous ankle dorsiflexion/gluteal tightening may aid quadriceps recruitment during this exercise.
- *Straight leg raise:* keeping the knee straight, lift the injured leg so that the heel is approximately 30cm from the ground
- *Inner range quads:* with a small ball under the knee, the athlete moves his/her knee into full extension.

Neuromuscular training/gait re-education
- *Weight transfers:* athlete stands on both feet, but with weight predominantly on the uninjured side. Within the limits of pain, slowly transfer weight on to the injured side. This should progress, until it is comfortable to stand solely on the injured foot.
- Walking with a controlled heel–toe gait pattern is encouraged.
- *Hydrotherapy/pool rehabilitation* will be useful in the majority of cases: the buoyancy of the water reduces the impact on the joints, and provides a better environment to restore normal movement patterns during rehabilitation. Hydrotherapy exercises include:
  - Walking using heel-toe gait.
  - Single leg balance.

- Mini squats.
- Knee flexion and extension in standing.

Biofeedback
EMG biofeedback may be useful, particularly in cases of extreme quadriceps inhibition. Surface electrodes placed over the muscle (usually the vastus medialis) provide the patient with real time feedback on muscle activity during rehabilitative exercises.

Before moving onto the middle stages of rehabilitation the athlete must have achieved:
- Good quadriceps recruitment with minimal to no inhibition.
- Ability to comfortably transfer weight onto the injured side.
- Full knee extension.

Post protection: weeks 2–3
Key aims
- Enhance neuromuscular control.
- Increase strength/ROM.
- Initiate weight-bearing exercise.

Mobility/strengthening/neuromuscular exercises
Single leg standing/balance
Standing on the injured side, the athlete tries to balance. At the start, the athlete is allowed to touch the ground with the uninjured side to regain balance when needed. As balance improves, they should be challenged to balance for a long as possible without touching the ground. This exercise can be progressed further by balancing with eyes closed or by balancing when undertaking additional physical tasks, e.g. an upper body movement which should progress from basic movements (bicep curl) to multijoint diagonal movement patterns.

Once the athlete is able to stand comfortably on one leg with his/her eyes closed, more advanced balance training can begin. A series of progressions should be undertaken using labile surfaces, visual stimuli, and skilled tasks. Progressions should also advance from double to single leg support.
- Athlete balances on the injured side, while throwing and catching a ball. Sports specific considerations could involve: varying the type of throw, e.g. underarm, overhead, side pass, chest pass; varying the direction of the pass received, e.g. in front, from side, overhead; varying the type of ball, e.g. tennis ball, medicine ball.
- Further progressions should be undertaken by balancing on dynamic surfaces, e.g. mini trampoline (rebounder), wobble board, balance pad/cushion, folded towel.

Strengthening
- *Mini squats:* ensuring an equal distribution of weight, the athlete should perform a 50% squat (to 45° knee flexion).
- *Drop squats:* as for a mini squat, except the speed is increased whilst maintaining control.
- Single leg squats.
- Lunges.

All these exercises can be progressed by increasing the demand on the neuromuscular system, e.g. the athlete must perform a single leg squat on a dynamic surface.

Cardiovascular
- Bike/cross trainer/upper body ergometer.

Post protection: weeks 3–6

To progress to the end stages of rehabilitation, the athlete must have full knee ROM, a good baseline of strength through all lower limb movements, be able to perform complex neuromuscular exercises in a pain free state and have good lumbopelvic/lower body control and alignment during squatting/advanced neuromuscular exercises.

In general, as the athlete progresses through the later stages of rehabilitation, the focus should become less joint-specific and more sport-specific.

Strength and conditioning
This may be progressed as follows:
- Squat.
- Deadlift.
- Hang clean.
- Clean.
- Snatch.

Ideally, the athlete should begin using the bar bell only. Their form and alignment should be monitored by a training partner, or strength and conditioning coach. The weight should be increased accordingly, building to their pre injury levels.

Plyometric exercises
Throughout all plyometric exercises, the athlete is encouraged to keep a 'soft' knee, using hips, knees, and ankles to cushion the impact. The athletes' ability to avoid 'corkscrewing' by keeping good pelvic, hip, knee, and toe alignment, is a good guide for their progress.
- *Jumping from two legs to one:* standing in a stationary position the athlete jumps vertically to land on the injured side.
- *Hop scotch:* this involves multiple jumps from two legs onto one, whilst moving forwards.
- *Jumping vertically while rotating:* e.g. from a stationary position, the athlete jumps vertically and turns 90° clockwise or anti-clockwise before landing. This can be progressed by using 180°, 270°, or 360° rotations.
- *Jumping to land from a height (e.g. Small step):* initially a 2-foot landing should be used. This exercise can be progressed as follows:
  - Athlete rotates 45° in air before landing.
  - Add 90°/180° rotation.
  - Single leg landing.
  - Landing on dynamic surface.
  - Immediately catching a ball on landing.
  - Therapist adds a light push on landing.

Running

Prerequisites
- Full knee ROM.
- Subject able to run on the spot.
- Able to undertake advanced balance (neuromuscular) exercises with good body control in a pain free state.

Straight line running
- Light jog, building from 30–50% (note: 100% pace is a sprint).
- Build up to 10–30min.

Begin progressive running
- This should be done on a flat surface, with cones dividing acceleration/maintenance/deceleration stages.
- For the first session athletes should accelerate from a standing start, up to 60% over the first 30m. They should then aim to maintain this pace over the next 30m, before decelerating slowly to a complete stop.
- Progress by decreasing the acceleration distance and increasing the maintenance distance (Table 22.1).

Functional running exercises
- *Athlete runs in a curved or figure of eight pattern:* this should initially involve gradual curves and progress to sharper/tighter curves.
- *Shuttle runs (doggies):* multiple sprints between cones or markers; athletes should be encouraged to slow into each turn, plant their foot, and accelerate out of the turn. The planting foot should vary between the injured and uninjured sides.
- *Run stops:* from a 60% run the athlete must come to a complete stop within 5 steps. To progress increase the speed of the run/minimize the number of steps needed to stop.
- *45°/90°cuts:* running forwards then side stepping to change direction at a 45° or 90°angle.
- *Full body spins/pivots:* running at 50% the athlete must spin 360° without slowing down.
- Agility drills.

Ladders or cones can be used to facilitate a series of running and footwork drills which challenge the athletes speed, balance, strength, and co-ordination, e.g. T-shuffle agility drill:
- Athlete sprints forwards 10m to touch cone A.
- Side shuffles to the left for 5m to touch cone B.
- Side shuffles to the right for 10 m to touch cone C.
- Turns and sprints back to the starting point.

Table 22.1 Progressive running: decreasing the acceleration distance, and increasing the maintenance distance

Acceleration	Maintenance	Deceleration
20m	40m	20m
10m	30m	20m
10m	40m	20m

Field testing
If available, field test results should be compared with pre-season or normative data. Useful tests might include:
- 10m/20m/30m sprint times.
- T-shuffle agility drill.
- Vertical jump.
- Standing broad jump:
  - Jumping from two feet/landing on two feet.
  - Jumping from injured/landing on two feet.
  - Jumping from injured/landing on injured.
- Sports specific task, e.g. kicking a ball, tackling.
- Back to play.

Lateral collateral ligament

History and examination
- Thinner than the MCL, a cord-like structure on the lateral aspect of the knee.
- Resists varus strain.
- Lateral collateral ligament (LCL) is separate from the lateral meniscus and the two are not so often injured in combination as on the medial aspect.
- LCL can be injured in combination with cruciate ligaments.
- Mechanism of injury—various loading of knee and hyperextension.
- Posterolateral complex injury can produce significant functional impairment and instability. (The posterolateral complex consists of the LCL, arcuate ligament, lateral head of gastrocnemius, biceps femoris tendon, and musculotendinous junction of popliteus muscle.)

Treatment
- LCL can be repaired or augmented, but this is usually in association with surgery to the other damaged tissues.

Anterior cruciate ligament

History and examination
- ACL is the primary restraint for anterior movement of the tibia on the femur.
- Also acts to stop antero-lateral rotation of the knee.
- Mechanism of injury is valgus force with a twisting motion (pivoting) or hyperextension of the knee.
- Injury usually occurs in contact situations, but non-contact ACL is frequently reported, particularly in females.
- Females are thought to be particularly prone to non-contact ACL injuries. Women playing basketball and soccer are 2–6 times more likely than men to sustain ACL rupture.
- Theories as to why women are so at risk include:
  - Women having a smaller intercondylar notch and ACL than men.
  - Lower limb mechanics.
  - Hormonal variations.
  - Joint laxity.
- Collateral ligament and meniscal damage often also occurs at time of cruciate injury.
- Symptoms of ACL rupture include immediate swelling of the knee joint due to haemarthrosis, and a 'pop' which may be heard at the time of contact.
- Haemarthrosis is very painful. With the above history, there is a 90% chance of an ACL tear.
- Clinically, there will be reduction of extension, and signs of ACL laxity (see p.212). Pivot shift test is often positive, but may be difficult to perform on an injured athlete. Medial joint line tenderness may suggest medial meniscus injury.
- ACL laxity on clinical examination (see p.212) does not mean that the knee is necessarily unstable.
- Recurrent episodes of instability will increase the risk of developing accelerated osteoarthritis of the knee (See Fig. 22.4).

Treatment

ACL repair
Most individuals involved in sports which involve pivoting will require surgical reconstruction of a torn ACL if they wish to continue in their sport.
Repair of an ACL tear is indicated if:
- There is associated meniscal or MCL tear.
- High level athletes (especially in pivoting sports).
- Lower level participants who wish to pursue sports which involve pivoting.
- Children/adolescents (giving way can cause significant damage to the joint).
- The knee remains unstable (i.e. gives way) after completion of rehabilitation protocol.
- Occupational factors (e.g. armed forces or police).

The aim of surgery to repair a torn ACL is to mimic the functional anatomy of the ligament. ACL repair can be undertaken using many techniques, although primary repair is not usually successful and currently the most commonly used reconstruction techniques involve harvesting:
- Semitendinosus and gracilis tendons.
- Middle third of the patellar tendon.
- The method of choice varies between specialist knee surgeons, and results appear to be very similar, although patellar tendon repairs have a higher incidence of post-operative anterior knee pain.
- The optimum time for ACL reconstruction is thought to be approximately 3 weeks post-injury, unless earlier repair is indicated by the clinical condition.
- There is no evidence that ACL repair reduces the long-term incidence of osteoarthritis of the knee.

ACL rehabilitation
- Standard protocols for ACL reconstruction post surgery, or as a conservative treatment approach have changed significantly over recent years.
- Early mobilization with brace protection allows commencement of strengthening and proprioceptive exercises within days, rather than the original periods of weeks or even months.
- With modern rehabilitation, return to sport is now usually possible (90%+) at 6 months post-operatively.

Posterior cruciate ligament

History and examination
- Less common than ACL injuries.
- PCL tears constitute less than 2% of acute knee injuries.
- PCL is the primary restraint for posterior movement of the tibia on the femur.
- Also acts as restraint of external rotation.
- Mechanism of injury involves falling on a bent knee, hyperextension of the knee, or torn with the ACL via a violent twisting movement.
- Posterolateral complex may be involved in PCL tears.
- Usually minimal swelling on examination. Posterior sag of the tibia may be seen.

Treatment
- Isolated PCL tears can generally be managed conservatively using a predominantly quadriceps strengthening programme.
- Surgical reconstruction is indicated if there is associated posterolateral complex damage (rotatory instability).
- PCL tears usually lead to long-term osteoarthritis.

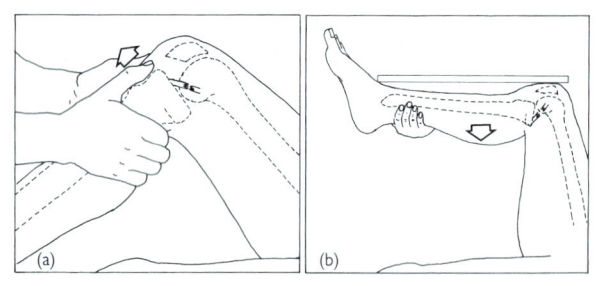

Fig. 22.4 (a) Anterior 'drawer' test; (b) 'sag' test. Reproduced with permission from MacKinnon P and Morris J. (2005). *Oxford Textbook of Functional Anatomy*, Vol. 1. Oxford University Press, Oxford. © 2005.

Meniscal injuries

History and examination
- Mechanism of acute injury involves a violent rotation of the knee.
- Tears may also occur without significant trauma due to repeated small injuries to the cartilage or degeneration of the tissue in older patients.
- Medial meniscus often injured in combination with MCL.
- Lateral meniscus is more likely to be damaged in isolation from the LCL, and is prone to degeneration secondary to biomechanical abnormalities.
- Meniscal tears are typically associated with pain along medial or lateral joint line of the knee.
- Mild to moderate joint effusion is noted.
- Symptoms of clicking, catching or locking of knee (the latter in extension rather than flexion) may be present.
- Knee may tend to give way.
- History often strongly suggestive of diagnosis.
- Cystic swelling of meniscus may be present at joint line.

Articular cartilage injury

This can be occult or involve chondral or osteochondral fractures (graded 1–4).

History and examination
- Can occur in association with cruciate or MCL tears, patellar dislocation, post-menisectomy, or in isolation.
- Medial femoral condyle often affected in ACL tears.
- Lateral tibial condyle and retro-patellar surface also commonly affected areas.

Investigations
- Diagnosed on MRI scan or at arthroscopy.
- Pain and swelling are usually acute symptoms.

Treatment
Articular cartilage receives its blood supply from sub-chondral bone. Healing is therefore slow and treatments include:
- Microfracture (drilling or using a curved awl to encourage healing with fibrocartilage from the sub-chondral area).
- Chondrocyte implantation.

Indications for surgery
- Younger patients with isolated grade 3–4 injury, intact menisci, and normal surrounding cartilage.
- Success of these procedures is greatly aided by correction of any existing biomechanical abnormalities.

Anterior knee pain

This is one of the commonest presenting symptoms in sport and exercise medicine. A precise diagnosis may be difficult and the term anterior knee pain describes symptoms without a specific cause identified.

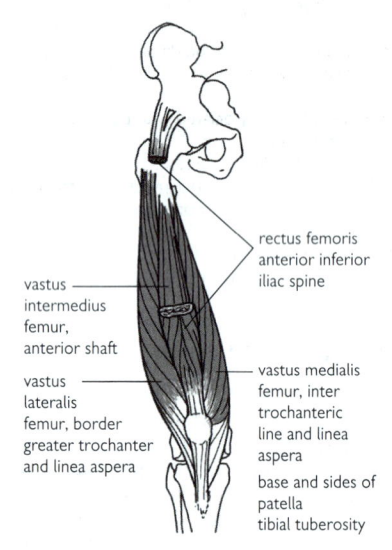

Fig. 22.5 Quadriceps femoris. Reproduced with permission from MacKinnon P and Morris J. (2005). *Oxford Textbook of Functional Anatomy*, Vol. 1. Oxford University Press, Oxford. © 2005.

Patellar dislocation

History and examination
- Usually a lateral displacement onto the lateral femoral condyle.
- Often traumatic and associated with haemarthrosis.
- Also in young girls with predisposing factors such as lower limb malalignments and generalized hypermobility.

Treatment
- Treatment aims to reduce the risk of recurrence with vastus medialis strengthening, although recurrent episodes will require surgery.

Hoffa's syndrome

History and examination
- Also known as fat pad impingement.
- Very painful, especially either side of the patellar tendon.
- Mechanism is usually a hyperextension injury.
- Haemarthosis often present.

Treatment
- Treat to reduce inflammation and taping if inferior tilting of patella is present.

Ilio-tibial band friction syndrome

History and examination
- Also called 'runners' knee'.
- Caused by friction of the ITB on the lateral femoral epicondyle usually at less than 30° of knee flexion.
- Causes pain over lateral aspect of knee during a run, especially on a cambered course.
- Tightness of the ITB may be present on Ober's test.
- Abnormal biomechanics (e.g. leg length discrepancy), excessive training load, downhill and distance running are other predisposing factors.
- Usually associated with bursitis at the site of pain.

Investigation
- Diagnosis usually on clinical findings.

Treatment
- NSAIDs.
- Myofascial tension massage to ITB.
- ITB stretching.
- Corticosteroid injection if bursitis present.
- Correction of biomechanical abnormalities/training errors.

Patello-femoral pain (syndrome)

- Often misnamed chondromalacia patella.
- Usually insidious onset, but can occur acutely.
- Vague, aching pain over anterior aspect of knee.
- Aggravated by activity especially distance running, squatting, lunging, going up or down stairs, or sitting for long periods.
- Patient may describe 'clicking' or 'grating' behind the patella on knee movement.
- Knee may give way due to pain and quadriceps inhibition.
- Clinical features may include tenderness in the retro- or infra-patellar areas, a small effusion, crepitus, and stiffness of patellar movement, and wasting of vastus medialis obliquus (VMO).
- There may be signs of squinting patellae, hyper-recurvatum, tibial torsion, or hyperpronation in standing.
- Usual causes are:
    - Over-use (excessive loading of patello-femoral joint—PFJ).
    - Lower limb malalignment—squinting patellae and femoral anteversion, hyperpronation (↑ PFJ forces).
    - Patellar maltracking (↓ PFJ contact area).

Patellar tracking

- During knee flexion, the patella moves from lateral to medial to travel within the intercondylar notch of the femur at end of range.
- The movement of the patella is dependent upon passive and active restraints.
- Any imbalance of these restraints is most likely to cause the patella to track more laterally, and during episodes of loading, patello-femoral symptoms may arise as a result.
- Some typical causes of this so-called patellar maltracking are:
    - Tightness of passive restraints (ITB, lateral retinaculum).
    - Weakness of active restraints (VMO).
    - Weakness of gluteus medius muscles, leading to increased internal rotation at the hips.
    - Muscle tightness—hamstrings and quadriceps (see Fig. 22.5).

NB If patello-femoral pain occurs on sitting, then it is unlikely to be caused by maltracking. Retro-patellar pressure is more likely.

The 'Q' angle

- Refers to the angle at the junction between two lines drawn from the anterior superior iliac spine to the middle of the patella and a line drawn to the same point from the tibial tubercle. (Normal is less than 20° and is increased in femoral anteversion.)
- A greater than normal angle is associated with patellar maltracking.
- Females tend to have a greater 'Q' angle than males, which will also predispose them to patellar maltracking, and therefore patello-femoral pain.

Investigation

- Diagnosis usually on clinical findings.

Treatment

Primary aim is to attempt to correct any abnormal biomechanics:
- Manual treatment and stretching of ITB, hamstrings, gastrocnemius and rectus femoris.
- Patellar taping to correct any malposition/tilt—can reduce pain by up to 50%.
- VMO strengthening (± biofeedback).
- Gluteus medius strengthening.
- Orthotics to correct hyperpronation.
- Proprioception.
- Modification of training regime to avoid over-use.
- Surgery for patello-femoral pain syndrome is not common due to improved rehabilitation techniques.

Patellar tendinopathy

History and examination
- Also known as 'jumper's knee'.
- Over-use injury.
- Underlying pathology is a degenerative tendinosis, not an inflammatory tendonitis.
- Commonest site is at the deep part of the tendon attachment to the inferior pole of the patella.
- Main complaint is of anterior knee pain aggravated by jumping, bounding, or hopping.
- Insidious onset usually, but tears can present acutely.
- Eccentric contraction usually reproduces symptoms.

Investigations
- US and MRI scanning are both very effective at confirming diagnosis.

Treatment
- Often very prolonged.
- *Physiotherapy:* transverse frictions and progressive strengthening to include eccentric exercises.
- Correction of biomechanical abnormalities/training errors.
- Dry needling and novel techniques such as autologous blood or platelet-rich plasma injection have limited evidence for use in patellar tendinopathy.
- High volume injection and lithotripsy treatments appear to be less successful than when used for Achilles tendinopathy.
- Surgical scraping of the tendon is rarely indicated and should only be considered after intensive rehabilitation.

The paediatric knee

Osgood-Schlatter disease

Clinical features
- Commonest traction apophysitis.
- Affects tibial tubercle.
- Boys > Girls (4:1).
- Presents between ages 10 and 14 (earlier in girls).
- Insidious onset of anterior knee pain (sometimes bilateral) in child involved in running and jumping sport.
- Pain worse during and after activity.
- Difficulty kneeling.

Examination findings
- Tenderness ± localized swelling over tibial tubercle.
- Quadriceps may appear wasted, depending on the duration of the symptoms.
- May be some restriction in knee flexion.
- Pain may be reproduced by resisted knee extension from the flexed position.
- May be associated biomechanical factors contributing to the condition, such as hyperpronation or lateral patella tilt/subluxation.

Investigations
- Not usually required.
- If performed, X-ray will show overlying soft tissue swelling (diagnostic) and may demonstrate fragmentation of the tibial tubercle apophysis.
- Only indications for X-ray in this group of children are:
  - If the diagnosis is in doubt.
  - If symptoms persist and calcification is suspected.
  - If an avulsion fracture of the tibial tubercle is suspected.

Treatment
- Child who has pain with daily living activities will need to avoid running and jumping until the pain subsides.
- Children with minimal symptoms may be able to continue running and jumping activities at a reduced level.
- Quadriceps flexibility program to ↓ traction force on TT.
- Biomechanical abnormalities such as hyperpronation and patella malalignment should be corrected with exercise programme, patella taping and orthotics.
- Quadriceps strengthening.
- Gradual resumption activity.

Prognosis
- Usually very good.
- In about 5% of cases, calcification can develop adjacent to the tibial tubercle, which causes persistence of symptoms and inability to kneel and may require surgical resection.

- Important to reassure child and parents that this condition does not cause long-term disability, but can be troublesome over one or two seasons during periods of rapid growth.

Sinding–Larsen–Johannsen disease ('jumper's knee')

Clinical features
- Traction apophysitis affecting inferior pole of the patella.
- Less common than Osgood–Schlatter disease, but similar presentation.
- Pain localized to inferior pole of the patella.
- Gradual onset of anterior knee pain exacerbated by activities that load the flexed knee, such as running and jumping.
- Focal tenderness inferior pole of the patella.
- Swelling rarely present.
- Resisted knee extension from flexed position usually reproduces the pain.
- Biomechanical factors such as hyperpronation, femoral anteversion, and patellar misalignment may be present.

Investigations
- Not required.

Treatment
- Similar to that in Osgood–Schlatter disease.
- Prognosis is good.

Juvenile osteochondritis dissecans

Aetiology
- Probably results from combination of minor repetitive trauma and microvascular compromise affecting the subchondral bone and articular cartilage.
- Bone becomes sclerotic, fragmented and loose bodies may form.

Sites affected
- Medial femoral condyle (MFC) 75%.
- LFC 20%.
- Patella and trochlear groove 5%.

Clinical features
- More common in boys than girls.
- Average age at diagnosis is 13.
- Present with knee pain ± swelling.
- May or may not have history of injury.
- May give history of locking 2° loose body.

Examination findings
- Effusion usually present.
- Tenderness usually localized to medial joint line (MJL).
- Quadriceps wasting if symptoms prolonged.

Investigations
- X-ray: look for irregularity in the lateral aspect of the MFC where 75–80% occur. May also see loose body.

- If X-ray is normal, but clinical history suggests OCD an MRI should be performed to confirm the diagnosis and to exclude a meniscal tear.

Differential diagnosis
- Inflammatory arthropathy.
- Meniscal tear.

Treatment
- Conservative treatment appropriate if articular cartilage intact.
- If loose bodies present, arthroscopy, and removal or reattachment of the loose body is indicated.

Prognosis
- Depends on site and size of the defect and age at presentation.
- The closer to skeletal maturity child is, the poorer the prognosis.

Bipartite patella and patellofemoral pain syndrome

Aetiology
- Bipartite patella results when secondary ossification centres at supero-lateral aspect of the patella fail to unite.
- May result from excessively tight lateral patellar retinaculum.

Clinical features
- Commonly asymptomatic.
- Can sometimes be palpated.
- May present with patellofemoral pain syndrome, i.e. anterior knee pain exacerbated by climbing stairs, squatting and prolonged sitting.
- May present with localized pain over superolateral aspect of the patella, where fibrous union between ossification centres lies.
- Trauma may precipitate the pain.

Investigations
- P-A X-ray will demonstrate bipartite fragment.

Treatment
- Strengthening vastus medialis oblique.
- Lateral retinacular releases (physiotherapy).
- Trial of medial patella taping.
- If pain persists at the superolateral border of the patella, surgical lateral retinacular release with or without excision of the bipartite fragment may be required.
- Bipartite patella rarely causes long-term disability.

Discoid lateral meniscus

When the lateral meniscus is D-shaped rather than normal C shape, it is predisposed to tearing.

Clinical features
- May present with a painless clunking in the knee.
- May present after a twisting injury, when child complains of lateral joint pain, swelling, clicking, and sometimes locking.

Examination findings
- Examination unremarkable if no tear has occurred.

- If associated with lateral meniscal tear, effusion is often present and restricted range of motion.
- Lateral joint line tenderness.
- May be a positive lateral McMurray's sign.

Investigations
- X-ray may demonstrate subtle widening of lateral joint space.
- MRI will confirm diagnosis.

Treatment
- Not required if condition is asymptomatic.
- If discoid meniscus is torn, usually requires excision of the torn lateral meniscal fragment and conversion of the meniscus to a C shape.
- Discoid lateral menisci may be bilateral.
- After partial lateral meniscectomy, prognosis is favourable.

Juvenile idiopathic arthritis (JIA)
Persistent arthritis of unknown aetiology which occurs before the age of 16yrs and persists for at least 6 weeks.

Aetiology
- Chronic inflammatory joint disease with probable genetic and environmental causes.

Clinical features
- Knee pain and swelling may be the first sign of oligoarticular JIA in an active child/adolescent.
- Frequently presents with swelling, but minimal or no pain.
- Symptoms often worse with inactivity.
- Morning stiffness.

Examination findings
- Knee effusion.
- Thigh muscle atrophy.
- Frequently have subtle reduction in range of motion (ROM).
- Examine other joints for effusions or ↓ ROM.
- Examine skin and nails for signs of psoriasis.

Investigations
- X-ray to exclude other causes of joint effusion/pain.
- Blood tests: inflammatory markers including FBC, ESR, CRP, antinuclear antibody (ANA) & RF (although ESR and CRP are usually normal in oligoarticular JIA).
- Synovial fluid analysis for definitive diagnosis.

Treatment
- Physical therapy including hydrotherapy, passive ROM exercises and isometric strengthening.
- Avoid heavy impact loading sports when joint disease is active.
- Oral NSAIDs.
- Referral to paediatric rheumatologist for consideration of intra-articular corticosteroid.
- Ophthalmology review to exclude asymptomatic uveitis (↑ risk if female & ANA +ve).

Chapter 23

Ankle and lower leg

Examination of the ankle 650
Special tests 653
Functional tests 653
Investigations 654
Acute ankle sprain 656
Persistent painful ankle 658
Rehabilitation after ankle sprain (grade 2) 660
Medial ligament injuries 665
Syndesmosis injury 666
Fractures 667
Lateral ankle pain 668
Medial ankle pain 672
Anterior ankle pain 674
Posterior ankle pain 675
Shin splints (chronic exertional leg pain) 676
Anterior compartment syndrome 678
Lateral compartment syndrome 679
Posterior compartment syndrome 680
Achilles tendinopathy 682
Achilles tendon rupture 683
Retrocalcaneal bursitis 683

Examination of the ankle

Inspection
The ankle contains three joints:
- Talocrural joint.
- Inferior tibiofibular joint.
- Subtalar joint.

With the feet in a symmetrical position the subtalar joint is in neutral; neither pronated or supinated. Pronation consists of:
- Eversion.
- Dorsiflexion.
- Abduction of the foot.

Supination consists of:
- Inversion.
- Plantar flexion.
- Adduction of the foot.

Look for evidence of abnormal biomechanics when standing, walking, supine, and prone:
- Excessive pronation.
- Excessive supination.
- Fore foot varus.
- Fore foot valgus.
- Rear foot varus.
- Rear foot valgus.
- Ankle equinus.
- Genu varum.
- Genu valgum.
- Leg length.

Palpation
See Fig. 23.1 for the bony anatomy of the ankle.

Anterior structures
- Ankle joint.
- Antero-inferior tibio-fibular ligament (AITFL).
- Talus.

Lateral structures
- Distal fibula.
- Lateral malleolus.
- Lateral ligaments (anterior talofibular ligament (ATFL), calcaneofibular ligament (CFL), posterior talofibular ligament (PTFL)).
- Peroneal tendons.
- Sinus tarsi.
- Base of fifth metatarsal.

Medial structures
- Medial ligament.
- Tibialis posterior.
- Flexor hallucis longus.

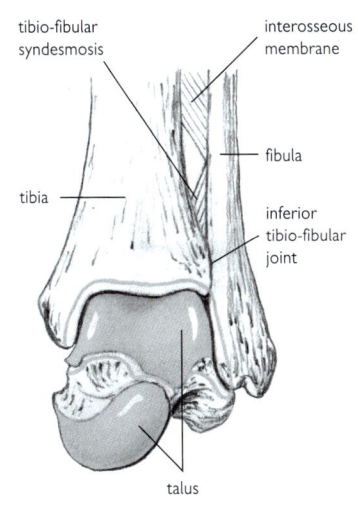

Fig. 23.1 Bony anatomy of ankle. Reproduced with permission from MacKinnon P and Morris J (2005). *Oxford Textbook of Functional Anatomy* Vol. 1. Oxford University Press, Oxford. © 2005.

- Sustentaculum tali.
- Navicular tubercle.
- Midtarsal joint.

Posterior structures
- Achilles tendon.
- Retrocalcaneal bursa.
- Posterior talus.
- Calcaneum.

Active and passive movements
- Ankle dorsiflexion (10–20°).
- Ankle dorsiflexion can be restricted by inflexibility of gastrocnemius and soleus.
- The minimum range of ankle dorsiflexion for normal locomotion is 10°.
- Ankle plantar flexion (35–50°).
- Dorsiflexion and plantar flexion take place between the talus and tibia and fibula.
- Subtalar inversion (10–20°).
- Subtalar eversion (5–10°).
- Inversion and eversion take place at the talocalcaneal, talonavicular, and calcaneocuboid joints. Perform with ankle dorsiflexed to limit lateral motion.
- Inversion is usually double that of eversion.

Resisted movements

Plantarflexion
- Gastrocnemius (knee extended).
- Soleus (knee flexed).
- Flexor digitorum longus, flexor hallucis longus (flex the toes against resistance). See Fig. 23.2.

Dorsiflexion
- Tibialis anterior (dorsiflex the foot against resistance).
- Extensor digitorum longus (dorsiflex the toes against resistance).
- Extensor hallucis longus (dorsiflex the big toe against resistance).

Inversion
Tibialis posterior (foot in plantar flexion, invert against resistance).

Eversion
Peroneus longus and brevis (foot in plantar flexion, evert against resistance).

Special tests

Ankle sprains are classified as:
- *Grade 1:* is painful without instability.
- *Grade 2:* demonstrates mild instability.
- *Grade 3:* complete rupture.

Anterior draw test

A positive anterior draw test in plantar flexion implies injury to the ATFL. It is performed by holding the heel and pulling the foot anteriorly, while applying a posterior force to the tibia. Alternatively, fix the foot to the examination couch and push the tibia posteriorly (knee flexed to relax gastrocnemius, foot in 10° plantar flexion). A positive anterior draw test in neutral suggests additional injury to the CFL and possibly the PTFL.

Talar tilt test

The talar tilt test examines for CFL instability. It is performed by holding the calcaneum and inverting the talus on the tibia. A talar tilt of 15° or 5° more than the opposite ankle is positive.

Tinels test

Tapping the posterior tibial nerve as it winds round the medial malleolus results in radiation of pain and paraesthesia along its course (heel and medial arch of the foot).

The squeeze test

Is positive when compression of the proximal tibia and fibula precipitates distal pain in the region of the interosseous membrane suggesting an injury to the syndesmosis.

External rotation test

Knee flexed 90°, foot held and rotated laterally with the ankle in neutral. Positive test—pain over the syndesmosis.

Functional tests

- Squat.
- Heel raise.
- Single leg stance.
- Single leg squat.
- Lunge.
- Hop.
- Jump.

Investigations

Radiographs
- The use of radiographs with acute ankle injuries is guided by the Ottawa rules.

Ankle radiograph—malleolar pain
- Inability to weight-bear after injury and in Emergency Department.
- Bone tenderness posterior edge or tip of medial malleolus.

Foot radiographs
- Bone tenderness base of 5th metatarsal.
- Bone tenderness navicular.
- Inability to weight-bear after injury and in Emergency Department.

Stress radiographs
May provide further assessment for ankle instability. Stress views include the talar tilt and anterior draw test views. Variables include patient co-operation, amount of force used, amount of laxity on the uninvolved side.
- CT may be useful for evaluating osteochondral injuries and stress fractures.
- MRI may be useful if evaluating ligament injuries, tendon injuries, osteochondral injuries or meniscoid lesions in patients with a history of recurrent ankle pain and discomfort.
- Musculoskeletal US images to evaluate associated tendon injuries.

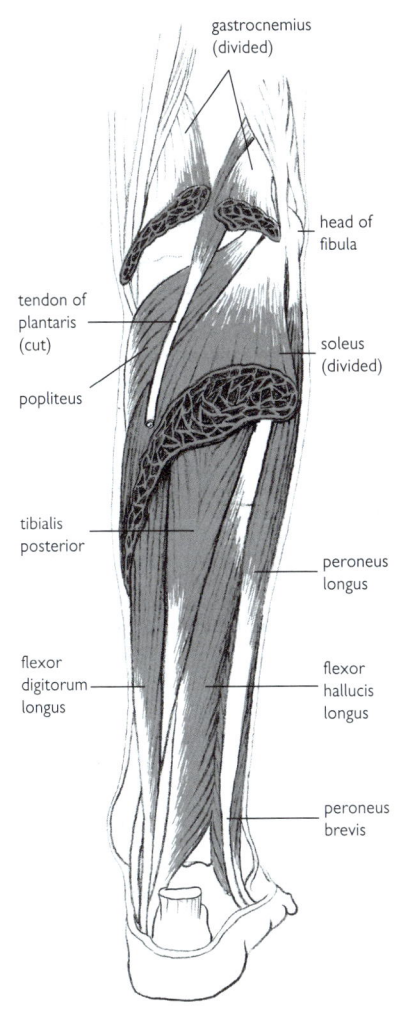

Fig. 23.2 Deep muscles of the calf (plantaris may or may not be present). Reproduced with permission from MacKinnon P and Morris J. (2005). *Oxford Textbook of Functional Anatomy*, Vol. 1. Oxford University Press, Oxford. © 2005.

Acute ankle sprain

History and examination

Acute ankle sprains can occur in any sport but are most common in sports that involve a change of direction or jumping e.g. football, rugby, basketball, netball, and volleyball. The lateral ligament includes the ATFL, CFL, and PTFL. The medial or deltoid ligament is composed of four bands—three superficial and one deep. The interosseous ligaments include the anterior tibiofibular ligament, posterior tibiofibular ligament, and interosseous ligament (see Fig. 23.3).

The mechanism of injury is important, an inversion injury suggests lateral ligament sprain, an eversion injury medial ligament sprain. Compression may suggest an osteochondral injury.

- Inversion injuries account for 70–85% of all ankle injuries. They occur when the foot is plantar flexed and inverted. Inversion injuries lead to sprains of the lateral ligament complex including the ATFL, CFL, and PTFL.
- The ATFL is most susceptible to injury. The CFL is injured in 40% of ATFL injuries. Complete tears of the ATFL, CFL, and PTFL result in ankle dislocation and are often associated with a fracture.
- The location of pain and swelling normally indicates the ligaments injured, most commonly the anterolateral aspect of the ankle joint involving the ATFL.
- Ability to weight-bear after the injury suggests a sprain and not a fracture.
- Clinical examination includes palpation of the ligaments, tendons, and also the lateral and medial malleoli, base of the fifth metatarsal, and proximal fibula to consider collateral injuries.

Investigations

- Radiographs are required if the patient cannot weight-bear or has point tenderness, particularly over the malleoli, tarsal navicular, base of the fifth metatarsal, or proximal fibular (Ottowa rules).
- Repeat radiographs should be considered if there is no improvement or progress is delayed.
- Radiographs should include the base of the fifth metatarsal to exclude a fracture.
- Anteroposterior, lateral, and mortis views are required. Fractures including osteochondral injuries to the medial and lateral talar dome should be excluded.
- Mortis views assess the distal tibial syndesmosis. Widening between the tibia and fibula (>5.5mm), and/or talus and medial malleolus (>4mm) indicates injury to the syndesmosis and deltoid ligament.
- MRI not usually indicated unless unusual features (severe swelling, bruising or pain) suggest an osteochondral injury not observed on plain radiographs.
- If symptoms persist 4–6 weeks after an apparently simple ankle sprain an MRI is indicated to exclude an osteochondral injury.

Treatment

- Initial treatment traditionally consisted of protection, rest, ice, compression, elevation and support (PRICES). More recently a modification of this acronym substitutes 'optimal loading' for rest and the acronym becomes POLICE. Optimal loading is more appropriate in facilitating early rehabilitation.
- Analgesics or NSAIDs for pain.
- Compression and elevation help reduce swelling.
- Protective devices include air splints or braces.
- *Surgery:* operative repair of Grade 3 AITFL injuries and medial ankle ligament injuries does not improve outcome. Surgery is required for injuries associated with a distal AITFL rupture with widening of the ankle mortise.
- Adequate rehabilitation is required to prevent functional instability and injury recurrence.
- Restore range of movement.
- Strengthen dynamic ankle stabilizers (ankle evertors and dorsiflexors).
- Proprioception, e.g. wobble board, mini-trampoline.
- Functional exercises, e.g. jumping, hopping, twisting.
- *Return to sport:* athletes can return to sport when they can perform sport specific actions without pain or instability.
- Functional bracing or taping may be required to prevent recurrence.
- The recurrence rate for lateral ankle sprains is as high as 80%

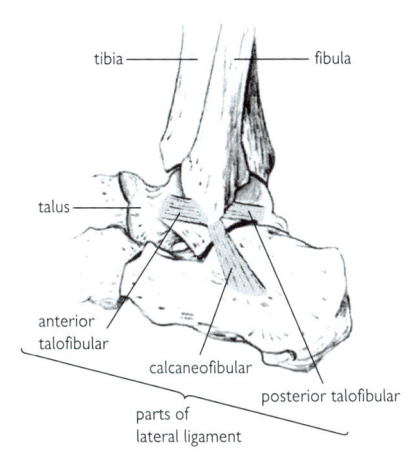

Fig. 23.3 Ligaments of ankle joint, lateral view. Reproduced with permission from MacKinnon P, Morris J. (2005). *Oxford Textbook of Functional Anatomy*, Vol. 1. Oxford: Oxford University Press, ©2005.

Persistent painful ankle

Pain, swelling, and impaired function may persist for 4–6 weeks after an acute injury. Secondary injuries may be overlooked at the time of the original injury. With persistent symptoms one should look for occult injury in addition to acute ankle sprain. Functional instability resulting from inadequate rehabilitation is the commonest cause, although there are a number of other possible causes.

Osteochondral injuries
- Initial radiographs may appear normal. Repeat radiographs or MRI are required for diagnosis.
- Osteochondral injuries occur most commonly at the following sites:
  - Superomedial talus.
  - Superolateral talus.
  - Tibial plafond.

Fractures
- Initial radiographs may appear normal. Follow-up radiographs or MRI may be required for diagnosis.
- Lateral talar process.
- Anterior calcaneal process.
- Posterior talar process.
- Os trigonum fracture.
- Fracture base of fifth metatarsal.

Impingement syndromes
- Anterior impingement syndrome.
- Anterolateral impingement syndrome.
- Posterior impingement syndrome.
- Capsular injury resulting in synovitis can present with anterior impingement on dorsiflexion.
- Synovium or ruptured ATFL becomes trapped between the lateral malleolus and talus provoking anterolateral impingement.
- Posterolateral process fracture or os trigonum injury may require CT or MRI to confirm the diagnosis.

Tendon dislocation and rupture
Peroneal tendons
- Radiographs may demonstrate a small bone chip.
- Resisted eversion in dorsiflexion precipitates tendon subluxation.

Tibialis posterior tendon
- Occurs with ankle dorsiflexion and inversion.
- Subluxation may be demonstrated by resisted plantar flexion.

Sinus tarsi syndrome
- Small osseous canal anterior and inferior to the lateral malleolus.
- Pain from subtalar ligament injury and fat-pad necrosis.
- Diagnosis confirmed by a local anaesthetic injection into the sinus tarsi.

Other causes
- Antero-inferior tibiofibular ligament
- Synovitis or ATFL scar tissue produces a meniscal lesion that impinges between the lateral talus and lateral malleolus.
- Post-traumatic synovitis.
- Calcaneocuboid ligament sprain (a bony fleck may be seen adjacent to the cuboid).
- Peroneal nerve or sural nerve injury.

Rehabilitation after ankle sprain (grade 2)

Time to return to sport is based largely on the quality of early management. Early, intermediate, and late rehabilitation objectives should be highlighted immediately after diagnosis. It is not possible to move on to the later stages of rehabilitation until all early stage goals are achieved. The athlete should be aware that progressive rehabilitation is necessary to minimize the chances of recurrence. Although rest is included in most guidelines, rehabilitation means progressive activity or optimal loading. Substituting rest in the PRICE guidelines creates the more appropriate POLICE. The anticipated time to return to sport after grade 2 injuries is 3–6 weeks. Note much of this programme is applicable for recovery after more minor, or severe injuries; however, the rate of progression will vary.

Early stage: days 1–7

Key aims
- Minimize swelling.
- Maintain range of movement and general ankle mobility.
- Begin controlled loading—optimal loading.
- Begin isometric strengthening.
- Challenge balance (neuromuscular control).
- Maintain upper body strength and cardiovascular fitness.

General exercises
- The athlete should be encouraged to weight-bear or partially weight-bear within the limits of pain. The use of crutches may be useful, but should not be to excess. A heel–toe gait pattern should be encouraged at all times. This will prevent the development of a toe-tap gait and minimize over activity/shortening of triceps surae.
- Ice, compression, and elevation can be of benefit after injury:
  - Applying focal compression around the malleolous may be most effective at preventing oedema accumulating around the healing ligaments.
  - Focal compression should be removed before cryotherapy is initiated, in order to prevent a barrier effect which can reduce the effectiveness of cooling.
- Gentle mobility exercises should be encouraged as soon as pain allows. Range of movement through dorsiflexion and plantar flexion should be followed by light circling exercises.
- The athlete may perform alphabet exercises—this involves using ankle movements to trace each letter of the alphabet in the air. This becomes more challenging with closed eyes and helps restore kinesthetic awareness (awareness of the foot and ankle in space) after joint injury. Kinesthetic training can also include matching or reproducing various joint angles or foot positions.
- Cryokinetics is a technique that involves performing mobility exercises immediately after or during cryotherapy. The pain relieving effect of cooling can reduce muscle spasm and inhibition, facilitating rehabilitative exercises.

REHABILITATION AFTER ANKLE SPRAIN (GRADE 2) 661

- The athlete should begin static stretching of the triceps surae as soon as pain allows. Stretching can be performed in a non-weight bearing position initially. For example, using a towel or belt around the foot to pull the ankle into dorsiflexion. If pain allows, gentle calf stretching can be performed in standing.
- In certain cases, stretching should also include the flexor hallucis longus complex; to do this, the athlete should replicate the triceps surae stretch position in bare feet, concomitantly stretching the 1st toe into extension.
- Other effective modifications to a triceps surae stretch include manually holding the heel in contact with the ground to maximally stretch the posterior joint capsule.
- Athletes complaining of anterior pain or restriction during weight-bearing dorsiflexion should be treated with additional manual therapy techniques to ensure that weight-bearing dorsiflexion is regained as soon as possible. The therapist could use a range of joint mobilizations such as posterior talar glides or Mulligan mobilization techniques.
- Static strengthening should be performed through all ankle movements. The non-injured foot can be used to provide counter pressure initially, e.g. push the outside borders of the feet together to activate and strengthen the ankle evertors. This can be progressed to counter pressure coming from the therapist.
- Electrotherapeutic modalities may be of the use in the acute and sub-acute stages after injury, e.g. low level laser therapy or electrical stimulation.
- *Massage:* this will have a role to play even at this early stage of management. Gentle massage techniques such as light finger kneading around the injured area can help disperse swelling. Deeper massage techniques can be used around the Achilles tendon; these can help to maintain tissue mobility, especially if used in conjunction with stretching exercises.
- *Hydrotherapy/pool rehabilitation:* the buoyancy of the water reduces the impact on the joints, and sometimes provides a better environment to restore normal movement patterns during rehabilitation.
  - For example, athletes with greater levels of pain on weight bearing may benefit from pool walking; again a heel-toe gait is encouraged.
  - The pool environment may also facilitate basic weight transfer or single leg standing exercises.
- *Upper body strength and conditioning:* athletes should be able to perform any upper body exercises in a supported position, e.g. shoulder press, arm ergometer.

Middle stage: weeks 2–3

Key aims
- Enhance neuromuscular control.
- Increase strength, ROM, ankle mobility.
- Initiate weight-bearing exercise.

Mobility/neuromuscular training
- *Weight transfers:* athlete stands on both feet but with weight predominantly on the uninjured side. Within the limits of pain,

slowly transfer weight on to the injured side. This should progress, until it is comfortable to stand solely on the injured foot.
- *Single leg standing/balance:* standing on the injured side, the athlete tries to balance. They should be challenged to balance for as long as possible without touching the ground. This exercise can be progressed by balancing with eyes closed or by incorporating additional physical task; this could include upper body movements which should progress from basic movements (bicep curl) to multi-joint, diagonal movement patterns.
- Athlete balances on the injured leg while throwing and catching a ball. Sports specific considerations could involve varying the type of throw, e.g. underarm, overhead, side pass, chest pass; varying the direction of the pass received, e.g. in front, from side, overhead; varying the type of ball e.g. tennis ball, medicine ball.
- Further progressions should be undertaken by balancing on dynamic surfaces, e.g. mini trampoline (rebounder), wobble board, balance pad/cushion, folded towel.

Strengthening
- Non-weight-bearing exercises can be undertaken using foot and ankle weights or therabands, and should incorporate all ankle ranges (D/F, P/F, inversion, eversion) and both concentric (shortening contractions) and eccentric (lengthening contractions) components. If more specific or functional strengthening is required, clinicians should consider using manual strengthening techniques such as PNF.
- *Heel to toes:* the athlete rocks from heel to toe. This requires good ROM though D/F and P/F with a good baseline of balance. This will begin initially with two legs. To progress:
  - Single leg heel to toes with upper body support (one hand resting against the wall).
  - Single leg heel to toe rock with no upper body support
- *Walking on heels and toes:* this should be undertaken in all directions (forwards/backwards/side to side).
- Other weight-bearing exercises are important prerequisites for jogging, e.g. March on the spot with high knees and swinging arms. To progress, a heel to toe push off is added on each step; jogging on the spot is a further progression.

Progressive strengthening
The athlete resists as the therapist or training partner applies manual pressure to the foot and ankle into D/F, P/F, inv, ev, or combinations of each. To progress, the athlete can close their eyes and activate the appropriate muscles based on the tactile stimulation.
- *Mini squats:* ensuring an equal distribution of weight, the athlete should perform a 50% squat (to 45° knee flexion).
- *Drop squats:* as for a mini squat, except the speed is increased whilst maintaining good body control and posture.
- *Single leg squats.*
- *Lunges:* the leading leg on the lunge should be varied using the injured and un-injured sides. Lunging direction should also vary; progressing from forwards (lead leg steps forward in the saggital plane towards 12 o'clock) to sidewards (lead leg steps sideways in the coronal plane

towards 3 o'clock/9 o'clock) to backwards (lead leg steps backwards in the saggital plane towards 6 o'clock)

All these exercises can be progressed by increasing the demand on the neuromuscular system, e.g. the athlete must perform a single leg squat on a dynamic surface.

Cardiovascular
- Bike/cross-trainer/upper body ergometer.

End stage: weeks 3–6

To progress to the end stages of rehabilitation, the athlete must have full ankle ROM, a good baseline of strength through all ankle movements, be able to perform complex balancing exercises in a pain free state and have good lumbopelvic/lower body control and alignment during squatting and advanced neuromuscular exercises.

In general, as the athlete progresses through the later stages of rehabilitation, the focus should become less joint-specific and more sport-specific.

Strength and conditioning
This may be progressed as follows:
- Squat.
- Deadlift.
- Hang clean.
- Clean.
- Snatch.

Ideally, the athlete should begin using the bar bell only. Their form and alignment should be monitored by a training partner or strength and conditioning coach. The weight should be increased accordingly. In many cases, this can progress quickly to their pre injury levels.

Plyometric exercises
Throughout all plyometric exercises, the athlete is encouraged to keep a 'soft' knee, using hips, knees, and ankles to cushion the impact. The athletes' ability to avoid 'corkscrewing' by keeping good pelvic, hip, knee, and toe alignment will act as a good guide for their progress.

Jumping from two legs to one
- Standing in a stationary position the athlete jumps vertically to land on the injured side.

Hop scotch
- This involves multiple jumps from two legs onto one, whilst moving forwards.

Jumping vertically while rotating
- For example, from a stationary position, the athlete jumps vertically and turns 90° clockwise/anticlockwise before landing. This can be progressed by using 180°, 270° or 360° rotations.

Jumping to land from a height
For example, small step. Initially, a two-foot landing should be used. This exercise can be progressed as follows:
- Athlete rotates 45° in air before landing.
- Add 90°/180° rotation.

- Single leg landing.
- Landing on dynamic surface.
- Immediately catching a ball on landing.
- Therapist adds a light push on landing.

Running

Prerequisites
- Full ankle ROM.
- Able to run on the spot
- Able to undertake advanced balance (neuromuscular) training with good body control and no pain.

Straight line running
- Light jog, building from 30%–50% pace (note: 100% pace is a sprint)
- Build up to 10–30min.

Begin progressive running
- This should be done on a flat surface.
- For the first session athletes should accelerate from a standing start, up to 60% pace over the first 30m. They should then aim to maintain this pace over the next 30m, before decelerating slowly a complete stop. Cones should be used to divide the acceleration/maintenance/deceleration stages

Progress by decreasing the acceleration distance and increasing the maintenance distance, see Table 23.1.

Functional running exercises

- *Running in a curved or figure of eight pattern*: should initially involve gradual curves over a long distance and progress to sharper/tighter curves.
- *Shuttle runs (doggies):* multiple sprints between cones or markers. Athletes should be encouraged to slow into the turn, plant their foot, and accelerate out of the turn. The planting foot should vary between the injured and uninjured sides.
- *Run stops:* from a 60% run the athlete must come to a complete stop within 5 steps. To progress increase the speed of the run/minimize the number of steps needed to stop.
- *45°/90°cuts:* running forwards then side stepping to change to direction at a 45° or 90° angle.
- *Full body spins/pivots:* running at 50% the athlete must spin 360° without slowing down.
- *Ladder or cone drills:* these can be used to facilitate a series of running and footwork drills, which challenge the athletes speed, balance, strength, and co-ordination.
- *T-Shuffle agility:* athlete sprints forwards 10m to touch cone A, side shuffles to the left for 5m to touch cone B, side shuffles to the right for 10m to touch cone C, turns and sprints back to the starting point

Table 23.1 Progressive running by decreasing the acceleration distance and increasing the maintenance distance

Acceleration	Maintenance	Deceleration
20m	40m	20m
10m	30m	20m
10m	40m	20m

Field testing
If available, field test results should be compared with pre-season or normative data. Useful test might include:
- 10m/20m/30m sprint times.
- Timed T-shuffle agility drill.
- Vertical jump or counter-movement jump height.
- Standing broad jump distance:
  - Jumping from two feet/landing on two feet.
  - Jumping from injured/landing on two feet.
  - Jumping from injured/landing on injured.
- Sports specific task, e.g. kicking a ball, tackling.

Back to play.

Medial ligament injuries

- The medial or deltoid ligament is injured as a result of an eversion injury, commonly external rotation of the tibia with the foot planted.
- The medial ligament is stronger than the lateral ligament and more often accompanied by additional injuries including fractures, e.g. medial malleolus, distal fibula, and talar dome.
- Radiographs are mandatory and widening of the ankle mortise (more than 2–4mm between the talus and tibia) may require surgery.
- Treatment of medial ligament injuries is similar to that of lateral ligament injury, however, recovery is much longer—often 6–12 weeks.

Syndesmosis injury

History and examination
- The tibiofibular syndesmosis consists of the anterior and posterior inferior tibiofibular ligaments, and interosseous membrane.
- Anterior ankle pain following a moderately severe ankle injury often with compression.
- The anterior inferior tibiofibular ligament is injured as a result of external rotation.
- Tenderness and swelling are maximal superomedial to the lateral malleolus.
- Provocation tests including the squeeze test and external rotation test (foot externally rotated on a fixed tibia) are positive.

The distal talofibular ligament and deltoid ligament are often injured
- *Grade 1 (stable):* no diastasis.
- *Grade 2 (unstable):* diastasis with stress.
- *Grade 3 (unstable):* diastasis and fibula fracture.
- Surgery is required for a distal talofibular ligament injury resulting in widening of the ankle mortise.

Investigations
- X-ray, CT, or MRI.

Treatment
- No diastasis: conservative treatment—recovery 6–12 weeks.
- Surgery is required for an injury resulting in widening of the ankle mortis (diastasis).

Fractures

- A fracture of the lateral, medial, or posterior malleoli is known as a Pott's fracture.
- Specialist orthopaedic opinion is required.
- Medial ligament injuries or medial malleolar fractures extending through the interosseous membrane and associated with a fracture of the proximal fibula are called Maisonneuve fractures. Palpate the proximal fibula to avoid missing this potentially unstable ankle injury.

Lateral ankle pain

The peroneus longus and brevis muscles dorsiflex, and evert the ankle to provide functional lateral ankle stability (Fig. 23.4). An injury often complicates an acute lateral ankle sprain. The patient may attend with an acute injury or a longer history of chronic subluxation. Rupture of the peroneal retinaculum may lead to subluxation of the peroneal tendons.

Peroneal tendinopathy

History and examination
- This is one of the commonest causes of lateral ankle pain behind, and distal to the lateral malleolus on exercise. Examination confirms tenderness and swelling posterior to the lateral malleolus. Passive inversion and resisted eversion reproduces symptoms.
- Precipitating factors include: rearfoot varus (supination), a history of ankle ligament sprains, a plantar-flexed first metatarsal, over pronation, and over-use, e.g. jumping sports.

Peroneal tendon subluxation
- Snapping along the lateral ankle, with pain and weakness.
- Pain with toe walking or change of direction.
- Subluxation results in recurrent inversion injuries and snapping over the lateral ankle (lateral ankle instability).

Peroneal tendon tears
- Acute injury, pain, swelling inferior and posterior to lateral malleolus.
- Chronic injury results from repeated inversion injuries, and damage to the retinaculum. Recurrent dislocation leads to chronic tears and lateral ankle instability.

Treatment
- Initial treatment is rehabilitation. Resisted eversion exercises in plantar flexion to strengthen the peroneals.
- Surgery is indicated for acute dislocation, peroneus brevis tendon rupture, and for peroneus longus tears associated with reduced function.

Investigation
- Musculoskeletal US or MRI can confirm the diagnosis. Real time musculoskeletal US can assess dynamic stability.
- Chronic injuries include longitudinal tears and recurrent subluxation.

Sinus tarsi syndrome

History and examination
A small osseous canal anterior and inferior to the lateral malleolus runs between the talus and calcaneum. It is part of the subtalar joint containing the subtalar ligaments. It may be injured in an acute inversion injury or by repetitive damage from excessive subtalar joint pronation. Athletes present with diffuse lateral ankle pain after an acute injury or of gradual onset. Symptoms result from subtalar ligament injury, synovial hypertrophy, peroneal nerve entrapment, or degenerative OA.

The symptoms include:
- Lateral ankle pain.
- Pain worse in the morning.
- Pain aggravated by eversion.
- Local tenderness over the sinus tarsi.
- Pain induced by forced passive inversion.

The clinical findings may include subtalar instability and a positive Tinel's test. The diagnosis is confirmed by injection of local anaesthetic.

Investigation
- Diagnosis is based on clinical findings, but the athlete will often have had an ankle X-ray and other investigations.

Treatment
- NSAIDs.
- Local injection.
- Rehabilitation.
- Biomechanical assessment.

Anterolateral impingement

History and examination
This usually results from an acute ankle sprain or recurrent ankle sprains. The patient complains of discomfort and catching at the anterior aspect of the lateral malleolus with a feeling of stiffness or restriction on dorsiflexion. Examination confirms tenderness over the ATFL and lateral gutter. The lunge test is positive and reproduces the discomfort. Swelling over the anterior aspect of the ankle may be present.

A meniscoid soft tissue lesion (soft tissue thickening and scar tissue) often develops.

Investigation
- Musculoskeletal US may be useful in identifying synovitic lesions.
- MRI is the imaging technique of choice (can be negative).
- Clinical assessment more important than MRI.

Treatment
- A local corticosteroid injection maybe helpful.
- Consider surgery if clinically suspicious in spite of normal MRI.
- Arthroscopic surgery (excision and debridement).

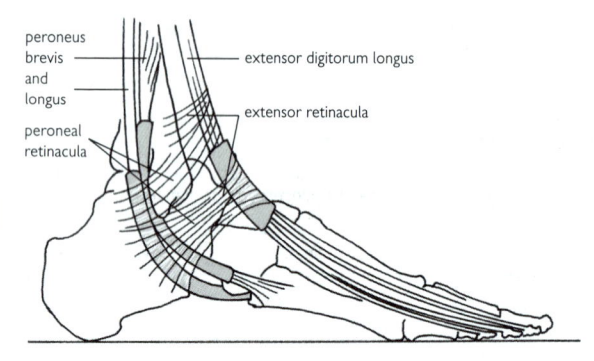

Fig. 23.4 Tendons, synovial sheaths, and retinacula on the lateral side of the ankle and foot. Reproduced with permission from MacKinnon P and Morris J (2005). *Oxford Textbook of Functional Anatomy* Vol 1. Oxford University Press, Oxford. © 2005.

Medial ankle pain

Tibialis posterior tendinopathy

History and examination

Medial ankle pain most often over the retinaculum postero-inferior to the medial malleolus although the patient may also complain of medial midfoot pain at the site of insertion of the tendon. Swelling is not always present. The pain is exacerbated by resisted inversion and passive eversion. Single heel raise demonstrates lack of hind foot supination. It may be associated with excessive pronation (rear foot valgus).

Rupture of tibialis posterior presents with posteromedial tibial pain extending around the medial malleolus to the navicular tubercle. Clinical examination reveals swelling and an inability to raise the heel. Immediate flattening of the medial arch may not be present. See Fig. 23.5 for anatomy.

Investigation
- US or MRI confirms the diagnosis.

Treatment
- *Physiotherapy:* concentric and eccentric exercise rehabilitation programme.
- *Immobilize:* (air cast) in severe cases.
- Conservative management fails or tendon rupture—surgery.

Flexor hallucis longus tendinopathy

History and examination

There is usually pain over the posteromedial calcaneum and sustentaculum tali with pain on plantar flexion. This pain is exacerbated by resisted flexion of the first toe with pain on passive extension of the first toe.
- It can be associated with posterior impingement syndrome.
- Triggering of the first toe in severe cases.
- Often secondary to over use, e.g. ballet (extreme plantar flexion).

Investigation
- Often a clinical diagnosis.
- MRI or US can confirm the diagnosis.

Treatment
- Physiotherapy.
- Soft tissue injection.
- Persistent triggering or synovitis—surgery.

Tarsal tunnel syndrome

History and examination
- The posterior tibial nerve becomes trapped in the fibro-osseous tarsal tunnel around the medial malleolus. This compression may be as a result of trauma, an inversion injury, over-use, excessive pronation, footwear, or chronic flexor tenosynovitis.
- The patient has medial ankle pain radiating into the arch of the foot, heel, and occasionally the toes. The pain is aggravated by prolonged standing, walking, and running. There is rarely paraesthesia and

numbness over the sole of the foot. Symptoms can be worse at night (similar to carpal tunnel syndrome).
- Examination confirms local tenderness and a positive Tinel's sign.

Investigations
- Radiographs may demonstrate a large os trigonum, which compresses the tibial nerve.
- Consider nerve conduction studies.
- MRI or US (ganglion, synovial cyst, tendinopathy, lipoma).

Treatment
- Footwear, orthotics.
- Steroid injection.
- Surgical decompression of the entrapped nerve.
- Also see 📖 p. 298.

Medial plantar nerve entrapment
- Also see 📖 p. 299.

History and examination
There is pain over the inferomedial calcaneum and this pain may radiate to the arch of the foot. Running aggravates the symptoms and it may be associated with pronation. Recently acquired orthotics can provoke symptoms. A branch of the posterior tibial nerve passes close to the calcaneonavicular ligament.

Examination confirms tenderness and a positive Tinel's sign is positive.

Investigation
- Nerve conduction studies confirm the diagnosis.

Treatment
- Modification of abnormal biomechanics, injection, or surgical decompression.

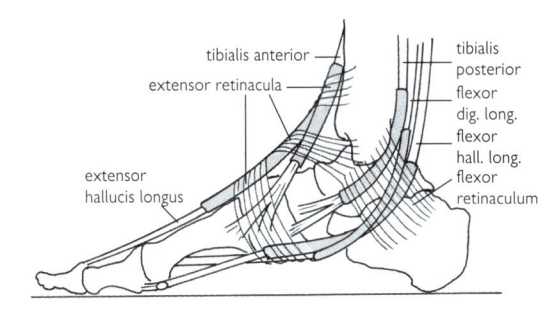

Fig 23.5 Tendons, synovial sheaths, and retinacula on the medial side of the ankle and foot. Reproduced with permission from MacKinnon P, Morris J. (2005). *Oxford Textbook of Functional Anatomy*, Vol. 1. Oxford: Oxford University Press, ©2005.

Anterior ankle pain

Tibialis anterior tendinopathy

History and examination
Tibialis anterior tendinopathy causes pain over the anterior ankle and midfoot. It is an over-use injury associated with excessive hill running and may be precipitated by footwear (tight laces or strapping). The athlete is tender over the anterior ankle joint and the pain is exacerbated by resisted dorsiflexion.

With tendonitis of the extensor hallucis longus there is pain on resisted dorsiflexion of the first toe and of extensor digitorum, there is pain on resisted dorsiflexion of the toes. Occasional swelling and crepitus.

Investigation
- MRI or US can confirm the diagnosis.

Treatment
- Eccentric strengthening, mobilization of ankle joint.
- Correction of biomechanics with orthoses

Anterior impingement ('footballer's ankle')

History and examination
Repetitive forced dorsiflexion impingement and plantar flexion of the ankle produces traction osteophytes at the margin of the joint capsule and exostoses develop on the anterior tibia and talus. 'Footballers ankle' is also seen in basketball, triple jump, long jump, and dance.

There is pain on running, lunging, or kicking with diffuse anterior ankle joint pain and swelling after activity. The pain is caused by impingement of soft tissues. Examination confirms local tenderness and pain on dorsiflexion. Anterior impingement test positive (active dorsiflexion with the heel on the ground).

Investigation
- X-ray: exostoses.
- US and MRI.

Treatment
- Conservative treatment, heel lift, modification of activity, NSAID, physiotherapy.
- Arthroscopic surgery to remove exostoses.

Posterior ankle pain

Posterior impingement syndrome

History and examination
Impingement of the os trigonum or posterior talus results from forced plantar flexion of the ankle.

This produces posterior ankle joint pain deep to the Achilles tendon. Ballet dancers, jumpers, and fast bowlers are at risk.

Confirmed by a positive posterior impingement test

Investigations
- X-ray and MRI.

Treatment
- NSAIDs, mobilization.
- Steroid injection.
- Surgery (removal of the posterior spur or os trigonum).

Shin splints (chronic exertional leg pain)

It is a general term used to describe shin pain, the most common are:
- Stress fractures.
- Medial tibial stress syndrome.
- Compartment syndromes.
- Popliteal artery entrapment syndrome.
- Nerve entrapment, e.g. superficial peroneal nerve

It is important to remember that these conditions may co-exist, e.g. stress fracture and medial tibial stress syndrome.

Stress fracture

These are micro-fractures associated with repetitive stress.
The bones are unable to adapt and breakdown is greater than repair.
- The history is of a crescendo type pain.
- The pain increases in severity with the duration of exercise.
- As the condition progresses the pain begins earlier in exercise.
- Night pain is a symptom of a severe stress fracture.
- Stress fractures occur most commonly in weight-bearing activities, such as running, jumping, or dancing.
- Stress fracture tibia.
- Middle third or junction of middle and distal third.
- Anterior stress fractures more resistant to treatment (increased non-union).

Examination
- Localized tenderness over the tibia.
- Biomechanical assessment.
- A stress fracture of the posterior tibia can present as calf pain.

Investigation
- X-ray may be normal.
- MRI most sensitive.
- CT or isotope bone scan.

Treatment
- Identify precipitating factors, e.g. excessive training.
- Biochmechanics.
- Rest.
- Pneumatic brace.
- ?Electrical stimulation.
- ?Bisphosphonates.

Stress fracture anterior tibia
- Prone to delayed union and complete fracture.
- 'Dreaded black line' on X-ray.
- MRI confirms.
- Delayed recovery: resistant stress injury.
- Delayed healing: surgical opinion required.

Stress fracture fibula
- Less frequent than tibia.
- Painful on weight bearing.
- Associated biomechanical abnormality, e.g. pronation or supination.
- Treat with rest until tenderness resolves.

Medial tibial stress syndrome
- Pain initially improves with exercise and recurs post-exercise.
- Diffuse pain is felt at the middle to lower 1/3 of the medial side of the tibia.
- The medial edge of the tibia may be swollen and tender.
- When symptomatic there is often a periostitis due to traction with repetitive stress.
- Biomechanics important
- The initial treatment is rest, although surgery with release of the fascia may be required.

Investigations
- *X-rays:* usually normal, occasional periosteal reaction.
- MRI.
- Isotope bone scan.

Treatment
- Physiotherapy, rest, ice, NSAIDs.
- Cross training (pain free activities).
- Taping to control foot pronation.
- Biomechanics.
- ?physiotherapy, injections.
- Surgical decompression.

Chronic exertional compartment syndrome
- Exertional pain.
- Increased pressure within a closed fibro-osseous space.
- Reduced blood flow and reduced tissue perfusion.
- Ischaemic pain.
- Increased discomfort and tightness with exercise.
- No rest pain.
- Resolves within 30min.
- Occasional paraethesia or weakness.
- Palpable tenderness with exercise.
- Swelling in the anterior compartment.
- Palpable tenseness with exercise.
- Muscle bulge or herniation with exercise.
- Pain on dorsiflexion of the ankle.
- There may be tenderness in the muscle on palpation with hypertrophy.
- There may be increased anterior compartment pressure.

Anterior compartment syndrome

History and examination

This affects the anterior compartment, which includes tibialis anterior, extensor digitorum longus, extensor hallucis longus, and peroneus tertius. The patient may describe exercise-induced discomfort or dull aching cramp-like pain lateral to the anterior border of the tibia. The symptoms develop within 10–30min of exercise and are often associated with an increase in the intensity. The athlete may describe a feeling of tightness. The symptoms are often reproducible, bilateral (50–60%), and resolve slowly on stopping exercise. As the syndrome becomes more severe, symptoms take longer to resolve but are usually gone by the next day. There may be numbness on the top of the foot (first web space) and weakness of ankle dorsiflexion suggesting nerve compression. It occurs most often in repetitive loading sports, such as running, football, and cycling.

Clinical examination is often normal. There may be tightness of the anterior compartment. Muscle herniation is sometimes seen in the distal third of the anterior compartment where the superficial peroneal nerve exits the compartment. Examination after exercise may demonstrate fullness of the compartment with discomfort on passive stretching. Tightness of the gastrocnemius and soleus may predispose to anterior compartment syndrome.

Lateral compartment syndrome

- The compartment consists of peroneous longus, brevis, and superficial peroneal nerve.
- Pain on exercises anterior to the fibula. Occasionally, paraesthesia over dorsum of foot.
- Examination confirms tightness of the lateral compartment.

Posterior compartment syndrome

History and examination
The posterior compartment consists of the deep (tibialis posterior, flexor hallucis longus, flexor digitorum longus) and the superficial (gastrocnemius, soleus) compartments. The deep compartment is affected more than the superficial. The patient describes a cramp like discomfort of the calf or medial border of the tibia and tightness that increases with exercise. Occasionally, sensory disturbance (tibial nerve compression). Small muscle hernias may be present along the medial border of the tibia. Muscle tightness may be less evident on examination. Active, passive, or resisted movement of these muscles may exacerbate pain.

Investigations
Chronic compartment syndrome consists of increasing pressure in the limited myofascial compartment, which causes reduced tissue perfusion and abnormal neuromuscular function.

Intracompartmental pressure studies
A catheter is inserted into the relevant compartment and the muscles exercised to reproduce the pain. Normal compartment resting pressures are between 0–10mmHg. The diagnosis of chronic compartment syndrome is supported by a pre-exercise pressure >15mmHg, maximum pressure during exercise >35mmHg, and a resting post-exercise pressure >20mmHg.

Treatment
- Conservative treatment often fails and surgical decompression is often necessary.
- Surgery fasciotomy (simple incision) and fasciectomy (removal of fascia tissue).
- Anterior and lateral chronic exertional compartment syndrome often respond to fasciotomy (90% success).
- Fasciectomy may be required for deep posterior chronic exertional compartment syndrome.
- Gradual return to exercise by 4 weeks.
- Return to training and sport by 6–8 weeks.

Nerve entrapment syndrome
- Superficial peroneal nerve in lateral compartment.
- Deep peroneal nerve in the anterior compartment.
- Tibial nerve deep posterior compartment.

Popliteal artery entrapment

History and examination
- Anatomical as it exits the popliteal fossa and medial head of the gastrocnemius.
- 'Functional' secondary to muscle contraction (hypertrophied gastrocnemius).
- Exercise-induced calf pain (claudication).
- Felt in the calf or anterior compartment.

- Disappears quickly on stopping exercise.
- Can be more severe walking than running.
- Examination: popliteal artery bruit with active ankle dorsi or plantar flexion.
- Examine immediately post-exercise.
- Peripheral pulses weak or absent immediately post-exercise.

Investigation
- Doppler US.
- Angiography.

Treatment
- Surgical decompression

Achilles tendinopathy

History and examination
The Achilles tendon is formed by the tendinous coalescence of gastrocnemius and soleus inserting into the calcaneal tuberosity. Plantaris inserts into the Achilles tendon. The tendons ability to glide is facilitated by the paratenon sheath (not a true synovial sheath). At first, there is gradual development of pain and stiffness after rest, which may occur, for example, in the morning. In the early stages the symptoms usually improve with exercise. As the condition progresses, there may be pain after exercise and, finally, pain during exercise. On examination, there is local tenderness and swelling. Predisposing factors include over pronation, lack of calf flexibility, and restricted dorsiflexion. Footwear may also contribute. Other contributory factors include a change in training pattern with increased exercise and reduced recovery.

Examination
Localization of tenderness differentiates between musculotendinous, intrasubstance and insertional tendinopathy. Paratenotitis presents with diffuse tenderness and swelling 2–4cm proximal to insertion. Crepitus may be felt. Tendinosis presents with a thickened tendon or nodule. Predisposing factors include over pronation; tight Achilles tendon, varus heel or forefoot, cavus foot, tibia vara and restricted dorsiflexion.

Investigation
- The diagnosis may be confirmed by US or MRI. X-rays are not usually helpful.

Treatment
- *Relative rest, ice, and elevation:* an eccentric exercise programme is most effective. The next stage is functional and sport-specific rehabilitation. It is important to correct predisposing factors. With delayed recovery some suggest US-guided injection. Surgery remains an option.
- Night resting splint (holds ankle to 5° dorsiflexion).
- Custom orthotics (refractory cases with over pronation).

The following treatments are subject to audit and evaluation. All procedures performed under US control:
- *Brisement:* inject saline and local anaesthesia into peritoneal sheath with US.
- Dry needling with US.
- PRP injections with US.
- Corticosteroid injections with US.
- *Surgery:* operative treatment if there are disabling or unacceptable symptoms after 6–12 months of conservative treatment.

A recent systematic review evaluated the evidence supporting eccentric exercise, extra-corporeal shock wave therapy (ESWT), topical GTN, and corticosteroid injections. Evidence-supported eccentric exercises and conflicting evidence for other treatment modalities.

Achilles tendon rupture

History and examination
- The Achilles tendon is the most frequently ruptured tendon.
- The patient has a sudden acute pain in the Achilles tendon with an audible snap or tear which is often described as 'like being hit or kicked in the back of the leg'.
- On examination there is swelling and a palpable defect.
- There is reduced function with an inability to plantar flex the ankle.
- Simmond's calf squeeze test positive.
- With a partial tear there is acute onset of pain, tenderness, and swelling but examination confirms no defect and normal function.

Investigations
- US or MRI confirms the diagnosis.

Treatment
- *Surgery:* either open or percutaneous repair. Surgery is probably the treatment of choice for physically active young adults.
- *Non-operative:* rehabilitation is prolonged.

Retrocalcaneal bursitis

History and examination
Inflammation of the bursa between the Achilles tendon and the calcaneum causing symptoms similar to Achilles tendinopathy. The patient is tender over Achilles tendon insertion. Retrocalcaneal bursitis can co-exist with Achilles tendinopathy. Haglund's deformity consists of Achilles tendinopathy, and retrocalcaneal bursitis associated with retrocalcaneal exostosis, or prominent calcaneum.

Treatment
- Physiotherapy, NSAIDs, and injection of corticosteroid.

Chapter 24

Foot

Fracture of the calcaneus 686
Fracture of the metatarsal bones 687
Lisfranc fracture: dislocations 688
Fat pad contusion 688
Midtarsal joint sprains 689
Turf toe 689
Hallux rigidus (footballer's toe) 690
Normal walking 691
Pronation 692
Supination 692
Footwear 693
Gait analysis 694
Plantar fasciitis 696
Extensor tendinopathy 698
Tarsal tunnel syndrome 698
Medial plantar nerve entrapment 699
Stress fractures of the calcaneus 699
Stress fractures of the navicular 700
Stress fractures of the metatarsals 701
Jones fracture 701
Metatarsalgia 702
Morton's (interdigital) neuroma 702
Sesamoid injury 703
Cuboid syndrome 703
Os naviculare syndrome 704
Sever's disease (traction apophysitis of the calcaneum) 704
Iselin's disease (traction apophysitis affecting base of fifth metatarsal) 705
Traction apophysitis of the navicular (insertion tibialis posterior tendon) 705
Tarsal coalition 706
Freiberg's disease (also called Freiberg's infraction or Freiberg's osteochondritis) 707
Kohler's disease 708
Sub-ungal haematoma 708
In-growing toenails 708
Callous 709
Verrucae 709

Fracture of the calcaneus

History and examination
Acute fractures usually occur as the result of a fall from a height and are therefore uncommon in sports.

Investigation
- X-ray.

Treatment
- Generally treated conservatively with a period of bed rest in the acute stage, followed by non-weight bearing on crutches, progressing to full weight bearing as tolerated.
- Fractures of the anterior process of the calcaneus can complicate an acute ankle sprain and, if displaced, may require open reduction and internal fixation.

Fracture of the metatarsal bones

History and examination
- Fractures occur commonly in many sports.
- May be caused by direct trauma (e.g. a kick in football) or a twisting injury (usually resulting in a spiral fracture).
- Avulsion fractures of the base of the 5th metatarsal may complicate acute ankle sprains.
- See also Jones fracture of the 5th metatarsal (p. 701).

See Fig. 24.1 for anatomy of the tarsal bones.

Investigation
- X-ray.

Treatment
- Generally respond well to conservative measures—strapping or use of a walking cast for a period of two or three weeks, followed by a return to sport in approximately six to eight weeks.
- Complications are rare—see Jones fracture of base of 5th metatarsal.
- Fitness should be maintained through non-weight-bearing activities, such as cycling, aqua jogging, or swimming.

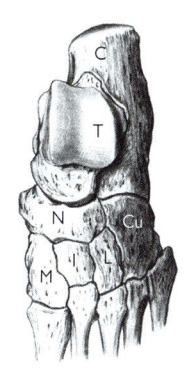

C = calcaneus
T = talus
N = navicular
Cu = cuboid
M = medial cuneiform
I = intermediate cuneiform
L = lateral cuneiform

Fig. 24.1 Tarsal bones: dorsal view. Reproduced with permission from MacKinnon P and Morris J. (2005). *Oxford Textbook of Functional Anatomy*, Vol. 1. Oxford University Press, Oxford. © 2005.

Lisfranc fracture: dislocations

History and examination
- Occurs at the tarsometatarsal joints and are rare in sports.
- Usually occur as the result of an acute plantar flexion injury.

Investigations
- Plain X-ray appearances are subtle and may be missed. Weight-bearing views may demonstrate a diastasis between the first and second metatarsal bases, and occasionally a bone fragment may be present.
- CT or MRI scan is very helpful in making the diagnosis.

Treatment
- Aimed at restoring the exact anatomical alignment and may be conservative for minor (grade 1 and 2 sprains) injuries or pinning of more severe, unstable injuries.
- Return to sport following these injuries is prolonged—often up to 1 year.

Fat pad contusion

History and examination
- Occurs either as a result of landing from a jump directly onto the heel, or due to repetitive heel strike on hard surfaces (especially in heavy individuals or those wearing inadequate footwear).
- Fat pad atrophy may be precipitated by steroid injection (e.g. for plantar fasciitis) and is irreversible.
- Tenderness is felt more proximally than with plantar fasciitis.

Investigations
- Not necessary.
- Diagnosis based on clinical findings.

Treatment
- Includes the use of shock-absorbing heel cushions, taping, and modification of training surfaces.
- Footwear with a firm heel counter should be worn to prevent splaying of the heel pad.

Midtarsal joint sprains

History and examination
Sprains may occur as a result of an acute injury or due to repetitive stress in an individual with an over pronated gait. They generally involve the calcaneonavicular ligament.

Investigations
- Diagnosis based on clinical findings.
- X-ray may be undertaken to exclude other causes of mid-foot pain.

Treatment
- Conservative treatment with electrotherapeutic modalities and taping/orthotic supports.
- Occasionally a cortisone injection is required if there is a persistent synovitis of one of the midtarsal joints.

Turf toe

History and examination
- An acute dorsiflexion sprain injury of the first metatarsophalangeal joint.
- Common on artificial surfaces where traction between the surface and the shoe is great, the foot moves forward pushing the toe upwards.
- Severe injuries may result in dislocation of the first metatarsophalangeal joint, but most are typical sprain injuries.

Investigation
- X-ray to exclude a fracture.

Treatment
- Managed conservatively with ice, analgesics, rest, and taping to limit joint movement on return to sport (generally after 2–4 weeks).
- These injuries can result in persistent discomfort on return to running.
- May result in the development of hallux limitus.
- Choice of footwear is important in preventing these injuries, with a rigid insole limiting excessive movement at the first metatarsophalangeal joint (MTPJ) (especially in those with hallux limitus).

Hallux rigidus (footballer's toe)

History and examination
- Occurs after repeated minor injuries to the 1st MTPJ resulting in early degenerative changes and restricted movement, especially dorsiflexion.
- Very common in sports such as soccer, where repetitive stress occurs during kicking and sprinting.
- This condition may cause the athlete to change his normal gait pattern to push off on the lateral border of the forefoot rather than at the hallux.

Investigation
- X-ray will show osteophyte formation and joint space narrowing.

Treatment
- Very difficult: NSAIDs and corticosteroid injection may give temporary relief.
- Referral to a podiatrist is indicated as orthotics may help unload the joint.
- Surgery to remove the osteophytes in more severe cases.

The term hallux limitus is used to describe less severe cases of this condition.

Normal walking

- The normal gait cycle consists of heel strike (usually towards the lateral border of the heel with the foot slightly supinated), stance phase and toe off with the gait cycle completed by the swing phase leading to heel strike once more.
- During distance running this gait cycle is maintained.
- In sprinting the stance phase tends to consist of a midfoot or forefoot rather than a heel strike (i.e. sprinters tend to run more on their toes).
- Following heel strike, the foot pronates (see Fig. 24.2 to allow full contact with the ground, subsequently supinating to form a rigid lever to allow toe off to occur.
- The subtalar joint is responsible for the conversion of the rotatory forces of the lower limb and is important in dissipating shock following foot strike. Stiffness of the subtalar joint will reduce the ability to absorb shock.

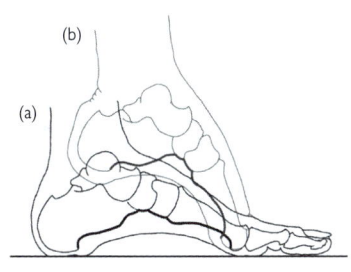

Fig. 24.2 (a) Medial longitudinal arch of the foot when standing. (b) Change in medial arch and dorsiflexion of metatarsophalangeal joint when standing on tip-toe and at the start of locomotion. Reproduced with permission from MacKinnon P and Morris J. (2005). *Oxford Textbook of Functional Anatomy*, Vol. 1. Oxford University Press, Oxford, © 2005.

Pronation

- Pronation is a tri-planar movement occurring at the subtalar joint.
- Pronation is a normal component of the gait cycle.
- Pronation consists of eversion, dorsiflexion, and abduction of the foot.
- Pronation should not occur past the latter stages of midstance, as the normal foot should then supinate in preparation for toe off.
- Excessive (over) pronation may contribute to, or be a consequence of, biomechanical anomalies elsewhere in the kinetic chain, placing abnormal stresses on other structures (e.g. will cause internal rotation of the lower limb and place abnormal stress on the medial structures of the foot and ankle).
- Over pronation or hyperpronation has been implicated as a causative factor in the development of many lower limb problems, including Achilles tendinopathy, plantar fasciitis, metatarsalgia, sesamoiditis, tibialis posterior tendinopathy, medial tibial periostitis, and stress fractures, patellofemoral pain, and ilio-tibial band friction syndrome.
- Over pronation can be corrected by the use of orthoses placed in the individual's shoe.
- Orthoses can be either preformed or (preferably) custom-cast to suit the individual athlete.
- Many asymptomatic athletes over pronate—there is little or no evidence for the use of orthoses to correct this as a preventative measure.

Supination

- Supination also occurs at the subtalar joint and normally occurs towards the end of the midstance phase of the gait to allow the foot to form a rigid lever in preparation for toe off.
- The supinated foot is plantar flexed, inverted, and adducted.
- Typically these individuals have a cavoid (high arched), rigid foot with poor shock absorption which predisposes to metatarsal stress fractures.
- Excessive supination may also contribute to the development of ilio-tibial band friction syndrome.
- Supination is much more difficult to correct with orthoses. Individuals should buy shoes with maximum shock absorption.

Footwear

- Different sports require different footwear and individuals also have different footwear requirements.
- Shoes consist of an upper (the part covering the foot) and sole (consisting of inner and mid-sole, wedge, and out-sole). Mid-sole is the main shock absorber and can be made of various materials with different inserts. Out-sole is designed for both traction and shock absorption, while the wedge increases heel height and aids shock absorption.
- Upper should have a toe box providing adequate room and a firm heel counter to stabilize the subtalar joint and prevent excessive pronation.
- The shape of the shoe can be straight or curved—a straight last shoe provides more stability.
- Board lasting and slip lasting describes the way the upper of the shoe is attached to the sole. In board lasting the upper is attached to a hard inner sole board and is heavier and more stable.
- Those with a tendency to over pronate require a running shoe providing more control—a straight (rather than curved) last construction, a combined last inner sole (i.e. board last to metatarsals, allowing more flexibility at the forefoot) with added medial support and a firm heel counter.
- Tennis and other court shoes are generally constructed to provide more control and will be of a full board last construction.
- Running shoes are not designed to allow sudden changes of direction and are unsuitable for sports involving a lot of twisting.
- A high heel tab should generally be avoided as this may cause impingement on the Achilles tendon when the ankle is fully plantar flexed.
- Shoes should be individual and sport-specific—those designed for distance running should provide stability and shock absorption, while those aimed at sports involving sudden changes in direction should provide good traction between the foot and the playing surface to avoid slipping.
- Running shoes lose their shock absorbing qualities after about 500km, and should be changed frequently. Using worn-out footwear may lead to injury.
- Football boots should allow the player to 'feel' the ball. Boots with 'blade' type cleats may increase the likelihood of some lower limb injuries, in addition to causing tibial lacerations.
- Shoes designed for aerobic classes become worn after approximately 100h of activity.
- Remember ask about the athletes leisure footwear as this may be a contributing factor as much as their sports footwear.
- There is a recent movement towards barefoot running. The biomechanics of running are altered when wearing shoes and, in particular, the pattern of ground reaction force. This has led to a new generation of thin flexible running shoes. Although enthusiasts suggest this will reduce chronic over-use injury there is, as yet, little evidence.

Gait analysis

A detailed description of the techniques used in formal gait analysis is beyond the scope of this book. However, from the above discussion it is clear that the physician should have some understanding of the normal biomechanics of walking and running, and should be able to recognize abnormal gait patterns and refer appropriately for more detailed podiatric assessment.

Pronation is a normal component of the gait cycle and there is no evidence supporting the prescription of foot orthoses as a preventative measure in asymptomatic athletes who 'over pronate'—these are generally individuals who have adapted and learnt to cope with their 'abnormal' gait and the introduction of orthoses into their shoes may cause considerable secondary problems.

- Athletes should first be assessed standing from the front and then the posterior aspect.
- Alignments such as persistent femoral anteversion will be obvious, producing a 'squinting patellae' appearance.
- A pelvic tilt may be due to a leg length discrepancy—this can be formally measured from the anterior superior iliac crest to the medial malleolus with the athlete supine.
- From the posterior aspect, the shape of the longitudinal arch and the angle between the Achilles and the calcaneus can be assessed—athletes who over pronate will tend to have a flat footed appearance with valgus heel position, producing the 'too many toes' sign.
- The athlete should be asked to perform a half squat with the heels flat—this will reproduce the position of the foot in the mid stance phase of running and will demonstrate any tendency to over pronate.
- The athlete should be observed walking in bare feet and if possible treadmill running in normal training shoes.
- The athlete who supinates excessively will typically have a rigid high arched foot with rear foot varus alignment.
- Core stability should be assessed, for example, by asking the athlete to perform a one leg squat and observing the degree of pelvic tilt and twisting that occurs during this manoeuvre.
- Any abnormal gait patterns identified in a symptomatic athlete should prompt referral to a podiatrist for more formal gait analysis.
- Several different types of orthoses are available, with the most appropriate usually being made from a cast of the athlete's foot taken in the 'subtalar neutral' position.

Plantar fasciitis

History and examination
- Plantar fasciitis is a chronic over-use injury resulting from repetitive traction on the plantar fascia attachment to the medial calcaneal tuberosity.
- It is often found in individuals with *pes planus* or a tendency to over pronate, and may be initiated by wearing sandals or soft shoes.
- Older or middle aged athletes are more commonly affected.
- The classical symptom is heel pain and stiffness which is worse in the mornings—individuals report that they have to walk on their toes for the first few strides, with their symptoms improving as they 'warm up'.
- Pain may be present during the day if walking long distances or after a period of sitting.
- Patients with plantar fasciitis have point tenderness at the plantar fascia attachment to the calcaneus anteromedially. They may also experience tenderness at the plantar fascia origin when the great toe is dorsiflexed.
- The differential diagnosis includes calcaneal stress fracture, tarsal tunnel syndrome, medial or lateral plantar nerve entrapment, Reiter's disease, and lumbar radiculopathy.
- Acute sprains of the plantar fascia are relatively common and generally respond quickly to a short period of rest.

Investigations
- X-ray often reveals a calcaneal spur in asymptomatic individuals (approximately 15% of the general population will have a heel spur) and the presence of a spur may be unrelated to the development of pain.
- US scan will confirm the diagnosis.
- There is an association with inflammatory conditions such as gout, RA, ankylosing spondylitis and Reiter's syndrome (especially if heel pain is bilateral), so further investigation may be appropriate.

Treatment
- A tension night splint is very useful in relieving morning pain and stiffness.
- Stretches for the calf/Achilles tendon and plantar fascia should be advised and heel cups or orthoses to correct abnormal foot biomechanics are indicated.
- Strapping techniques to support the plantar fascia are very useful in providing short term symptomatic relief. Taping begins at the level of the metatarsal heads and continues to the heel, forming a fan to support the plantar fascia. It is quick and easily applied by the patient and may also be used on return to impact activities.
- Intrinsic foot exercises should be advised—easily performed using a towel on the floor and instructing the athlete to pull this towards him using his toes. Physiotherapy advice is often useful.
- Extracorporeal shock wave therapy has recently been reported as being a promising treatment option.
- Electrotherapeutic modalities are usually ineffective.

- Cortisone injections may be useful, but can cause rupture of the plantar fascia or fat pad atrophy which may lead to permanent heel pain. The preferred technique is to use a medial approach, rather than inject directly through the heel pad, which has a plentiful nerve supply. US guidance will ensure accurate placement of the injection at the plantar fascia attachment. Injection is usually reserved for patients who have failed to respond to other conservative measures.
- Surgery is occasionally required for refractory cases (i.e. at least 12 months duration)—results are generally good, although long-term problems following surgery have been reported.

Extensor tendinopathy

History and examination
- Over-use of the extensor tendons is reportedly caused by uphill running, and in some cases an acute peritenonitis can occur, causing crepitus and swelling. The tibialis anterior tendon is most commonly affected and may be caused by a sudden increase in training.
- Pain can also arise from ill-fitting shoes or laces tied too tightly.

Treatment
- Pay attention to footwear; soft padding may prevent excessive pressure.
- Steroid injection along the tendon sheath is often helpful in cases of peritenonitis. Other injection therapies commonly used in tendinopathies (platelet rich plasma or autologous blood injections) have not been studied in this condition.
- Referral for physiotherapy, including eccentric strengthening exercises is indicated.
- Surgery is very rarely necessary.

Tarsal tunnel syndrome

See also 📖 p. 698.

History and examination
- This describes an entrapment of the posterior tibial nerve or one of its branches (medial calcaneal or lateral plantar nerve) in the tarsal tunnel just below the medial malleolus.
- More likely to occur in the over pronated athlete, where increased load on the flexor tendons results in swelling and increased pressure.
- May also be associated with anatomical variations such as ganglions and varicosities.
- Athletes feel pain and occasionally paraesthesia from the medial aspect of the heel and along the medial longitudinal arch.
- Symptoms can occur at night and may disturb sleep.
- Tinel's sign may be positive over the entrapped nerve at the level of the flexor retinaculum.

Investigation
- EMG and nerve conduction studies may be positive.

Treatment
- Orthoses to correct over pronation.
- Cortisone injection to the tarsal tunnel can provide temporary relief of symptoms.
- Surgical release of the entrapped nerve usually gives permanent cure and return to sport is possible approximately 2 months post-surgery.

Medial plantar nerve entrapment

History and examination
- Entrapment occurs in the midfoot, especially in athletes who over pronate or have a valgus heel alignment. May also be found secondary to chronic ankle instability.
- Athlete experiences pain in the medial longitudinal arch, radiating to the toes.
- Often aggravated by running uphill or around bends.
- May be accompanied by numbness affecting the medial border of the foot.
- Tenderness is found at the medial plantar aspect of the longitudinal arch.

Treatment
- Correct over pronation with orthotics.
- Cortisone injection may provide temporary relief of symptoms.
- Surgery may be necessary in resistant cases.

Stress fractures of the calcaneus

History and examination
- Stress fractures of the calcaneus are relatively uncommon, having been described mostly in military populations.
- The history is of an insidious onset of heel pain on impact activities.
- On clinical examination there will be pain compressing the calcaneus from the sides.

Investigations
- X-rays usually show a sclerotic line parallel to the posterior margin of the calcaneus on the lateral view.
- Isotope and/or MRI scanning may be necessary to make the diagnosis.

Treatment
- Treatment is conservative with return to impact activities as the symptoms and signs permit (usually 6–8 weeks). There is no need to advise a period of non-weight bearing.
- Fitness can be maintained through non-impact training—aqua jogging and cycling.
- On return to impact activities, footwear that provides adequate shock attenuation should be worn.

Stress fractures of the navicular

History and examination
- The exact cause of navicular stress fractures is unclear.
- They occur through the sagittal plane of the central third which is felt to be relatively avascular.
- Impingement and shearing of the navicular between the talus and first, second, and third rays is thought to occur in sprinting and jumping activities.
- Occur most commonly in sprinters and jumping athletes, but also in footballers.
- Usually present insidiously with mid-foot pain and localized tenderness to palpation over the proximal, dorsal surface of the navicular (the so-called 'N' spot).

Investigations
- Plain X-rays are often negative and the diagnosis should be confirmed with isotope, CT, or MRI scanning.

Treatment
- These fractures are prone to non-union and require aggressive treatment—initially strictly non-weight-bearing in a cast for 6–8 weeks. Fitness can be maintained through cycling during this phase.
- Once the cast is removed the 'N' spot is palpated—if there is residual tenderness then a further 2-week period of immobilization is employed.
- If there is no localized tenderness at this stage then gradual weight-bearing activities can be resumed, with return to full training over the next 6–8 weeks.
- Repeat imaging is of limited value, with CT or MRI having poor correlation with clinical findings.
- Non-union or delayed union is a major problem and surgery may be required for those fractures that fail to unite with conservative treatment.
- Recovery from these injuries is often prolonged. A gradual return to impact activities is required and footwear should be carefully checked to ensure that it is appropriate to the individual.
- Orthoses are indicated for those athletes who have an excessively over pronated gait.

Stress fractures of the metatarsals

History and examination
- These are very common—most often involving the second ('March fracture') and third metatarsal shafts.
- Stress fractures or the second metatarsal are especially common in ballet dancers.
- These fractures present with increasing pain on impact activities and localized tenderness over the affected bone.

Investigation
- Plain X-rays may not be positive for 3 or 4 weeks.
- Isotope or MRI scans are used to make an earlier diagnosis.

Treatment
- Conservative—strapping or use of a cast brace/walker with return to impact activities over a period of 6–8 weeks.
- Fitness can be maintained with low-or non-impact exercise such as aqua jogging.
- Return to full activity to be expected over eight to ten weeks.

Jones fracture

History and examination
- This is a stress fracture at the junction of the metaphysis and diaphysis of the proximal 5th metatarsal (although this fracture can also occur acutely as the result of an inversion/plantar flexion injury).
- These fractures represent a special group, as they are prone to non-union due to the relative avascularity of this area.

Investigation
- In stress fracture, plain X-rays may not be positive for 3 or 4 weeks.
- Isotope or MRI scans are used to make an earlier diagnosis in this situation.

Treatment
- These fractures should be immobilized in a short leg cast, non-weight bearing for 8 weeks—subsequent non-union is treated with intra-medullary screw fixation or bone grafting.
- Early surgical intervention should be considered in the professional or elite athlete.

Metatarsalgia

History and examination
- Forces while walking are normally transmitted through the 1st and 5th metatarsal heads.
- Loss of the transverse arch of the forefoot will result in excessive stress being placed on the other MTPJs causing synovitis and pain.
- The second and third MTPJs are commonly affected and there may be callous formation in this area reflecting the excessive stress.

Investigation
- Diagnosis is based on clinical examination. There is pain compressing the metatarsal heads and manipulation of the affected joints.

Treatment
- Includes the use of a metatarsal pad (this must be placed on the plantar surface of the foot, proximal to the MTPJs to restore the normal transverse arch), and orthoses to correct any over pronation.
- Occasionally a cortisone injection into the affected MTPJ may give good relief.

Morton's (interdigital) neuroma

History and examination
- Swelling and scar tissue around the interdigital nerve due to compression between the metatarsal (MT) heads.
- Typically occurs between the third and fourth metatarsal heads and causes pain and interdigital numbness and paraesthesia.
- On clinical examination there will be pain compressing the metatarsal heads and a click (known as Mulder's click) may be felt between the MT heads, representing compression of the swollen nerve and scar tissue. Normal feet may have this click so; it is diagnostic only if reproducing the pain.

Investigation
- Diagnosis is clinical, but can be confirmed by MRI scan.

Treatment
- Treatment is the same as that for metatarsalgia and cortisone injections to the affected area may give temporary relief of symptoms.
- Metatarsal pads and orthotic correction of any abnormal gait pattern should be advised.
- Surgical excision is the definitive treatment.

Sesamoid injury

History and examination
- The medial and lateral sesamoid bones lie within the tendon of flexor hallucis brevis and injuries are frequent in sport. They act to increase the efficiency of the tendon and to stabilize the first MTPJ.
- The medial sesamoid is most commonly affected due to repetitive loading leading to the development of sesamoiditis/osteonecrosis or stress fracture. Athletes who over pronate are particularly vulnerable to these problems.
- On clinical examination there will be tenderness to direct palpation over the medial sesamoid and the patient may tend to walk on the lateral border of the foot in an attempt to unload the painful area.

Investigation
- Specific 'sesamoid views' on plain X-ray may show fragmentation or fracture of the involved bone—however, a bipartite sesamoid is a common finding and differentiation from a stress fracture may be difficult (the fibrous joint of a bipartite sesamoid is also prone to injury).
- Isotope or MRI scanning can be used to make the diagnosis.

Treatment
- These stress fractures are prone to non-union and initial treatment should be in a non-weight bearing cast for 6 weeks followed by gradual resumption of impact activities if bony tenderness is no longer present. Over-pronation should be corrected with orthoses and padding may be used to unload the area on return to training.
- Sesamoiditis may occasionally respond to a cortisone injection.
- Generally excision of the sesamoid bones should be avoided as there can be significant problems following such procedures (although excision of a partial fragment can produce good results).

Cuboid syndrome

- Occasionally, the lateral aspect of the cuboid may be subluxed dorsally due to excessive pull of the peroneus longus tendon. This results in lateral foot pain when weight bearing.
- Treatment is by manipulation of the subluxed cuboid and taping may be used post-reduction to hold the cuboid in place.
- Any biomechanical problems, such as over pronation, should be corrected.
- Stress fractures of the cuboid are uncommon and usually respond to a 4–6-week period of non-weight-bearing immobilization in a cast followed by a gradual return to activity. Displaced fractures may require surgical treatment.

Os naviculare syndrome

- An accessory ossicle at the tuberosity of the navicular occurs in approximately 10% of people and is generally asymptomatic.
- Pain may occasionally occur due to traction from the tibialis posterior tendon, especially in an individual with an over pronated gait.
- Treatment is aimed at reducing the traction with activity modification and orthoses to correct the abnormal gait pattern.
- A traction apophysitis may occur at this site in the adolescent athlete—treatment is along similar lines (see p. 704).

Sever's disease (traction apophysitis of the calcaneum)

History and examination
- 2nd commonest traction apophysitis after Osgood–Schlatter disease.
- Usually presents in children between 10 and 13yrs.
- Unilateral or bilateral heel pain related to running and jumping activity.
- Pain may be associated with limping.
- Heel pain often worst on rising from bed.
- In severe cases, swelling develops over the posterior calcaneum.
- Hyperpronation and flat feet may be associated.
- Calf and hamstring flexibility usually poor.
- Focal tenderness at posterior border of the calcaneum at the insertion of the Achilles tendon.
- Ankle dorsiflexion may be reduced.
- Differential diagnosis includes a calcaneal stress fracture.

Investigations
- Rarely required.
- X-rays will demonstrate fragmentation of the calcaneal apophysis.

Treatment
- Limit running and jumping activities.
- Heel raise in shoe will ↓ pain.
- Ice heels after activity.
- Calf and hamstring stretching programme implemented.
- Calf strength programme.

Prognosis
- There are generally no long-term complications.
- Activity may need to be modified during vulnerable periods.

Iselin's disease (traction apophysitis affecting base of fifth metatarsal)

History and examination
- Presents with pain over lateral aspect of foot at site of insertion of peroneus brevis tendon into base of fifth metatarsal.
- Pain reproduced by passive foot inversion and resisted eversion.

Investigation
- Not required.

Treatment
- Unloading tendon with standard ankle taping in eversion (as is done for the prevention of lateral ligament injuries).
- Exercise programme to stretch and strengthen the peroneal muscles.
- Prognosis is good.

Traction apophysitis of the navicular (insertion tibialis posterior tendon)

History and examination
- Presents with medial mid-foot pain.
- Pain reproduced by passive foot eversion and resisted inversion.
- Flat feet and hyperpronation commonly associated.
- No investigations are required.

Treatment
- Unload tibialis posterior tendon with orthotic device.
- Programme to stretch and strengthen tibialis posterior.
- Prognosis is good.

Tarsal coalition

- Congenital abnormality resulting in bony, cartilaginous, or fibrous fusion of two tarsal bones.
- Causes abnormal mechanics around affected bones.
- Most common coalitions are calcaneo-navicular followed by talo-calcaneal and calcaneo-cuboid.
- In 40% of cases, tarsal coalition is bilateral and a family history of tarsal coalition is common.

History and examination

- Can present in several different ways depending on bones involved.
- Common presentations include recurrent ankle sprains, mid-foot pain, or a painless, rigid, asymmetric flat foot.
- May be asymptomatic in childhood and only present in adult life as a result of degenerative changes caused by altered foot mechanics.

Investigations

- X-rays useful when appropriate views are requested.
- A 'Harris–Beath' view will show bony coalition of middle subtalar facet in bony talocalcaneal coalitions.
- Lateral views useful for diagnosing talocalcaneal coalitions (continuous 'C' sign) and for identifying talonavicular spurring, which results from altered mechanics at the subtalar joint.
- Bony calcaneonavicular coalitions are often seen with an oblique foot X-ray.
- CT scanning will usually identify cartilaginous and fibrous unions, which cannot be detected on plain X-ray.

Treatment

- Depends on site of coalition and symptoms.
- Orthotics for symptom relief.
- Immobilization in neutral or inverted position in child with pronounced peroneal spasm.
- If symptoms severe and unresponsive to conservative measures or if indications of degenerative changes occurring in other joints, surgical excision of the bar may be required.

Prognosis

- Tarsal coalition is commonly missed in childhood and presents as severe arthritic change in the tarsal joints of adults.

Freiberg's disease (also called Freiberg's infraction or Freiberg's osteochondritis)

History and examination
- Freiberg's disease is an avascular necrosis of the metatarsal head, most commonly presenting between the ages of 12 and 18yrs.
- Initial synovitis is followed by sclerosis, resorption, and collapse of the metatarsal head, leading to secondary degenerative changes.
- The second metatarsal head is most commonly affected, although the third can also be involved.
- Usually seen in running athletes and dancers, probably secondary to compressive forces at the metatarsal heads.
- This is the only ostechondrosis more common in females, perhaps due to preponderance of females in dancing.
- Gradual onset forefoot pain, worse with push-off and dancing *en-pointe*.
- Focal tenderness and ↓ ROM over involved metatarsal head.
- Morton's foot (foot in which second metatarsal is longer than first) is commonly associated and increases the load on the second metatarsal head.

Investigations
- X-ray often normal initially.
- Later shows fragmentation of epiphysis, followed by flattening of metatarsal head.
- If the X-ray is normal, early in course of symptoms, a bone scan or MRI will confirm the diagnosis.

Treatment
- In the acute phase rest from all impact activity is necessary.
- Limit activity and modify footwear (use metatarsal bar to unload metatarsal head and avoid high-heeled shoes).
- In severe cases, immobilization may be required.
- Persistent pain may necessitate surgical intervention, but this should be delayed until after re-ossification has occurred.
- If symptoms do not resolve with conservative measures, excision of the metatarsal head is sometimes required.
- Freiberg's disease may cause long-term disability.

Kohler's disease

- Avascular necrosis of navicular.
- More common in boys than girls.
- Ischaemia and stress have been implicated as causative factors.

History and examination
- Presents earlier than other osteochondroses (around age 3–5).
- Presents with a painful limp and focal tenderness over the navicular.
- Passive eversion and resisted inversion often reproduce the pain.

Investigation
- X-ray shows patchy sclerosis of the navicular, followed by compression and collapse.

Treatment
- Symptomatic.
- Analgesia.
- Rest from running activities.
- Medial arch-support orthotic improves pain by unloading the navicular.

Prognosis
- Excellent prognosis.
- Despite marked abnormalities on initial imaging, navicular returns to its normal shape before growth is complete.

Sub-ungal haematoma

- Painful condition. Should be drained by piercing the nail with a needle or heated paper clip to prevent loss of the nail, which would otherwise occur in 2 or 3 weeks. Dress to avoid infection.
- Black nails can also occur as the result of wearing poorly fitting shoes.

In-growing toenails

- Usually affects the great toe and is caused by ill-fitting shoes or injudicious nail clipping.
- Can readily become infected and require antibiotic treatment.
- May require wedge resection of part of the nail and ablation of the nail bed with phenol to prevent re-growth.
- Prevention through proper and regular nail care is the best solution.

Callous

- Skin thickens in response to pressure, forming callous, which can be painful.
- Common at heel and over the second metatarsal head.
- Hard skin can be pared back with a sharp scalpel.
- Attention should be paid to footwear to prevent recurrence.

Verrucae

- Verrucae (warts) are viral infections and can be spread, especially in shower areas or around pools.
- Can be self-treated by paring back and applying a proprietary wart remover.
- May require to be burnt using podophyllin or frozen with liquid nitrogen.
- Recurrence is common.

Chapter 25

The team physician

Introduction: the team physician *712*
The medical kit bag *714*
Basic medical equipment *716*
Drugs and medications *718*
Security and insurance issues *720*
Team travel *722*
Managing your medical service *728*
Multi-sport events *732*
The holding camp *733*
The games *734*
The return home *735*
Professional and ethical considerations *736*
Organizing a major sporting event *738*

Introduction: the team physician

The medical care of a team or squad of athletes is an integral part of the role of the sports medicine specialist, and potentially one of the most rewarding aspects of sports medicine practice.

The specifics of the team physician role will depend on a variety of issues including the sport involved, the nature of the event, e.g. single sport or multi-sport, and the level of competition or ability of the athletes. There are, however, a number of general principles that are relevant to team medical support in general, and some special circumstances.

The medical kit bag

The medical kit bag is of central importance in enabling a clinician to practice. The equipment that you take to an event will depend on a number of factors.

Experience of practitioner

Carry equipment that you are competent to use. If covering a sport that might require a particular piece of equipment then seek appropriate training before agreeing to cover that event. If your level of knowledge and experience is not commensurate with that required to provide a duty of care for those you are looking after, then you should not be there, no matter how attractive the opportunity.

Medical risk assessment

A vital part of team coverage is medical risk assessment. This means identifying what problems you are likely to encounter, what facilities will be at your disposal to deal with such events, and what additional equipment will you need to provide or arrange to have provided. A number of issues will govern the medical risk associated with a particular event.

Sport

Different sports clearly carry different injury profiles, e.g. the high risk of contact trauma associated with rugby union compared with the low risk associated with tennis. You must have an appreciation of the injury profile of the sport to be able to adequately plan. It would, for example, be indefensible if you could not adequately immobilize the cervical spine when covering a rugby match, whereas serious cervical injury would be highly unlikely on a tennis court. That said there are core skills which all doctors covering sport must maintain, and emergency medical skills including the management of cervical injury are such skills no matter how unlikely such an injury.

Venue or event

The venue will influence the equipment that you carry. The equipment you will personally need to arrange, for example, to provide medical cover at rugby international at Twickenham will be very different from that required to cover a game at a local rugby club. Similarly consider the role of the medical officers for the London marathon, run over the same distance as another on the foothills of Mount Everest. The following list, although not exhaustive, covers many of the important factors:
- Will you be a single handed practitioner or part of a team of clinicians? If part of a team what is their experience, what equipment are they likely to bring?
- What medical equipment will be provided by the venue (e.g. is there a fully equipped medical room)?
- Emergency medical support (will there be a paramedic ambulance on site) and what equipment will they have at their disposal?
- Where will you be situated in relation to the field of play and what access to the field of play do you have?
- Where are the nearest emergency care/hospital facilities?

- What is the transfer time to these facilities and how might that change on the day of competition?
- Environment and climate considerations.

The team you are covering
Most athletes are by definition healthy, however, they may have medical conditions, e.g. diabetes, asthma, or disabilities that will influence what equipment you require. Furthermore, you will almost certainly be responsible for the health of those individuals supporting the athletes, e.g. performance directors, coaches, medical and paramedical staff. In some circumstances you may even have responsibility for family members including children. Support staff may have a variety of chronic illnesses and medical requirements and you should be prepared. If you are travelling with a team with whom you don't usually work it is useful to send out a questionnaire prior to departure requesting key current and past medical history, medications, and allergies. Even if you do work regularly with athletes there may be athletes, support staff, or additional party members to with whom you are unfamiliar.

Touchline kit bag
The key to a basic first aid kit is to only put in what you know how to use. It should be hands-free, carried on the shoulder or waist and should be clean, compact, and secure.

Suggested contents will depend on the sport you are covering, but might include:
- Squirty water bottle or ampoule: this allows pressure to be exerted when irrigating wounds. Pressurized canisters are commercially available.
- Gauze swabs.
- Disposable gloves.
- Tape.
- Scissors, forceps, tweezers.
- Stethoscope, BP cuff, torch/opthalmoscope, tongue depressor.
- Assorted plasters, sterile wound dressings and bandages.
- Antiseptic spray and wound congealer.
- Insect sting/bite relief spray.
- Analgesia, antihistamines, buccal anti-emetic.
- Emergency drugs, e.g. adrenalin (epipen), ventolin, GTN, glucose, aspirin.
- Pocket facemask, oral and nasopharyngeal airway, petroleum jelly.
- Pen and paper or copies of a suitable incident report form.
- Clinical waste bag.
- Telephone.

Basic medical equipment

In addition to a touchline carry on bag there is a basic level of equipment to which every doctor covering sport should have immediate access and, of course, be able to use. The following list is included as a guide.

- Stethoscope.
- Portable sphygmomanometer.
- Oto/opthalmoscope/spare batteries.
- Scissors.
- Nail clippers.
- Tongue depressors.
- Thermometer.
- Oropharyngeal airways (e.g. Guedel sizes 2, 3, 4).
- Nasopharyngeal airways (6–8mm).
- Petroleum gel.
- Pocket mask with mouthpiece and O_2 inlet (e.g. Laerdal).
- Alcohol wipes.
- Antimicrobial soap/gel.
- Cleaning fluid (e.g. chlorhexidine, betadine sachets).
- Semipermeable dressing (e.g. Tegaderm) various sizes.
- Low adherence dressing (e.g. Mepore) various sizes.
- Sterile gauze swabs and cotton wool.
- Tubular bandage (e.g. Tubigrip).
- Elastic/adhesive bandage (e.g. crepe).
- Cohesive bandage.
- Permeable adhesive tape.
- Blister pack.
- Sterile and non-sterile gloves.
- Adhesive strips (e.g. Steri-strip).
- Tissue adhesive (e.g. 2-octyl cyanoacrylates).
- Suture kit.
- Scalpel and blades.
- Razor.
- Sharps bin.
- Assorted needles and syringes.
- Tourniquet.
- Blood and specimen bottles.
- Peak flow meter and disposable mouthpieces.
- Assorted cannulae and giving set.
- 500ml bag of dextrose/saline (emergency use only).
- Adjustable hard collar.
- Safety pins.
- Tape measure.
- Urinalysis testing strips (e.g. clinitest).
- Eye kit.
- Glucose testing meter and test strips.
- BNF or access to BNF online.

Don't forget the obvious non-medical items, e.g. pen, paper, mobile telephone, and useful contact numbers. A driving license is often helpful.

Drugs and medications

If providing medical support to a large team or squad competing internationally you may need an extensive drug list to cover most medical situations. Irrespective of what drugs you have available at a main base there are basic drugs/medication that you should aim to have easy access to. This list is only a guide as it will be influenced by the medical history of your team members.

Emergency management
- Epinephrine (adrenaline) (1/1000) 1mg in 1mL pre-filled syringe and Epipen.
- Parenteral antihistamine, e.g. chlorpheniramine (10mg/mL).
- Hydrocortisone IV 100mg vial.
- Oral steroid.
- Concentrated (40%) glucose or dextrose gel.
- Furosemide (IV and oral) depends on circumstances.
- Midazolam 1mg/mL as 50mL vial (optional).
- Parenteral opiate analgesia (e.g. pethidine 25mg/1mL amp or morphine) depends on circumstances.
- Naloxone (optional, if carrying opiate analgesia essential).
- Nitrolingual spray.
- Aspirin oral.

General
- Anaesthetic, e.g. lidocaine, bupivacaine.
- Intra-articular steroid, e.g. triamcinolone, methylprednisolone.
- Sterile water ampoules for injections/irrigation.
- Antihistamine (oral and topical).

Analgesia
- Paracetamol.
- Compound analgesic (e.g. co-codamol).
- Parenteral analgesia (e.g. IM diclofenac).
- Oral NSAID, e.g. ibuprofen, diclofenac.
- Topical NSAID, e.g. diclofenac patch and gel.
- Aspirin 75mg dispersible.

Antibiotics
- Penicillin (IV and oral).
- Non-penicillin broad spectrum IV antibiotics.
- Other oral antibiotics, e.g. azithromycin, augmentin, amoxycillin. metronidazole, ciprofloxacin, acyclovir.
- Topical anti-bacterial and anti-fungals.
- Antibiotic drops suitable for ocular and aural use.

Gastrointestinal
- Antacid, e.g. gaviscon.
- PPI, e.g. omeprazole.
- Diarrhoea, e.g. loperamide.
- Constipation, e.g. senna.
- Bowel spasm agent, e.g. mebeverine.

- Rehydration sachets, e.g. diarrolyte.
- Anti-emetic, e.g. prochlorperazine, buccal and IV/IM.

Respiratory and ear, nose, and throat/eyes
- Beta-2 agonist/steroid inhaler for oral/nasal use.
- Throat lozenge (e.g. merocaine, strepsil).
- Steroid drops suitable for ocular and aural use.
- Fluorescein/amethocaine eye drops.
- Decongestant/cold remedy.
- Acyclovir cream.
- Mouth ulcer treatment, e.g. Bonjela.

Topical
- Flamazine or equivalent.
- Hiridoid or equivalent.
- Antiseptic, e.g. Savlon.
- Sunscreen.
- Topical steroids.

CNS
- Migraine treatment.
- Diazepam.
- Sleeping tablet, e.g. zopiclone.

Obstetrics and gynaecology/contraception
- Mefenamic acid.
- Anti-fungal treatment.
- Contraception.

You must be up-to-date with current doping regulations and which apply to the athletes under your care, e.g. in/out competition, IOC, WADA, International Federation. Some of the medications on this list require the completion of a TUE. Carry some blank forms.

Security and insurance issues

Increased security has restricted the ease with which a doctor can transport medical equipment and medication. I would encourage you to consider taking practical steps to preempt or avoid difficulty.

- Itemize in full the contents of your medical bag.
- Write to the Embassy of the country of destination detailing your travel arrangements and seek approval for the carriage of your medical equipment being sure to include your list.
- Do not take strong opiate-based analgesia, e.g. morphine unless absolutely necessary, and then seek prior agreement. Many countries restrict even moderate or weak opiates not intended for personal medical use.
- Where possible source medications in the country of destination, and certainly plan how you will replenish supplies locally.
- Consider writing to the airline concerned detailing your medical luggage.
- Carry a copy of your itemized medical bag and a letter confirming your medical role.
- Ensure that any prohibited 'dangerous' (or potential prohibited) items are stored in the hold.
- Do not take pressurized containers, e.g. oxygen, entanox.
- Ensure that you have appropriate travel insurance.
- Ensure that you have appropriate medical insurance and indemnity in order to practice in the country of destination.
- Carry separately a photocopy/jpeg of your passport.

Team travel

Providing medical support to a traveling team presents the sports physician with additional challenges and adequate and timely preparation is essential. The following considerations should help you prepare for your team travel experience.

Selecting a medical team

You may be responsible for a team of medical officers. In these circumstances you should be involved in the appointment of your medical team and it is vitally important to get your team right from the start. This process should be just as any other professional appointment with a job description (including essential and desired criteria), application process with open job advert, short-listing and interview. Your interview panel should be multi-disciplinary and might include the team manager/head coach/chef de mission (or equivalent), chief physiotherapist, and a medical colleague (not involved with the sport or event in question). The appointments panel should meet prior to the interview to identify key questions that will allow the interviewee to demonstrate that they possess the necessary essential and desired qualities. In particular the ability to work effectively within a multidisciplinary team should be assessed.

It may be useful to have, within a team; doctors of differing sports medicine backgrounds, e.g. primary care, musculoskeletal, emergency care. In the future with specialty recognition and certified training programmes, doctors certifying in sports and exercise medicine (SEM) will have similar backgrounds and such distinctions may no longer hold true.

Medical preparation

Adequate preparation is essential whether you are the Chief Medical Officer to the Olympic team or the medical officer to an amateur team going on a club tour. The preparation will, of course, reflect the particular circumstances, but should follow good medical practice and applies irrespective of the stature of your athletes.

Team building

Get to know your team ahead of departure. In many circumstances you will already be part of a well-established team or squad. However, for major events, the headquarters staff may be from different backgrounds and you will almost certainly be working with a number of 'strangers'. For this reason organizations arrange team building sessions, usually residential and often at weekends, which you should attend whether medical team leader or medical officer. They are invaluable opportunities to get to know other team members and facilitate preparation and planning. You should be prepared to advise your team on relevant medical issues including the ubiquitous 'what if' scenarios, e.g. what do we do if one of the team brings into camp a highly contagious form of viral gastro-enteritis?

You may attend training or preparation camps. These will serve a number of purposes, not least is the opportunity to ensure effective team working and meet any athletes or support staff who are new to a squad.

If you are part of the HQ medical team it is impossible to get to know all the athletes and support staff who will form a countries delegation at a major games. Training, preparation, or holding camps may provide an opportunity to get to know some individual squads.

Pre-travel medical assessment
Providing medical support during competition can be challenging with the additional complications of being in a foreign country with all the cultural, environmental, and linguistic differences that may exist. It helps to have as much information about your destination and team members as possible.

You may have had the luxury of a pre-games visit or training camp, in which case you should perform a medical risk assessment as described previously. If not, contact non-medical colleagues who are going on a pre-games visit, other medical colleagues who may have been to your destination previously, and try and make contact with local medical services. Internet and email facilitate communication.

Your appreciation of the team's previous medical history may vary from having a detailed knowledge of a team through years of working with the same individuals, to having virtually no prior knowledge. In either case a pre-travel questionnaire is essential and should be a pre-requisite of inclusion in the team, something that you should clarify with the team manager or equivalent. The following should be included within your pre-games questionnaire:

- Demographic information (full name, date of birth, address, telephone and email contacts, GP name and contact details, national governing body (NGB) medical team members contact details, and the names and contact details of 2 independent adult next of kin).
- Current health and injury status.
- Previous medical and injury history.
- Vaccination history.
- Current and accurate list of medications and supplements.
- Documented confirmation of TUE.
- Allergy history.
- Recent drug test record (date, event, testing body within 6 months).
- Travel history: e.g. problems with jetlag, GI upset.
- Dental and optician check: encourage athletes to ensure they have visited their dentist and optician prior to major tournaments. Equally, if a team member has a chronic medical problem encourage them to attend for a specialist review prior to departure.

Such questionnaires often reveal important and relevant information and being aware of this information prior to travel can be very helpful.

Most sports will have a NGB medical officer. In addition to asking athletes to complete the pre-games questionnaire, if you are not the NGB then contact the NGB doctor and ensure you have his/her contact details.

Team education
Invest time in educating your team prior to competition. Hopefully, you will have the opportunity to meet your team at team building sessions, preparation, or holding camps. These will usually be arranged to replicate some of the environmental challenges that may be encountered and thus provide an ideal learning opportunity for athletes and support staff. You may wish to consider a medical fact sheet, which can be sent to those on your team who you are not able to attend.

The following are some of the issues that you might wish to cover:
- Your contact details (and those on the medical team).
- Jet lag and travel sickness.
- Environmental advice (dealing with heat, humidity, cold, altitude, insects).
- Hygiene (in particular the prevention of travel related illness).
- Fluid and nutrition.
- Immunization advice.
- Locality advice: e.g. details of how to access local pharmacy, opticians, hospital services, dentist with relevant names and contact information.
- Emergency advice, e.g. what to do if you are involved in a car crash.
- Medical insurance cover (what cover is provided as a member of a team and what additional cover will individuals have to arrange).
- General travel advice.

Immunization and vaccination

Exact immunization requirements depend on your destination and you must ensure that you are aware of the latest advice. The 'Yellow book' available in paper and online from the department of health is a useful resource.

Assuming that the normal vaccination program against TB, measles, mumps, rubella, pertussis, Hib, meningococcus, and polio has been completed, you may up date immunization against hepatitis A and tetanus. Vaccination should take place as early as possible to allow sufficient time to get over any reaction.

Tetanus

The initial vaccination is a 3-injection course (usually given as a baby). Two booster injections are then required to a total of 5 injections (5th injection is likely to be by the age of 18). While further injections are only required at the time of injury, for those who have not had a booster within 10yr a booster is recommended before foreign travel.

Hepatitis A

It is strongly recommended that athletes are vaccinated against Hepatitis A. This is a very debilitating illness, which can easily be passed through food, drinks, and via hand to mouth. A single injection will provide protection for 12 months, however a course of 2 injections over the 6 months prior to travel will provide protection for 10yrs.

The journey

Your role as a team doctor goes far beyond normal medical practice, you are very much a member of a team, and may be able to help with other tasks including travel logistics, e.g. helping with luggage and assisting with check in.

Ensure that you have a small medical bag in your hand luggage. It may be useful to include the following:
- Letter of authority confirming your medical role and requirement to carry medical equipment (and a list of that equipment).
- Paracetamol.
- Ibuprofen.
- Prochlorperazine (buccal).
- Loperamide.

- Antihistamine.
- Throat lozenges.
- Salbutamol inhaler.
- GTN spray.
- Aspirin.
- Migraine treatment.
- Epinephrine (Epipen®).
- Laerdal pocket mask.
- Any specific medications depending on the regular prescriptions of team members.

Jet lag

Most of us have experienced jet lag, an almost indescribable feeling of utter uselessness. It is characterized by:
- Altered sleep pattern with daytime sleepiness and nighttime insomnia.
- Poor concentration.
- Fatigue and malaise.
- GI disturbance.

In addition to these generic symptoms it will impair athletic performance for several days.

Jet lag is thought to be caused by disrupted circadian rhythms in those flying across 3 or more time zones (a time zone is defined by a 1h time change for every 15° travelled in either direction from the Greenwich meridian. There are, of course, 24). Although jet lag cannot be prevented it can be modified and its impact reduced by taking fairly simple measures:
- Ensure adequate rest and sleep prior to departure. You may want to start adjusting your time zone prior to departure, e.g. going to bed and getting up an hour earlier or later.
- Aim to arrive late afternoon.
- Maintain good hydration. Avoid excess alcohol.
- Synchronize your watch to the destination time zone upon departure.
- Ensure adequate relaxation during the flight. Try to eat and sleep in concordance with your new time zone.
- Upon arrival try to remain active during any remaining daylight hours and adjust meal and bedtimes to new time zone.
- Avoid stimulants (e.g. caffeine) at times when you should be resting.
- Try to adopt a flexible routine upon arrival: a rigid routine will prolong the effects of jet lag.
- Be prepared to allow one day of recovery for each time zone crossed (e.g. if travelling from London to Sydney you should expect to modify your normal training and expect altered performance for up to 10 days).

Melatonin is a hormone secreted in the evening by the pineal gland. It has been used in experiments to modify the symptoms of jet lag. Current evidence to support its use in reducing the symptoms of jet lag is inconclusive and there is a lack of data on its long-term safety.

Arrival—getting started

Upon arrival, check that your team and their medical equipment have arrived complete and undamaged. Once appropriately refreshed and rested (if time permits) establish a well-organized base from which to

operate from, be it the hotel room, medical room, or medical suite. You should have considered the location of your medical room prior to arrival, but be flexible if the situation requires it. Issues to consider when planning the location of your medical room are:
- Confidentiality and privacy.
- Accessibility.
- Security.
- Space:
  - An examination couch should be accessible from all sides.
  - In an ideal world you will need a desk, 2 chairs, storage space including secure storage and a fridge.
- Proximity to colleagues, e.g. physiotherapy.
- Environment, e.g. air conditioning, natural light.
- Power, communication, computer, and IT connections.
- Mobile telephone with appropriate network coverage.
- Access to washing and toilet facilities.
- Drug testing facility.
- Isolation room.
- Your own privacy, ideally avoid your own room becoming the medical room although all too frequently this is what happens.
- In addition the medical team should have access to a designated car.

Managing your medical service

Organization is essential for a successful medical service. Despite best made plans, medical support in a competitive environment will constantly throw up new problems; require changes in plan, flexibility, and unreasonable deadlines which have to be met. If you are organized then managing change becomes more achievable.

Medical consultations

Athletes train and compete, eat, and rest at varying times, and your accessibility should reflect this. A flexible drop-in approach to appointments suits most athletes—this usually means being available from early morning to late evening. However, you also need some rest to remain fresh and enthusiastic (and don't feel guilty about it). If single-handed make everyone aware of your availability for that day, structure any down time around the likely quiet periods, e.g. athletes will frequently want to see you before and after training and competition, they are less likely to need your services during their rest time. You will of course need to provide 24h contact details in the case of an emergency.

You will almost certainly be required to provide cover at training and competition. This is challenging in a multi-games environment. If you are part of a team then arrange a rota.

In medical consultations, remember:
- Your ethical code of practice (see 📖 GMC Good Medical Practice, p. 736).
- An athlete's right to confidentiality.
- Do not practice beyond your scope of practice. If you have prepared properly you will have made arrangements to seek specialist advice when appropriate.
- The ability to ask for a second opinion. Even if you are a single-handed practitioner there is always someone somewhere available to ask advice.
- You must have professional indemnity and insurance to allow you to practice medicine in the country you are working in.
- Accurate medical record keeping is essential. The development of a web-based electronic record (e.g. injury zone (IZ), performance profiler) has made an important contribution to our ability to maintain an accurate medical record for UK athletes as patients who are constantly on the move. If it isn't documented it didn't happen.
- Most consultations reflect a primary care problem, e.g. URTI, GI upset, skin rashes.
- You must have contingency plans in the event of contagious illness.
- Any prescribing must be within the IOC, WADA, games organizing body or International Federation out/in competition doping regulations and you must be aware of which applies. If you prescribe or use a regulated substance then you must complete and submit the relevant documentation (e.g. TUE) and ensure copies are retained by you, the athlete, and scanned into any electronic record.

- Good team work and communication. You are part of a medical team and all members of that team, acknowledging any limitations imposed by respecting an athlete's confidentiality, should be included in a multidisciplinary approach to management. You are also part of a wider athletic team and in many circumstances the coach and performance director should also be kept informed although this must be with the athlete's full consent.

Medical review

Pre-competition knowledge of the athletes under your care will vary. A medical review offers a valuable opportunity to introduce yourself and seek the following:
- Accurate demographic details including local mobile telephone number and next of kin.
- Current injury status.
- Current medical status.
- Documentation of previous relevant past injury and medical history.
- Current and complete list of all medications and supplements.
- Confirmation that relevant TUEs have been completed and that you and the athlete have either a copy of the submitted forms, or confirmation from the relevant authority (UK Sport, International Federation, IOC) that the TUE has been acknowledged.
- Allergy history.

Welcome meeting

The medical component of a generic welcome meeting or team gathering with your athletes and support staff should cover:
- Introduce yourself if not known to all.
- Your contact details including emergency telephone number.
- Arranging routine medical consultation.
- Arranging emergency medical consultation.
- What to do in the event of an emergency, e.g. road accident.
- Drug testing procedure.
- Medical review.
- 'What if...' scenarios, e.g. what to do if a team member develops a contagious illness.
- Advice on avoiding problems, e.g. hydration, sun protection, insect problems, fluid and nutrition hygiene.
- Questions: make it clear that you will try to accommodate your teams individual needs as far as is possible.

Drug testing

Your athletes will be required to have in or out of competition drug testing. Establish a procedure in the event of a request for a drugs test. As part of this you should identify:
- Appropriate drug testing room (within limits imposed by available facilities).
- Who should be informed upon arrival of drug testing officials?
- Your role? Will you always be available as an athlete representative? If not who will stand in should the athlete request a representative?
- What to do in the event of a positive test.

Before competition has started:
- Visit the competition or athlete village medical centre. Introduce yourself to reception staff and the lead physician if possible. Find out what facilities are on site and how to organize those tests that are not immediately available, e.g. MRI.
- Where possible visit the venues you are likely to be using and assess their facilities.
- Establish where the nearest bank, telephone card sales, supermarket, opticians, dentist, pharmacist are located. You'll be amazed how much athletes rely on the doctor and physiotherapist for day to day information.

Medical management

Whether you are a single-handed medical officer or the chief medical officer (CMO) of a team of medics you will have management meetings to attend. These meetings are valuable opportunities for receiving or communicating information.
- Team leader meetings, meetings with leads within your squad or team, e.g. chef de mission, camp director, individual team leaders (at a games there will be leads for a number of areas, e.g. transport, nutrition, competition, media, security, etc), performance director, senior coaching staff, chief physiotherapist.
- Team meetings, meetings with all members of your team.
- Medical Meetings. As CMO you should arrange to meet with the rest of your medical team on a regular basis. This should include meetings with the chief physiotherapist and physiotherapy colleagues.
- Competition medical meetings. At major competitions there will usually be an opportunity for the games/competition medical committee to meet with medical representatives from competing teams/nations. This is a valuable opportunity to receive information on host medical protocols, but more importantly to feed back on areas that require attention, e.g. fluid and nutrition issues, drug testing procedure, access to investigations.

Multi-sport events

The role of a medical officer is very different if you are responsible for a team at a multi-event competition.

As a medical officer to a team at a single sport competition your focus is only on one sport, albeit with the different individual demands of those athletes under your care. This might vary from a team of cricketers all training/playing the same sport at the same time to an athletics squad with very different athletic disciplines training and competing at different times.

Prioritizing

If working at a multi-sport event you will have to balance the requirements of individual athletes (and their support staff) and different sports.

The key to a successful games is communication and prioritizing. Most performance directors and coaches will appreciate that you have competing demands on your time.

- Ask individual teams what medical support they would like and ask them to prioritize the training and competition elements of their programme.
- Once you have an appreciation of each sport's requirements go through the same exercise sport by sport from a medical view point. This will reflect:
  - Risk of serious injury of that sport, e.g. gymnastics vs. tennis.
  - Availability of NGB medical support.
  - Physiotherapy support. It is vital that you discuss your plans with physiotherapy colleagues as there will be the option of a certain amount of cross-cover.
  - Training vs. competition. Usually, competition support is prioritized, however, there may be local medical services supporting competition that is not available for training, e.g. gymnastics training.
  - Local medical services, e.g. venue medical provision (as above), athletes village medical centre.
  - Requirement to provide medical consultations for those athletes not competing or training. In a games situation you will have to provide cover at the athletes village or equivalent.
  - Logistical issues: e.g. ability to communicate with team, access to transport. You may be able to cover adjacent venues if travelling times are short and communication via mobile telephone is easy. A distant venue may require that you have to travel with that squad, however, be conscious that then removes one member of the medical team from any cross-cover.
- This process should be flexible enough to accommodate sudden changes in circumstances, e.g. medical emergency, athletes progressing to final stages of competition.

The holding camp

There is an increasing tendency for athletes to go to a holding camp prior to major competition. This is valuable for a number of reasons:
- Environmental acclimatization (time zone, heat, humidity).
- Opportunity to fine tune technical aspects.
- Team building.
- Tapering, focus, rest, and relaxation.

You may travel with the team onwards to competition or alternatively you may be employed solely to work at the holding camp. Working at a holding camp provides a unique opportunity to contribute to the preparation of elite athletes in a slightly more relaxed environment than you will find at a games or championships. Your medical management has to be tailored to the situation and the proximity to competition means that the time frames you have to work within are very tight and your practice may be modified accordingly.

The games

Caring for athletes at a championship or during an event is a privilege, but is also the most demanding aspect of medical care because of the importance of the timing of any health issue. You may be faced by an athlete whose sole focus for the last 4yrs has been Olympic competition and who may only have this one opportunity. Even simple problems may assume mammoth proportions in the athletes mind.

Maintaining your focus

The pressure cooker environment of athletic competition puts an additional strain on relationships.
- Ensure you are working as a team.
- Communicate a concern before it becomes a problem; don't bottle things up.
- As far as is possible take adequate down time.
- Be supportive of others taking their down time.
- A hasty word can do irreparable harm. If tensions rise, walk away and figuratively count to 10.
- Appreciate the stress of the situation and give colleagues some slack.
- A simple thank you, a smile or a hug (whichever is appropriate), costs nothing, but makes a world of difference.

Rest and relaxation (down time)

You will work long and unsociable hours so it is vital that you take downtime when you can. Establish a rota so that you can cross-cover. If you are single-handed then ensure that you and your physiotherapy colleague/s cover each other leaving emergency contact details.

The return home

The evening after competition is usually celebrated by any closing ceremonies and time with your team. This is an important opportunity for everyone to unwind, but may have medical implications.

The journey home

You are still responsible for the medical care of those in your team so ensure that you have access to appropriate equipment for all stages of the journey home.

Compile a short medical report even if you are not required to do so as part of your medical officer responsibilities. It may help improve future trips and prove useful for successors.

- Your arrival at home can be quite challenging for yourself and your partner and family. There is usually a feeling of deflation when your trip comes to an end.
- You will almost certainly be physically and more importantly mentally tired in addition to any jet lag.
- You may be making the rapid transition from an exciting period of work in a new environment back to 'the day job' with all the mundane roles and responsibilities that that involves (and all too often a backlog of work that has accumulated in your absence).
- Be appreciative and balance recounting exciting moments from your travels with showing an interest in what others have been up to.
- Allow yourself adequate time to recover from jet lag before returning to work.

Professional and ethical considerations

Medical work within sport is governed by exactly the same considerations and responsibilities that govern any other form of medical work. You have a duty of care to those that you are looking after and you must execute that duty of care within the framework of the GMC's Good Medical Practice. This encompasses all aspects of your work as a team doctor, but has particular relevance to respecting patient confidentiality. The Faculty of Sports Medicine Code of Practice also provides helpful guidance on maintaining your professional standards and responsibilities.

In addition to the medical work you carry out while away with a team, you have to comply with requirements for appraisal, revalidation, clinical governance, and your own continuing professional development.

Chief Medical Officer's role

If you are the CMO then you will have additional responsibilities as a medical team leader.

- It is your responsibility to ensure that all in your team are medically qualified and appropriately trained. If you were not involved with the interview process then ensure you have seen proof of GMC registration and relevant qualifications of anyone not known to you.
- Code of Conduct: establish a code of conduct for all members of the medical team. The UK Faculty of Sport and Exercise Medicine (FSEM UK) has produced a professional code of conduct for SEM physicians available from their website. There may well be a generic team code of conduct, which the medical team code of conduct has to incorporate. Issues to consider are:
  - *Medical duties*—ensure that everyone has the same team philosophy.
  - *Line management*—as CMO you are responsible for all aspects of medical care and you need to ensure that your colleagues report any problems to you before they get out of hand. You will probably be responsible to a non-medical colleague, e.g. chef de mission, camp director, and you should equally keep them informed without breaching confidentiality.
  - *On-call arrangements*—you have a duty to provide 24h emergency medical cover or make clear what alternative arrangements are in place.
  - *Rest and relaxation*—you should ensure that all members of your team are taking adequate down time.
  - *Alcohol consumption*—squads and teams may have their own generic views on alcohol consumption and you must abide by the team code of conduct if a dry philosophy is adopted.
  - *Wearing of team kit.*
- Medical representation at governing body, competition, games, and delegation management meetings.
- Clinical governance issues of your team.
- Mentoring and professional development. Be mindful that you may have considerably more experience than some of your colleagues and

particularly if this is their first games. Be supportive to ensure that their experience is a positive one.

Patient confidentiality

Athletes have the same right to confidentiality as any other patient.

Medical indemnity

Ensure that your medical insurance and indemnity covers your scope (contact your provider to confirm you have the appropriate cover).

Organizing a major sporting event

A major sporting event is a place of employment, of entertainment, and of competition and hence entails an unusually large and diverse number of potential areas of risk. It is vital to be able to deal with these crowds in a safe and efficient manner.

Accidents at sporting events have precipitated the development of guidelines to ensure crowd safety. The sources include the Safety of Sports Grounds Act, the Taylor report and the Green Guide. Guide to safety at sports grounds:

If a ground holds a safety certificate consultation through a local authority this will give information regarding:
- The limit to number of spectators.
- Duration of cover.
- Details of exits, entrances, means of access, crush barriers, and means of escape in case of fire.

First aid minimum requirements
- No event should have fewer than 2 first aiders.
- If seated and standing spectators there should be 1 first aider per 1000 spectators.
- If all seated, 1 first aider per 1000 up to 20,000, then 1 per 2000.
- If more are anticipated then consult local ambulance service.
- First aider holds standard certificate of first aid issued by voluntary aid societies. Health and Safety (first aid) regulations 1981.
- Should be 16yrs or older with no other duties at ground.
- At ground prior to spectators and remain until all spectators have left the ground.
- Responsibility to provide room(s) for spectators in addition to other medical facilities.
- Should compliment the facilities provided by the ambulance services.
- Consultation with ambulance, local authority, the crowd doctor, and appropriate voluntary aid services.
- Non-smoking area.
- Minimum size 15m^2, increase to 25m^2 if >15,000.
- To hold a couch, area for sitting casualties, extra couch if necessary.
- Sufficient room for equipment and materials.
- Blankets, pillows, stretchers, buckets, bowls, trolleys, and screens.
- Suitable disposal facilities for sharps and waste.
- Defibrillator if >5000 expected. Provided by other agency if required.
- Appropriate design for access and egress, fittings and facilities. Should have appropriate location.

Crowd doctor

If >2000 present there should be a crowd doctor trained in immediate care with appropriate qualifications, skills, experience, and support.

Knowledge of cardiopulmonary resuscitation, airway maintenance, spinal fracture immobilization, and treatment of anaphylaxis. Training in ALS and paediatric life support. Governing body rules will give recommendation regarding level of qualification.
- The first duty of the 'crowd doctor' is to the spectators.

- Their whereabouts should be known to first aid, ambulance, and control point personnel, and they be contactable.
- Equipment levels and clinical protocols used should conform to guidelines published by the relevant sporting body.
- They should be in position before and remain until all spectators leave the ground.
- If <2000 spectators there should be arrangements to summon a suitably trained and experienced crowd doctor.
- Be aware of the location and staffing arrangements of the first aid room, and ambulance cover and emergency plans for major incidents.

Ambulance provision
- One fully equipped ambulance if >5000 spectators and sourced from approved group.
- Relationship of an ambulance, if not supplied by the NHS, to access NHS facilities should be known to management.
- Access for ambulance personnel to control point.
- Ambulance present before and after spectators access and egress ground.
- With 5000–25,000 spectators, there should be 1 accident and emergency ambulance with a paramedic crew. 1 ambulance officer, paramedic holds certificate of proficiency in ambulance paramedic skills issued by IHCD and has access to equipment including drugs.
- With 25,000–45,000 spectators, 1 accident and emergency ambulance with a paramedic crew, 1 ambulance officer, 1 major incident equipment vehicle and a paramedic crew, and 1 control unit.
- 45,000 or more 2 accident and emergency ambulances with paramedic crews otherwise as above.

Major incident plan
- Plans compatible with the local emergency services major incident plan.
- Identify areas for dealing with casualties in multiple situations, may include fire, accident, crowd disturbance, bomb scare, adverse and inclement weather.
- Identify access and egress routes and rendezvous point for vehicles.
- Agreed plan of action by all interested parties.
- Briefing of all first aid and medical staff on role in the major incident plan per event. Copy kept in the first aid room.
- Risk assessments should be performed.

International governing body check lists
- Includes review of all medical arrangements.
- Includes safety measures outside stadia.
- Will define high risk event.
- Assesses size of stadium, and provision of safety and medical cover.
- Reviews risks of trouble including ticket forgery.
- Fire brigade, ambulance, and security measures.
- Practical issues regarding floodlights, etc.
- General rules where appropriate regarding access of medical staff and stabilization of injuries on the field of play.

- *Additional cover:* temporary insurance can often be arranged with a foreign defence organization, however, there will be an application process and it can be lengthy and very expensive.

Media issues

One of the biggest challenges of a major tournament is dealing with the media. Think very carefully before discussing any issues pertaining to the health of an athlete or group of athletes. Ideally, your team will be supported by a media representative who will guide you. Leave it to the experts who will release well scribed press statements that have been cleared with all concerned, most importantly the athlete. Issues to consider are:
- Beware the quiet news day—schedules still need filling.
- Requests for interviews are made to make news not to find out what life as a doctor is like. Ideally, you should say nothing in saying something.
- Recorded interviews will be edited!
- Live interviews are less likely to be misrepresented at the time (they can be edited later for recorded news), but are extremely dangerous—interviewers are trained to produce a result.
- The media will work covertly and may pretend to be an interested fan.

Index

6 minute walk test 289
10 × 5m speed/agility test 146
12 minute run test 150
20m shuttle test 150

A

abdominal injuries 548
abrasions 44
abscess 340
absolute rest 40
acetabular labral tears 609
acetazolamide 191
Achilles tendon 682–3
acne vulgaris 340
acromioclavicular joint 456
 degenerative disease 496
 separations 484
 testing 467
actin filaments 129
actioners 107
active knee extension test 143
active rest 40
acupuncture 237
acute hot joint 246
acute injury, management 36, 38
acute renal failure 556
adaptation 124
adhesive capsulitis 496
adrenaline
 anaphylaxis 30
 cardiac arrest 14
adrenogenital syndrome 369
Adson's manoeuvre 468
adult basic life support 6, 11
adult congenital heart disease 272–6
advanced adult life support 14, 17
aerobic-anaerobic threshold 140–1
aerobic base training 154
aerobic capacity 144, 149, 148–9
aerobic conditioning 125
aerobic endurance training 154, 155
aerobic metabolism 127–8
aerobic power 125
afterload 289
ageing
 bone metabolism 59
 fitness deterioration 378
 muscle changes 78, 378
 osteoarthritis risk 229
 successful ageing 372
 see also older people
airway management 16
albuterol 306
allergic asthma 300
allocation concealment 120
alphabet exercises 660
altitude acclimatization 190
altitude sickness 191
alverine citrate 321
ambulances 739
amenorrhoea 352–3, 355
American footballers 386
amiodarone 14
amphetamines 200
amputees 220
anabolic steroids 198, 341
anaerobic capacity 144
anaerobic glycolysis 126
anaerobic metabolism 126
anaerobic power 125, 144
anaerobic training 162
anaphylaxis 30–1
 exercise-induced 305
androgen insensitivity syndrome 369
ankle
 active and passive movements 624
 anterior impingement (footballer's ankle) 674
 anterior pain 674
 anterolateral impingement 669
 bony anatomy 651
 examination 650
 flexor hallucis longus tendinopathy 672
 fractures 658, 667
 functional tests 653
 impingement syndromes 658
 inspection 650
 investigations 654
 lateral pain 668, 670
 ligaments 657
 medial ligament injuries 665
 medial pain 672–3
 medial plantar nerve entrapment 673
 osteochondral injuries 658
 palpation 650
 peroneal tendinopathy 668
 persistent pain 658
 posterior impingement syndrome 675
 posterior pain 675
 resisted movements 652
 sinus tarsi syndrome 658, 668
 special tests 653
 sprains 653, 656–7, 660, 665
 strapping and taping 72
 syndesmosis injury 666
 tendon dislocation and rupture 658
 tibialis anterior tendinopathy 674
 tibialis posterior tendinopathy 672–3
ankylosing spondylitis 448
anterior apprehension test 464
anterior compartment syndrome 678
anterior cruciate ligament 626, 636
anterior draw test 626, 638, 653
anterior inferior iliac spine avulsion 594
anterior interosseous syndrome 524
anterior slide test 468
anterior superior iliac spine, avulsion 594
anthropometric measurement 143
Anti-Doping Administration and Management System (ADAMS) 206
anti-inflammatory drugs 50
antioxidants 203
anti-platelet therapies 262
aortic stenosis 294
ApoE4 385, 416–17
arrhythmias 295
arteriovenous difference 138
arthritis, juvenile idiopathic 647 *see also* inflammatory arthritis; osteoarthritis

INDEX

aspirin 50
asteatotic dermatitis 332
asthma, intrinsic/
  allergic 300, 308
asthma therapies, TUE 201
asystole 14–15
atheromatous plaques 260
athlete's foot 336
athletic
  pseudoanaemia 134, 178
athletic
  pseudonephritis 554
atopic dermatitis 331
ATP 126
atrial fibrillation 135
atrial septal defect 276
atropine 15
augmentation test 464
automated external
  defibrillators (AEDs) 12,
  18, 21
autonomic dysreflexia 225
autonomic nervous
  system 124
avascular necrosis 500
AVPU scale 23
avulsion fracture
  anterior superior iliac
    spine 594
  hip 615

B

back
  acute injuries 433
  fracture dislocation 433
  fractures 433
  muscles 427
  red flags for back
    pain 424
  sprains and strains 433
  see also spine
backpacker's
  neuropathy 468
bacterial skin infections 340
bag-mask ventilation 10
balance 68
balance exercises 90, 376
balance testing 389
Bankart lesion 472
banned drugs 207
barefoot running 693
barrier contraception 356
basal metabolic rate 174
basic life support
  adults 6, 11
  paediatric 12–13
Bath Ankylosing Spondylitis
  Disease Activity Index
  (BASDAI) 449
behaviour change 106
behavioural determinants of
  physical activity 103

belly-press test 466
benign exertional
  headache 414
benign sex headache 414
Bennett's fracture 534
beta alanine 205
beta blockers 262
beta-hydroxy-beta-
  methylbutyrate 204
beta-2 adrenoceptor
  agonists 201, 307
biceps
  distal biceps tear/
    rupture 516
  special tests 467, 506
  tendinopathy 494, 522
  tendon dislocation 488
  tendon rupture 487
biceps load test II 467
bicipital groove 456
biological therapies 249
biomechanical
  assessment 80
biopsychosocial
  approach 99
bitolterol 306
black dot syndrome 327
black globe 186
black heel 327
black toe 327, 708
bladder rupture 551
bleeding 26
blinding 120
blisters 326
blood-borne infection
  control 317
blood doping 208
blood pressure 134
blood testing 144, 211
blood viscosity 134
body fat 143, 164, 378
body mass 143, 164
body mass index 143, 173
body temperature 182
bodyweight 173
boils 340
bones 58
  ankle 651
  biomechanics 59
  carpal 531
  density and osteoarthritis
    risk 360
  effect of physical
    activity 60
  functions 58
  lower limb and pelvic
    girdle 561–2
  mass 359
  metabolism 58
  shoulder girdle 457,
    459, 483
  tarsal 687
  types of 58

upper limb 457, 459
vertebrae 439, 459
see also fractures
boosting 225
Boutonniere deformity 538
bowel rupture 552
bowstring sign 429
boxer's fracture 534
boxer's knuckle 538
boxing 416
brachial plexus 470
Brugada syndrome 296
bruises 44
bulla 324
bursitis
  ischial (ischiogluteal) 612
  olecrannon 525
  radial head 525
  retrocalcaneal 683
  trochanteric 574

C

caffeine 200, 205
calcaneus
  fracture 686
  stress fracture 699
calcific tendinopathy of
  hip 608
calcific tendonitis of
  shoulder 495
calcium 59, 178
calcium channel
  blockers 262
calcium pyrophosphate
  crystals 245
calf muscles 655
calluses 326, 709
cancellous bone 58
capitellum, osteochondritis
  dissecans 514
capsaicin 238
carbohydrate 176, 202
carbohydrate loading 177
carbuncle 340
cardiac arrest 14, 17
cardiac arrhythmias 295
cardiac failure
  aetiology 286
  central
    haemodynamics 286
  classification 286
  clinical presentation 286
  definition 286
  drug treatment 288
  effects of exercise 290
  epidemiology 286
  exercise capacity 289
  exercise testing 289
  exercise training 291
  investigations 287
  left ventricular failure 286
  lifestyle modification 288

right ventricular failure 286
cardiac output 134
cardiac rehabilitation 265–6
cardiac tamponade 22
cardiac work 135
cardiopulmonary resuscitation, see resuscitation
cardiorespiratory fitness tests 76
cardiovascular drift 134
cardiovascular system
 ageing 378
 gender differences 165
 response to exercise 124, 132, 135
L-carnitine 204
carotid pulse 7
carpal bones 531
 dislocation 536
carpal tunnel syndrome 540
case–control studies 120
cauda equina syndrome 435
cellular recovery after exercise 172
cellulitis 342
centre of gravity 164
cercarial dermatitis 339
cerebral oedema 191
cerebral palsy 220–1
cervical radiculopathy 500
cervical spine
 disc herniation 434
 primary survey 4
 sideline assessment 388
cervicogenic headache 413
chain of survival 6, 18
Channel swimmers 183
chemical radiculitis 434
chest compressions 8, 10, 12
chest injuries 22
chicken pox 347
Chief Medical Officer 736
chilblains 334
children
 automated external defibrillators (AEDs) 12, 19
 body composition 169
 choking 25
 exercise prescription 170
 exercise testing 168
 first aid situations 2
 flexibility 169
 groin pain 586–7
 growth plate injuries 570, 594
 heat-related illness 187–8
 hip problems 614
 knee problems 644
 limbus vertebra 454
medial collateral ligament instability 508
 overweight and obese 116–17
 resistance training 166
 resuscitation 12–13
 Scheuermann's disease 446, 453
 skin-fold thickness 169
 spondylolysis and spondylolisthesis 443, 452
 sports injuries 62
 strategies to increase exercise by 118
 VO$_2$ max 168
 wrist problems 544
Chlamydia infection 240, 256
choking 24–5
cholinergic urticaria 333
chondroitin sulphate 238
choreo-athetoid cerebral palsy 221
chromium 204
chronic exertional compartment syndrome 677
chronic exertional leg pain 676
chronic traumatic encephalopathy 386
ciprofloxacin 321
citrullinated protein antibodies 243
clavicle
 fracture 489
 osteolysis 497
cleaning wounds 46
clinical epidemiology 120
clinical interventions 110
clunk test 468
coarctation of aorta 276
codeine 321
Code of Conduct 736
cold cures 200
cold-related injuries
 hypothermia 182
 skin 334
cold shock response 93
cold sore 348
cold therapy 41, 92
cold water immersion 92
Colles' fracture 532
community acquired methicillin-resistant *Staphylococcus aureus* 342
community interventions 110
compact bone 58
compartment syndrome
 anterior 678
 chronic exertional 677
 forearm 525
 lateral 679
 posterior 680
 pressure studies 680
competition medical meetings 730
compression 42
compression-only CPR 9
concentric exercise 70
concentric left ventricular hypertrophy 293
concussion, see sports concussion
concussive convulsions 397, 408
condyloma acuminatum 346
confidentiality 737
congenital adrenal hyperplasia 368
congenital heart disease 272–6
contemplators 107
continuous jump test 145
contraception 356
contractility 289
contusions 44
coolant sprays 41
Cooper 12 minute run test 150
core stability 90
coronary artery anomalies 293
coronary artery bypass 262
coronary artery disease 260
 aetiology 261
 exercise 263
 investigations 261
 pathophysiology 260
 physical inactivity 264
 secondary prevention 268
 sudden death 296
coronary heart disease
 clinical presentation 260
 treatment 262
cortical bone 58
costoclavicular manoeuvre 468
court abrasions 327
court shoes 693
COX2 inhibitors 50
crank test 468
C-reactive protein 242
creatine supplements 179, 203
cromolyn sodium 307
crossover test 467
cross-sectional studies 120
crowd doctor 738
cruciate ligaments 623
 anterior 626, 636
 posterior 626, 638

crusts 325
cryokinetics 660
cryotherapy 41, 92
crystal arthropathy 254 see also gout; pseudogout
cuboid syndrome 703
cuts 44
cycle ergometer test
  maximal 150
  sub-maximal 148–9
cytomegalovirus (CMV) 315

D

dactylitis 256
daily stretching 66
Dal Monte sprint test 145
deaflympics 216
deep vein thrombosis 225
dementia pugilistica 416
dependent oedema 225
De Quervain's tenosynovitis 541
dermatology 323–49
  abscesses 340
  acne vulgaris 340
  ageing skin 378
  atopic dermatitis 331
  bacterial infections 340
  blisters 326
  boils 340
  calluses 326, 709
  carbuncles 340
  cellulitis 342
  cercarial dermatitis (swimmer's itch) 339
  chilblains 334
  cholinergic urticaria 333
  cold-induced urticaria 335
  cold-related injuries 334
  cold sore 348
  community acquired MRSA 342
  condyloma acuminatum (genital warts) 346
  court abrasions 327
  erysipelas 342
  erythrasma 343
  felon 343
  folliculitis 341
  friction-related problems 326
  frostbite 334
  frostnip 334
  fungal infections 336
  furuncle 340
  heat-related problems 330
  herpes gladiatorum (traumatic herpes) 349
  herpes labialis 348
  herpes simplex virus 348
  herpes zoster 348
  hyperhidrosis 332
  impetigo (ecthyma) 341
  intertrigo 339
  miliaria rubra 331
  molluscum contagiosum (water warts) 347
  onychocryptosis 343
  paronychia 343
  photodermatitis 331
  piezogenic pedal papules 329
  pitted keratolysis 343
  plantar petechiae 327
  shingles 348
  striae distensae 329
  sub-ungual haematoma 327, 708
  sunburn 330
  terminology 324
  tinea corporis (ringworm/ scrum pox) 337
  tinea cruris (jock itch) 336
  tinea gladiatorum 337
  tinea pedis (athlete's foot) 336
  tinea unguium (onychomycosis) 338
  tinea versicolor (pityriasis versicolor) 338
  turf burns 327
  varicella (chicken pox) 347
  verruca 346, 709
  viral infections 346
  warts 346
  xerosis 332
dermatomes 563
determinants of physical activity 102
diarrhoea 320, 553
diet 176
dietary supplements 177, 202
diffuse cerebral swelling 404
disability (primary survey) 4
disabled athletes 213–26
  amputees 220
  barriers to physical activity 215
  boosting 225
  cerebral palsy 220–1
  choosing a sport 214
  classification groups for competition 219–21
  deaflympics 216
  definition of disability 214
  doping issues 226
  elite sport talent identification and profiling 224

history of sports participation 214
  injury issues 224
  intellectual disability 222
  les autres 222
  limb deficiency 220
  organization of sport 216
  Paralympic Games 216
  prosthetic limbs 218
  recommended levels of physical activity 214
  Special Olympics 217
  spinal cord-related disability 220
  technological advances 218
  thermoregulation 224
  travel issues 225
  visual impairment 222
  wheelchairs 218
  Winter Paralympic Games 217
disc
  degeneration 434
  herniation 433–4
disease-modifying agents
  inflammatory arthritis 248
  osteoarthritis 239
dislocation
  biceps tendon 488
  carpal 536
  elbow 516
  1st metacarpophalangeal joint 536
  hip joint 607
  interphalangeal joints 537
  lunate 536
  patella 641
  scapholunate 536
  shoulder 472–82
distal biceps
  tear/rupture 516
  tendinopathy 522
distal interphalangeal joint dislocation 537
distal radial physeal stress injury 544
documentation 33
doping 206
  disabled athletes 226
dose–response curve 98
drop arm test 466
drop sign 467
drowning 32
DRS ABC 4
drugs
  basic drugs list for team physician 718
  performance-enhancing 198
  prescribing for athletes 208
  prohibited drugs 207

therapeutic use exemption (TUE) 201
drug testing 210, 729
dry bulb 186
dry powder inhalation test 304
dynamic stability 72
dynamic stretching 66
dysautonomic cephalgia 410
dysmenorrhoea 355

E

eating disorders/distress 358
eccentric exercise 70
eccentric patellar tendon loading 90
ecthyma 341
education
 osteoarthritis management 236
 sports concussion 386
 team education 723
effort headache 414
ejection fraction 289
elbow
 acute injuries 516
 chronic injuries 522
 dislocation 516
 examination 504–5
 history 504
 inspection 504
 lateral condylar fracture 518
 lateral epicondylitis 506, 510
 lateral pain 525
 medial collateral ligament injury 507
 medial collateral ligament instability 508
 medial epicondylitis 506, 512
 Monteggia fracture 520
 osteochondritis dissecans 514
 palpation 504
 Panner's disease 515
 radial head bursitis 525
 radial head and neck fracture 518
 special tests 506
 supracondylar fracture 518
 traction apophysitis medial humeral epicondyle (Little Leaguers' elbow) 509
electromechanical dissociation 14–15
electron transport chain 127

electrophysical therapies 84
elevation 42
empty can test 466
endurance 128, 130
energy 126, 174
energy expenditure for activity 174
enteric arthritis 256
enthesitis 256
environment
 body metabolism 182
 determinant of physical activity 102
epidemiology 120
epilepsy 397, 408–9
Epstein-Barr virus 315
ergogenic aids 198–202
ER lag sign 467
erysipelas 342
erythema nodosum 257
erythrasma 343
erythrocyte sedimentation rate (ESR) 242
erythropoietin 199
ethical issues 736
eucapnic voluntary hyperpnoea 201, 304
event management 38
event organization 738
exercise
 advice on starting 97
 at altitude 188
 benefits 270
 capacity measurement 142
 cellular recovery after 172
 energy for 126
 environmental conditions 182
 food 176
 in heat 186
 immunity 312
 intensity and type of in specific sports 298
 menstrual cycle 352, 355
 muscle adaptation to 78
 negative interpretation of term 97
 physiological response to 124
 recovery after 180
 strategies to increase exercise in children 118
exercise-induced anaphylaxis 305
exercise-induced asthma 201, 300
exercise-induced bronchoconstriction 300
 aetiology 300
 albuterol 306

 anti-doping rules 308
 bitolterol 306
 bronchodilator test 302
 clinical clues 303
 clinical presentation 301
 cromolyn sodium 307
 definition 300
 diagnosis 302
 differential diagnosis 304
 dry powder inhalation test 304
 epidemiology 300
 eucapnic voluntary hyperpnoea 201, 304
 exercise challenge 137, 144, 201, 303
 exercise programmes 306
 formoterol 307
 general management principles 308
 glucocorticosteroids 306
 histamine challenge 302
 history 302
 hyperosmolar saline test 304
 ipratropium bromide 307
 isocapnic hyperventilation test 304
 late phase reaction 302
 leukotriene inhibitors 307
 long-acting beta2 agonists 307
 mannitol test 304
 mast cell stabilizers 307
 metaproterenol 306
 methacholine challenge 302
 monitoring lung function 308
 montelukast 307
 nedocromyl sodium 307
 nutrition 306
 osmotic challenge tests 304
 prevention 308
 pulmonary function tests 144, 302
 refractory period 302
 salbutamol 306
 salmeterol 307
 short-acting beta2 agonists 306
 sports associated with 300
 stimulants contributing to 303
 terbutaline 306
 theophylline 307
 treatment 305
 zafirlukast 307
 zileuton 307
exercise induced rhabdomyolysis 556

exercise referral 270
exercise testing
  adult congenital heart disease 272
  children 168
  heart failure 289
  older people 380
exercise therapy 83
experimental studies 120
exposure 4
extensor carpi ulnaris tendinopathy 542
external rotation test 653
external rotator test 466
extracranial vascular headache 410
extradural haematoma 402
eye injuries 421

F

Faber test 566
Fallot's tetralogy 276
falls 68
Fartlek training 163
fast twitch fibres 77, 129
fast twitch oxidative-glycolytic fibres 77, 129
fat pad contusion 688
fat pad impingement 641
FEF_{25-75} 301
felon 343
female athletes, see women
female athletic triad 60, 358
femoral neck stress fracture 572
femoral nerve test 429
femoral shaft fractures 568
femoroacetabular impingement 610, 617
FEV_1 301
FEV_1/FVC 301
fibrodysplasia ossificans progressiva 580
fibula, stress fracture 677
fingers, see wrist and hand
Finkelstein's test 541
first aid 2
  general approach to athlete 3
  primary survey 4
  required number of first aiders 738
  roles and responsibilities of first aiders 2
  venue facilities 3
1st metacarpophalangeal joint dislocation 536
fish oils 204
Fitch test 429, 438
fitness 125, 378
fitness tests 76
FITT principle 97

flat bones 58
flexibility 90, 125, 143, 164, 169
flexibility exercises 376
flexor hallucis longus tendinopathy 672
folliculitis 341
Fontan circulation 277
food 176
food supplements 177, 202
foot 685–709
  calluses 326, 709
  cuboid syndrome 703
  extensor tendinopathy 698
  fat pad contusion 688
  fractures 701, 686–7
  hallux rigidus (footballer's toe) 690
  ingrowing toenail 343, 708
  Lisfranc fracture: dislocation 688
  medial plantar nerve entrapment 699
  metatarsalgia 702
  midtarsal joint sprain 689
  Morton's neuroma 702
  os naviculare syndrome 704
  piezogenic pedal papules 329
  pitted keratolysis 343
  plantar fasciitis 696
  plantar petechiae 327
  sesamoid injury 703
  stress fractures 700
  subungual haematoma 327, 708
  tarsal coalition 706
  tinea pedis 336
  turf toe 689
  verrucae 346, 709
football boots 693
footballer's ankle 674
footballer's migraine 410
footballer's toe 690
footwear 237, 693
forearm
  compartment syndrome 525
  muscles 517, 519
formoterol 307
fractures
  ankle 658, 667
  back 433
  Bennett's 534
  boxer's 534
  calcaneus 686
  clavicle 489
  Colles' fracture 532
  distal radius/ulna 532
  femoral shaft 568

hamate 533
Jones fracture 701
lateral condylar 518
Lisfranc fracture: dislocation 688
Maisonneuve fracture 667
mandibular 420
metacarpal bones 534
metatarsals 687
Monteggia 520
nasal 420
phalangeal 535
physeal 570
pisiform 534
Pott's fracture 667
proximal humerus 489
radial head and neck 518
scaphoid 532
scapular 489
skull 420
supracondylar 518
zygomatic 420
see also stress fractures
free radicals 172
Freiberg's disease 707
frostbite 334
frostnip 334
frozen shoulder 496
fulcrum test 464
functional performance tests 76
fungal skin infections 336
furuncle 340
FVC 301

G

gait analysis 85, 694
gait cycle 691
gamekeepers' thumb 539
ganglion 542
gas exchange 137
gender
  osteoarthritis risk 229
  performance and 164
  verification 368
gene doping 209
genital warts 346
Gerber's lift off test 466
Gillet test 429
Gilmore's groin 585
glandular fever 315, 549
Glasgow Coma Scale 392
glenohumeral joint 456, 458, 465
  dislocation 472
  instability 472, 490
  stability testing 464
glenoid labrum tears 486
Global Advocacy for Physical Activity (GAPA) 109
globe perforation 421

globe temperature 186
glucocorticosteroids 306
glucosamine 238
glutamine 204
golfers' elbow, see medial epicondylitis
gout 245, 254
grazes 44
greater tuberosity of the humerus 456
groin
  hernia 585
  pain 586, 587
growth hormone 199
growth plate injuries 570, 594

H

haematin 556
haematocrit (Hct) 135
haematoma 44
haematuria 550, 555
haemochromatosis 230, 243
haemoglobin 138–9
haemoglobinuria 556
haemothorax 22
hallux rigidus (footballer's toe) 690
hamate fracture 533
hamstring injury 598
  conservative treatment 598
  history and examination 598
  physiotherapy 599
  predisposing factors 598
  prevention 600
  rehabilitation programme 602
  return to play 600, 605
  surgical management 599
hand, see wrist and hand
Hawkin's sign 466
headache 412
  post-traumatic 410
headache overlap syndrome 410
head injuries
  advice card 405
  boxing-related 416
  diffuse cerebral swelling 404
  extradural haematoma 402
  fractures 420
  indications for CT 396
  intracerebral haematoma 400
  prevention 385
  scalp wounds 397
  subarachnoid haemorrhage 403
  subdural haematoma 401
  traumatic brain injury 395
  see also sports concussion
head protectors 407
health and physical activity 98
heart block 295
heart failure, see cardiac failure
heart rate 133
heart rate monitors 135
heart valve disease 294
heat acclimatization 186
heat loss 182
heat-related problems
  hyperthermia 184
  illness in children 187–8
  skin 330
heatstroke 184
height, see stature
helmets 407
hepatitis A 316, 724
hepatitis B 316–17
hepatitis C 316–17
hernia 585
herpes gladiatorum 349
herpes labialis 348
herpes simplex virus 348
herpes zoster 348
hidradenitis suppurativa 332
high altitude 188
high-fat diet 176
Hill–Sach's lesion 472
hip and pelvis 559–617
  acetabular labral tears 609
  active and passive movements 560
  avulsion fracture 615
  avulsions around ilium 594
  calcific tendinopathy 608
  dislocation and subluxation 607
  dysplasia 616
  examination 560–2
  femoral neck stress fracture 572
  femoroacetabular impingement 610, 617
  growth plate injuries 570
  inspection 560
  irritable 615
  ischial (ischiogluteal) bursitis 612
  loose bodies 611
  movements, muscles and innervation 564
  myositis ossificans 578, 580
  obturator nerve entrapment 606
  osteoarthritis 232, 582
  paediatric problems 614
  palpation 560
  piriformis syndrome 567, 595
  pubic bone stress injury 584
  rehabilitation of over-use injuries 588, 592–3
  resurfacing 583
  slipped upper capital femoral epiphysis 614
  snapping hip syndrome 596
  special tests 566
  sports hernia 585
  traction apophysitis of the ischial tuberosity 616
  trochanteric bursitis 574
histamine challenge 302
historical cohort studies 120
'hitting the wall' 127
HIV 317
HLA-B27 449
HMB 204
Hoffa's syndrome 641
holding camp 733
hormones
  menstrual cycle 352
  placental 362
  response to exercise 124
hot tub folliculitis 341
H-substance 49
humanistic approach 99
humerus
  bony landmarks 456
  epiphysiolitis 494
  fracture of proximal humerus 489
hyaluronic joint injections 238
hyperabduction manoeuvre 468
hyperbaric oxygen therapy 139
hyperhidrosis 332
hypermobility 230
hyperosmolar saline test 304
hypertension
  aetiology 282
  diagnosis 282
  exercise capacity 284
  natural history and prognosis 283
  prevalence 282
  symptoms and signs 283
  treatment 284
hyperthermia 184

hypertrophic
cardiomyopathy 292
hypothermia 182
hypoxia 189

I

ice therapy 41
ilio-tibial band
assessment 567, 627
ilio-tibial band friction
syndrome 627, 641
ilio-tibial band
syndrome 576
ilium, avulsions around 594
immediate energy 126
immunization 724
impaction syndromes 543
impact seizures 397
impetigo 341
impingement (syndrome)
ankle 658, 669, 674–5
femoroacetabular 610, 617
rotator cuff 486, 490, 493
impingement sign 465
impingement test 466
impulse energy 126
incident reports 2
infection 311–21
common viral
infections 315
control of blood-borne
infections 317
effects of exercise on
immunity 312
increased risk in
athletes 313
skin, see under
dermatology
transmission risk during
CPR 7
upper respiratory
tract 314
infectious
mononucleosis 315, 549
inflammation 48
inflammatory arthritis 240, 251
biological therapies 249
blood tests 242
Chlamydia infection 240, 256
crystal arthopathy 254
see also gout; pseudogout
dactylitis 256
disease-modifying
drugs 248
enteric arthritis 256
enthesitis 256
examination 241
history 240
investigations 242

joint rehabilitation 250
management 248
monoarthritis 250
multidisciplinary care 250
oligoarthritis 250
psoriatic arthritis 256
radiology 243
reactive arthritis 256
red flags 240, 257
rheumatoid arthritis 252
septic arthritis 246, 499
seronegative 251, 256
spondyloarthropathy 250
steroid therapy 249
synovial fluid analysis 244
synovitis management 248
inflammatory
response 48–9
informed sport 202
in-growing toenail 343, 708
insurance 720, 737
intellectual disability 222
intensity of exercise 298
interdigital neuroma 702
interferential therapy 84
internal bleeding 27
international governing
body check lists 739
International Liaison
Committee on
Resuscitation (ILCOR) 7
International Paralympic
Committee (IPC) 216
interphalangeal joint
dislocation 537
intersection syndrome 541
intersex 368
intertrigo 339
interventions, increasing
physical activity 110
intracerebral
haematoma 400
intradiscal electrothermal
annuloplasty 434
intraosseous access 16
intravenous access 16
intrinsic asthma 300, 308
'Investments that work for
physical activity' 109
ipratropium bromide 307
IR lag sign 469
iron
deficiency 144
endurance athletes 137
normal requirements 178, 204
iron deficiency anaemia 178
irregular bones 58
irritable hip 615
ischaemic necrosis 500
ischial (ischiogluteal)
bursitis 612
ischial tuberosity

avulsion 594
traction apophysitis 616
Iselin's disease 705
isocapnic hyperventilation
test 304
iso-inertial strength
measurement 146
isokinetic contraction 78
isokinetic strength
measurement 147
isometric contraction 78
isometric strength
measurement 146
isotonic contraction 78
isotonic strength
measurement 146

J

jaw thrust 7
jersey finger 538
jet lag 725
Jobe's manoeuvre 466
jock itch 336
joint hypermobility 230
joint pain 233
joint rehabilitation 236, 250
joint stability, static and
dynamic 72
Jones fracture 701
jumper's knee 643, 645
juvenile idiopathic
arthritis 647
juvenile osteochondritis
dissecans 645

K

Kibler test 468
kidney trauma 550
Kienbock's disease 545
kit bags
hand luggage for team
travel 724
medical kit bag 714
touchline kit bag 715
knee 619–47
active and passive
movements 624
anterior cruciate
ligament 626, 636
anterior pain 640
articular cartilage
injuries 639
bipartite patella 646
discoid lateral
meniscus 646
examination 622, 623
fat pad impingement 641
history 620
ilio-tibial band friction
syndrome 627, 641

inspection 622–3
investigations 628
jumper's knee 643, 645
lateral collateral
  ligament 626, 635
medial collateral
  ligament 54, 626,
  629–30, 634
meniscal injuries 627, 639
osteoarthritis 232
paediatrics 644
palpation 624
patellar dislocation 641
patellar tendinopathy 643
patellar tracking 642
patellofemoral pain
  syndrome 642, 646
posterior cruciate
  ligament 626, 638
resisted movements 624
special tests 626
Kohler's disease 708

L

labral tears 467, 566
Lachman's test 626
lactate response
  profiling 155
lactate threshold 140–1
lactate threshold
  training 154
lactic acid 205
Lasegue test 429
laser therapy 84
lateral collateral ligament
  tests 626, 635
lateral compartment
  syndrome 679
lateral condylar
  fracture 518
lateral epicondylitis 506,
  510
L-carnitine 204
left ventricular failure 286
left ventricular
  hypertrophy 283
  concentric 293
Leger and Lambert 20m
  shuttle test 150
leg length discrepancy 80,
  560
legs, see lower limb
les autres 222
leucocytes 49
leukotriene inhibitors 307
lichenification 325
lift off test 466
ligaments 54
  ankle 657
  shoulder girdle 483
limb deficiency 220
limbus vertebra 454

Lisfranc
  fracture:dislocation 688
Little Leaguer's elbow 509
Little Leaguer's
  shoulder 494
liver damage 549
load 78
load and shift test 464
loading 159
long-acting beta2
  agonists 307
long bones 58
long-term energy 127
loose bodies 611
loperamide 321
lower limb
  bones 561–2
  dermatomes 563
  muscles 579, 655
  nerve roots 565
  thigh contusion 578
  see also ankle; foot; knee
Ludwig's angina 342
lunate dislocation 536
lung function tests 136,
  143, 301
lung volumes 136
luxatio erecta 473
Lyme disease 315

M

McMurray's test 627
macrominerals 177
macule 324
Maddocks questions 388
magnesium 204
maintainers 107
Maisonneuve fracture 667
major emergencies 23
major incident plan 739
malaria 318
mallet finger 537
management meetings 730
mandibular fractures 420
manipulation 83
mannitol test 304
manual therapy 82
marathon running 127
Marfan syndrome 278, 293
Margaria stair climbing
  test 145
Martin Gruber
  anastamosis 522, 524
mast cell stabilizers 307
maximal cycle ergometer
  test 150
maximal oxygen uptake
  (VO_2 max) 140, 168
maximum accumulated
  oxygen deficit 146
media issues 740
medial collateral ligament

elbow 507–8
knee 54, 626, 629–30, 634
medial epicondylitis 506,
  512
medial humeral epicondyle
  traction apophysitis 509
medial ligament injuries 665
medial plantar nerve
  entrapment 673, 699
medial tibial stress
  syndrome 677
mediators 49
medical bag 714, 724
medical equipment, basic
  requirements 716
medical records 33, 728
medical risk assessment 714
melatonin 725
menarche 353
meniscal injuries 627, 639
  discoid lateral
    meniscus 646
menstrual cycle 352
  amenorrhoea 352–3, 355
  dysmenorrhoea 355
  effects of exercise 352,
    355
  irregularities 354, 357
  manipulation 357
  menarche 353
  oligomenorrhoea 352
  polymenorrhoea 352
  premenstrual
    syndrome 356
mental fitness 125
metabolic response to
  exercise 124
metacarpal fractures 534
metaproterenol 306
metatarsal fractures 687,
  701
metatarsalgia 702
methacholine challenge 302
methicillin-resistant
  *Staphylococcus
  aureus* 342
microminerals 177
migraine 410, 413
miliaria rubra 331
military brace position 468
minerals 177
minute ventilation 137
mitral valve prolapse 295
mixed-type cerebral
  palsy 221
modafinil 200
molluscum
  contagiosum 347
monoarthritis 250
Monteggia fracture 520
montelukast 307
Morton's neuroma 702
motor units 77

mouthguards 406
mouth to nose ventilation 10
MRSA 342
Mulder's click 702
muscles
  adaptation to exercise 78
  ageing 78, 378
  arm 517, 519
  cellular adaptation 172
  contractions 78
  endurance 130
  excitation-contraction coupling 129
  fibre types 77, 129
  function 130
  gender differences 164
  hip joint 564
  lower limb 579, 655
  motor units 77
  power 130
  repair and recovery 172
  shoulder girdle and back 427
  strength 130
  tension s 78
  training 78
musculoskeletal screening/profiling 87
Mustard repair 276
myelography 430
myocarditis 294
myoglobin 138-9
myoglobinuria 556
myosin filaments 129
myositis ossificans 578, 580
myositis ossificans progressiva 580

N

nasal fractures 420
navicular stress fracture 700
near-drowning 32
neck check 314
neck muscle conditioning 407
nedocromil sodium 307
Neer's sign 465
nerve entrapment
  medial plantar nerve 673, 699
  obturator nerve 606
nerve entrapment syndrome 680
neuromuscular control training 90
neuromuscular coordination 125
neuropsychological assessment 389
neutrophils 49

nicorandil 262
nitrates 262
nodal osteoarthritis 232
nodule 324
non-shockable rhythms 14-15
non-ST elevation myocardial infarction (non-STEMI) 260
non-steroidal anti-inflammatory drugs (NSAIDs) 50, 239
  topical 51, 237
Nordic (Norwegian) hamstring curls 89, 604

O

Ober's test 567, 627
obesity
  children 116-17
  osteoarthritis risk 229
O'Brien test 468
observational studies 120
obturator nerve entrapment 606
O'Donoghue's triad 629
older people 371-81
  aerobic exercise 375
  evidence for adopting exercise 372
  exercise testing 380
  fitness deterioration 378
  flexibility/balance exercise 376
  primary prevention 373
  resistance exercise 375
  secondary prevention 373
  successful ageing 372
olecrannon bursitis 525
oligoarthritis 250
oligomenorrhoea 352
omega-3 oils 204
one-legged hyperextension 429
onychocryptosis 343
onychomycosis 338
opiate analgesia 239
oral contraceptive pill 356
orgasmic cephalgia 414
orthotics 81, 237
Osgood-Schlatter disease 644
osmotic challenge tests 304
os naviculare syndrome 704
osteitis pubis 584
osteoarthritis 228
  acupuncture 237
  age 229
  bone density 230
  capsaicin 238
  chondroitin sulphate 238
  compound analgesia 238

definition 228
diet 237
disease-modifying agents 239
examination 231
exercise and sport 230
exercise prescription 236
footwear 237
gender 229
glucosamine 238
hand 231
heritability 229
hip 232, 582
history 230
hyaluronic joint injections 238
hypermobility 230
joint rehabilitation 236
joint shape 229
knee 232
local risk factors 228
management 236
nodal 232
non-pharmacological management 236
NSAIDs 237, 239
obesity 229
occupation 229
opiate analgesia 239
orthotics 237
pain 230
paracetamol 238
pathogenesis 228
patient education 236
pharmacological management 237-8
plain X-rays 233
prevalence 228
RICES 237
smoking 230
spine 232
steroid joint injections 238
surgical treatment 239
synovitis 231
systemic illness 230
systemic risk factors 229
walking aids 237
weight management 236
osteochondritis dissecans 514
  juvenile 645
osteochondroses 62
osteogenesis 359
osteoid osteoma 257
osteolysis, distal clavicle 497
osteonecrosis, shoulder 500
osteoporosis 59, 358
otitis externa 317
overhead exercise test 469
overload 152

INDEX

overtraining syndrome 124, 194
overuse injuries 36
  hip and pelvis 588, 592–3
  shoulder 490, 493
overweight, see obesity
oxidative phosphorylation 127
oxygen consumption 140
oxygen free radicals 172
oxygen transport 138–9

P

paediatrics, see children
pain 49
pancreatic damage 549
Panner's disease 515
Panton-Valentine leukocidin (PVL) 317
papule 324
paracetamol 238
Paralympic Games 216–17
paronychia 343
pars interarticularis 438, 442
patella
  bipartite 646
  dislocation 641
  tendinopathy 643
  tracking 642
patellofemoral pain syndrome 642, 646
patient confidentiality 737
peak expiratory flow rate (PEFR) 301
pelvic girdle 561–2
pelvic pain 366
pelvis, see hip and pelvis
percutaneous coronary interventions 262
perforated globe 421
performance-enhancing drugs 198
pernio 334
peroneal tendinopathy 668
personality 103
Perthes' disease 614
phagocytosis 48
phalangeal fracture 535
Phalen's test 540
phenotypic sex disorders 368
phospho-creatine system 126
photodermatitis 331
physeal fractures 570
physical activity 97
  determinants 102
  disability 214
  effect on bones 60
  health and 98

humanistic/biopsychosocial approach to 99
  increasing participation in 109
  interventions 110
  recommended levels 98, 270
physical environment 102
physical inactivity 96, 100, 264
physiological response to exercise 124
physiotherapy 82
piezogenic pedal papules 325
pigmented villonodular synovitis 257
piriformis syndrome 567, 595
piriformis test 566
pisiform fracture 534
pitted keratolysis 343
pityriasis versicolor 338
pivot shift test 627
placental hormones 362
plantar fasciitis 696
plantar petechiae 327
plantar warts 346
plaque 325
plyometrics 70
pneumothorax 22
POLICE 40
policy 103
polycystic ovary syndrome 354
polymenorrhoea 352
polymorphs 49
Popeye defect 487
popliteal artery entrapment 680
post-concussion syndrome 418
posterior apprehension 464
posterior compartment syndrome 680
posterior cruciate ligament 626, 638
posterior draw test 626
posterior element injury 438–9
posterior element pain 426
posterior impingement sign 466
posterior impingement syndrome 675
post-traumatic epilepsy 397, 408
post-traumatic headache 410
post-traumatic migraine 410
Pott's fracture 667

power 130, 146
pre-activity stretching 66
precontemplators 107
precordial thump 14
pre-event diet 177
pre-event meal 177
pregnancy 362
prehabilitation 56, 89
preload 289
premenstrual syndrome 356
preparers 107
pre-participation screening for sudden death 292
prescribing for athletes 208
pressure epiphyses 594
prevention of injuries 86
PRICES 40
prickly heat 331
primary amenorrhoea 353
primary angioplasty 262
primary survey 4
Prime test 506
probiotics 43
professional issues 736
profiling 87
progression 152
prohibited drugs 207
prolonged QT syndrome 296
pronation 692
pronator syndrome 523
proprioception 68
proprioneurofacilitation 71
prospective cohort studies 120
prostaglandins 49
prosthetic limbs 218
protect 40
protective equipment
  head injury prevention 385
  helmets and head protectors 407
  mouthguards 406
  risk compensation 385
protein 176, 202
proteinuria 554
proximal interphalangeal joint dislocation 537
pseudoanaemia 134, 178
pseudogout 231, 245, 254
pseudonephritis 554
psoriatic arthritis 256
psychological component of fitness 125
pubic bone, stress injury 584
pubic rami, stress fracture 608
pulmonary function tests 136, 143, 301
pulmonary oedema 191

pulmonary stenosis 276
pulseless electrical activity 14–15
pulseless ventricular tachycardia 14
punch drunk syndrome 416
pure gonadal dysgenesis 368
pustule 324
PWC170 test 148-9

Q

Q' angle 642
QT prolongation 296

R

radial head
  bursitis 525
  osteochondritis dissecans 514
radial head and neck fracture 518
radial nerve lesions 524
radial tunnel syndrome 541
radio-ulnar joint 527
randomization 120
range of passive movement 80
reactive arthritis 256
record keeping 33, 728
recovery after exercise 180
recruitment 77
rectus abdominus rupture 548
reflex sympathetic dystrophy 499
rehabilitation, principles 74
relapse 107
relative humidity 186
relative rest 40
relaxin 362
relocation test 464
renal failure, acute 556
renal physiology 554
renal trauma 550
rescue breaths 9
resistance 78
resistance exercise 158, 166, 375
resistance reaction 124
respiratory-derived anaerobic threshold 141
respiratory system
  ageing 378
  response to exercise 124, 136–7, 139
rest 40, 152
resuscitation
  adult basic life support 6, 11
  advanced adult life support 14, 17
  automated external defibrillators (AEDs) 12, 18, 21
  children 12–13
retrocalcaneal bursitis 683
retrospective studies 120
return to play
  acute injuries 39
  bleeding injuries 26
  concussion 389
  hamstring injury 600, 605
  renal trauma 550
  shoulder dislocation 480
  wounds 47
rhabdomyolysis, exercised-induced 556
rheumatoid arthritis 252
right ventricular dysplasia 294
right ventricular failure 286
ringworm 337
risk assessment 714
risk compensation 385
Roos test 469
rotator cuff 456
  impingement 486, 490, 493
  tears 492, 493
  testing 466
rule changes, concussion prevention 407
runner's knee, see ilio-tibial band friction syndrome
runner's toe 327, 708
runner's trots 553
running shoes 693

S

sacro-iliac joint 447, 613
sag test 638
salbutamol 201, 306
Salmeterol 201, 307
Salter–Harris classification 570
sarcomeres 129
sartorius avulsion 594
scales 325
scalp wounds 397
scaphoid fracture 532
scapholunate dislocation 536
scapular fracture 489
scapulothoracic joint 456
scarf sign 467
SCAT2 388, 390
Scheuermann's disease 446, 453
Schmorl's nodes 446, 454
Schrober's test 426, 429
sciatica 434
sciatic nerve tests 429
Scottie Dog sign 430
screening
  ligament injuries 56
  musculoskeletal 87
  pre-participation screening for sudden death 292
scrotal injuries 551
scrum pox 337
scuba diving 300, 356
secondary amenorrhoea 352
secondary survey 22
second impact syndrome 385
security 720
seed oils 204
seizures 397, 408–9
septic arthritis 246, 499
sesamoid injury 703
Sever's disease 704
sex chromosome disorders 368
sex development disorders 368
shingles 348
shin splints 676
shock 26
shockable rhythms 14
short-acting beta2 agonists 306
short bones 58
short-term energy 126
shoulder 455–501
  acromioclavicular degenerative joint disease 496
  acromioclavicular joint separations 484
  active and passive movements 462
  acute trauma 472
  adhesive capsulitis (frozen shoulder) 496
  anatomy 456–7, 459
  articulations 456
  bursae 458
  calcific tendonitis 495
  causes of disorders 471
  cervical radiculopathy 500
  differential diagnosis of disorders 471
  dislocation 472–82
  epidemiology of disorders 471
  examination 462–3
  fractures 489
  glenoid labrum tears 486
  history 460
  inspection 462
  ligaments 483
  muscles 427
  nerves 470

osteolysis of distal clavicle 497
osteonecrosis 500
over-use disorders 490, 493
palpation 462–3
proximal humeral epiphysiolisis (Little Leaguer's shoulder) 494
referred pain 501
reflex sympathetic dystrophy 499
septic arthritis 499
SLAP lesion 486
special tests 464–5
sternoclavicular joint separations 485
tumours 500
shoulder-hand syndrome 499
side strain 557
Sinding–Larsen–Johannsen disease 645
single leg standing 90
single stage jog test 148
single stage walk test 148
sinus tarsi syndrome 658, 668
sit and reach test 143
six minute walk test 289
skeletal muscle, see muscles
skier's thumb 539
skill 125
skin, see dermatology
skin-fold thickness 169
skull fractures 420
SLAP lesion 486
slipped disc (herniation) 433–4
slipped upper capital femoral epiphysis 614
slow twitch fibres 77, 129
slug nutty 416
slump test 429
snapping hip syndrome 596
soccer specific tests 151
social environment 102
sodium bicarbonate 205
soft tissue inflammation 36
soft tissue injuries 40
solar purpura 331
solar urticaria 331
spastic cerebral palsy 220
Special Olympics 217
specific adaptations to imposed demand (SAID) principle 70
speed 125
Speed's test 467
spinal cord-related disability 220
spine 423–54

active and passive movements 426
acute injury 432
ankylosing spondylitis 448
disc disease 434
examination 426–8
fractures 433
history taking 424
immobilizing spine 432
inspection 426
investigations 430
limbus vertebra 454
neurological examination 426
osteoarthritis 232
palpation 426
pars interarticularis 438, 442
primary survey 4
red flags 424
sacro-iliac joint 447
Scheuermann's disease 446, 453
sideline assessment 388
special tests 429
spondyloarthropathy 250
spondylolisthesis 442, 452
spondylolysis 438, 443, 452
see also back
spiromentry pre- and post-exercise challenge 201
splenic bleeding 549
spondyloarthropathy 250
spondylolisthesis 442, 452
spondylolysis 438, 443, 452
spongy bone 58
sports concussion 384
acute concussion management 388
balance testing 389
education 386
history and examination 384
long-term problems 386
Maddocks questions 388
management algorithm 392–3
neck muscle conditioning 407
neuropsychological assessment 389
return to play 389
rule changes 407
SCAT2 388, 390
severity grading 389
sideline evaluation 388
symptoms 384
sports hernia 585
sports injuries
acute soft tissue injuries 40
children 62

clinical examination 39
disabled athletes 224
general management of acute injuries 36, 38
history taking 38
initial management 36
prevention 86
return to play 39
women 370
sports-specific fitness tests 76
sprains 52
ankle 653, 656–7, 660, 665
back 433
midtarsal joint 689
sprint training 162
squeeze test 653
stable angina pectoris 260
stamina 125
Standardized Concussion Assessment Tool 2 (SCAT2) 388, 390
Staphylococcus aureus, methicillin-resistant 342
starting exercise 97
static stability 72
stature 143, 164, 378
ST elevation myocardial infarction (STEMI) 260
Stener lesion 539
sternoclavicular joint 456
separations 485
steroids
anabolic steroids 198, 341
exercise-induced bronchoconstriction 307
folliculitis 341
inflammatory arthritis 249
osteoarthritis 238
stimulants 200
stinky foot 343
stork test 438
straight leg raise 88, 429
strains 52
back 433
strapping 72
strength 125, 130, 146
strength training 79, 89
stress fracture 59
anterior tibia 676
calcaneus 699
cuboid 703
femoral neck 572
fibula 677
lower leg 676–7
metatarsals 701
navicular 700
pubic rami 608
stress reaction 124
stretching 66
stretch marks 329
stretch-shortening cycle 70

striae distensae 329
stroke volume 133
subacromial bursa 458
subarachnoid haemorrhage 403
subcoracoid bursa 458
subdeltoid bursa 458
subdural haematoma 401
sub-maximal cycle ergometer test 148–9
sub-maximal two-stage jog test 148–9
subscapular bursa 458, 469
subungual haematoma 327, 708
successful ageing 372
sudden death 292
sulcus sign 464
sunburn 330
sun poisoning 331
superior labrum anterior to posterior (SLAP) lesion 486
supination 692
suppleness 125
support 42
supracondylar fractures 518
sweating, excessive 332
swelling 48
swimmer's itch 339
sympathomimetics 200
syndesmosis injury 666
synovial fluid analysis 244
synovitis
 inflammatory arthritis 248
 osteoarthritis 231
 pigmented villonodular 257

T

talar tilt test 653
talon noir 327
taping 72
tarsal bones 687
tarsal coalition 706
tarsal tunnel syndrome 672, 698
team physician 712
 drug and medication provision 718
 drug testing 729
 ethical issues 736
 holding camp 733
 insurance issues 720, 737
 list of basic medical equipment 716
 maintaining focus 734
 management meetings 730
 managing the medical service 728
 medical consultations 728
 medical kit bag 714
 medical review 729
 medical risk assessment 714
 multi-sports events 732
 patient confidentiality 737
 precompetition orientation 730
 prescribing for athletes 208
 professional issues 736
 record keeping 728
 rest and relaxation 734
 return home 735
 security issues 720
 touchline kit bag 715
 welcome meeting 729
team travel
 disabled athletes 225
 immunization and vaccination 724
 jet lag 725
 journey home 735
 medical kit for journey 724
 medical preparation 722
 medical room provision 725
 medical team selection 722
 pre-travel medical assessment and questionnaires 723
 team building 722
 team education 723
10 × 5m speed/agility test 146
tendinopathy
 Achilles 682
 biceps 494, 522
 calcific tendinopathy of hip 608
 calcific tendonitis of shoulder 495
 extensor carpi ulnaris 542
 flexor hallucis longus 672
 patellar 643
 peroneal 668
 rotator cuff 490, 493
 tibialis anterior 674, 698
 tibialis posterior 672–3
tendon dislocation and rupture
 ankle 658
 biceps 487–8
tennis elbow, see lateral epicondylitis
tennis shoe foot 343
tennis shoes 693
tennis toe 327, 708
tension pneumothorax 22
tension-type headache 413
terbutaline 306
Terry Thomas' sign 536
testicular feminization 369
testicular injuries 551
tetanus 47, 724
tetralogy of Fallot 276
theophylline 307
therapeutic use exemption (TUE) 201
thermoregulation
 children 187
 gender 165
 spinal injury 224
thigh contusion 578
Thomas' test 566
thoracic outlet syndrome 468, 498
thrombolytic therapies 262
Thurston–Holland sign 570
tibia
 anterior stress fracture 676
 medial tibial stress syndrome 677
tibialis anterior tendinopathy 674, 698
tibialis posterior tendinopathy 672–3
tinea corporis 337
tinea cruris 336
tinea gladiatorum 337
tinea pedis 336
tinea unguium 338
tinea versicolor 338
Tinel's test 653
toenails
 in-growing 343, 708
 subungual haematoma 327, 708
toes, see foot
toe touching 426
topical NSAIDs 51, 237
Toronto Charter for Physical Activity: A Global Call for Action 100
touchline kit bag 715
toxoplasmosis 315
trabecular bone 58
traction apophysitis 62
 base of fifth metatarsal 705
 calcaneum 704
 ischial tuberosity 616
 medial humeral epicondyle 509
 navicular 705
traction epiphyses (apophyses) 594
training
 aerobic endurance training 154, 155
 ageing and response to training 379
 anaerobic/sprint training 162
 basic principles 152–3
 resistance training 158, 166
transfer 33
transposition of great arteries 276

INDEX **755**

transsexual athletes 369
traumatic brain injury 395
traumatic herpes 349
trauma-triggered migraine 410
traveller's diarrhoea 320
travelling, see team travel
Trendelenburg test 566
triangular fibro-cartilage complex tears 544
tricarboxylic acid cycle 127
triceps tear/rupture 516
trigger finger 542
triple X female 368
trochanteric bursitis 574
tumours, shoulder 500
turf burns 327
turf toe 689
Turner's syndrome 368
12 minute run test 150
20m shuttle test 150
two-stage jog test 148–9
type I and type II muscle fibres 77
type A and type B exercise 298

U

UK Anti-Doping (UKAD) 206
ulcer 324
ulnar collateral ligament injuries 539
ulnar neuropathy 506, 522, 540
ultrasound therapy 84
unconscious athlete 23
unstable angina 186
upper respiratory tract infections 314
urate crystals 245
ureteric avulsion 551
urethral rupture 551
uric acid 243
urine
 haematuria 550, 555
 haemoglobinuria 556
 myoglobinuria 556
 proteinuria 554
 spurious causes of red urine 556
urticaria
 cholinergic 333
 cold-induced 335
 solar 331

V

vaccination 724
Valsalva manoeuvre 137
valvular disease 294
varicella 347

ventilation 136–7
ventricular fibrillation 14, 184
ventricular septal defect 276
ventricular tachycardia 14
verrucae 709
 verruca plantaris 346
 verruca vulgaris 346
vertebrae 428, 439
vertebral body compression fracture 433
vertical jump test 145
vesicle 324
viral hepatitis 316
viral infections 315, 346
visual impairment 222
vitamin D 205, 359
vitamins, normal requirements 177
VO_2 140
VO_2 max 140, 168
vocal cord dysfunction 304

W

waist to hip ratio 143
walking 691
 gait analysis 85, 694
 gait cycle 691
walking aids 237
warts 346
 genital 346
 plantar 346
 water warts 347
Watson's test 536
weight gain 173
weight loss 173
welcome meeting 729
wet bulb 186
wet bulb globe temperature 186
wheal 324
wheelchairs 218
winded athlete 548
Wingate test 145
Winter Paralympic Games 217
Wolff–Parkinson–White syndrome 295
Wolff's law 59
women 351–70
 contraception 356
 female athletic triad 60, 358
 gender and performance 164
 gender verification 368
 menstruation, see menstrual cycle
 pelvic pain 366
 pregnancy 362
 sports injuries 370
World Anti-Doping Agency 206

World Anti-Doping Code 206
World Health Organization, recommended levels of physical activity 98
wound care 44
wound stress 55
Wright's manoeuvre 468
wrist and hand 529–45
 biomechanics of wrist 531
 Boutonniere deformity 538
 boxer's knuckle 538
 carpal tunnel syndrome 540
 De Quervain's tenosynovitis 541
 dislocations 536–7
 distal radial physeal stress injuries 544
 epidemiology of injuries 530
 extensor carpi ulnaris tendinopathies 542
 fractures 532–5
 gamekeepers' thumb 539
 ganglion 542
 impaction syndromes 543
 intersection syndrome 541
 jersey finger 538
 mallet finger 537
 movements, muscles and innervation of wrist joint 527
 osteoarthritis 231
 paediatric problems 544
 radial tunnel syndrome 541
 triangular fibro-cartilage complex tears 544
 trigger finger 542
 ulnar collateral ligament injuries (skier's thumb) 539
 ulnar nerve compression 540

X

xerosis 332
XXX female 368

Y

Yergason's test 467

Z

zafirlukast 307
zileuton 307
zygomatic fractures 420